Duplex sonography of the brain-supplying arteries

Bernhard Widder • Gerhard F. Hamann
Editors

Duplex sonography of the brain-supplying arteries

Springer

Editors
Bernhard Widder
Expert Opinion Institute
District Hospital
Guenzburg, Germany

Gerhard F. Hamann
Clinic of Neurology and Neurological Rehabilitation
District Hospital
Guenzburg, Germany

ISBN 978-3-662-65565-8 ISBN 978-3-662-65566-5 (eBook)
https://doi.org/10.1007/978-3-662-65566-5

This book is a translation of the original German edition „Duplexsonographie der hirnversorgenden Arterien" by Widder, Bernhard, published by Springer-Verlag GmbH, DE in 2018. The translation was done with the help of artificial intelligence (machine translation by the service DeepL.com). A subsequent human revision was done primarily in terms of content, so that the book will read stylistically differently from a conventional translation. Springer Nature works continuously to further the development of tools for the production of books and on the related technologies to support the authors.

This Springer imprint is published by the registered company Springer-Verlag GmbH, DE, part of Springer Nature.
The registered company address is: Heidelberger Platz 3, 14197 Berlin, Germany

Preface to the Seventh Edition

Despite the great progress made in neuroradiological procedures, especially MRI and CT and MR angiography, ultrasound diagnostics of the vessels supplying the brain is still one of the core competencies of neurologists, neurosurgeons, neuroradiologists, angiologists, vascular surgeons, and cardiologists in clinics and practices. The high significance of the method is due to its broad availability, also as a "bedside" examination, the lack of stress and risk to the examined patients, and the high sensitivity and specificity in the detection of pathological findings in the hands of the trained examiner.

In the 33 years since the first edition was published, this book has changed both its content and its appearance several times. The current seventh edition is a new edition, which in particular has the claim to be a practice book that presents in detail everything that is currently important in ultrasound diagnostics of the vessels supplying the brain. We want to provide our colleagues with the tools to quickly and completely record the individual vascular situation of the patient. On the other hand, we have deliberately refrained from using procedures and techniques that are only of historical interest or are only used scientifically but are no longer clinically relevant today, for example, microembolic detection or contrast-enhanced duplex sonography.

In addition, the book is intended to be a working aid for both beginners and those already experienced. The modular structure makes it possible to familiarize oneself with the method quickly and in a structured manner. Those experienced in ultrasound diagnostics will find numerous practical tips and frequent sources of error and problems are pointed out so that not everyone has to go through them again. The book is supplemented by many case studies, which present illustrative—even rare and unusual—cases from the respective problem areas.

In addition to the editors, the authors Prof. Georg Gahn, Prof. Max Nedelmann, and Prof. Dirk Sander have been recruited to work on individual chapters with their special expertise. The editors would like to thank them for their timely and competent chapter editing. We would also like to express our special thanks to Springer-Verlag and the editor in charge, Dr. Lerche, who continued to motivate us to tackle the new edition.

We would be pleased to receive feedback and criticism in order to be able to include it in a possible eighth edition.

Guenzburg, Germany
Spring 2018

Bernhard Widder
Gerhard F. Hamann

Notes on the Use of the Book

For didactic reasons, the entire book has a modular structure. Markings in the margin of the text make it easier to find the different modules.

Basics	The first module describes the anatomy and physiology of cerebral blood flow and introduces the technical basics of the various sonographic techniques. It is aimed at both to the sonographic beginner who wants to get acquainted with the method and the experienced one who receives information about anatomical variations and new technical procedures.
Analysis technique	This module is primarily intended for the sonographic beginner. It covers the methodological principles of extra- and transcranial Doppler and duplex examinations, but also the qualitative and quantitative sonographic assessment of cerebral hemodynamics.
Findings with stenoses and occlusions	Since the detection of stenoses and occlusions of the arteries supplying the brain is the main focus of sonographic vascular diagnostics, detailed information on the various constellations of findings, including their accuracy and possible errors, can be found here.
Constellations of findings for special questions	This module, which is to be used as a reference book, describes all relevant cerebrovascular diseases with their most important clinical findings and discusses the contribution of sonographic examination in the care of disease patterns in the context of other examination methods. In addition, the individual chapters contain numerous case studies.
Glossary and standard values	In this section you will find practical standard value tables, which are prerequisites for the definition of pathological findings, and a glossary for sonographic diagnostics.

Contents

Editors and Authors

Editors

Bernhard Widder Expert Opinion Institute, District Hospital, Guenzburg, Germany

Gerhard F. Hamann Clinic of Neurology and Neurological Rehabilitation, District Hospital, Guenzburg, Germany

Authors

Georg Gahn Department of Neurology, Community Hospital Karlsruhe gGmbH, Karlsruhe, Germany

Max Nedelmann Regio Kliniken GmbH, Clinic for Neurology, Pinneberg, Germany

Dirk Sander Department of Neurology, Benedictus Hospital, Tutzing, Germany

Part I

Basics

1 Anatomical Basics

Bernhard Widder and Gerhard F. Hamann

1.1 Classification of Supraaortic Arteries

In neuroradiology, a division into segments has become established (Fig. 1.1, Table 1.1), which has also found its way into ultrasound diagnostics. In addition, Table 1.2 provides an overview of the most important jargon terms used in neurovascular diagnostics.

1.2 Aortic Arch Branches

1.2.1 Normal Anatomy

The first and most powerful branch of the aortic arch is the brachiocephalic trunk, the second is the left common carotid artery, the third is the left subclavian artery (Fig. 1.2). The right common carotid artery does not have a direct outflow from the aortic arch, but originates from the brachiocephalic trunk, which itself flows into the right subclavian artery. This asymmetry is of clinical significance, as occlusive processes near the aorta can have a different effect on the right than on the left.

> **Note**
> **Since the first vascular branches of the aortic arch lead to the brain, emboli coming from the cardiac system spread preferably cranially.**

Another sonographically noteworthy feature is the fact that the **thyrocervical trunk** emerges from the subclavian artery few millimeters distal to the vertebral artery. Its main branch, the inferior thyroid artery, can be quite large in caliber (Table 1.3) and initially runs over a distance of usually 3–4 cm next to the vertebral artery in a cranial direction until it runs in an arc in a caudal direction to the lower pole of the thyroid gland. The other vessels of the thyrocervical trunk and the costocervical trunk, which also originates from the subclavian artery, are so thin, at least normally, that they cannot be followed sonographically over a longer distance.

> **Practical Tips**
> In the case of a extended vessel diameter, the initial section of the inferior thyroid artery can be sonographically confused with the terminal section of the vertebral artery. Decisive for the differentiation is the traceability of the vertebral artery further cranially to the sonographically well recognizable transverse processes.

1.2.2 Anatomical Variations

Variants of Aortic Arch Branches

Anatomical variations in the area of the aortic arch branches are relatively rare compared to the intracranially located vessel sections and are found "only" in 25–30% of all cases (Lang 1991; Lippert 1969). The most important are (Fig. 1.3):

- Origin of the left common carotid artery from the brachiocephalic trunk (25%)
- Origin of the left common carotid artery from the left subclavian artery(7%)
- Origin of the left vertebral artery from the aorta (5%)
- Origin of the vertebral artery from the thyrocervical trunk (1–2%).

B. Widder (✉)
Expert Opinion Institute, District Hospital, Guenzburg, Germany
e-mail: bernhard.widder@bkh-guenzburg.de

G. F. Hamann
Clinic of Neurology and Neurological Rehabilitation, District Hospital, Guenzburg, Germany

B. Widder, G. F. Hamann (eds.), *Duplex sonography of the brain-supplying arteries*, https://doi.org/10.1007/978-3-662-65566-5_1

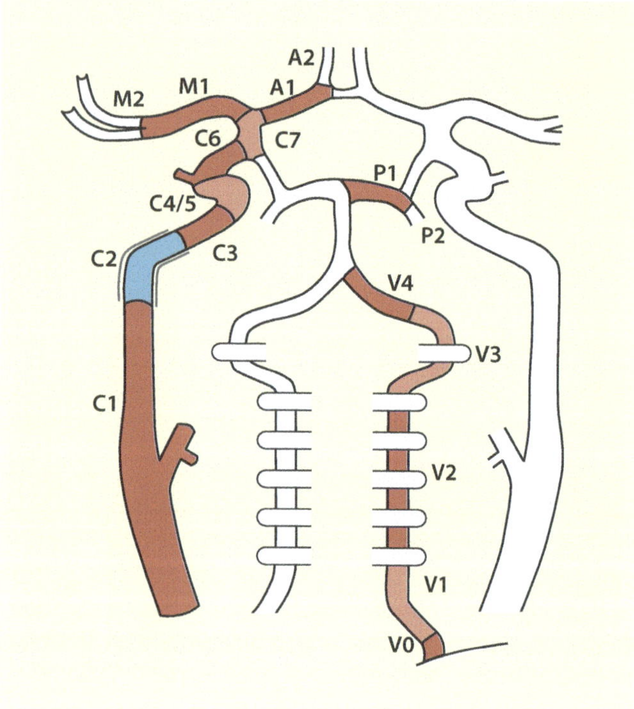

Fig. 1.1 Segmentation of the brain-supplying arteries (further details Table 1.1)

Other varieties, such as a bicarotic trunk or the direct exit of the right common carotid artery from the aortic arch, are in the range of less than 1%.

> **Note**
> **The frequency of anatomical variations in the arteries supplying the brain increases from caudal to cranial.**

Kinkings and Coilings

Stronger elongations of the common carotid artery are among the rarities and are usually noticed by the affected persons themselves with increasing age, when a pulsating "tumor" – preferably on the right side of the neck – slowly develops. The cause of the development of such vascular changes, which according to clinical experience are coincidentally often the result of colds with persistent coughing, is not known. In contrast, kinkings and coilings at the origin of the vertebral artery occur in about 50% of all normal persons and thus do not represent a fundamentally pathological finding (Trattnig et al. 1993). Information on the diameter varieties of the vertebral artery can be found in Sect. 20.3.

Summary
The first vascular outlets from the aorta lead to the brain. They are usually asymmetrically arranged (on the right side in upstream position the brachiocephalic trunk). Anatomical variants of the aortic arch branches are found in 20–30% of cases.

1.3 Extracranial Course of the Carotid Arteries

1.3.1 Normal Anatomy

The common carotid artery runs cranially to the side of the trachea and divides into the internal carotid artery and the external carotid artery approximately at the level of the thyroid cartilage. The localization of the bifurcation is subject to considerable individual variations in each case. In young people in particular, there is a bifurcation which is still located far cranially and can hardly be detected sonographically below the jaw angle, whereas in older people it is usually located much more caudally. In relation to the cervical spine, the point of division is at the level of the vertebral body C4 in almost 70% of all cases, C3 in 20% and C5 in about 10% (Lang 1991). The origin of the internal carotid artery, usually referred to as **carotid bulb** or **carotid sinus**, regularly shows a dilatation of the vascular lumen (Fig. 1.4).

> **Practical Tips**
> The location of the carotid bifurcation – usually in the middle of the fourth cervical vertebra – can serve as a rough "guide" for the assignment of the cervical transverse processes when examining the vertebral artery.

Normally, the internal carotid artery is largely straight until the base of the skull, without significant branches, while the external carotid artery branches out into various branches shortly after its origin. The first branch is regularly the superior thyroid artery, which, on its way to the thyroid gland, usually runs ventral of the common carotid artery, a short distance against the direction of flow (Fig. 1.5, Table 1.4).

Other important branches are the occipital artery, the facial artery, and the superficial temporal artery, all three of which supply the scalp and muscles with blood, the maxillary artery, which gives off branches to the upper and lower jaw

Table 1.1 Segmentation of the brain-supplying arteries

Vessel	Segment	Segment description	Ultrasound
Internal carotid artery	C1	Cervical section from the carotid bifurcation to the skull base	To be recorded by Doppler or duplex sonography between the carotid bifurcation and the jaw angle
	C2	Petrous section through the petrous bone	**Not detectable by sonography**
	C3	Lacerous section with the passage through the foramen lacerum	To be recorded in coronary section by transcranial duplex sonography at the exit from foramen lacerum
	C4	Cavernous section through the cavernous sinus ("**carotid siphon**"), S-shaped course	To be recorded transorbital with transcranial Doppler and duplex sonography
	C5	Clinoidal section between the proximal and the distal dural ring	**Not detectable by sonography**
	C6	Ophthalmic segment from distal dural ring up to the origin of the posterior communicating artery	To be recorded with transcranial duplex sonography
	C7	Distal section between the origin of the posterior communicating artery and the carotid T	To be recorded with extra cranial Doppler- and duplex sonography
Vertebral artery	V0	Origin of vessel	To be recorded with extracranial duplex sonography
	V1	Course up to the entry in the transversal foramina	To be recorded with extracranial duplex sonography
	V2	Course between the transversal foramina to HWK2	To be recorded with extracranial duplex sonography between the foramina
	V3	"**Atlas loop**"	To be recorded with extracranial duplex sonography
	V4	Intracranial section with origin of the posterior inferior cerebellar artery	To be recorded with transcranial duplex sonography
Middle cerebral artery	M1	Main trunk with origin of the lenticulostriatal vessels	To be recorded with transcranial duplex sonography
	M2	Main branches	**Not detectable by sonography**
Anterior cerebral artery	A1	Precommunical section proximal to the anterior communicating artery	To be recorded with transcranial duplex sonography
	A2	Post-communical cranial section	**Not detectable by sonography**
Posterior cerebral artery	P1	Precommunical section proximal to the posterior communicating artery	To be recorded with transcranial duplex sonography
	P2	Post-communical course at the cerebral peduncle	To be recorded with transcranial duplex sonography

According to Runge (2017)

Table 1.2 Important jargon terms of supraaortic vascular anatomy

Term	Meaning
Carotid bulb	Dilatation of the internal carotid artery at the exit from the common carotid artery
Carotid siphon	Convex arch of the internal carotid artery after passing through the skull base including the exit of the ophthalmic artery
Carotid T	Branching of the internal carotid artery into the middle and anterior cerebral artery
Atlas loop	Suboccipital elongation of the vertebral artery to allow for pitching and rotating movements
Basilaris head	Branching of the basilar artery into the posterior cerebral arteries

and the meninges, and the ascending pharyngeal artery. The diameter of the large branches of the external carotid artery is normally 1.5–2 mm, but can also be up to approximately 3 mm (Lang 1991). A smaller branch is the posterior auricular artery, which supplies the base of the skull in the area of the mastoid and can be considerably hyperperfused in dural arteriovenous malformations.

1.3.2 Anatomical Variations

Internal Carotid Artery

In the area of carotid bifurcation as well as in the course of the internal carotid artery there are numerous anatomical variations which can lead to uncertainties in the sonographic assessment. Due to the essential importance of the internal

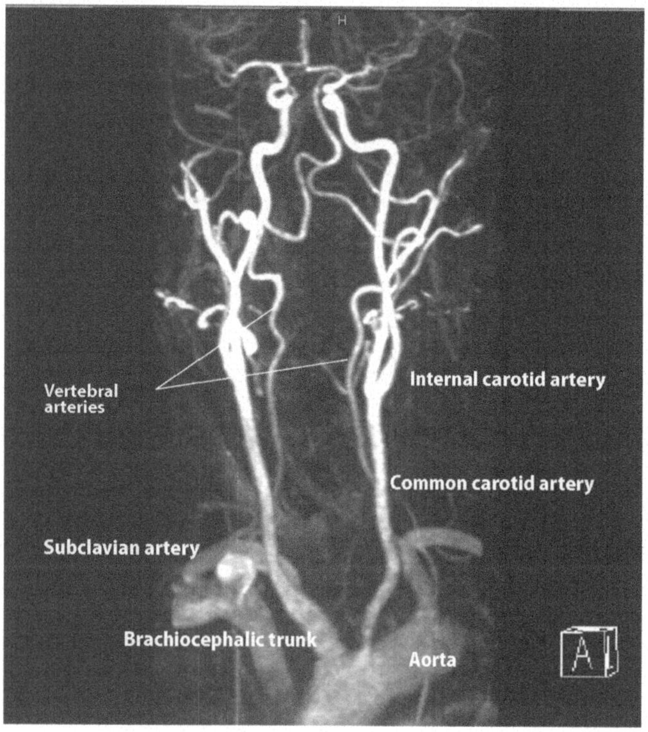

Fig. 1.2 Aortic arch and cervical arteries in MRA

carotid artery in vascular diagnostics, these should be familiar to the examiner.

Bifurcation Variants

In almost 90% of all cases (Prendes et al. 1980) the internal carotid artery is located dorsally to the external carotid artery, but in almost 20% of these cases the external carotid artery is located laterally to the internal carotid artery (Fig. 1.6). In almost 10% of cases, the internal and external carotid arteries are completely superimposed in lateral view, whereby both the internal and external carotid arteries can be the more superficial vessel. In rare cases, a rostral exit of the internal carotid artery can also be found. ◄

Variants of the Carotid Bulb

In duplex sonographic differentiation of the carotid branches, variants of the carotid sinus can cause confusion in individual cases. Although in the majority of cases the typical dilatation at the exit of the internal carotid artery is evident, there may also be an isolated dilatation at the origin of the external carotid artery or a completely missing "bulb" (Fig. 1.7, Table 1.5). ◄

Practical Tips
A missing carotid bulb or sinus is mainly found in connection with elongations and kinking of the internal carotid artery, which usually can be found 1–3 cm distal to the bifurcation.

Kinkings and Coilings

In 2/3 of all cases, the internal carotid artery runs in direct extension of the common carotid artery, in the remaining third there are more or less strongly kinked courses. Bends toward the skin surface ("lateral") and inward ("medial") occur with about the same frequency (Fig. 1.8). In about 15% of the cases the angle is 30° and more. In connection with, but also independently of a kinking at the origin of the internal carotid artery, further kinking and looping can occur in the course of the vessel up to the base of the skull. These are relatively rare in young people, but increase significantly with age (Fig. 1.9). In most cases, such vascular processes are then visible on both sides. Elongations, kinkings, and coilings can be distinguished by their shape (Sect. 20.1). ◄

Background Information
Two factors can be assumed to be the cause of elongations and kinkings that occur more frequently at an advanced age: On the one hand, there is a reduction in body size with "too long" vessels in the course of life, mainly due to the reduction in height of the intervertebral discs, on the other hand, there may be a hypertension-associated cranial displacement of the aortic arch.

Table 1.3 Standard values (mean value and range of variation) of diameter and length of the proximal cervical arteries in the anatomical preparation

	Diameter in mm	Length in mm
Brachiocephalic trunk	15 (10–22)	45 (20–74)
Subclavian artery (until vertebral outflow)	10.5 (7–15)	Right 20 (0–48) Left 35 (16–50)
Common carotid artery	9 (6–12)	Right 100 Left 120
Inferior thyroid artery	3.5 (2.0–4.7)	32 (10–58)

According to Lang (1991)

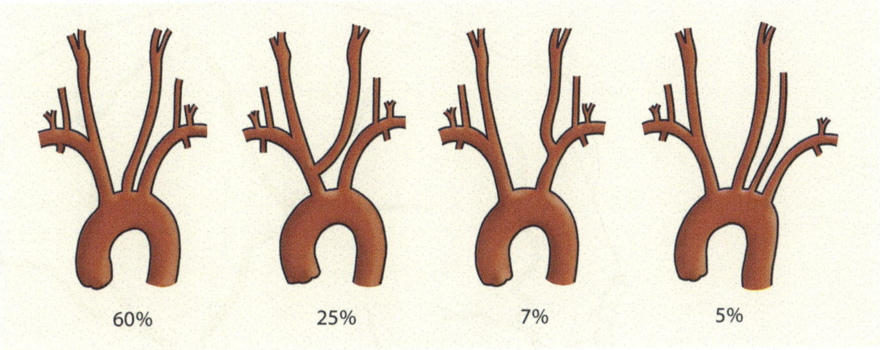

Fig. 1.3 Anatomical variations of the aortic arch

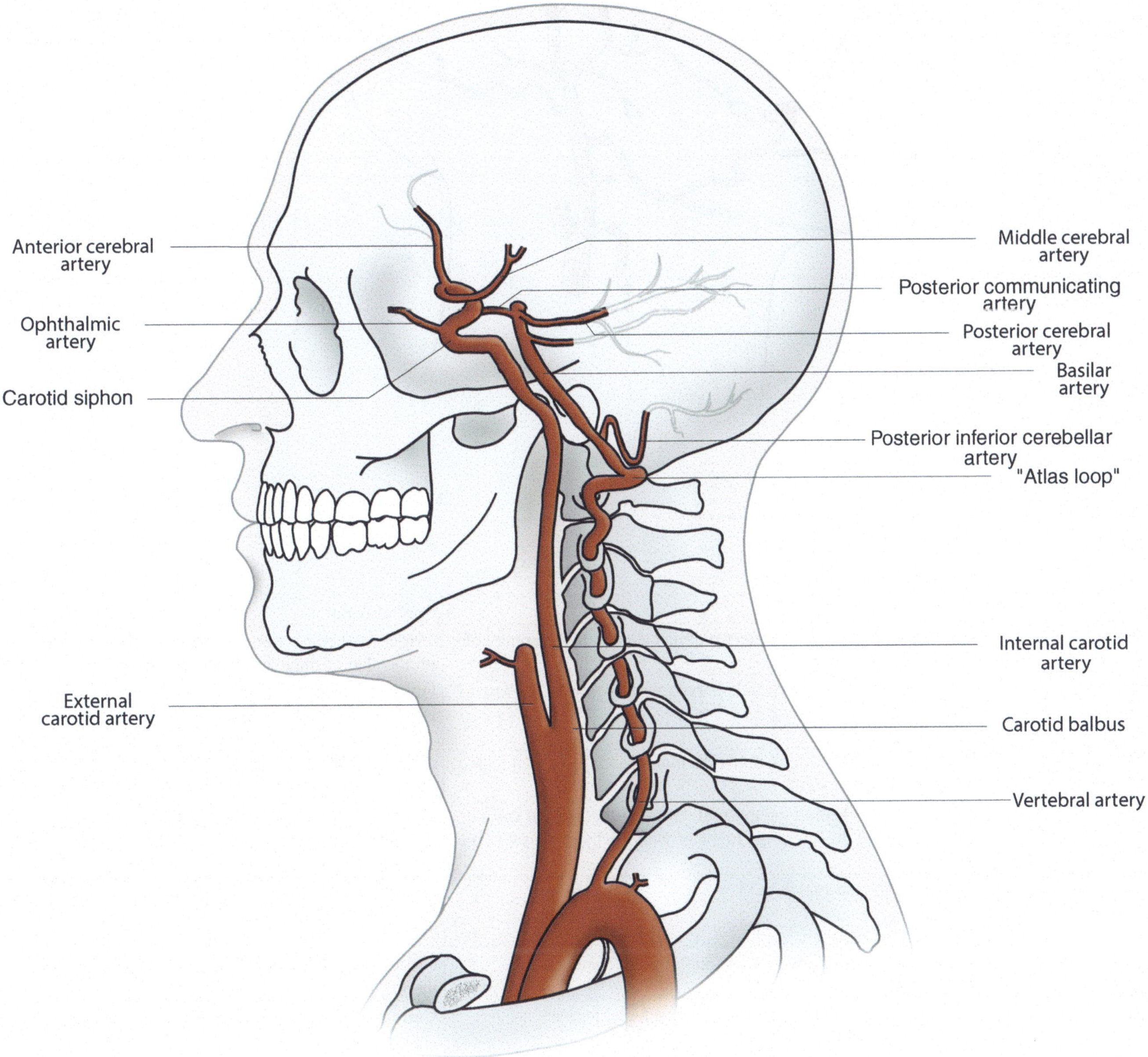

Fig. 1.4 Course of the large brain-supplying arteries in the area of the neck and the skull base in lateral view

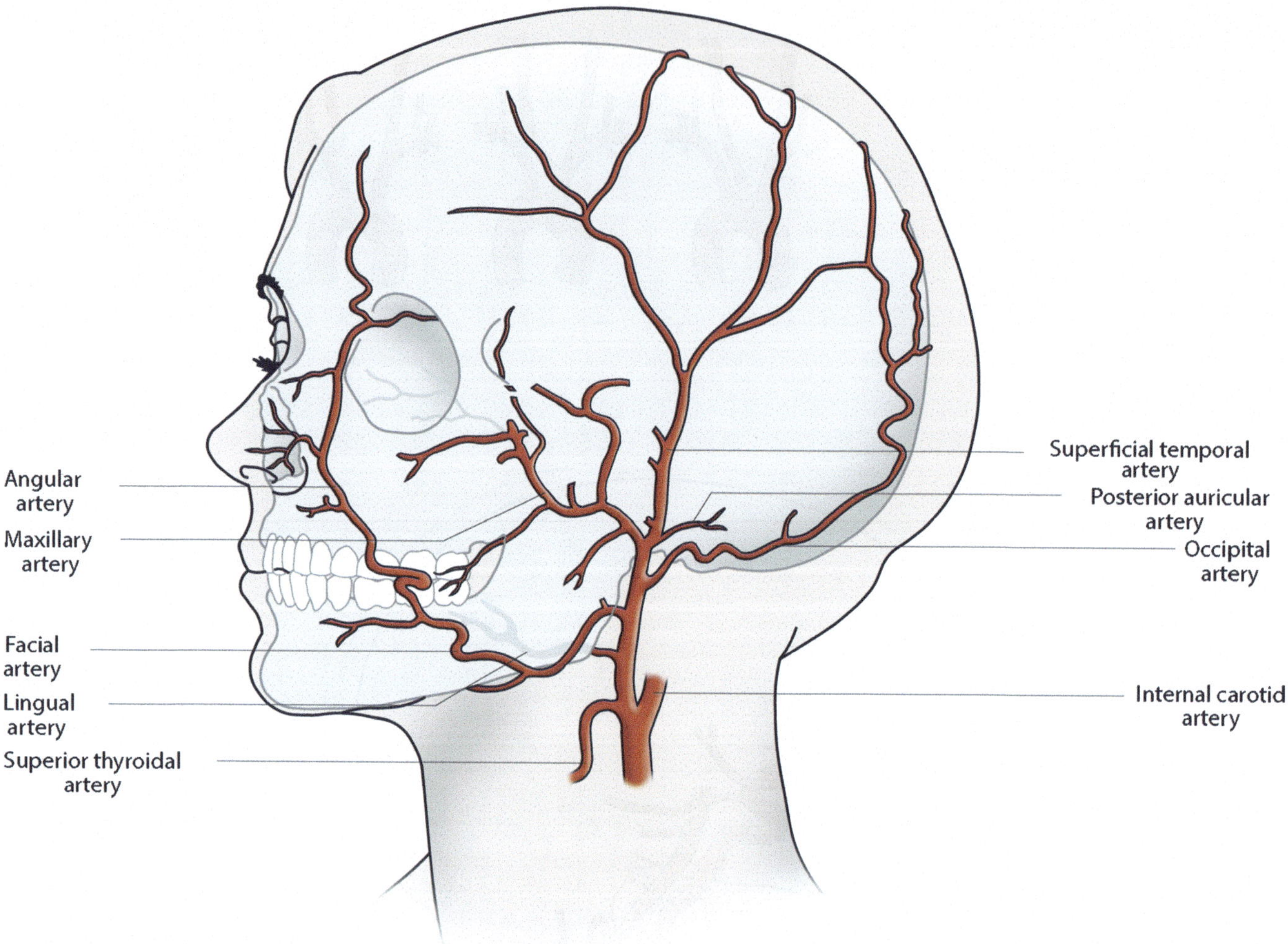

Fig. 1.5 Branches of the external carotid artery in lateral view

Table 1.4 Branches of the external carotid artery

	Course	Special features
Superior thyroid artery	In front of the common carotid artery pulling caudally to the upper pole of the thyroid gland	Origin frequently from the common carotid artery, but on the side of the external carotid artery
Ascending pharyngeal artery	Between internal carotid artery and pharynx pulling toward the base of the skull	Originates in 5% of cases from the internal carotid artery or directly from the carotid bifurcation
Lingual artery	With a strongly tortuous course under the lower jaw with cranialmedial course to the tongue	**Cannot be detected sonographically**
Occipital artery	Craniodorsal course behind the mastoid, crossing the internal carotid artery in the area of the jaw angle together with the hypoglossal nerve	Hyperperfusion can be confused by Doppler sonography with a stenosis of the internal carotid artery, e.g., as a result of an AV fistula
Posterior auricular artery	Pulling behind the mastoid at the jaw angle	Sonographically normally not detectable, but may be hyperperfused due to an AV fistula
Facial artery	Wraps around the lower jaw bone cranially to the cheek muscles	Can be sonographically displayed on the cover around the lower jaw
Maxillary artery	From the parotid gland forward into the deep facial region	**Cannot be detected sonographically**
Superficial temporal artery	Pulling cranially from the jaw angle	In front of the ear on a distance of 1–2 cm sonographically representable

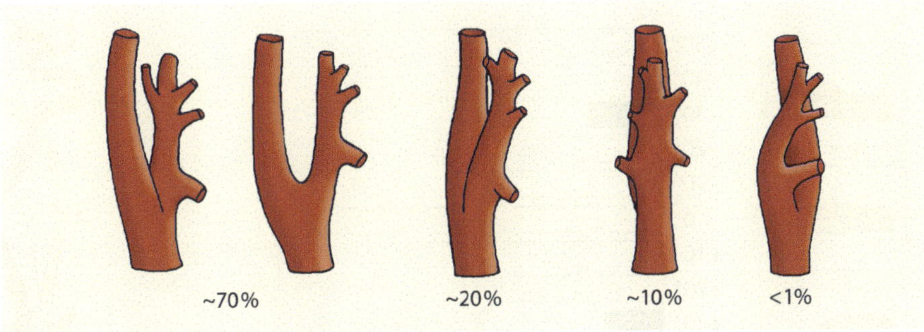

Fig. 1.6 Positional variants of the internal carotid artery (ICA) when looking laterally at the right carotid bifurcation. (according to Prendes et al. 1980)

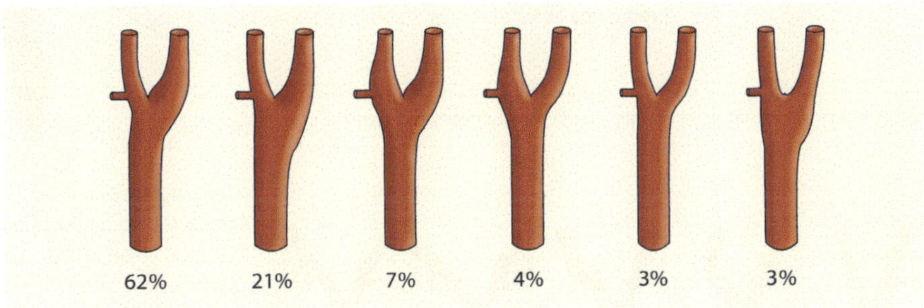

Fig. 1.7 Frequency of the different types of carotid sinus/ Carotid bulb at the carotid bifurcation

Table 1.5 Standard values (mean value and range of variation) of the diameter of the large cervical arteries in the anatomical preparation (Lang 1991)

	Diameter in mm
Common carotid artery	9 (6–12)
Internal carotid artery (carotid bulb)	9 (4–11)
Internal carotid artery (course)	5 (3.5–7)
External carotid artery	5 (3–7)
Vertebral artery	3.5 (0–5.5)

Practical Tips
When using the simple Doppler probe without B-mode image control, kinkings can cause false results due to the increased or decreased Doppler frequencies compared to standard values (Fig. 5.2).

Additional Carotid Artery Branches

In about 5% of the cases, the cervical section of the internal carotid artery shows further arterial branches. These include above all the ascending pharyngeal artery, but also the occipital artery. Furthermore, "primitive" connections between the internal carotid artery and the vertebrobasilar vascular system can persist from the embryonic period (Fig. 1.10). There is also evidence of an origin of the anterior inferior cerebellar artery from the internal carotid artery (Bykowski et al. 2011). ◀

Practical Tips
Cervical vessel outlets can, in the case of an intracranially located occlusion of the internal carotid artery, produce the image of a partially recanalized dissection with apparently typical string sign (Sect. 18.1), if a thin vessel runs cranially with an open initial section of the internal carotid artery.

Variations of the Vessel Diameter

The width of the carotid artery is physiologically subject to considerable fluctuations (Table 1.5) and depends on the body size, but also on the general constitution. A clear distinction from pathological phenomena such as dilated arteriopathy on the one hand, or narrowing of the vessels in long-term smoking or vascular dysplasia on the other hand, is therefore only possible if the measured values clearly fall below or exceed normal values. ◀

External Carotid Artery
The branches of the external carotid artery show a high degree of variety. For example, vessels that are not attached or duplicated, as well as vessels originating from another artery, are the rule rather than the exception. Sonographically, it should be noted that the superior thyroid

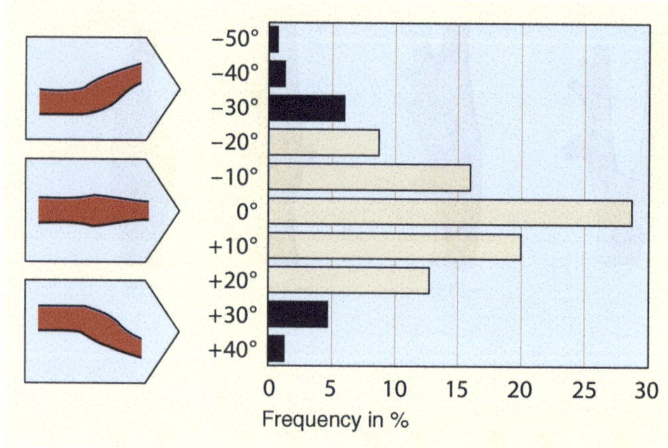

Fig. 1.8 Frequency of "lateral" (top) and "medial" (bottom) deflections of the internal carotid artery at its exit from the common carotid artery

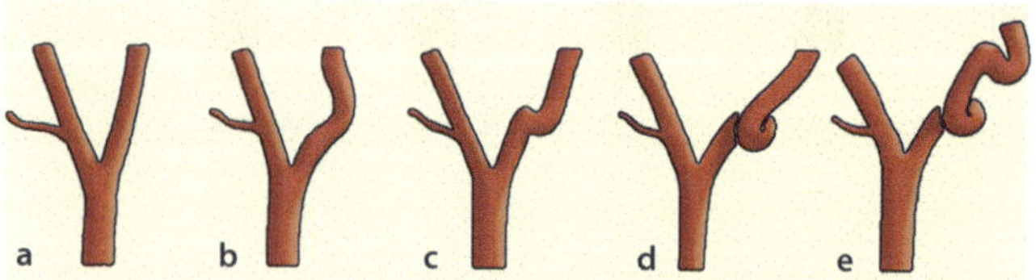

	0 – 20 Years	21 – 50 Years	51 – 74 Years
Straightforward **a**	86%	72%	34%
Crooked **b**	8%	12%	29%
Buckled **c**	4%	10%	22%
Loop **d**	2%	5%	13%
Double loop **e**	—	1%	2%

Fig. 1.9 Frequency of kinkings and coilings of the internal carotid artery. (Huber et al. 1982)

artery only emerges from the external carotid artery in slightly more than half of all cases, otherwise it emerges at the carotid bifurcation – but then almost always on the side of the external carotid artery.

Summary
The common carotid artery is usually divided into the internal carotid artery and the external carotid artery at the level of HWK4. The internal carotid artery rarely gives off cervical branches, while the external carotid artery usually divides into eight branches. Elongations and kinkings of the internal carotid artery are more frequent with increasing age.

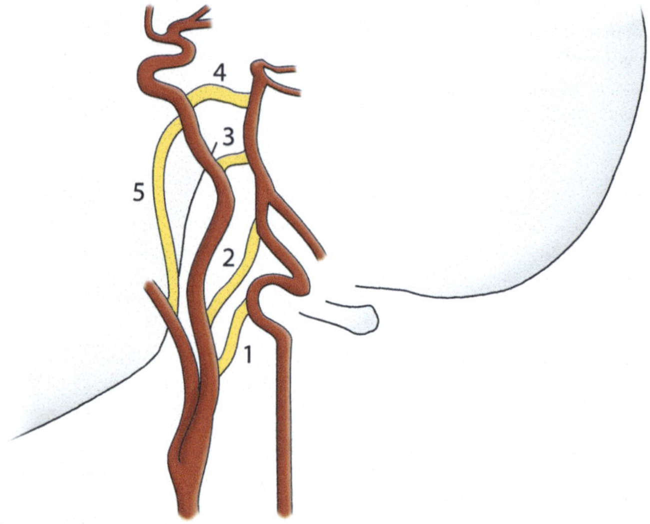

Fig. 1.10 Persistent primitive connections of the internal carotid artery with the vertebrobasilar vascular system and the external carotid artery. 1 proatlantal artery, 2 primitive hypoglossal artery, 3 Primitive auditory artery, 4 primitive trigeminal artery, 5 ascending pharyngeal artery. (According to Siqueira et al. 1993)

1.4 Cervical Course of the Vertebral Artery

1.4.1 Normal Anatomy

Coming from its origin, the vertebral artery usually enters the transverse processes at the sixth cervical vertebra and then runs largely stretched together with the vertebral vein – more precisely a network of several veins – through the foramina of the transverse processes in a cranial direction. In order to ensure head rotation between axis and atlas, a loop formation dorsolateral is found in the cervical segment HWK 1/2. After passing through the atlas, the vertebral artery initially bends back almost at right angles and runs almost horizontally dorsally for approximately 1 cm, then bends medially toward the foramen magnum. This so-called **atlas loop** enables above all the pitching movement of the head in the atlantooccipital joint (Fig. 1.11).

Practical Tips
Sonographically, the loop of the vertebral artery is usually derived in the segment HWK 1/2. Although formally not quite correct, it has also become common practice here to derive from atlas loop to speak.

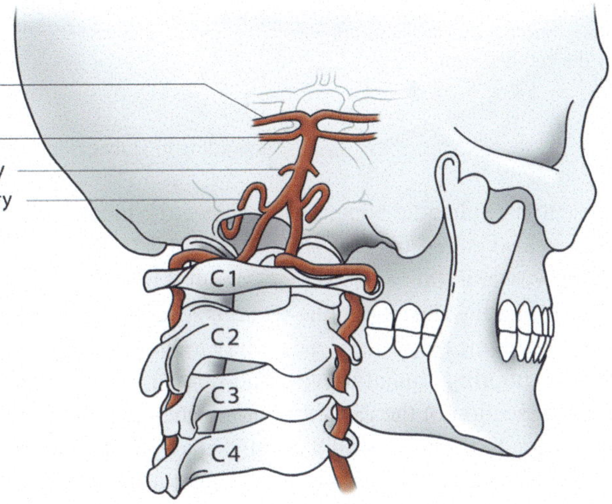

Fig. 1.11 Vertebrobasilar transition area when viewed from the rear

1.4.2 Anatomical Variations

In the area of the vertebral artery, three anatomical variants are of sonographic importance.

Variants of Origin

The exit of the vertebral artery from the subclavian artery shows a more or less distinct elongation (Fig. 1.12). It is also not uncommon for the vertebral artery to form kinkings and coilings, which – comparable to the internal carotid artery – increase with age.

Entry Variants in the Transverse Foramina

In 12% of all people the vertebral artery does not enter the transverse foramina at HWK 6, in individual cases an extraforaminal course up to HWK 4 is even possible (Table 1.6).

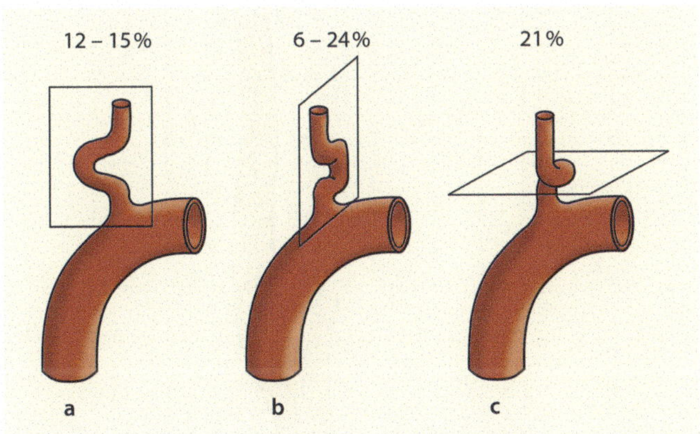

Fig. 1.12 (**a–c**) Frequency of kinkings and coilings at the exit of the vertebral artery. (**a**) lateral elongation, (**b**) sagittal elongation, (**c**) horizontal kinking. (According to Trattnig et al. 1993)

Variations of the Vessel Diameter

Caliber asymmetries of the vertebral artery are the rule rather than the exception, and even more pronounced hypoplasia is to be expected in as many as 9% of cases (Sect. 20.3). In most cases, however, compensatory hyperplasia of the contralateral vertebral artery is present. Heavily hypoplastic vertebral arteries often show no or only insufficient connection to the basilar artery and end in the posterior inferior cerebellar artery (PICA) or possibly only in a branch leading to the neck muscles. If both vertebral arteries are hypoplastic (2%), the supply of the posterior cerebral artery (and the distal basilar artery) is via the circle of Willis from the anterior cerebral circulation, in individual cases also via an postoccipital artery originating from the external carotid artery or a primitive hypoglossal artery (Lang 1991).

> **Summary**
> The vertebral artery usually begins its course through the transverse foramina at HWK 6. In HWK 1/2, elongations of the vessel are found, which are called "atlas loop." Caliber asymmetries of the vertebral artery are frequent, in individual cases hypoplasia can also occur on both sides.

1.5 Intracranial Course of the Internal Carotid Artery

1.5.1 Normal Anatomy

After entry into the skull base, the internal carotid artery runs in the 25–35 mm long carotid canal of the petrous bone in medioventral direction **(petrous section).** The vessel then enters the cavernosus sinus **(cavernous section)** and shows,

Table 1.6 Entry of the vertebral artery into the transverse foramina of the cervical spine

HWK 4	5%
HWK 5	7%
HWK 6	88%
HWK 7	5%

According to Huber et al. (1982)

close to the sphenoid bone, a sharp forward convex arch. This bow is also called **carotid siphon** (Fig. 1.14). The diameter of the vessel in this area averages about 3 mm (Table 1.7).

On entering the cavernous section, several small vascular branches come off, which lead mainly to the tentorium and to the neighboring cranial nerves. The first larger branch in the anterior section of the carotid siphon is the ophthalmic artery (diameter 1–1.5 mm), which supplies the eye, the largest part of the orbital cavity and the medial, supraorbital part of the forehead skin with blood via its end branches.

After exiting the cavernosus sine, the internal carotid artery turns over 10–20 mm craniolaterally. This part is called the **subarachnoid** or **cerebral part** and is directly assessable by sonography. Here, the second larger vascular outlet of the internal carotid artery is the posterior communicating artery. Immediately above it (2–4 mm), the third major vascular branch is the anterior choroidal artery, which supplies parts of the visual pathway and the dorsal leg of the internal capsula (Fig. 1.15). On average 5 mm further cranially, the internal carotid artery divides into its two main branches, the middle cerebral artery and the anterior cerebral artery, which are responsible for the blood supply to the largest part of the brain. The site of division is usually referred to as **carotid T**.

Practical Tips

Since short-stretch embolic occlusions can only affect the segment between two vessel outlets, knowledge of the sequence of vessel outlets and their anatomical variants is of great clinical importance.

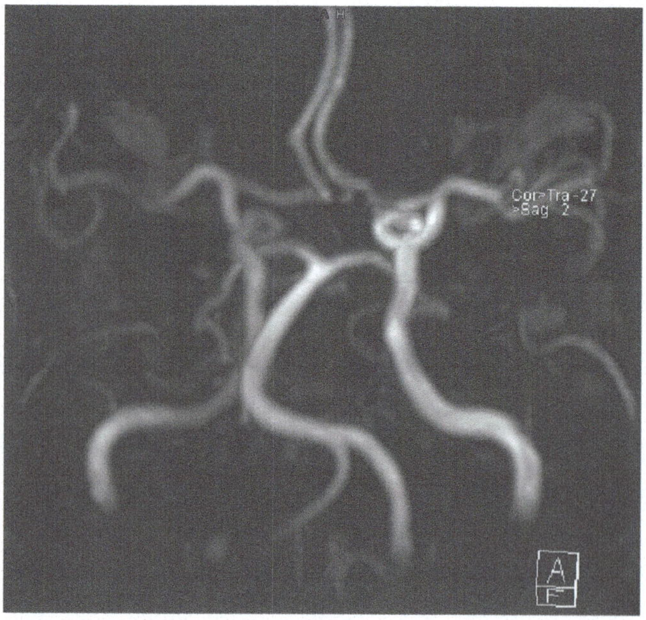

Fig. 1.13 MR angiography for hypoplasia of the right vertebral artery. Typical is the deflection of the basilar artery in an arc to the hypoplastic side

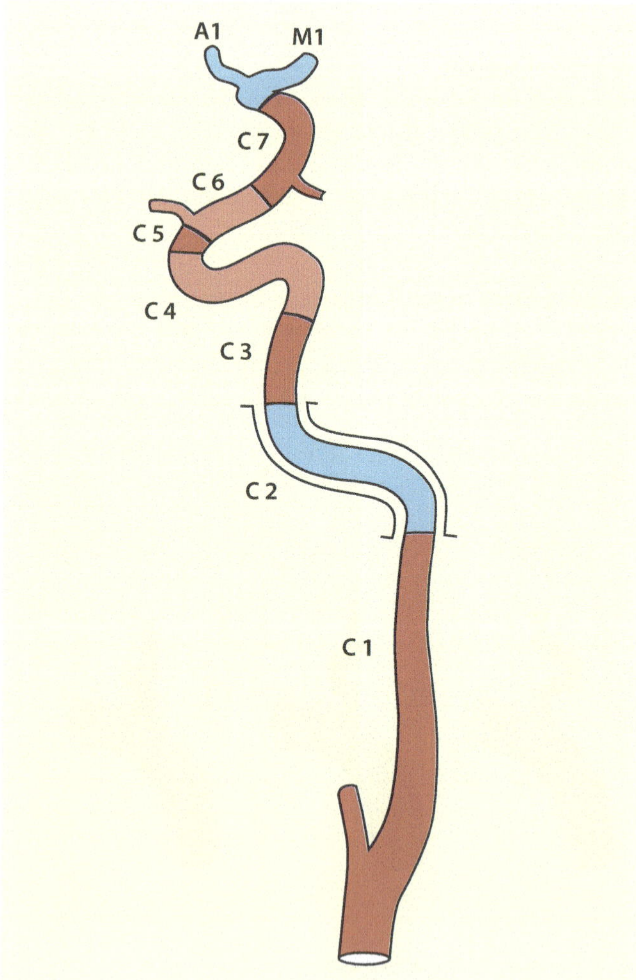

Fig. 1.14 Course of the internal carotid artery with segmentation in lateral view

Table 1.7 Standard values (mean value and range of variation) of the diameter of the main intracranial arteries in the anatomical preparation

	Diameter in mm	Length in mm
Distal internal carotid artery	3 (1.6–3.8)	13 (8–18)
Ophthalmic artery	1–1.5	–
Anterior choroidal artery	Approx. 0.5	–
Middle cerebral artery (M1)	2.7 (1.5–3.5)	16 (5–24)
Anterior cerebral artery (A1)	2.1 (0.5–4)	13 (8–18)
Posterior cerebral artery (P1)	2.1 (0.7–3)	6 (3–9)
Anterior communicating artery	2–2.5 (often as plexus)	2.5 (0.3–7)
Posterior communicating artery	1.2 (0.5–3)	14 (8–18)
Basilar artery	3 (2–4)	32 (15–40)

According to Lanz and Wachsmuth 1955; Riggs and Rupp 1963)

1.5.2 Anatomical Variations

Similar to the extracranial internal carotid artery, elongations are also found in the carotid siphon of older people. However, pronounced kinkings are relatively rare at about 4% (Huber et al. 1982). Sonographically significant is the fact that in about 4% of cases it must be expected that the ophthalmic artery does not originate from the carotid siphon but from the middle meningeal artery. Among the numerous varieties of posterior communicating artery, see Sect. 1.7.2.

Practical Tips
Indirect Doppler sonography of the supratrochlear artery fails in the case of an ophthalmic artery originating from the middle meningeal artery (branch of the external carotid artery), which is based on the evaluation of the pressure equilibrium between the internal carotid artery and external carotid artery.

Summary
After passing through the bony skull, the carotid artery runs in a forward convex arc, the "carotid siphon." It can be sonographically detected cranially from this arc over a short distance and here it gives off the posterior communicating artery and the anterior choroidal artery. Anatomical variations are rarely found here.

1.6 Vertebrobasilar Arteries

1.6.1 Normal Anatomy

The vertebral artery together with the brainstem passes through the foramen magnum into the interior of the skull, where usually the posterior inferior cerebral artery (known as the **PICA** abbreviated) origins, who supplies the dorsolateral medulla oblongata and caudal cerebellum with blood (Fig. 1.15). The posterior inferior cerebellar artery shows a pronounced caudal loop in its course, which facilitates its sonographic identification. In addition, the anterior spinal artery, although very thin and generally not detectable by sonography, is detached medially a few millimeters before it joins the basilar artery.

At the lower edge of the pons the two vertebral arteries meet to form the unpaired basilar artery. The basilar artery releases numerous small, paramedian vessels and, as larger branches, the anterior inferior cerebellar artery, the labyrinthine artery, and the superior cerebellar artery. At the upper edge of the pons, the basilar artery divides into its two end branches, the posterior cerebral arteries (neuroradiologically known as **basilaris head**). These normally supply the dorsal, mediobasal part of the brain.

1.6.2 Anatomical Variations

The intracranial section of the vertebral and basilar arteries regularly shows numerous anatomical variations that can lead to uncertainties during sonographic examination.

Vertebral Artery
While young people predominantly demonstrate a "textbook-like", stretched course of the vertebral artery, older people show "normal" conditions in less than 20% of cases (Lanz and Wachsmuth 1955). In about half of the cases there are elongations of both vertebral arteries of different kinds. In about 1/3 of cases only one vertebral artery shows a more or less strong elongation, while the other vessel is stretched. The basilar artery lies at its beginning regularly laterally shifted toward the vertebral artery with a smaller caliber (Fig. 1.13).

The most important branch of the vertebral artery, the posterior inferior cerebellar artery, is not build in about 20% of all people (Huber et al. 1982). In about 10% of cases it emerges from the basilar artery. In individual cases, it already originates from the vertebral artery in the area of the

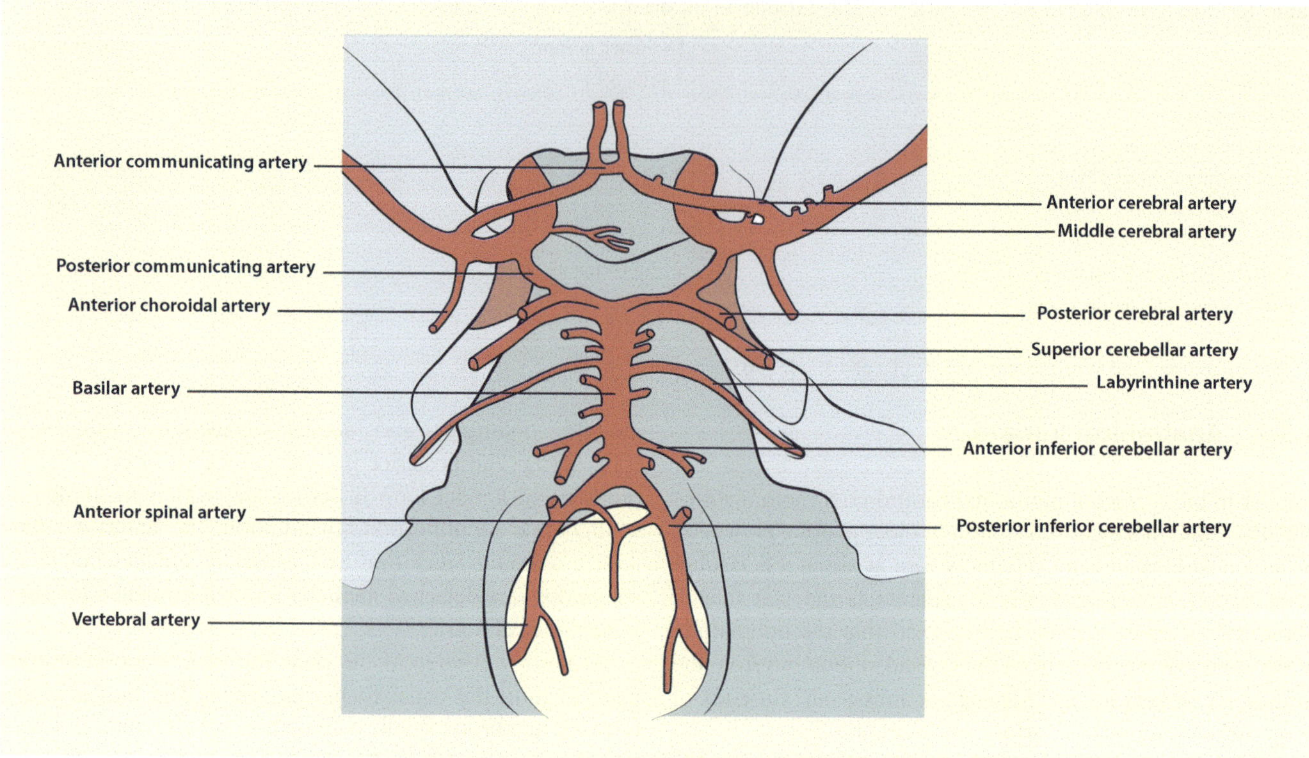

Fig. 1.15 View from above to the arteries at the skull base

atlas loop. Its diameter is usually 1–1.5 mm, which is just sufficient for duplex sonographic imaging.

Basilar Artery

Figure 1.16 gives an overview of the most common varieties in the area of the basilar artery. These range from aneurysmatic dilatation ("ectasia") to pronounced hypoplasia, in rare cases also to a complete or almost complete absence of the basilar artery with vertebral arteries separated up to cranially. Fenestrations (short-distance double-branched basilar artery) are also frequent, especially in the area of the proximal basilar artery (Fig. 1.17).

Summary

The vertebral artery passes together with the brainstem through the foramen magnum, then the paired vessels meet at variable locations to form the basilar artery. The most important branch of the vertebral artery is the posterior inferior cerebellar artery (PICA). In elderly people the vertebral artery frequently show an elongated course. Anatomical variations in the vertebrobasilar transition area are very common.

1.7 Intracerebral Arteries

1.7.1 Normal Anatomy

Middle Cerebral Artery

The middle cerebral artery is the largest intracranial vascular branch with an average diameter of 2.5–3 mm. According to its origin from the distal internal carotid artery in the area of the **carotid T** it initially continues the course of this vessel at its origin, which underlines its importance as the cerebral main vessel (Fig. 1.18). The first segment called the main stem (**"M1 segment"**) is 10–20 mm long on average and runs in the subarachnoid space of the skull base largely horizontally outward. The only vascular outlets here are the lenticulostriatal branches which run vertically to the cranial side and are not recognizable by sonography.

After their division into usually 2–5 so-called main branches, the **M2 segment** begins. Here the vascular branches initially run further in the direction of the M1 segment, which is why they can usually be visualized sonographically. In the insula area they bend almost at right angles to cranial and supply the predominant part of the cerebral cortex.

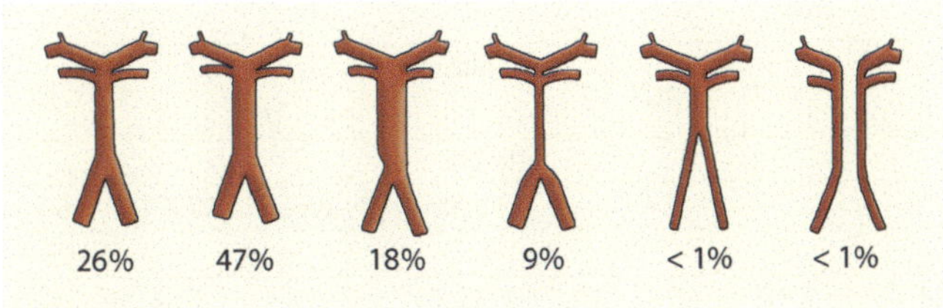

Fig. 1.16 Anatomical variants of basilar artery. (According to Huber et al. 1982)

Anterior Cerebral Artery

The anterior cerebral artery also originates in the area of the **Carotid T** in a short medial arc and then runs initially almost horizontally for an average of 10–15 mm medially (A1). The A2 segment begins after the anterior communicating artery has left, and the vessel moves cranially in the interhemispheric gap, where it supplies medial and frontal brain structures.

Posterior Cerebral Artery

The posterior cerebral artery continues in the area of the **basilar head** from the basilar artery and winds in an arc just above the pons around the cerebral peduncle. The first section (P1) extends to the posterior communicating artery, which is usually reached after 5–10 mm. The posterior cerebral artery supplies parts of the brain base including the base of the temporal lobe as well as the occipital region.

Anterior Communicating Artery

In the midline above the optic chiasma, the anterior communicating artery connects the two anterior cerebral arteries. The anterior communicating artery represents the anterior part of the circle of Willis and is the most important anastomosis in unilateral internal carotid artery occlusions. Its average length is 2.5 mm, its diameter is comparable to that of the large cerebral arteries (Table 1.7).

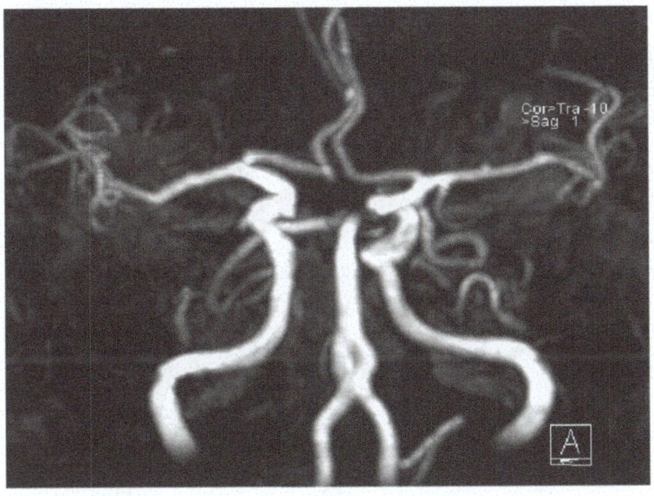

Fig. 1.17 MR angiography for fenestration of the basilar artery

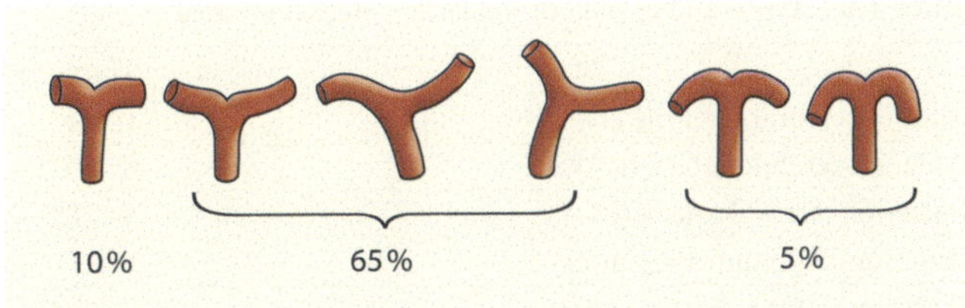

Fig. 1.18 Anatomical variants of the carotid T with the origins of the middle and anterior cerebral artery – seen from the front (a.p. view), corresponding to the sonographic view in the coronary section. (According to Huber et al. 1982)

Posterior Communicating Artery

The posterior communicating artery connects the distal internal carotid artery and the proximal posterior cerebral artery and forms the posterior part of the circle of Willis. Compared to the anterior communicating artery, it is considerably longer (14 mm in diameter) and usually has a smaller caliber, which is why it is often of only minor hemodynamic importance in the case of vascular occlusion.

1.7.2 Anatomical Variations

Middle Cerebral Artery

The main stem of the middle cerebral artery is the only intracranial vessel that is almost always "textbook-like." According to the literature, a non-existent middle cerebral artery is found in only 0.3% of all investigated cases (Table 1.8). However, in 0.2–3% of the cases it is duplicated, which can lead to confusion during ultrasound examination (Lanz and Wachsmuth 1955). While in younger people the main stem of the middle cerebral artery runs largely horizontally, in older people the vessel regularly runs downward at an angle of up to approximately 30°. The distance to the division into its branches is relatively constant. Only in 2% of cases is there branching less than 10 mm after its origin (Fig. 1.19).

Anterior Cerebral Artery

In contrast, this vessel shows a considerable number of anatomical variations. Only in about 2/3 of all cases is there a symmetrical formation of the initial section. In all other cases, hypoplasia of varying degrees must be expected (Fig. 1.20). In rare cases (1–2%) there is a complete aplasia of the proximal A1 section and a complete restoration of the distal anterior cerebral artery via the contralateral side.

Table 1.8 Hypo- and aplasia of the large cerebral arteries

	Hypoplasia	Aplasia
Middle cerebral artery (M1)	0.3%	–
Anterior cerebral artery (A1)	1–9%	1–2%
Posterior cerebral artery (P1)	9–22%	"Fetal supply type" in 17% (10–36%)
Anterior communicating artery	9% (1–40%)	1%
Posterior communicating artery	22% (16–40%)	2–12%

According to Hoksbergen et al. (2000); Lanz and Wachsmuth (1955); Riggs and Rupp (1963)

Posterior Cerebral Artery

The most intracranial varieties can be found for the posterior cerebral artery. This is due to the fact that the vessel initially emerges from the internal carotid artery during the fetal period. Only with the later "degeneration" of this vascular connection the posterior cerebral arteries are connected to the basilar artery. This results in two clinically important supply variants:

- **Fetal supply type** in 10–36% of cases with (almost) exclusive supply of the posterior cerebral artery via the internal carotid artery. In this constellation, hypoplastic vertebral arteries are often found (Sect. 20.3). This situation can occur on one or both sides.
- **Mixed supply type** in 8–15% of the cases with supply of the posterior cerebral artery via both the internal carotid artery and the basilar artery

Practical Tips

Due to the frequent supply of the posterior cerebral artery via the anterior cerebral circulation, a possible cause of occipital cerebral infarction by carotid artery embolization must be considered.

Anterior Communicating Artery

The anterior communicating artery as the anterior part of the circle of Willis is "textbook-like" in about 3/4 of all cases. More pronounced hypoplasia is present in only about 10% of cases. However, it should be taken into account that the anterior communicating artery is not always a single vessel, but a collection of several small vessels or even a network of vessels (Huber et al. 1982).

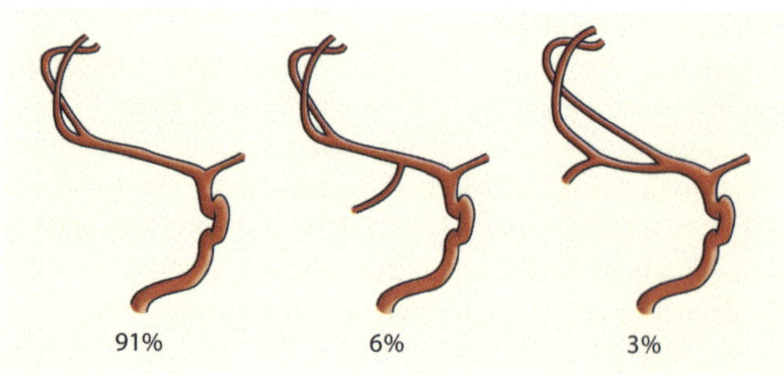

Fig. 1.19 Variants of middle cerebral artery. (According to Huber et al. 1982)

Posterior Communicating Artery

The numerous varieties of the posterior communicating artery are due to its embryonic development. For details see above.

Summary

The three large cerebral arteries middle, anterior, and posterior cerebral artery are interconnected via the anterior communicating artery and the two posterior communicating arteries (circle of Willis). While the anterior communicating artery is relatively rarely hypoplastic or not created, the posterior communicating artery shows numerous variants. In about 1/4 of the cases, the posterior cerebral artery is even supplied exclusively by the anterior circulation ("fetal supply type").

1.8 Collateral Connections

1.8.1 Extracranial Collaterals to the Anterior Cerebral Circulation

The most important anastomoses between the internal and external carotid artery run through the ophthalmic artery, which is in contact with both vessels. However, due to the larger diameter of the internal carotid artery, the intracranial perfusion pressure is higher, so that the ophthalmic artery is

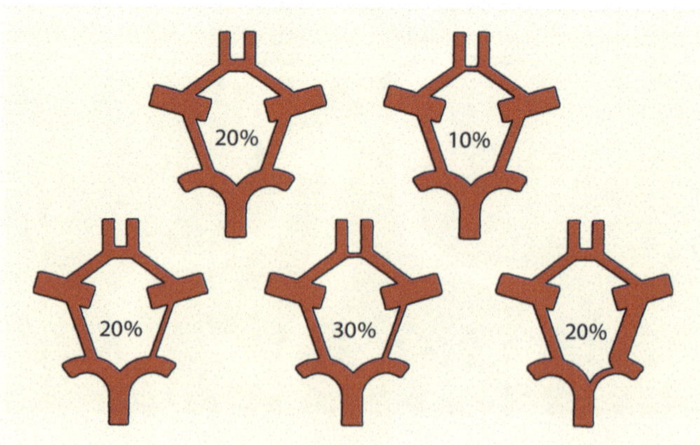

Fig. 1.20 Overview of the most important anatomical variations of the circle of Willis (according to Riggs and Rupp 1963)

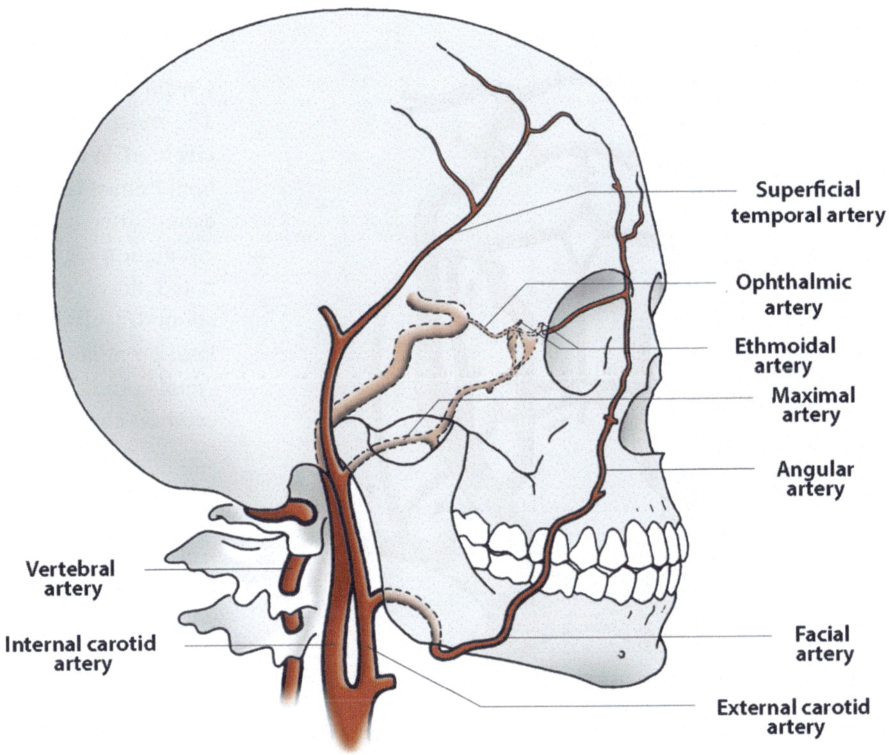

Fig. 1.21 Important collateral connections between the external carotid artery and internal

normally perfused from the inside to the outside. However, in occlusive disease of the internal carotid artery, the flow in the ophthalmic artery can be reversed and the collaterals via the external carotid artery can contribute to the blood flow in the anterior cerebral region. To be mentioned are three so-called **ophthalmic collaterals** between the internal carotid artery and the external carotid artery (Fig. 1.21):

- Facial artery → Angular artery → Supratrochlear artery → Ophthalmic artery,
- Superficial temporal artery → Supratrochlear artery (and orbital) → Ophthalmic artery,
- Maxillary artery → Ethmoidal arteries → Ophthalmic artery.

Practical Tips
It is important for the ultrasound examination that both the facial and the superficial temporal arteries run in significant sections outside the skull bone and are therefore both palpable and compressible, whereas this is not possible with the maxillary artery inside the maxillary sinus.

Background Information
When the common carotid artery is occluded, it is not uncommon for the internal carotid artery to remain open, with the vessel being filled via the external carotid artery, which in turn is supplied retrogradely from the opposite side or from the ipsilateral thyrocervical trunk. A relatively rare collateral is an ascending pharyngeal artery which opens into the distal internal carotid artery (Fig. 1.10). This can cause confusion during the sonographic examination if it is mistaken for an non-occluded internal carotid artery. Since in such a case the distal internal carotid artery may still be slightly perfused, thrombi may form in it and lead in particular to ophthalmic ischemia. Other external branches such as the occipital artery or the middle meningeal artery can also form anastomoses to the internal carotid artery. Finally, there are also collaterals between the two ophthalmic arteries via the dorsal nasal arteries, which can "jump in" in hypoplasia of the anterior communicating artery.

1.8.2 Extracranial Collaterals to the Posterior Cerebral Circulation

In occlusive disease of the proximal vertebral artery (V0/V1 segment), three collateral connections are particularly relevant, which can guarantee perfusion of the vessel in the V2 or V3 segment (Fig. 1.22):

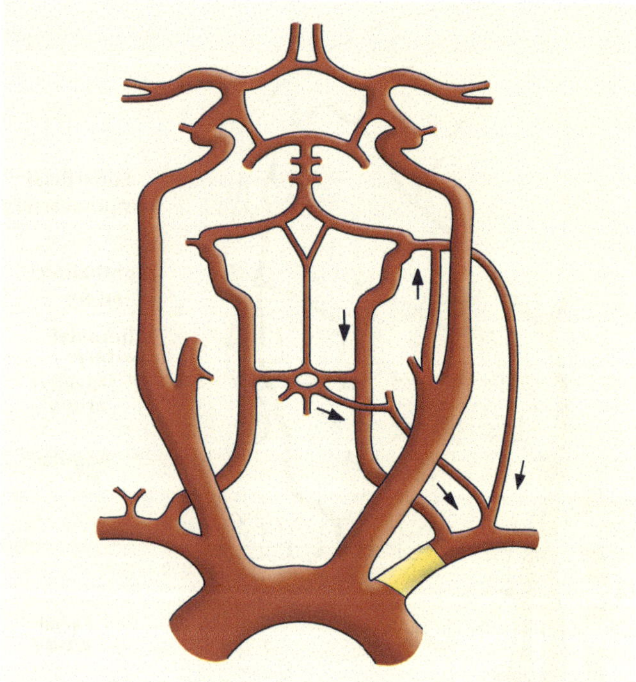

Fig. 1.22 Collaterals in occlusions of the proximal subclavian artery

- Thyrocervical trunk → Ascending cervical artery → Vertebral artery,
- Contralateral vertebral artery → Spinal arteries → Ipsilateral vertebral artery,
- External carotid artery → Occipital artery → Vertebral artery.

Of particular importance are also the spinal arteries, which are often very large in caliber but rarely present in all segments and are then usually impressively visible in color coded duplex sonography.

Background Information
Collaterals between the proximal internal carotid artery and the vertebrobasilar system are very rare (<1%), but can lead to considerable confusion (Gasecki et al. 1994; Siqueira et al. 1993). These are persistent primitive vessels of the embryonic period, which connect the internal carotid artery with the distal vertebral artery and basilar artery at different localizations (Fig. 1.10). In stenoses of the internal carotid artery, paradoxical embolisms can thus occur in the vertebrobasilar vascular system.

1.8.3 Intracranial Collateral Connections

Circle of Willis
The most important intracranial collateral connection is the **circle of Willis**, located at the base of the skull. It connects both hemispheres with each other via the anterior communicating artery and the hemispheres with the vertebrobasilar circulation via posterior communicating arteries. It should be noted, however, that the circle of Willis is only "textbook" in about 1/5 of all people. In all other cases there are more or less pronounced hypoplasias and/or the afore mentioned "fetal" origin of the posterior cerebral artery from the anterior cerebral circulation (Fig. 1.20).

Leptomeningeal Anastomoses
The second most important collateral connection is the network via the vessels of the cerebral convexity (Fig. 11.1). However, in acute vascular occlusions, these anastomoses are generally insufficient to ensure sufficient collateral supply.

Practical Tips
A sonographic evaluation of leptomeningeal anastomoses is only indirectly possible by means of the increase in flow in the other large cerebral arteries.

Rare Anastomoses
For the ultrasound examiner, in individual cases also rare collateral compounds are of importance, since they can develop relevant vessel diameters >1 mm, especially in slowly developing occlusive diseases, and thus – at least under good examination conditions – can be detected with transcranial color coded duplex sonography.

The three most important ones are:

- The so-called **Heubner's artery** (recurrent artery of Heubner) originates from the A1 segment of the anterior cerebral artery and runs "backward" from there to the middle cerebral artery. If the middle cerebral artery is occluded, it can contribute to collateral supply and, if the lumen is wide enough, can simulate an open vessel.
- **Choroidal anastomoses** run between the distal internal carotid artery and the posterior cerebral artery at the skull base, in individual cases also transversely from one side to the other, which can lead to confusing images in the ultrasound image.
- In slowly developing (or already existing) occlusive disease in the carotid T-region, small vascular anastomoses are often found, which are angiographically described as **moyamoya network** and in individual cases can also be detected by duplex sonography (Sect. 19.2).

1.8.4 Collaterals in Subclavian Artery Occlusions

When the proximal subclavian artery is occluded, the vertebral artery is often retrogradely perfused and contributes to the blood supply of the affected arm (Fig. 1.22). This situation is called **subclavian steal effect.** Another connection to the subclavian artery is via the thyrocervical trunk, which anastomoses with thyroid branches and via the skin vessels of the neck with the external carotid artery.

Summary
Collateral connections play an essential role in cerebral vascular disorders. The most important extracranial collateral to the anterior cerebral circulation runs from branches of the external carotid artery via the ophthalmic artery (ophthalmic collateral). Almost all dorsal cervical vessels lead to the posterior circulation. The circle of Willis and leptomeningeal anastomoses are mainly responsible for the intracranial collateral supply.

1.9 Cerebrovascular Territories

Since sonographic examinations should never be performed isolated, but always in the context of the clinical picture, the following section will briefly discuss the brain areas supplied by the described arteries and their variants, as they are of importance in daily routine.

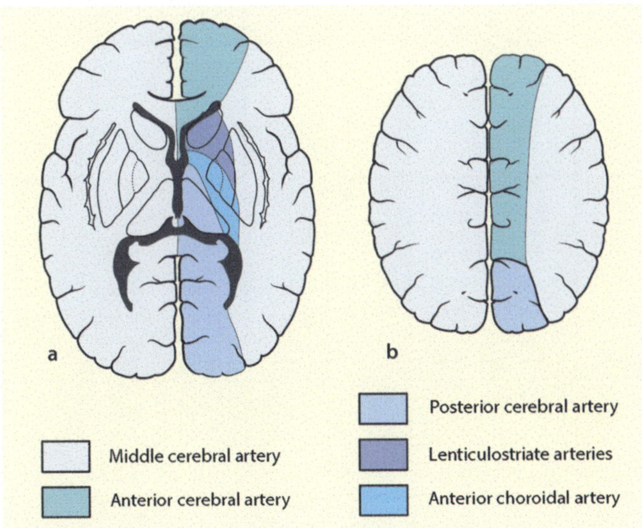

Fig. 1.23 (**a, b**) Topographical assignment of the supply areas of the major cerebral arteries on two characteristic axial sections through the brain. (**a**) Section at the level of the internal capsula, here both the anterior and posterior horn of the lateral ventricles are shown. (**b**) Section a few centimeters below the vertex (Centrum semi-ovale). Note in particular the paramedian borderline running from front to back between the middle cerebral artery and the other two major cerebral arteries

1.9.1 Normal Anatomy

The reference for the differentiation of the supply areas of the three major cerebral arteries is the ventricular system. As a rule, the borderline between the middle and anterior cerebral artery as well as between the middle and posterior cerebral artery is in extension of the anterior or posterior horn

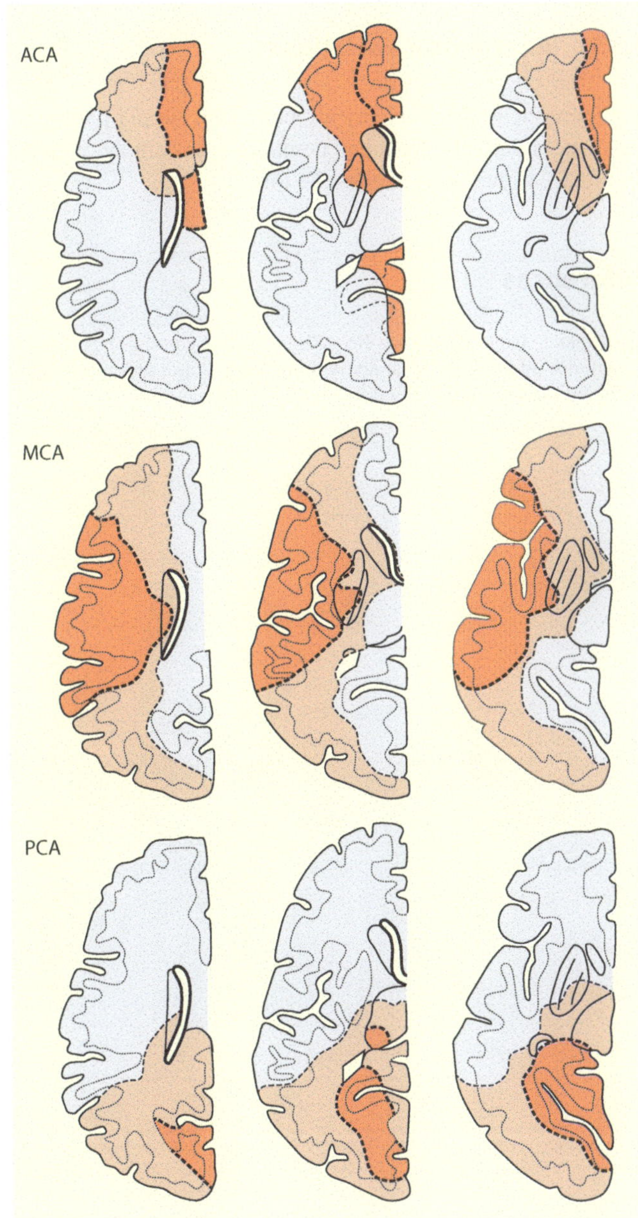

Fig. 1.24 Most important varieties of the cerebral vascular supply areas. Dark red minimum supply area, light red maximum possible supply area; ACA anterior cerebral artery, MCA middle cerebral artery, PCA posterior cerebral artery. (According to van der Zwan et al. 1992)

(Fig. 1.23). On the higher layers, there is an paramedian boundary line, with the majority of the midline structures being supplied by the anterior cerebral artery.

The supply area of the anterior choroidal artery is of special importance, since it is normally the only larger cerebral vessel that emerges directly from the internal carotid artery before the intracranial vessel bifurcation. Lesions in this area therefore give important indications of an occlusive disease in the upper section of the internal carotid artery. In contrast, lesions involving the area supplied by the lenticulostriate arteries indicate a process in the main stem of the middle cerebral artery.

1.9.2 Anatomical Variations

Not least due to the above mentioned "fetal supply patterns," there are relatively frequent deviations in supply pattern. Figure 1.24 gives an overview of this.

References

Bykowski J, Jahan R, Pakbaz RS (2011) Variant carotid origin of left anterior inferior cerebellar artery mimicking infarct on angiography. J Neurointerv Surg 3:279–281

Gasecki AP, Fox AJ, Lebrun LH, Daneault N (1994) Bilateral occipital infarctions associated with carotid stenosis in a patient with persistent trigeminal artery. Stroke 25:1520–1523

Hoksbergen AW, Legemate DA, Ubbink DT, Jacobs MJ (2000) Collateral variations in atherosclerotic population assessed by means of transcranial color-coded duplex ultrasonography. Stroke 31:1656–1660

Huber P, Krayenbühl H, Yasargil MG (1982) Cerebral angiography. Thieme, Stuttgart

Lang J (1991) Über die Lagebeziehungen der Hirnnerven zu benachbarten Gefässen und deren ärztliche Bedeutung. Zentralbl Neurochir 52:165–183

Lanz T, Wachsmuth W (1955) Praktische Anatomie. Springer, Berlin

Lippert H (1969) Arterienvarietäten. Klinische Tabellen. Beilagen in Med Klin 18–32

Prendes JL, McKinney WM, Buonanno FS, Jones AM (1980) Anatomic variations of the carotid bifurcation affecting Doppler scan interpretation. J Clin Ultrasound 8:147–150

Riggs HE, Rupp C (1963) Variation in form of circle of Willis. Arch Neurol 8:24–30

Runge VM (2017) Imaging of cerebrovascular disease. Thieme, Stuttgart

Siqueira M, Piske R, Ono M, Marino R (1993) Cerebellar arteries originating from the internal carotid artery. AJNR Am J Neuroradiol 14:1229–1235

Trattnig S, Matula C, Karnel F, Daha K, Tschabitscher H, Schwaighofer B (1993) Difficulties in examination of the origin of the vertebral artery by duplex and colour-coded Doppler sonography: anatomical considerations. Neuroradiology 35:296–299

Van der Zwan A, Hillen B, Tulleken CAF, Dujovny M, Dragovic L (1992) Variability of the territories of the major cerebral arteries. J Neurosurg 77:927–940

2 Physiological Basics

Bernhard Widder and Gerhard F. Hamann

2.1 Regulation of Arterial Blood Flow

The majority of organs in the human body have the ability to actively regulate the amount of blood circulation. This is controlled mainly by varying the width of the arterioles and capillaries (so-called **resistance vessels**), the reaction time is in the range of a few seconds. In contrast, the larger arteries contribute relatively little to the control of blood flow by of slow tone regulation which changes the vessel diameter.

2.1.1 Demand Regulation

The simplest form of blood flow regulation is found in the muscles where there is only a low blood requirement at rest. Accordingly, the resistance vessels are largely narrowed (**high peripheral resistance**). During physical load, however, the blood requirement can increase significantly. This is achieved by dilatation of the resistance vessels (Fig. 2.1).

2.1.2 Autoregulation

The regulation of blood flow in the brain is much more complex, but also in various other organs such as the kidney. Although an increased blood requirement – for example, in the case of augmented brain activation – also leads to an increase in blood flow, this is only in the order of 30–40%. The main task of the so-called autoregulation is to keep the blood flow rate largely constant regardless of the prevailing system blood pressure. In order to be able to compensate for blood pressure changes both upward and downward, the resistance vessels are set at a medium width for "normal" systemic blood pressure values (Fig. 2.1). In this case, one speaks of an already at rest (relative) **low peripheral resistance.**

Summary
The regulation of blood flow in the various organs is achieved by adjusting the diameter of the arterioles and capillaries. A distinction must be made between autoregulation with the aim of keeping perfusion largely constant and demand regulation adapted to current consumption.

2.2 Cerebral Blood Flow Characteristics

2.2.1 Cerebral Blood Supply

Due to the brain's low tolerance for hypoxic conditions, its blood supply is remarkably secure or even "oversized." Provided that the collateral connections are intact, each of the 4 large arteries supplying the brain is sufficient to maintain the entire blood supply of the brain with a volume of 600–800 ml/min (Table 2.1). Accordingly, the failure of one or more brain-supplying arteries is usually tolerated without neurological deficits.

Background Information
Assuming a "normal" diameter of the internal carotid artery of 5 mm and the vertebral artery of 3.5 mm on each side, the total cross-sectional area of the brain-supplying arteries is approx. 60 mm^2 through which an average of 700 ml/min of blood flows. The average

(continued)

B. Widder (✉)
Expert Opinion Institute, District Hospital, Guenzburg, Germany
e-mail: bernhard.widder@bkh-guenzburg.de

G. F. Hamann
Clinic of Neurology and Neurological Rehabilitation, District Hospital, Guenzburg, Germany

B. Widder, G. F. Hamann (eds.), *Duplex sonography of the brain-supplying arteries*, https://doi.org/10.1007/978-3-662-65566-5_2

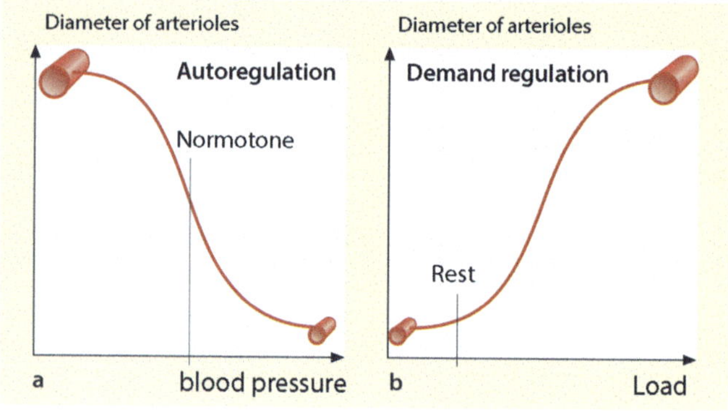

Fig. 2.1 (**a, b**) **Response** of the resistance vessels during autoregulation and demand regulation. Autoregulation with medium dilatation of the arterioles at "normal" blood pressure values (**a**); narrowed resistance vessels at rest during demand regulation with the possibility of dilatation in case of increased blood demand (**b**)

flow velocity in theses arteries is usually in the order of 50 cm/s. If an increase in average flow velocity in the large neck vessels to at least 120–150 cm/s is taken into account, which is still tolerable from a hemodynamic point of view without occurrence of relevant turbulence, the required vessel cross-sectional area for sufficient cerebral blood flow is approx. 20 mm^2 which corresponds to the normal diameter of a single internal carotid artery. This does not yet take into account the numerous collaterals via the external carotid artery, through which another 100–150 ml/min of blood can flow into the brain. Correspondingly, if the collaterals are intact, even one normal sized vertebral artery appears to be sufficient to ensure sufficient blood supply of the brain if the other three vessels fail.

Note

If the circle of Willis is sufficiently developed, one of the four large brain-supplying arteries is sufficient to maintain the blood supply of the brain.

2.2.2 Regulation of Cerebral Blood Flow

In addition to the four major arteries, the brain has two further protective mechanisms to maintain cerebral metabolism.

Autoregulation

As already mentioned in the Sect. 2.1.2 above, the brain is able to keep its blood flow (largely) independent of fluctuations in cerebral perfusion pressure by means of autoregulation. If the cerebral perfusion pressure drops, compensatory dilatation of the cerebral arterioles occurs, in the opposite case, these vessels constrict (Fig. 2.2). As expected, the system of autoregulation finds its limit at maximum dilatation or maximum constriction of the arterioles, however, the extent of vascular width regulation can be limited in cerebral microangiopathies.

Background Information

A special case arises with maximum constriction of the resistance vessels. If there is a further increase in perfusion pressure, the autoregulation breaks down. In this case the cerebral arterioles lose their tone and dilate, which then leads to a more or less pronounced cerebral hyperperfusion with increased capillary permeability and the formation of an edema as well as an increased risk of cerebral bleeding. This situation is found in the so-called **hypertensive crisis**.

Oxygen Extraction Rate

If the intracerebral arterioles are already at maximally dilatated (abolished cerebrovascular reserve capacity, Chap. 12), a (further) drop in perfusion pressure leads to a proportional drop in cerebral blood flow, but cell metabolism can still be maintained over a wide range by increasing the oxygen extraction rate from the blood (Fig. 2.2). According to experimental studies by Strandgaard (1976) in patients with just maximum dilatation of the intracerebral arterioles, a drop in blood pressure of 40–50% of the initial value is tolerated before neurological deficits occur.

Note

Even when autoregulation is largely abolished, the brain still tolerates a drop in blood pressure by 40–50% without neurological deficits by increasing the extraction of oxygen from the blood.

If cerebral blood flow drops below 20–22 ml/100 g/min, which corresponds to a total blood flow of approx. 300 ml/min at a brain weight of 1400–1500 g, neurological deficits may occur (Fig. 2.3). These are initially completely reversible. Although the **functional metabolism** of the nerve cells is no longer guaranteed, the blood circulation is still sufficient to maintain **structural metabolism**. However, in the case of a further drop to values below approx. 16 ml/100 g/min, reversibility of functional loss is only maintained for a period

Table 2.1 Flow volumes in the large brain-supplying arteries and in collateral connections

Flow volumes (each side)	
Internal carotid artery	200–300 ml/min
Vertebral artery	50–150 ml/min
Possible flow volumes in collateral vessels	
Ophthalmic artery	50–100 ml/min
Anterior communicating artery	150–200 ml/min
Posterior communicating artery	100–150 ml/min

of a few hours. In the worst case of a drop in blood flow below 8–10 ml/100 g/min, irreversible cell death can be expected within a few minutes.

2.2.3 Cerebral Perfusion Pressure

The cerebral perfusion pressure (usually abbreviated to "CPP") is not to be equated with the systemic arterial blood pressure. Although there are approximately identical values in healthy individuals, in pathological cases two essential case constellations must be taken into account which reduce the regional cerebral perfusion pressure:

- **Upstream flow obstructions** in the form of stenoses or occlusions of the brain supplying arteries. The remaining perfusion pressure in this case is determined by the degree of stenosis and/or by the "quality" of the collaterals.
- **Increase in intracranial pressure,** e.g., due to a cerebral edema or a cerebral lesion expansion. In this case the CPP is calculated as
  CPP = ABP – ICP
  with
  CPP Cerebral perfusion pressure
  ABP Arterial blood pressure
  ICP Intracranial pressure

Summary
To avoid hypoxia, the brain has two protective mechanisms: cerebral autoregulation and the ability to increase oxygen extraction from the flowing blood. If the cerebral blood flow drops below critical values, the resulting neurological deficits are initially reversible, depending on the residual perfusion.

2.3 Arterial Flow

The flow in vessels essentially obeys three physical laws.

Ohm's Law
Ohm's law is particularly common in electrical engineering, where the formula U = R × I defines the relationship between voltage U, resistance R and current I. With minor modifications, this relationship can be applied to cerebral blood flow:

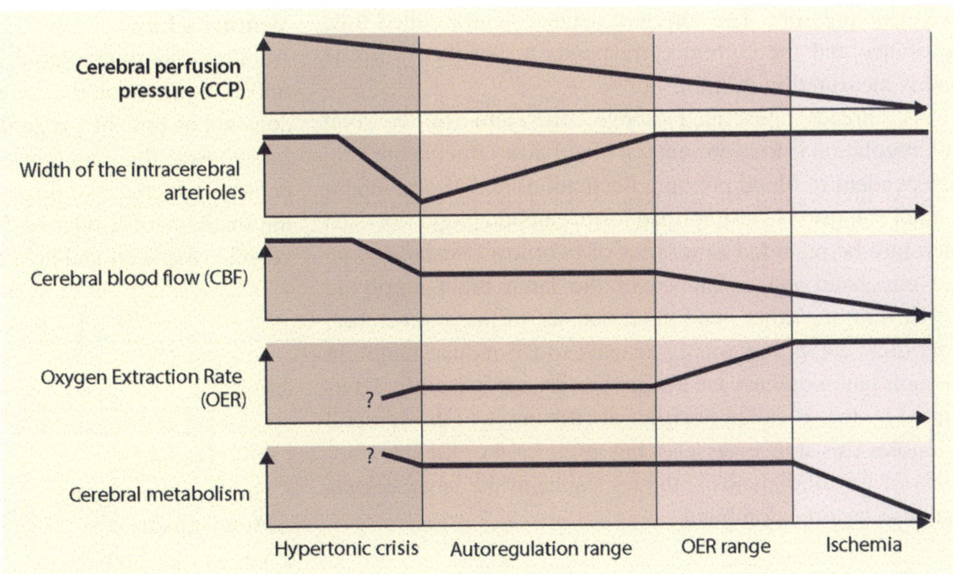

Fig. 2.2 Regulatory parameters of cerebral blood flow. Relationship between cerebral perfusion pressure, the width of the intracerebral arterioles, cerebral blood flow (CBF), oxygen extraction rate (OER) and cerebral metabolism

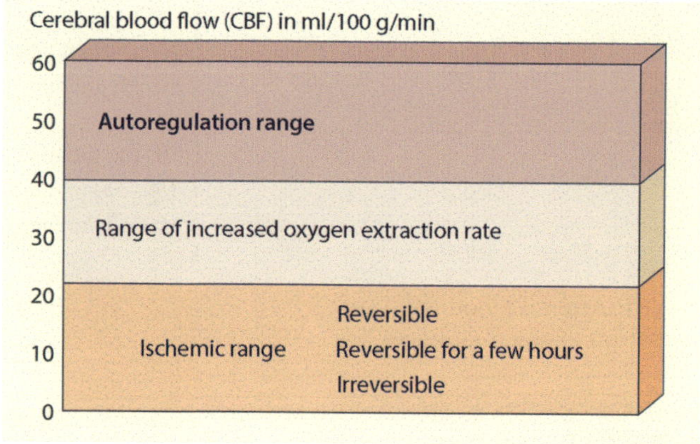

Fig. 2.3 The three areas of cerebral blood flow. Autoregulation range: normal range with relatively small fluctuations in cerebral blood flow, adapted to the requirements; range of increased oxygen extraction rate (OER): maintenance of cell function by increasing the O_2-extracion from the blood; ischemic area: loss of functional metabolism of the brain cells, but depending on the residual blood flow, maintenance of structural metabolism for a more or less long period of time

$$\Delta p = R \cdot I$$

respectively

$$I = \Delta p / R$$

with

I Flow volume
Δp Pressure gradient
R Flow resistance

Voltage is replaced by the pressure gradient, which – with reference to the entire brain – corresponds to the cerebral perfusion pressure. The current resistance is now called flow resistance and the current corresponds to the **flow volume** and is measured in ml/min.

As already described above, the aim of cerebral autoregulation is to keep cerebral blood flow largely constant, independent of blood pressure fluctuations and also independent of stenoses. In a simplified form, cerebral blood flow can therefore be regarded as a series of two flow resistances, on the one hand the resistance of the large brain-supplying arteries, on the other hand the resistance of the intracerebral arterioles, which is variably adapted to the requirements. In the non-pathological case the flow resistance is mainly determined by the so-called **peripheral resistance** of the cerebral arterioles (resistance vessels), but in the case of the development of vascular stenosis, the resistance in the large vessels can also become dominant.

Hagen-Poiseuille Law

The somewhat more complex law of Hagen-Poiseuille is particularly relevant when it is necessary to understand the influence of stenoses on the flow resistance. Although this law only applies to rigid tubes with laminar flow, it can also be used for blood vessels in a rough approximation. Assuming a constant blood viscosity, the flow resistance of a stenosis can be calculated as:

$$R \sim l/d^4$$

with

l Length of the stenosis
R Flow resistance of the stenosis
d Vessel diameter

The flow resistance becomes higher the smaller the residual lumen is, whereby a decrease in vessel diameter increases the flow resistance with the fourth power. In a comparatively small, "merely" linear amount, the length of a stenosis also contributes to the flow resistance. This has 2 practical consequences:

- Only very severe stenoses lead to hemodynamic effects due to the "explosive" increase in flow resistance. Thus, in comparison to a 50% stenosis, the flow resistance increases eight-fold in a 70% stenosis, 40-fold in an 80% stenosis and 600-fold in a 90% stenosis.
- The flow resistance of longpath stenoses is higher than that of shortpath stenoses. According to Ohm's law, this leads to a higher flow velocity in shortpath atherosclerotic stenoses compared to long-path dissections, for example.

Venturi's Law

Another important relationship results from the already mentioned requirement that cerebral blood flow should be kept as constant as possible, regardless of the presence of a stenosis. In stenoses, this requirement can only be achieved by compensatory increase of flow velocity within the stenosis. Using the mathematical relationship between the flow volume, the vessel cross-sectional area and flow velocity:

$$I = F \cdot v = \pi/4 \cdot d^2 \cdot v$$

with

I Flow volume
F Cross-sectional area
v Flow velocity
d Vessel diameter

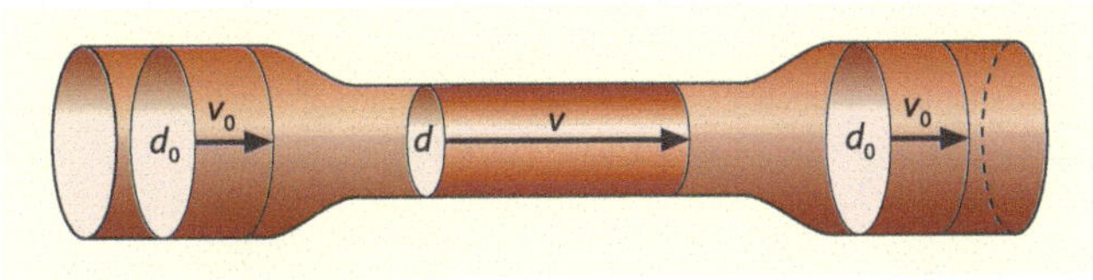

Fig. 2.4 Venturi'law of continuity for constant flow volume in the unstenosed and stenosed vessel

flow volume ist maintained by increasing flow velocity in the presence of a stenosis (Fig. 2.4):

$$I = \pi/4 \cdot d_0{}^2 \cdot v_0 = \pi/4 \cdot d^2 \cdot v = \text{constant}$$

If flow velocity v_0 and the diameter d_0 are constant in the unstenosed vessel, the flow velocity within a stenosis depends on the square of the diameter reduction

$$v \sim 1/d^2$$

This relationship has practical significance for the Doppler and duplex detection of stenoses (Fig. 5.4). However, it is only valid as long as the flow resistance of the stenosis can be compensated by increasing dilatation of the cerebral arterioles, which is usually the case up to a stenosis degree of maximum 80%. At higher degrees of stenosis, the flow velocity increases only moderately – not least also depending on the length of the stenosis – and finally even shows a decrease.

> **Summary**
> The flow in vessels is essentially characterized by three relationships: Ohm's law characterizes the relationship between pressure gradient, flow resistance and current. Hagen-Poiseuille's law defines the variables influencing vessel resistance – especially the vessel diameter. Venturi's law describes the quadratic relationship between the degree of stenosis and flow velocity in a stenosis.

2.4 Flow Disturbance

In arteries, the behavior of blood flow in non-pathological cases is characterized by two factors: Firstly, all blood particles flow toward the periphery, and secondly, the blood velocity ist much faster in the middle of the vessel than near the vessel wall. This is caused by friction losses at the vessel wall resulting in a rotationally symmetrical flow profile that is reminiscent of a parabola (Fig. 2.5). This type of flow is usually called **laminar**.

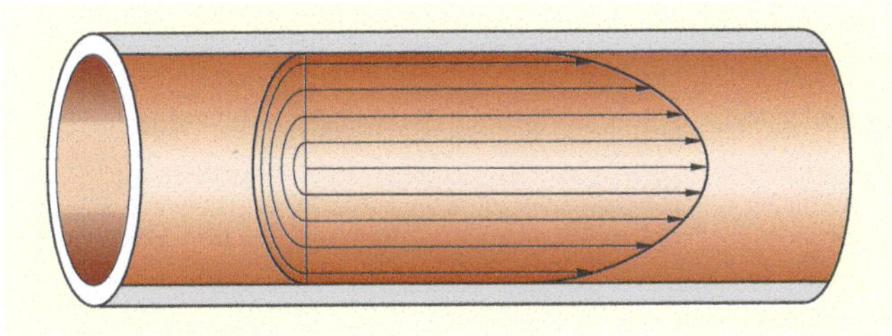

Fig. 2.5 Laminar flow in a vessel with approximately parabolic, rotationally symmetrical distribution of the flow velocity components (flow filaments) and parallel flow direction

In contrast to this are flow disturbances, which occur when the rotationally symmetric flow profile is distorted. In terms of fluid mechanics, a distinction must be made between turbulence and flow separation (Table 2.2).

2.4.1 Turbulence

As already mentioned above, blood flow velocity near the vessel wall is relatively low due to friction losses. If for any reason the flow velocity increases, this also results in increased friction on the vessel wall. If this velocity exceeds a certain value, which is physically defined by the so-called **Reynolds number, turbulence** occurs which expands further and further toward the center of the vessel as flow velocity increases (Fig. 2.6). However, up to filiform stenoses, a laminar "residual flow" remains in the center of the vessel, which, due to the high flow velocity prevailing there, is referred to in jargon as "**jet flow.**"

Reynolds Number

$$Re \sim d \cdot v/\eta$$

with

d Vessel diameter
v Flow velocity
η Blood viscosity

> **Background Information**
> In individual cases the blood viscosity is also important. For example, in the case of pronounced anemia, the reduced blood viscosity can cause the Reynolds number to be exceeded even without stenosis or hyperperfusion, which can lead to turbulence.

Table 2.2 Types of flow disturbances and their causes

Type	Definition	Cause
Turbulence	Flow disturbance exceeding the Reynolds number	Stenosis Hyperperfusion Distinctive anemia
Flow separation	Flow disturbance by deflecting the flow filaments from their straight course towards the vessel wall	Curved vessel Vessel junction (post-stenotic) vascular dilatation Aneurysm

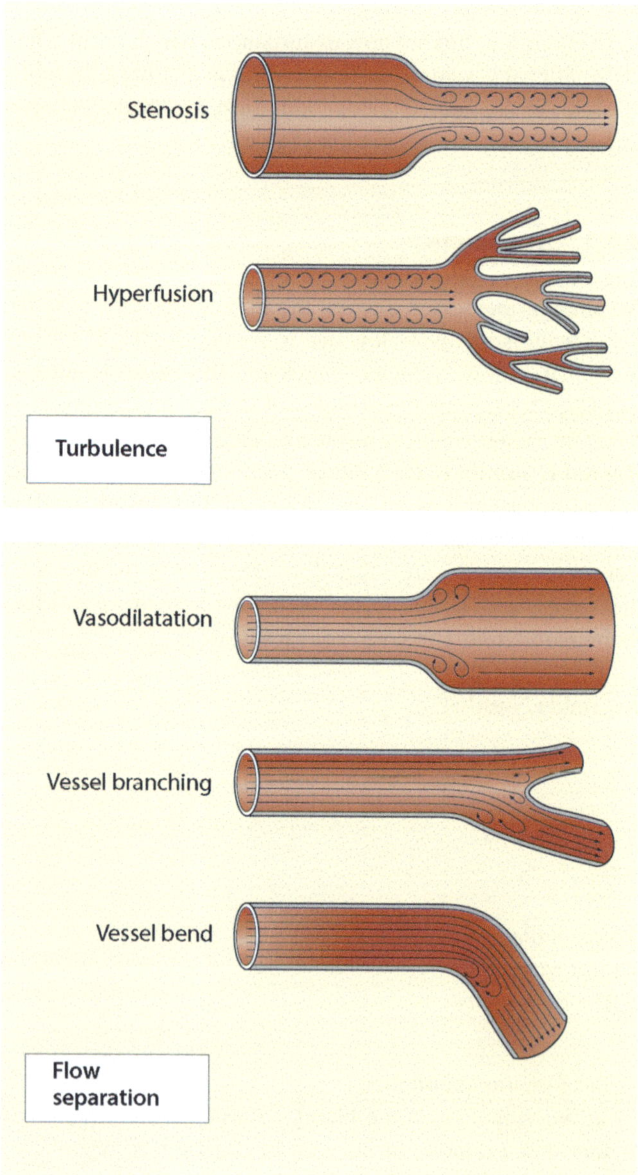

Fig. 2.6 Occurrence of flow disturbances. Turbulence due to exceeding the Reynolds number in stenoses and hyperperfusion; flow separation in vasodilatation, vascular junctions, and curved vascular course

2.4.2 Flow Separation

Although belonging to flow disturbances, flow separation has a fundamentally different cause than the turbulence. They always occur when the vessel wall abruptly changes its (largely) straight course. These can be a curved vessel course, vessel dilatations or vessel junctions (Fig. 2.6). In all these cases, the "flow filaments" require a certain distance to adapt to the changed conditions and to run in a straight line again.

Practical Tips
Both types of flow disturbances are regularly found in higher grade vascular stenoses. While turbulence prevails at the stenosis maximum (in addition to the "jet flow"), poststenostic flow separation occur due to the "jump" in caliber from the stenosed to the unstenosed lumen (Fig. 2.7). These are more pronounced the more severe and the shorter the stenosis is.

Summary
Disturbances of the normally laminar blood flow can be caused by turbulence as well as by flow separation. The former occur at high flow velocities together with the so-called "jet flow," the latter are found with abrupt changes in the vessel width or the vessel course.

2.5 Pulsatile Flow in Arteries

All data given so far assumed a continuous flow. In fact, however, pulsatile flow is present in arteries. This is caused by the rapid rise in blood pressure p during systole and the subsequent drop during diastole (Fig. 2.8). Due to the elasticity of the aortic arch, however, the pressure never reaches zero – at least not in healthy vessels – even during diastole.

According to Ohm's law (see above), the decisive factor for the formation of the flow curve in vessels not the course of

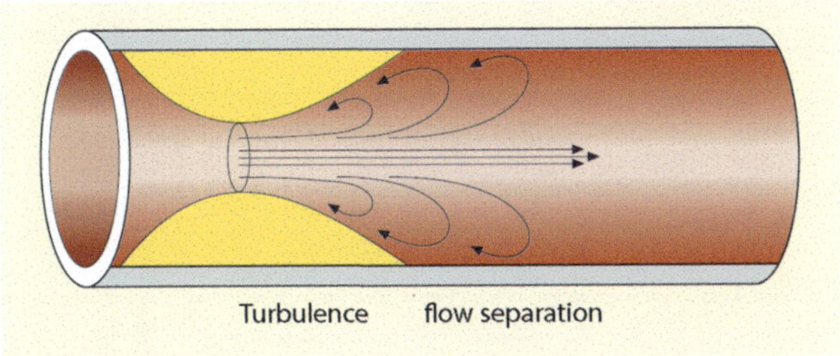

Fig. 2.7 Flow phenomena around stenoses. In the middle of the stenosis maximum there is a fast "jet flow," which is surrounded by turbulence. In the poststenotic course, flow separation appears

the blood pressure, but the respective pressure gradient Δp in each vessel section. In pulsatile flows, this pressure gradient is additionally determined by reflection phenomena of the pulse wave.

The reflection of the pulse wave depends on the level of the peripheral resistance. In narrow arterioles (high peripheral resistance), the reflected pulse wave is essentially identical to the pulse wave emitted from the heart, since only a small part of the blood passes through the narrow arterioles. If the two pulse waves meet with the time delay caused by peripheral reflection, partial extinction by subtraction occurs. The resulting pressure gradient or **flow pulse curve** (also called the "Doppler curve" in the jargon) shows a steep systolic rise and an equally steep early diastolic fall **(early diastolic backflow)** that goes below the zero line. In this case one also speaks of a **high pulsatility.**

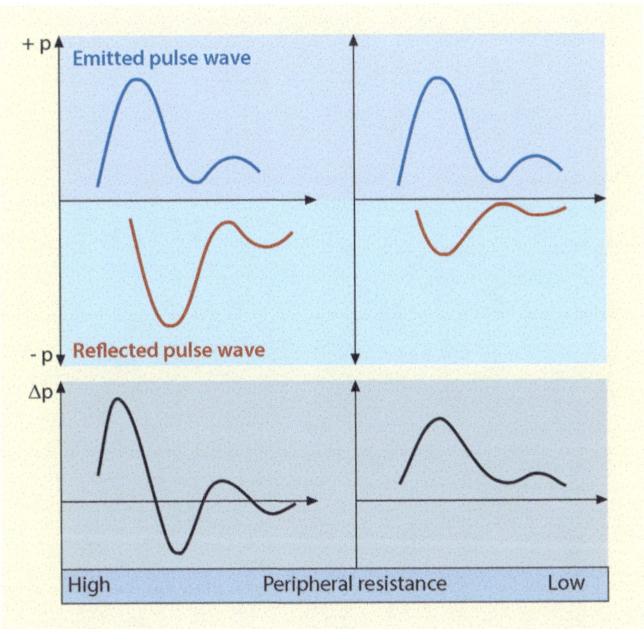

Fig. 2.8 Formation mechanism of flow curves in vessels with high (left) and low (right) peripheral resistance. Subtraction of the emitted (top, above zero) and reflected pressure pulse curves (top, below zero) results in the pressure gradient Δp (below), which is directly proportional to the flow velocity according to Ohm's law

Table 2.3 Relationship between the peripheral resistance and parameters of the (Doppler sonographic) flow pulse curve

Peripheric resistance	Pulsatility	Diastolic flow
High	High	Low
Low	Low	High

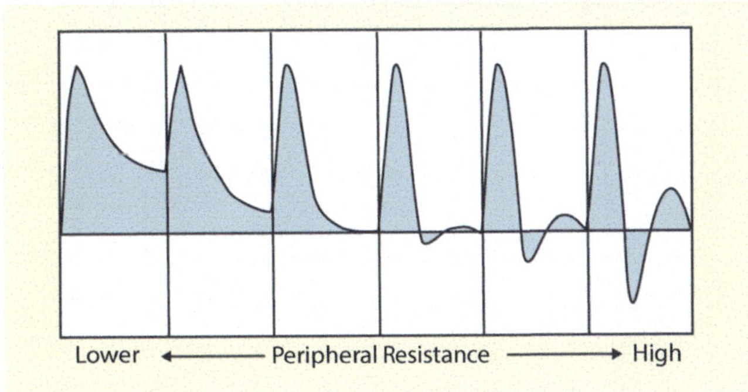

Fig. 2.9 Typical flow pulse curves with different peripheral resistances

At low peripheral resistance, however, the reflected pulse wave is significantly reduced in amplitude. If this wave is superimposed on the emitted pressure pulse curve, a rapid systolic increase of the pressure gradient is also obtained, but during diastole the flow pulse curve never reaches the zero line **(low pulsatility)** (Table 2.3).

Since the peripheral resistance can vary in all types of vessels, arteries not only have the extreme forms shown in the Fig. 2.8, but also smooth transitions between high and low diastolic flow velocity (Fig. 2.9).

Practical Tips

The assessment of the pulsatility of flow curves is of great importance in sonographic vascular diagnostics, as it is one of the most important Doppler sonographic criteria and provides information not only about the type of vessel but also about upstream and downstream flow obstacles (Sect. 5.2.4).

Summary

Depending on the peripheral resistance, arterial pulse curves show a different systolic-diastolic course, which is called pulsatility. A high peripheral resistance is associated with a high pulsatility, a low peripheral resistance with a low pulsatility.

Reference

Strandgaard S (1976) Autoregulation of cerebral blood flow in hypertensive patients. Circulation 53:720–727

3 Basics of Ultrasound Technology

Bernhard Widder and Gerhard F. Hamann

3.1 Basic Concepts of Diagnostic Ultrasound

3.1.1 Ultrasound Frequencies

From 16–18 kHz, the upper limit of the frequency range audible to humans, we speak of ultrasound. However, the frequencies used in diagnostic ultrasound are much higher, usually 2–15 MHz, and for special dermatological questions even up to 50 MHz. The choice of high sound frequencies is caused by the fact that otherwise no sufficient image resolution could be achieved. This is closely coupled to the wavelength of ultrasound (Sect. 3.3.2), which in view of the relatively "slow" sound propagation in the tissue of approx. 1500 m/s is usually in the order of 0.1–1 mm at the mentioned ultrasound frequencies (Table 3.1):

$$\lambda = c/f$$

with

c Sound propagation speed
λ Wavelength of the ultrasound oscillation
f Ultrasound frequency

3.1.2 Methods of Sound Transmission

All diagnostic ultrasound procedures are based on the principle that ultrasound is irradiated into the tissue via a "loudspeaker" and the sound components reflected from tissue structures are recorded with a "microphone" and electronically processed. There are two fundamentally different techniques.

Continuous Wave Technique
The simplest ultrasound technique is the so-called **continuous wave (CW) Doppler** (Fig. 3.1). Here, there are two piezoceramic transducers in the sound probe, one of which continuously emits a sinusoidal ultrasound wave of constant frequency, the other continuously receives it. Since sound is received from all depths of the tissue, this method is only suitable for use in simple Doppler devices with pin probes, in which the entire backscattered signal is analyzed for the presence of Doppler frequency shifts (Sect. 4.1.3).

Pulsed Wave Technique
The majority of the ultrasound devices available today operate according to the **pulsed wave (PW) or pulse-echo technique**. With this technique there exists only one transducer, which is used alternately as a transmitter and as a receiver. The transit time between sound transmission and reception of an echo provides information about the depth from which the echo originates in the tissue. This is enabled by the fact that the speed of sound in the soft tissues of the human body is sufficiently constant and fluctuates by less than 10% (Table 3.2).

3.1.3 Sound Probes

Piezoelectric Effect
Ceramic disks are used as "microphones" or "loudspeakers", whose piezoelectric effect is exploited. This means that certain materials have the ability to change their shape when a voltage is applied to them. The change in shape can be used to emit sound waves when an alternating voltage is applied. Conversely, such disks generate an electrical voltage between the surfaces coated with a thin conductive layer when they

B. Widder (✉)
Expert Opinion Institute, District Hospital, Guenzburg, Germany
e-mail: bernhard.widder@bkh-guenzburg.de

G. F. Hamann
Clinic of Neurology and Neurological Rehabilitation, District Hospital, Guenzburg, Germany

B. Widder, G. F. Hamann (eds.), *Duplex sonography of the brain-supplying arteries*, https://doi.org/10.1007/978-3-662-65566-5_3

Table 3.1 Wavelength in body tissue at different ultrasound frequencies. The wavelength corresponds approximately to the maximum axial resolution (Sect. 3.3.2)

Frequency in MHz	Wavelength in mm
1	1.50
2	0.75
5	0.30
10	0.15

are mechanically deformed by incoming sound waves. It goes without saying that these deformations are in the range of a few μm.

One-Dimensional Sound Probes
Sound probes with a single ultrasound transducer are used to detect blood flow in extra- and transcranial Doppler devices without imaging. Due to the typical design with a cable attached to the back, the term **pin probe** or – for Doppler applications – simply **Doppler probe** is used. The sound propagation of the one-dimensional sound beam is in the direction of the longitudinal axis of the probe.

Two-Dimensional Sound Probes
If several piezoceramic sound transducers are arranged next to each other and electrically controlled sequentially, a two-dimensional sound field is created from individual sound beams, which are described as **scan lines** (Fig. 3.2).

For diagnostic ultrasound applications, three two-dimensional sound probe types are mainly used today (Fig. 3.3):

- **Linear-array probes** with linear arrangement of a large number of separately controlled piezoceramic transducers. The sound field has a rectangular character. Linear-array transducers are mainly used for imaging superficial structures such as extracranial neck vessels and the thyroid gland.
- **Curved-array probes** with transducers placed on a circular section, which produce a trapezoidal sound field. Such probes are mainly used in the abdominal area.
- **Phased-array probes** with sound transducers that are located linearly close to each other, which produce a sector-shaped sound field due to the special electronic control. Due to the small contact surface, these probes are mainly used when there is little space available for sonographic coupling. This situation arises in transcranial duplex sonography due to the often very small temporal sound window (Sect. 9.3.1) and in cardiology when the sound is applied through the intercostal spaces. A disadvantage is the significantly reduced resolution compared to the other transducer types due to the small transducer area (Sect. 3.3.2).

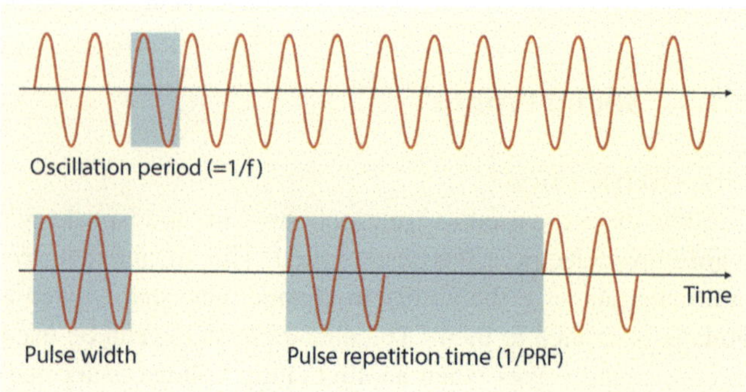

Fig. 3.1 Continuous wave (CW) (top) and pulsed wave (PW) technique (bottom) with associated wave parameters

Background Information
In contrast to the so-called "electronic" transducers with differently shaped transducer arrays, some manufacturers also offer so-called "mechanical" transducers. These usually consist of 1–3 single transducers that oscillate or rotate in an oil bath. The electronic control of mechanical transducers is considerably simpler, why they are still found in low-cost duplex devices. However, they have serious disadvantages. Due to the extremely slow image build-up rate, they are not suitable for color coded duplex sonography.

3.1.4 Ultrasound Investigations

The procedures used in diagnostic ultrasound can be distinguished according to two fundamentally different objectives with little uniform terminology (Table 3.3).

Table 3.2 Propagation velocity of ultrasound and sound attenuation in various media

Medium	Speed in m/s	Approximate damping in dB/MHz × cm
Air	340	0
Fat tissue	1480	0.5
Water	1500	0.5
Blood	1510	0.5
Brain tissue	1520	0.5
Musculature	1580	1
Bones	3400	5–10

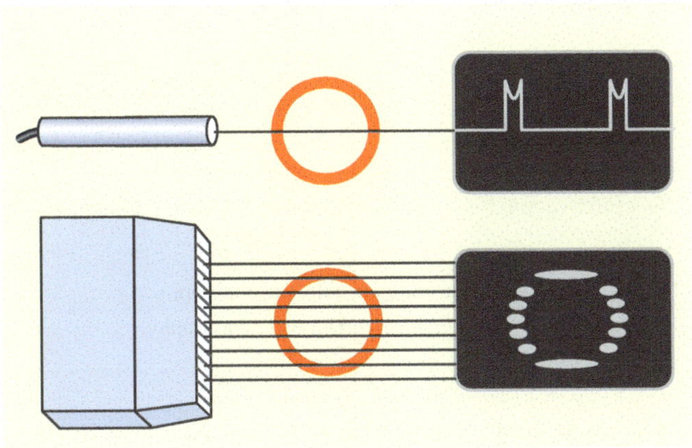

Fig. 3.2 Principle of A- and B-mode technology. While in the former the reflection amplitudes of the one-dimensional sound beam are directly visible as amplitude values on the y-axis of the screen (A means "amplitude"), in the two-dimensional B-mode image with its numerous scan lines these are represented as light points of different brightness (B means "Brightness") (below)

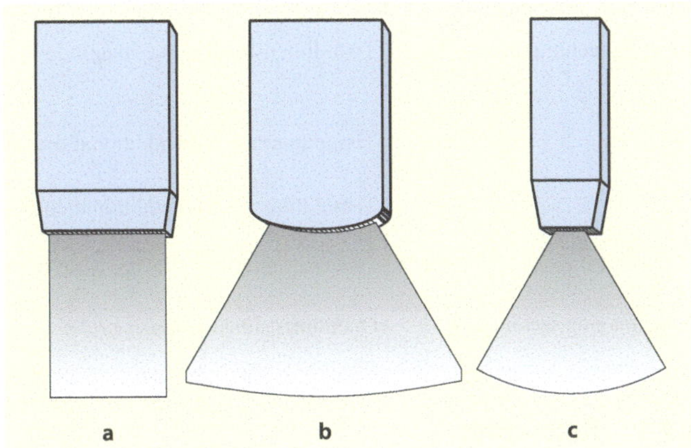

Fig. 3.3 (**a**–**c**) Different types of transducers. (**a**) linear array, (**b**) curved array, (**c**) phased array

Tissue Imaging

If an array of adjacent transducers is driven by the pulse-echo method, an almost anatomically correct image of the tissue structures in the sound plane can be achieved if the propagation times in the tissue are correctly taken into account. Since the amplitudes of the received ultrasound echoes are made visible on the screen by light spots of different brightness, this method is also known as **B-mode sonography** (**B** for "Brightness") or as **B-mode imaging** (Fig. 3.2).

Background Information

Besides B-Mode other "modes" are known in ultrasound technology. For example, the one-dimensional sonographic imaging of brain tissue (Sect. 10.3), the so-called echoencephalography, was also known as A-mode sonography (A for "Amplitude"). Similar to transcranial Doppler sonography, this is a single ultrasound beam whose reflection amplitudes (y-axis) are displayed on the screen above the penetration depth (x-axis) (Fig. 3.2). In cardiology, the so-called M-mode sonography (M such as "Motion"), in which the amplitudes of a one-dimensional sound beam are displayed in a brightness-coded manner over time. For example, pulsations of the extracranial vessel walls can be displayed in this way (Fig. 5.25).

Blood Flow Assessment

If blood flow is detected, this is mainly done according to the Doppler principle (Sect. 4.1). In a somewhat arbitrary manner, Doppler flow measurement with a single Doppler sound beam within a two-dimensional B-mode image is generally regarded as (conventional) **duplex sonography,** the additional combination with color coded flow detection is called as **color coded duplex sonography**. In addition, however, short terms for this are also found in the literature, such as **color duplex** or **color Doppler.**

The term "**Doppler**" is used in a very confusing way, sometimes even in textbooks. In neurological terminology, for example, it refers to one-dimensional Doppler sonography with the pen probe, but in internal medicine it is often used for duplex sonography as well.

Summary

Diagnostic ultrasound with frequencies of usually 2–15 MHz is based on the principle of reflection and backscattering at different tissue structures in the body. The techniques used differ mainly in 3 categories:

- Continuous (CW) and discontinuous (pulse-echo) sound transmission
- Imaging (B-mode imaging and duplex sonography) and non-imaging (Doppler sonography) methods
- Procedures for assessing anatomical structures (B-mode sonography) or blood flow (Doppler sonography) or both (duplex sonography).

3.2 Biological Ultrasound Parameters

The biological effects of ultrasound are essentially characterized by three parameters that are interrelated and that are also relevant to safety aspects mentioned in Sect. 3.5.

Table 3.3 Sonographic examination techniques and terms used for them in the literature

Imaging techniques	Two-dimensional tissue imaging	Ultrasonography B-mode sonography B-mode imaging
	Tissue imaging with additional one-dimensional Doppler sound beam	(conventional) duplex sonography Doppler sonography
	Tissue imaging with additional color-coded flow information	Color-coded duplex sonography Color duplex Color Doppler Triplex sonography
Non-imaging techniques	One-dimensional Doppler probe	Doppler sonography Doppler

3.2.1 Reflection

Every structure of the human body has a typical sound resistance, which is physically called **impedance**. In analogy to the optical laws of reflection and refraction, sound transmission through body tissue at interfaces between two impedances causes both partial reflection of the waves and deflection through refraction of the sound beam, depending on the size of the impedance difference (Fig. 3.4).

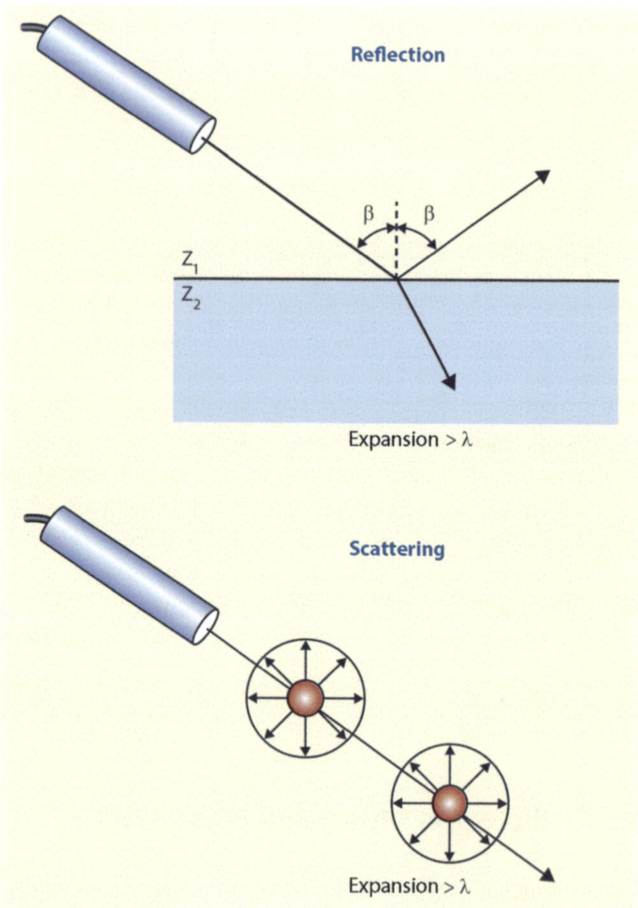

Fig. 3.4 Reflection and scattering of ultrasound waves at structures of different sizes with respect to the ultrasound wavelength λ. Z_1, Z_2 different impedances

For ultrasound applications, reflection can only be decisive if the interface is (largely) perpendicular to the sound beam. Otherwise the reflected beam will not reach the transducer. Furthermore, reflection only occurs if the expansion of the structure insonated is at least equal to the wavelength of the ultrasound beam (usually 0.2–1 mm). Reflection is of particular practical importance when assessing the so-called intima-media thickness (Sect. 16.1.1).

3.2.2 Scattering

Since structures perpendicular to the sound beam occur relatively rarely in the body, the majority of the reflected ultrasound energy is based on a different effect. This is a diffuse, omnidirectional scattering at tissue cell clusters, which, however, only has a low backscattered energy. Correspondingly, structures perpendicular to the sound beam appear more signal-intensive than oblique structures despite having the same ultrasound impedance. This is particularly impressive in the case of transverse sections through vessels, where the lateral structures are only represented relatively poorly (Fig. 3.5).

> **Practical Tips**
> In clinical practice, for the sake of simplicity, all types of reflected ultrasound signals are usually referred to as "reflection," although this is only partly physically correct for the reasons mentioned above.

3.2.3 Attenuation

Ultrasound signals are attenuated with increasing penetration depth in the tissue. This attenuation caused by reflection, scattering and friction losses is called attenuation and is tissue-specific (Table 3.2). For fatty and brain tissue it is in the order of 0.5 dB/MHz × cm and increases to 10 dB/MHz × cm for bone. As it can already be seen from the dimensioning, it also increases exponentially (definition of

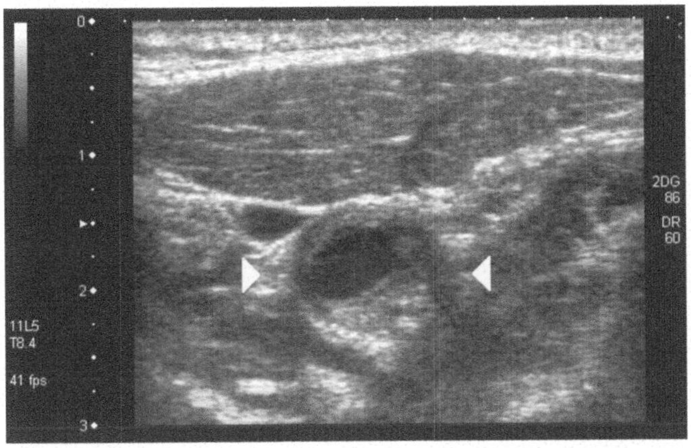

Fig. 3.5 Transversal section through the common carotid artery in a moderate, semi-circular stenosis. Note the clearer representation of the vessel wall perpendicular to the sound propagation (reflection), while the lateral parts are only diffusely visible (scattering)

dB see below) with the penetration depth and the ultrasound transmission frequency. As a result, when using higher frequencies of 7–10 MHz from tissue depths exceeding 4–5 cm, almost nothing reaches the sound probe even in the case of total internal reflection (Table 3.4). In practice, attenuation is therefore the most important obstacle to the use of higher ultrasound frequencies, and the selection of the ultrasound frequency must be based on the required penetration depth of the ultrasound in the tissue.

Note
The greater the required penetration depth of the ultrasound in the tissue, the lower the ultrasound transmission frequency used must be.

For transcranial examination, the bony skull must also be transmitted, which is virtually impermeable to higher ultrasound frequencies due to its impedance and generally only allows investigations of intracranial structures to a practically usable extent at transmission frequencies below 3 MHz. However, even at a transmission frequency of 2 MHz, approx. 80% of the sound energy is already lost when passing through the skull (Aaslid 1986).

Table 3.4 Proportion of the signal power absorbed by the transducer after complete reflection at different depths in soft tissue

	Reflected ultrasound power [%] after total reflection in a depth from	
Transmission frequency in MHz	1 cm	5 cm
2	40	1
5	10	0.001
7	4	0.00001
10	1	0.00000001

Table 3.5 Ratio of two signal intensities P_1 and P_2 (e.g., signal-to-noise ratio) when dB values are specified

dB value	2	3	10	20	30
P_1:P_2	1:1.7	1:2	1:10	1:100	1:1000

Background Information
The decibel (dB) is a parameter frequently used in physics to characterize the relative relationship between two signal intensities. The logarithmic relationship is particularly useful when the expected signal intensities have a very wide range, but even smaller differences in intensity are relevant and should be recorded. In each case 10 dB more means a tenfold increase of the original signal (Table 3.5). A so-called signal-to-noise ratio of, for example, 30 dB is defined as a gain difference of 1:1000 between noise and the possible useful signal.

Summary
Reflected ultrasound signals are mainly caused by diffuse scattering at cell assemblies. Reflection is only found on larger structures rather perpendicular to the sound beam. The sound attenuation in the tissue (attenuation) increases exponentially with increasing ultrasound transmission frequency. Image resolution, which depends on transmission frequency, and penetration depth are opposite variables. The choice of transmission frequency therefore results from the desired examination depth.

3.3 Technical Parameters of Diagnostic Ultrasound

3.3.1 Parameters of the Pulse-Echo Technique

The use of the pulse-echo method is linked to a number of technical parameters that are important in practical application, including the question of the biological safety of ultrasound.

Pulse Width

The length of the ultrasound pulse used depends on the application. To achieve the best possible local resolution (e.g., for B-mode imaging), a very short pulse must be used (Fig. 3.6). In Doppler applications, on the other hand, the ultrasound pulse must cover several cycles of a sinusoidal

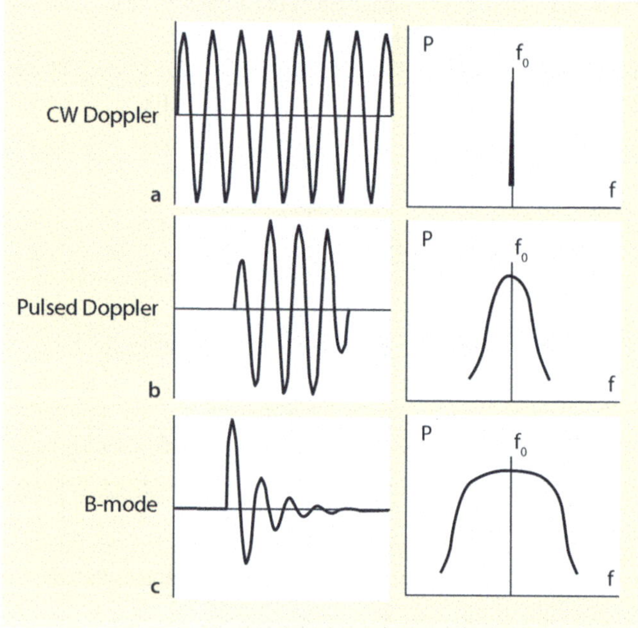

Fig. 3.6 (**a–c**) Different techniques of ultrasound transmission (left) with the respective bandwidth of the ultrasound signal (right). Continuous wave (CW) with a single transmission frequency (**a**); pulsed ultrasound with relatively long transmission pulse for pulsed Doppler applications (**b**); pulsed sound for B-mode imaging technique with the shortest possible transmission pulse and a resulting large frequency bandwidth (**c**). P Sound energy ("Power"), f_0 central frequency

oscillation, otherwise frequency differences between the transmitted and the reflected signal cannot be calculated.

Bandwidth

The shorter the emitted sound pulse, the greater the so-called **bandwidth.** This term, which originates from physics, refers to the fact that any curve can be converted into a more or less large number of individual sinusoidal oscillations **(harmonic Fourier analysis)** (Fig. 3.7). The shorter an impulse is, the more individual oscillations with different frequencies must overlap to cause it to decay within a short time. In this case one speaks of a "wide bandwidth" of the ultrasound frequency components. In contrast to this, the CW Doppler application with continuous sound radiation has only a single frequency component (bandwidth = 0). The bandwidth of the ultrasound signal in multifrequency transducers (Sect. 3.3.3) plays an important role.

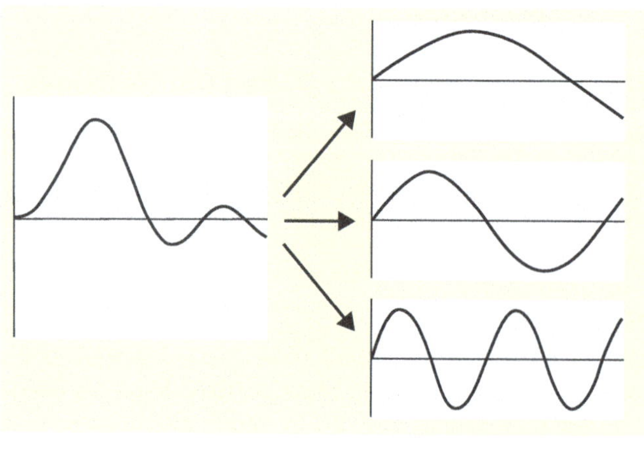

Fig. 3.7 Decomposition of a complex curve function (left) into three sinusoidal single oscillations using Fourier analysis (right)

Pulse Repetition Frequency (PRF)

By using pulse-echo technique an acoustic pulse is emitted and afterwards the sound probe is switched to receive reflected sound waves. The frequency at which sound pulses are emitted is called pulse repetition frequency (PRF). In Doppler applications it is essential for the maximum Doppler frequencies that can be displayed (Sect. 5.34).

Pulse-Pause Ratio

The relationship between the period of transmission of an ultrasound pulse and the subsequent detection period is particularly important for thermal ultrasound effects (Sect. 3.5.1). In common diagnostic applications, the pulse-pause ratio is well below 1%.

Acoustic Performance

The acoustic power of ultrasound equipment for B-mode sonography is usually in the range of less than 1 W/cm^2. In color coded duplex sonography and especially in pulsed Doppler applications, however, local peak intensities of up to 8 W/cm^2 may be measured. In the particularly critical "suction phase" of the ultrasound wave, negative sound pressures of up to 5 MPa are reached for a short time (Jenne 2001). 1 MPa corresponds to the value of approx. 150 PSI, which is better known from the tyre pressure of a car. This can result in both thermal and non-thermal (cavitation) biological effects with possible hazard potential (see Sect. 3.5). The term **mechanical index** (MI) ist used as a measure of acoustic performance.

Mechanical Index (MI)

In addition to its original meaning as a measure of the probability of cavitation (Sect. 3.5.2), the MI is considered a 'normalized' value for acoustic performance. It is calculated as the quotient of the negative peak pressure and the emitted ultrasound frequency:

Mechanical Index (MI).

$$MI = p- / \sqrt{f}$$

with

p– Negative peak pressure
f Ultrasound frequency

Table 3.6 Rating sound energy using the Mechanical Index (MI)

MI <0.1	Low sound energy
MI 0.1–0.5	Middle sound energy
MI >1.0	High sound energy

For most ultrasound devices, the current MI is displayed on the screen. The lower the MI, the lower the sound energy emitted (Table 3.6).

Middle Frequency

The frequency information displayed on the screen of most ultrasound devices gives the impression a single, clearly defined transmission frequency. However, as mentioned above, pulse-echo applications always include a more or less broadband frequency spectrum, and the transmission frequency displayed on the device corresponds only to the **middle-** or **central frequency** f_0 (Fig. 3.6).

Frame Rate

Fundamentally different to the above mentioned frequency values is the frame rate. This defines how often a new image with changed content is built up on the screen of the ultrasound device and thus provides information on whether the ultrasound display is actually in "real time." In the case of pure B-mode imaging applications and by using not too many focal points (Fig. 3.14), the frame rate is significantly higher than the image fusion rate of 16 Hz known for the human eye. Color coded imaging, however, slows down the frame rate – especially with low-cost devices down to below 3–4 Hz -, which can be very disturbing when examining agitated patients.

Time Gain Compensation (TGC)

By using a runtime-dependent amplification, the so-called **time gain compensation** (TGC), an attempt is made to compensate for the effect of attenuation mentioned in the Sect. 3.2, so that identical structures from different depths lead to identical echo amplitudes, at least in theory (Fig. 3.8). The reason for the limited penetration depth of ultrasound is that noise artifacts increase, if an augmented electronic amplification of the low signals reflected by deep tissue layers is required. The extent of possible amplification up to the occurrence of significant noise is described as **dynamic range** and is expressed in decibels (dB). Ultrasound devices today have a dynamic range of around 100 dB.

3.3.2 Resolution

Resolution means the ability to discriminate two structures in the examined tissue. A fundamental distinction is made between axial and lateral resolution.

Axial Resolution

The resolution in the direction of sound depends exclusively on the length of the emitted sound pulse. Since sound pulses, at least in B-mode sonography, consist of only 1–2 sinusoidal oscillations (Fig. 3.6), an axial resolution in the order of the wavelength can be achieved (Fig. 3.9). Depending on the transmission frequency used, this is 0.2–1 mm (Table 3.1).

Lateral Resolution

Much more complex is the lateral resolution, that is, the possibility of discriminating between two points perpendicular to sound propagation (Fig. 3.10). Although this also depends on the transmission frequency respectively on the resulting ultrasound wavelength, two additional factors play a significant role.

1. **Dependence on the focus range.** The sound beam reaches its maximum sensitivity only in a narrowly defined area, the so-called **focus.** In the **near-** and **far field** the resolution is much worse (Fig. 3.11). Furthermore, in the near field so-called **side lobes** play a role leading to considerable artifacts. "High-end devices" often try to suppress these artifacts with considerable technical effort.

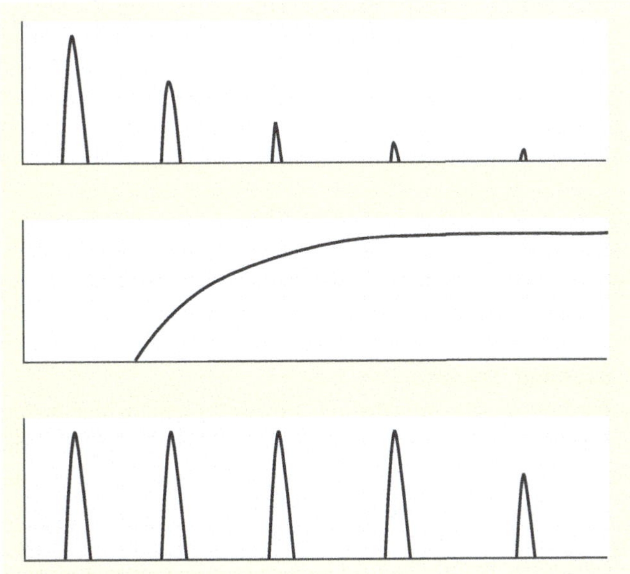

Fig. 3.8 Principle of runtime-dependent gain compensation (time gain compensation, TGC). Due to an amplification (middle) that increases with increasing propagation time of the sound pulse, weak reflections from deeper tissue layers are amplified disproportionately

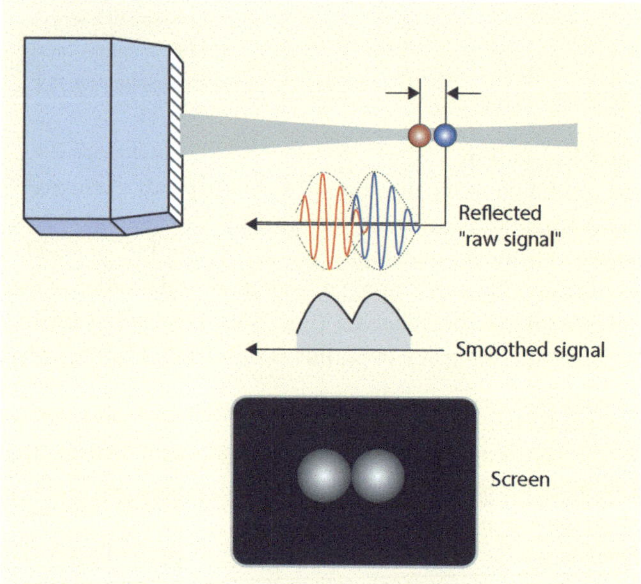

Fig. 3.9 Definition of the axial resolution. A discrimination of two structures located in the direction of sound propagation is possible if the two reflected sound signals arriving in series can be kept sufficiently apart

2. **Dependence on the transducer area.** The larger the propagation area of the transducer, the better the lateral resolution at the focal point, but the further away from the transducer the focal point moves.

> **Practical Tips**
> Due to the close relationship between transducer propagation area and lateral resolution, transducers with a small contact area (e.g., phased-array transducers) always have a poorer resolution than, for example, large linear or curved-array transducers for physical reasons.

3.3.3 Measures to Improve Ultrasound Image Quality

Broadband Transducer

According to the information already given on the bandwidth, the shorter the transmitted ultrasound pulse, the greater the bandwidth. In recent years, it has been possible to generate very short ultrasound pulses with a correspondingly broad frequency spectrum by using special piezoelectric materials (Sect. 3.1.3). As a result, the above mentioned center frequency of an ultrasound transducer becomes less important and it is possible to process certain sound frequencies preferentially within the bandwidth of the ultrasound pulse by means of appropriate electronic control (see

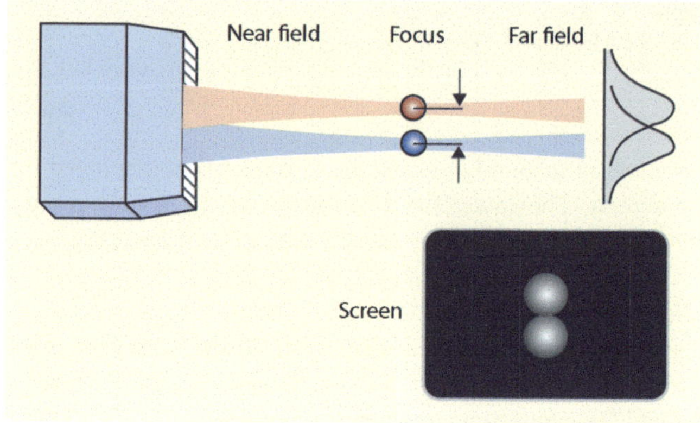

Fig. 3.10 Definition of the lateral resolution. A sufficient discrimination of two structures transverse to the direction of sound propagation is only possible in the focus area

below). Broadband transducers have the advantage that the resolution in the near range is improved due to the high frequency components. With deeper structures, the low-frequency components contained in the broadband spectrum become relevant, with which even deeper structures can still be displayed – albeit with reduced resolution.

Multifrequency Technology

In recent years, the development of broadband ultrasound transducers has led to the fact that a variable weighting of the transmission frequency has become possible in most duplex devices. This means that, for example, in the case of a 7.5 MHz transducer, the center frequencies emitted can be shifted between 5 and 10 MHz. To a limited extent, the maximum penetration depth can be improved in this way when the lower frequency range is selected – but with a reduction in resolution – whereas when switching to the higher frequency range, structures lying just below the skin surface can be detected with improved resolution.

However, the use of multi-frequency technology is only a moderately suitable compromise for covering several areas of application with a single ultrasound probe. In fact, the

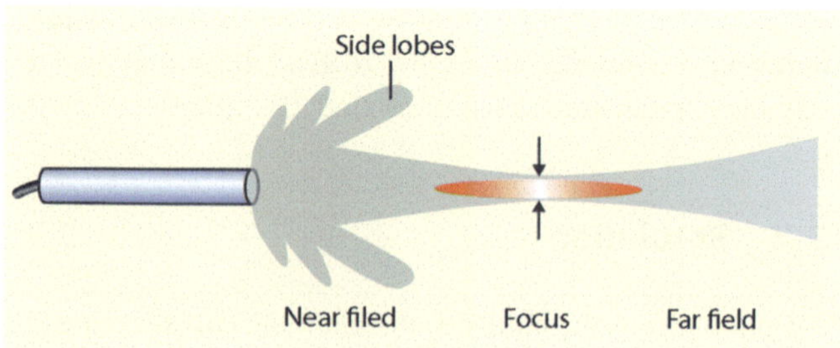

Fig. 3.11 Different sensitivity of the ultrasound transducer in the near and far field and in the focus range. In the near range, the resolution is additionally impaired by "side lobes"

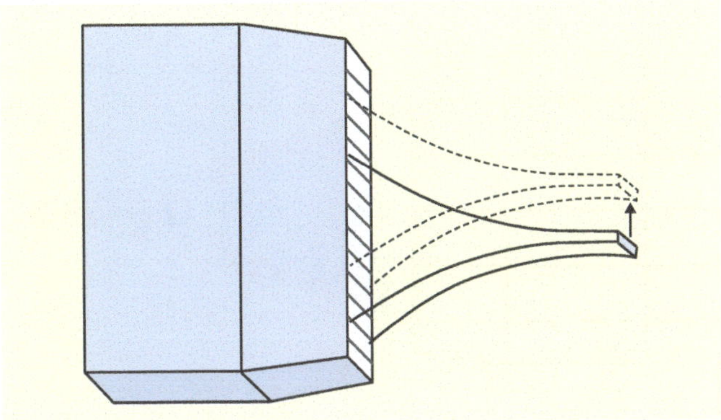

Fig. 3.12 Improvement of the lateral resolution of a linear array transducer in the long axis by joint control of several ultrasound transducers resulting in an increase of the propagation area. Note the unchanged poor resolution on the narrow side of the transducer

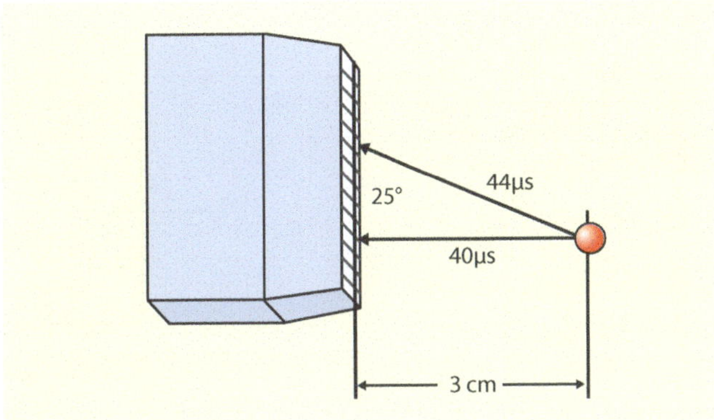

Fig. 3.13 Runtime differences of the ultrasound for a reflector at a depth of 3 cm. If different transducers are activated, the transit times can vary by up to approx. 10%

performance of a transducer is always best in the range of its physically specified resonant frequency, so that a "real" 7.5 MHz transducer, for example, will provide better results in terms of both penetration depth and resolution than a 10 MHz transducer "tuned" to 7.5 MHz.

Control of Several Transducers

If, as shown in the Fig. 3.10, transducer arrays are used to generate an ultrasound image, poor lateral resolution is to be expected due to the small area of each individual transducer (Sect. 3.2.2). This disadvantage can be compensated for by the fact that the electronics do not only control one transducer at a time, but always several at the same time and this "transducer package" is continuously shifted one transducer at a time (Fig. 3.12). Thus a good resolution can be achieved at least in the longitudinal axis of the transducers, whereas this resolution is less satisfactory on the narrow side of the transducer.

Background Information

In recent years, attempts have been made to compensate for this deficiency in "high-end devices" by dividing the transducers on the narrow side as well and controlling them separately. According to the principle of dynamic focusing mentioned below, the lateral resolution in this plane can be improved considerably in this way. With fan-shaped control in the sense of a "phased-array transducer," 3D reconstruction can also be made possible in this way.

Dynamic Focusing

Reflections, especially from superficial tissue structures, arrive at slightly different times at the transducers of the above mentioned "transducer package" due to the different distances travelled (Fig. 3.13). This fact can be used to achieve additional focusing – independent of the "natural" focus mentioned in Sect. 3.3.2 – by including delays in the control of the individual transducers.

If different delays are selected, the examiner can – at least in theory – use them to control several focus points in succession. This method is called dynamic focusing and is used today in most ultrasound devices (Fig. 3.14). The different focal points are usually marked by a dot or an arrow at the edge of the B-mode image. In "high-end" devices, this type of focusing occurs both during transmission and reception of the ultrasound signals.

Practical Tips

Due to the improvement in resolution that can be achieved by dynamic focusing, it seems obvious to set as many focus points as possible on the device in order to achieve optimum resolution in the entire image. However, the individual focus points are "processed" one after the other, so that the frame rate slows down with an increasing number of these points. Since the slowdown only becomes noticeable below a frequency of approx. 10 Hz, the use of 2–3 focus points in B-mode sonography usually represents a good compromise. In color coded duplex sonography, however, the possibilities are very limited due to the already slow frame rates.

Tissue Harmonic Imaging (THI)

Harmonic frequencies are well known from music and are responsible for the sound character of the different musical instruments. They are integer multiples of the fundamental frequency (for a fundamental frequency of 440 Hz, for example, 880, 1320, 1760 Hz, etc.). In medical ultrasound technology, on the other hand, only the **second harmonic wave** has practical significance.

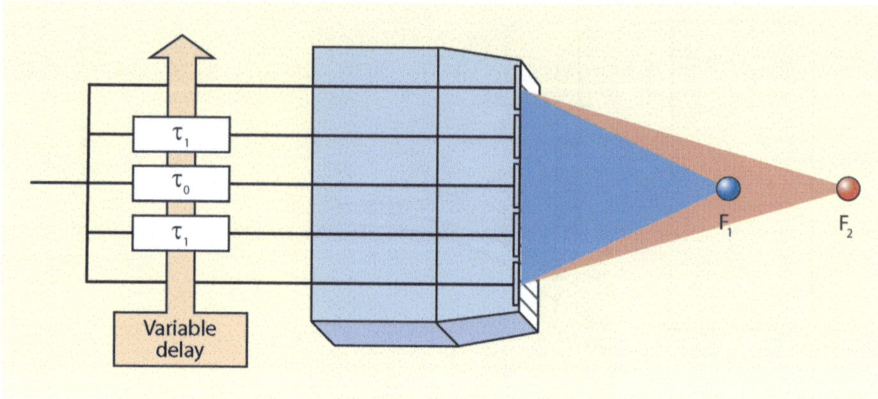

Fig. 3.14 Principle of electronic focusing by delayed control (τ_0, τ_1 ...) of the transducers located toward the center. If the delay times are kept variable, several focal points F_1, F_2 ... can be set

During their propagation in the tissue, ultrasound pulses are increasingly deformed (Fig. 3.15). The distortion of the waveform of the transmitted pulse means that the signals picked up again by the transducer contain not only the transmitted frequency spectrum, but also its harmonics. These harmonics can be filtered out and used to generate a sectional image of tissue (**tissue harmonic imaging**).

The process is based on two physical effects:

1. The occurrence of harmonics has a quadratic relationship to sound intensity. In practice, this means that strong ultrasound signals are additionally amplified, while weak signals are increasingly lost. Since, by definition, the ultrasound energy is strongest in the focal area of the sound field, additional focusing can be achieved in this way and the side lobes of the sound field (Fig. 3.11) can be suppressed.
2. Harmonics only occur when the ultrasound passes into deep tissue. Accordingly, artifact signals originating from the near field of the ultrasound signal and reverberations from the skin surface can be significantly reduced in this way. Conversely, however, this means that in slim patients with already ideal examination conditions, the use of tissue harmonic imaging leads to a deterioration in image quality compared to "conventional" techniques.

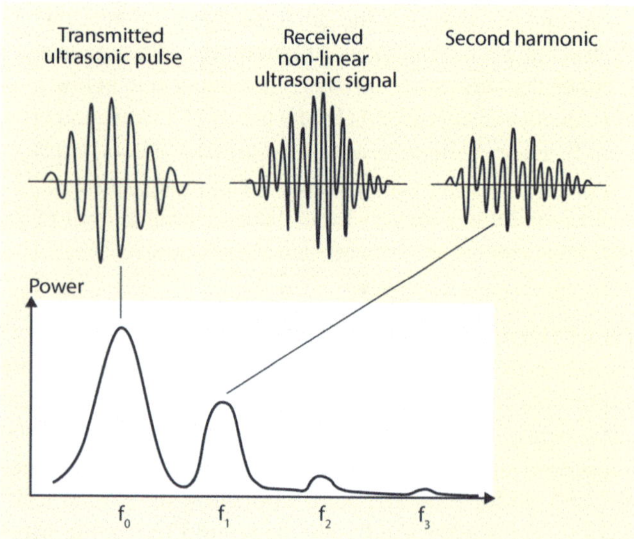

Fig. 3.15 The reflected ultrasound signal contains harmonics that can be analyzed by comparing them with the transmitted pulse

Practical Tips

The use of "tissue harmonic imaging" leads to an improvement of the lateral resolution and image contrast as well as to a reduction of image artifacts (e.g., reverberations and "ghost images") in B-mode ultrasound in the case of primarily unfavorable examination conditions.

3.4 Contrast-Assisted Procedures

3.4.1 Signal Amplified Doppler and Duplex Sonography

The increased backscatter of ultrasound contrast-enhancing agents (Fig. 3.16) can be used with all Doppler-dependent ultrasound procedures to better visualize blood flow in comparison to the surrounding tissue. The application of such agents has been intensively researched over a long period of time to enable the examination of the cerebral arteries especially in the absence of a temporal sound window, and to improve the image quality in deep-seated cervical vessels. However, due to the constant improvement of ultrasound technology, the high costs of the ultrasound contrast agents and other techniques such as CT and MR angiography, which are now available almost everywhere, disillusionment has set in here. Therefore such procedures no longer play a relevant role in the practical application of ultrasound diagnostics of the cerebral arteries.

Low sound energy	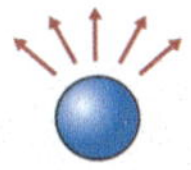	Increased ultrasonic reflection or scattering
Medium sound energy	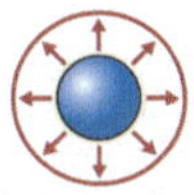	Non-linear oscillation of the contrast medium bubbles (contrast harmonic imaging)
High sound energy	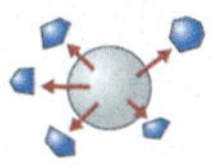	Destruction of the contrast medium bubbles (stimulated acoustic emission)

Fig. 3.16 Behavior of gas-containing contrast medium bubbles when exposed to ultrasound of different acoustic/sound energy. Further explanations in the text

3.4.2 Contrast Harmonic Imaging

This method is used to visualize slow blood flow in tissue capillaries by resonance effects of the contrast medium bubbles. It was hoped that this method would enable to assess perfusion deficits in brain tissue in acute stroke. However, since the method is limited to one diagnostic slice, it could not prevail over CT and MR perfusion imaging and has since been largely abandoned.

3.4.3 Stimulated Acoustic Emission (SAE)

Since contrast agent vesicles are destroyed at high sound energy, this effect can also be used to visualize perfusion in brain tissue. However, the method has not been used in practice for this purpose. Already used is this technique for applying cystostatic drugs precisely especially in liver tumors.

Summary
The resolution in the direction of sound propagation (axial resolution) of ultrasound devices is frequency-dependent in the order of the wavelength of the emitted sound. The lateral resolution transverse to the direction of sound propagation is best in the area of the focal point. Overall, however, it is always worse than the axial resolution and depends in particular on the size of the transducer crystals. In addition to the physically based focusing of the transducer, the resolution of the ultrasound image can be improved by time-delayed control of the transducers ("dynamic focusing"). Tissue harmonic imaging (THI) uses the non-linear distortion of the ultrasound waves occurring during reflection in body tissue to suppress image artifacts by detecting the second harmonic. Ultrasound contrast agents no longer play a significant role in the cerebrovascular sonography.

3.5 Safety Aspects of Ultrasound Diagnostics

A significant advantage of ultrasound diagnostics is its largely risk-free nature, especially in comparison to X-ray applications. Under certain conditions, however, sonographic applications can also be potentially hazardous. For the user, knowledge of the most important parameters and bioeffects of ultrasound therefore appears essential.

3.5.1 Thermal Effects

In ultrasound applications tissue heating may occur, although tissue perfusion contributes to a continuous heat dissipation. From a technical point of view, especially pulsed Doppler applications lead to local temperature peaks due to their narrow focus on the sample volume, whereas thermal effects are negligible in B-mode sonography. Color coded duplex sonography lies between these two applications with regard to thermal problems. The following overview mentions the risk factors for thermal effects:

Technical Risk Factors
1. Pulsed Doppler application
2. Long examination times
3. High sound energy (acoustic power).

In ultrasound devices the thermal risk is characterized by the **thermal index** (TI), which defines the conditions for an expected temperature increase. With newer devices, the TI is usually displayed continuously on the screen.

As a general rule, up to a TI of 1 (= 1 °C), no significant thermal hazard is to be expected, except in the case of poorly perfused tissue. This includes the lens of the eye, specifically heat-sensitive tissue such as in the fetus, or an already pre-existing temperature increase in the case of febrile diseases (see overview below).

Biologically Induced Risk Factors

1. Tissue with high ultrasound absorption (bone 10–20 times higher than soft tissue)
2. Tissue with poor blood supply (e.g., lens and cornea of the eye)
3. Specific heat-sensitive tissue (e.g., fetus)
4. Already existing high body temperature (fever).

Temperature increases may also occur in tissues with high sound absorption such as bones. The TI concept attempts to take this situation into account by specifying different TI values for different constellations (Table 3.7).

Due to a number of uncertainties in the calculation of the TI, a division into two hazard classes is favored:

- **Class A devices** without significant risk potential, provided that the duration of the exposure does not exceed 15 min, that the body temperature is normal and that no contrast medium is used.
- **Class B devices** with possible thermal hazards, for which a risk-benefit analysis should be carried out and the exposure times should be kept as short as possible.

Practical Tips

In extracranial Doppler and duplex applications, no relevant thermal stress is generally to be expected, not least because of the high dissipation of thermal energy in the vessels. However, the basic rule should be to keep examination times as short as possible, especially in pulsed Doppler mode ("as little as possible, as much as necessary"). The situation is somewhat more problematic in transcranial ultrasound diagnostics, where the heating of the skull bone is the most important feature. Both Doppler and duplex devices can achieve relevant temperature increases of the skull by 3–4 °C. The duration of the exposure to ultrasound plays a remarkably small role, since according to studies by Barnett (2001) 75% of the maximum temperature increase is already reached after 30 s. In principle, therefore, the lowest possible sound transmission energy (power) should be used, and it is better to try to set the ultrasound gain as high as possible. In the case of particularly critical transorbital insonation, where damage to the lens of the eye can occur, an attempt should also be made to keep the examination time to well below 30 s without moving the probe or switching off the Doppler mode.

Table 3.7 Definition of the thermal index (TI) for different constellations

TIB	"Bone"	Bones at focus point of ultrasound field
TIS	"Soft tissue"	Soft tissue at ultrasound field
TIC	"Cranial"	Transmission of cranial bone to the surface

3.5.2 Mechanical Effects (Cavitation)

Cavitation means the formation of small gas bubbles in liquid media. Animal experiments have shown that cavitation can cause tissue lesions and microbleeding as well as the formation of free radicals. The occurrence of cavitation depends both on the characteristics of the ultrasound pulse (frequency, pulse duration and pulse repetition frequency) and on the properties of the liquid medium (e.g., density, viscosity, thermal conductivity and gas content). At usual sound pressures of diagnostic ultrasound, the risk of cavitation is minimal. However, cavitation can occur when using ultrasound contrast agents, which by definition contain small gas bubbles. Such techniques, however, are no longer used in cerebrovascular ultrasound, at least not in routine diagnostics.

A measure for the probability of cavitation effects occurring is the "Mechanical Index" (MI) already mentioned in Sect. 3.3.1. "Normal" MI are below a value of 1, the maximum MI recommended for diagnostic ultrasound equipment is 1.9.

Summary

Risks from ultrasound applications are possible due to two effects:

1. Thermal effects occur particularly during prolonged use of pulsed Doppler sonography and can lead to relevant temperature increases, especially in bones and in the eye.
2. Mechanical effects (cavitation) are mainly found in connection with the use of ultrasound contrast agents, which must be taken into account when using them.

References

Aaslid R (ed) (1986) Transcranial Doppler sonography. Springer, Berlin Heidelberg New York

Barnett SB (2001) Intracranial temperature elevation from diagnostic ultrasound. Ultrasound Med Biol 27:883–888

Jenne J (2001) Kavitation in biologischem Gewebe. Ultraschall Med 22: 200–207

Basics of Sonographic Flow Detection

4

Bernhard Widder and Gerhard F. Hamann

4.1 Doppler Dependent Procedures

4.1.1 Doppler Effect

The Doppler effect, named after the mathematician Christian Doppler from Vienna (1803–1852), describes the frequency shift that occurs when there is relative movement between the transmitter and receiver of a wave front – for example, light or sound. The correctness of the relationship, which had been only theoretically derived, was proven by the Dutchman Buys Ballot in 1845 for sound waves by means of a practical experiment using the railway. For example, the whistle emitted by the steam pipe of a locomotive appears higher in frequency when the observer is standing in the driving direction (Fig. 4.1). The wave front is therefore "compressed" when the sound is moving in the direction of propagation. Conversely, the frequency appears lower when the locomotive moves away from the observer. Here the wave front is "pulled apart" accordingly.

If, as in the case of the mentioned locomotive, the movement of the sound transmitter is significantly slower than the propagation speed of the wave front (340 m/s in air), the originally quite complex physical relationship is simplified considerably, since in this case there is a directly proportional relationship between the speed v of the sound transmitter and the frequency shift Δf.

4.1.2 Application of the Doppler Effect to Blood Vessels

If there is blood flow in the sound field of an ultrasound Doppler device, the sound scattered back by the erythrocytes will have a slightly different frequency than the sound reflected by unmoving structures. Since the blood flow velocity with a maximum of 5 m/s is significantly lower than the sound velocity in the body with about 1500 m/s even in high-grade stenoses, a simple correlation in the form of the so-called **Doppler equation** can be determinated:

$$\Delta f = 2/c \cdot f_0 \cdot v \cdot \cos \alpha$$

Δf (Doppler) frequency shift
f_0 Emitted ultrasound frequency
c Sound velocity in the body tissue
v Blood flow velocity
α Angle between the ultrasonic beam and the vessel (insonation angle)

The factor 2 is due to the fact that, in contrast to the above mentioned example with the locomotive, the sound has to travel twice the distance due to the fixed sound source and the moving reflector. In addition to the largely invariable sound velocity in body tissue, however, there are various influencing variables which will be discussed in more detail in the following.

Emitted Ultrasound Frequency f_0
Since different ultrasound frequencies must be used in diagnostic ultrasound for different examination conditions, it must be taken into account that different Doppler frequency shifts are generated for the same blood flow velocity at different sound frequencies (Table 4.1).

B. Widder (✉)
Expert Opinion Institute, District Hospital, Guenzburg, Germany
e-mail: bernhard.widder@bkh-guenzburg.de

G. F. Hamann
Clinic of Neurology and Neurological Rehabilitation, District Hospital, Guenzburg, Germany

B. Widder, G. F. Hamann (eds.), *Duplex sonography of the brain-supplying arteries*, https://doi.org/10.1007/978-3-662-65566-5_4

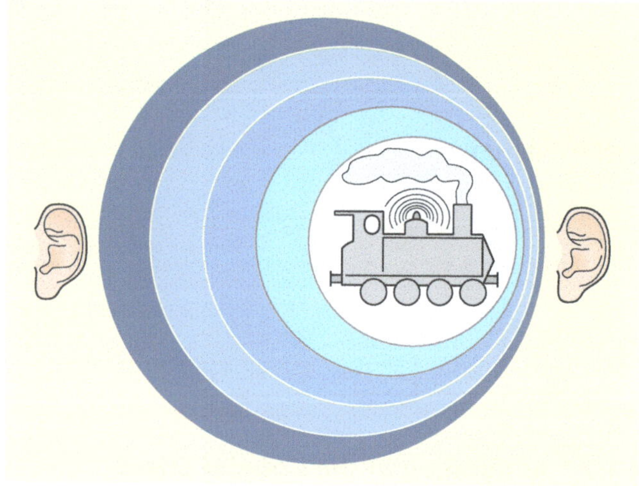

Fig. 4.1 Doppler effect using the example of a whistling locomotive moving to the right. The sound waves are "pressed together" in the driving direction, and "pulled apart" against the driving direction. Correspondingly, you hear a higher tone than the signal frequency actually emitted when the locomotive approaches you. When the locomotive is moving away, the frequency is lower

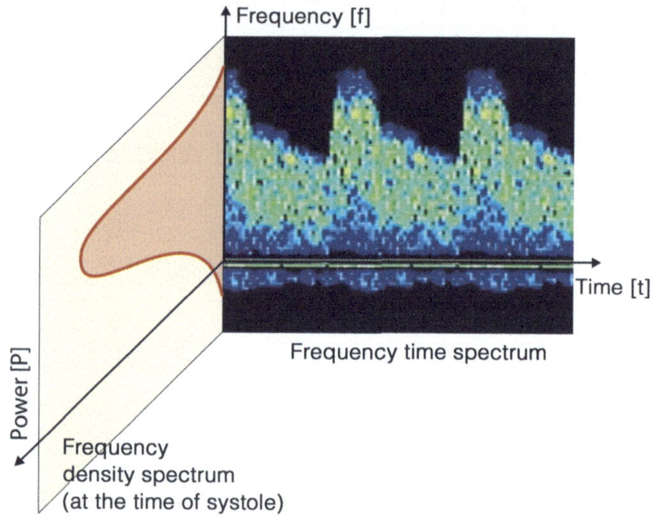

Fig. 4.2 Time course of the Doppler frequencies in the systolic-diastolic cycle with color coded representation of their frequency (frequency-time spectrum) as well as frequency distribution of the different frequencies (frequency-density spectrum) at the time of systole

Practical Tips

Using angle-corrected display of flow velocity in duplex devices, different emitted ultrasound frequencies are automatically included. The emitted ultrasound frequency is therefore particularly important when using simple Doppler probes. In this case it is not possible to indicate specific flow velocities due to a lack of knowledge of the insonation angle.

Blood Flow Velocity V

As already shown in Sect. 2.4, the velocity in blood vessels is not uniform, but at least in laminar flow it is distributed approximately parabolically over the vessel cross section. This means that not only one flow velocity v, but a wide range of different flow velocities must be considered, which also change considerably over the systolic-diastolic cycle. Correspondingly, when applying the Doppler effect to vessels, not only a single frequency shift is obtained, but a spectrum of different shift frequencies. This spectrum can be represented in two ways.

Table 4.1 Doppler frequency shift in kHz at different sound transmission frequencies in MHz, related to a (single) flow velocity of 150 cm/s at an insonation angle of 60°

2 MHz	2 kHz
4 MHz	4 kHz
8 MHz	8 kHz

- **Frequency time spectrum.** In this case the spectrum is recorded over the course of time, and the incidence of the distinct frequency components (power) at every point is displayed "color coded" or with different gray levels (Fig. 4.2). This type of display is the standard method in diagnostic ultrasound today. All Doppler and duplex devices available today have as a standard feature the possibility of continuous display of the Doppler frequency time spectrum, abbreviated in the jargon as **Doppler spectrum**. Details on the technical and diagnostic parameters can be found in Chap. 5.
- **Frequency density spectrum.** In addition, the distribution of the different frequency components can be displayed as a curve at any time during the systolic-diastolic cycle. This method is of practical importance in color coded duplex sonography, in which the various frequency components are displayed in different colors.

Insonation Angle α

In the transcutaneous Doppler assessment of blood flow, in most cases the axis of the sound beam does not lie in the flow axis of the vessel, but runs at an angle to it called "insonation angle". From a physical point of view, blood flow velocity v must be divided into 2 parts (vectors) – the part v_{axial} which is responsible for the Doppler frequency shift, and the component $v_{tangential}$ (Fig. 4.3), which has no significance for the Doppler spectrum. In extreme cases, with the Doppler probe perpendicular to the blood vessel, the measurable fraction v_{axial} completely disappears, so that despite the sound beam

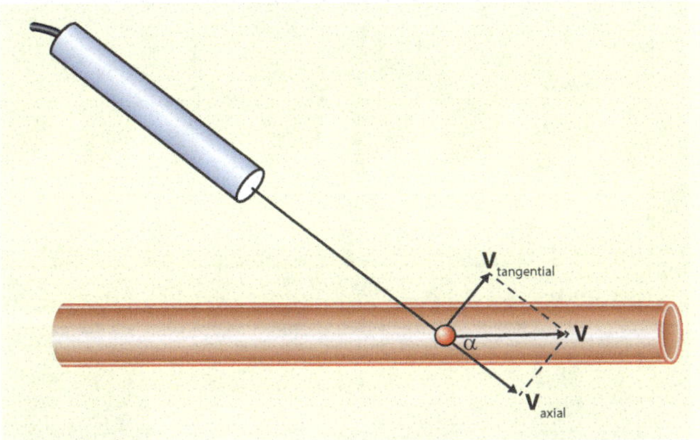

Fig. 4.3 Application of the Doppler effect for transcutaneous assessment of the blood flow velocity with oblique ultrasound insonation. Measurable component v_{axial} and non-recordable portion $v_{tangential}$

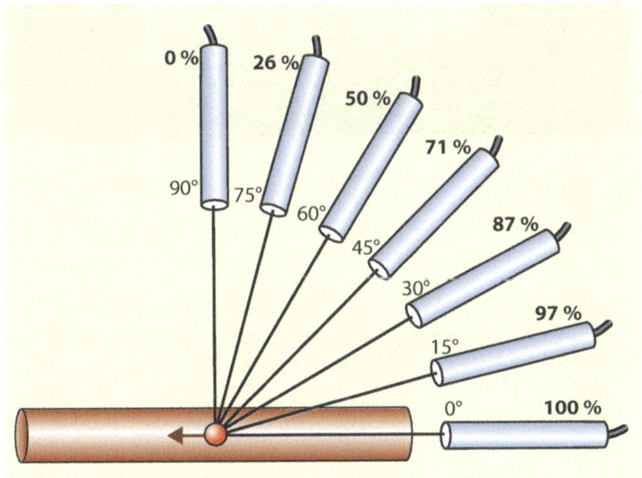

Fig. 4.4 Dependence of the measured Doppler frequency shift on the cosine of the angle between the sound beam and the vessel course (insonation angle)

directed at the blood vessel, no Doppler frequency shift can be obtained. Mathematically, this relationship is described by the cosine of the angle α between the sound beam and the blood vessel (Fig. 4.4). This has the value 1 at an angle of 0°, at 90° it reaches the value 0.

4.1.3 Doppler Techniques

As already briefly mentioned in Sect. 3.1.4, Doppler-dependent methods are used in various device constellations. Fig. 4.5 gives an overview of the different techniques.

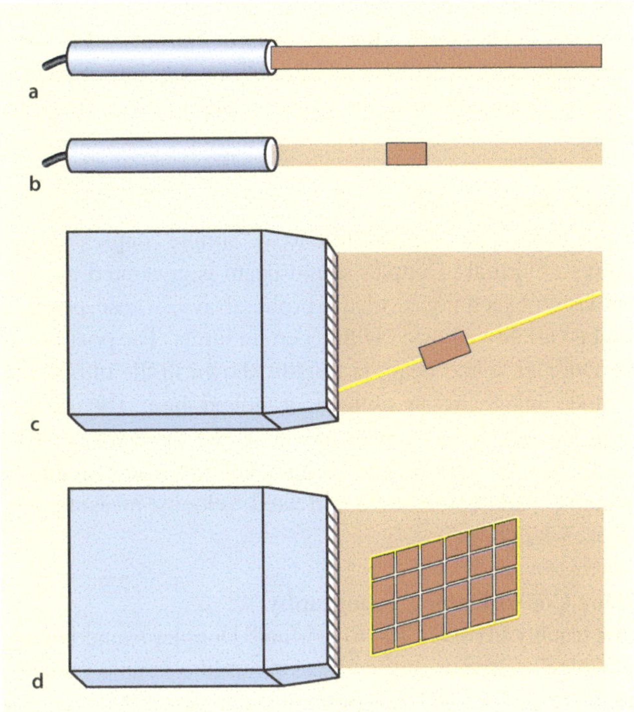

Fig. 4.5 (**a–d**) Overview of the different Doppler techniques. (**a**) CW Doppler pin probe without distinct sample volume, (**b**) pulsed Doppler pin probe with sample volume, (**c**) duplex sonography with single sample volume on a "virtual" Doppler sound beam, (**d**) color coded duplex sonography with numerous sample volumes in a two-dimensional "color window"

CW Doppler Pin Probe

With this technically simplest method, ultrasound of a constant frequency is continuously emitted and the reflected signal received from an ultrasound transducer located close by is analyzed for Doppler frequency shift. This method is still used today in extracranial Doppler sonography of the cervical vessels. An advantage of this method is the high signal quality due to a low noise level. The disadvantage of the method is that it is not possible to define a distinct sample volume. Therefore all vessels located in the direction of propagation of the sound beam are detected together, so that discrimination problems can occur.

Pulsed Doppler Pin Probe

By using pulsed ultrasound technology (pulse-echo method, Sect. 3.3.1), a specific region along the sound beam can be variably defined ("**sample volume**"), in which Doppler frequency shifts are to be evaluated. This procedure is used primarily in transcranial Doppler sonography, since the different depth position of the sample volume (Sect. 5.3.1) is the most important criterion for differentiating intracerebral arteries. In principle, the procedure can also be used extracranially, but without additional imaging information it has no advantages over the above mentioned CW Doppler probe.

Duplex Sonography

In this technique, often referred to as "simple" duplex sonography, a "virtual" Doppler sound beam is generated by special control techniques of the probe arrays, whose position can be variably adjusted within certain limits. The position of the Doppler sound beam is usually shown in the ultrasound B-mode image as an oblique or dotted line. The sample volume (Sect. 5.3.1) can be moved in the same way and its length can be varied. The sample volume also contains a rotatable paddle for angle-corrected velocity measurement (Sect. 5.3.2).

Color Coded Duplex Sonography

This usually involves 20–40 "virtual" Doppler sound beams, on which numerous, more or less point-like sample volumes are found, which are analysed by the ultrasound device for the presence of Doppler frequency shifts. The two-dimensional measurement field is called the "color window" and is made visible in the ultrasound B-moder image (see Sect. 6.1).

4.1.4 Acoustic Presentation of Doppler Signals

The evaluation of the flow information obtained with the above mentioned techniques can be done graphically by different methods (Fig. 4.6), but also acoustically.

Since the Doppler shift frequencies in medical ultrasound applications are in the range up to a maximum of approx. 20 kHz, there is the possibility to make the Doppler spectrum audible via loudspeakers. This can also result in a separation of directions into flows toward and away from the sound beam, which is why most devices have stereophonic loudspeakers.

Background Information

In the early days of Doppler diagnostics, the acoustic evaluation of the Doppler signal was of major importance, as the possibilities of graphic representation were inadequate at that time. This changed with the general availability of spectrum analysis. Compared to acoustic evaluation, the graphical representation of the Doppler spectrum has the advantage that measurable criteria such as maximum frequency can be used. In addition, the spectrum is accessible for documentation and thus also for subsequent review. In the following text, acoustic phenomena are therefore described only exceptionally (e.g., **Seagull crying phenomenon**, see Fig. 5.8) is not described further.

a

b

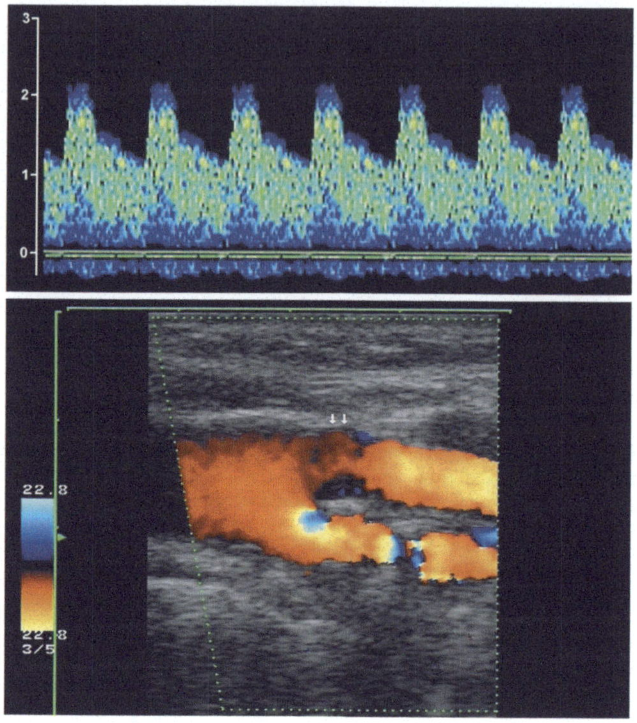

Fig. 4.6 (**a–b**) Display of Doppler-dependent flow information. (**a**) Doppler frequency time spectrum, (**b**) color coded two-dimensional flow display

Summary

The Doppler effect describes the frequency shift that occurs when there is a relative movement between a sound emitter and receiver. Doppler-dependent examination techniques (Doppler and duplex sonography) make use of this frequency shift in order to obtain information on blood flow parameters. The Doppler frequency shift is directly proportional to the blood flow velocity. Other influencing variables are the angle between the sound beam and the vessel as well as the emitted sound frequency.

4.2 Doppler Independent Techniques

In the past decades, various techniques for flow detection have been developed that are not based on the Doppler effect. However, all of these methods have not become generally accepted, mainly for cost reasons. The only exception is currently **B-flow technology,** which is based on the displacement of moving reflectors.

4.2.1 B-Flow Technique

If the reflected signals of two ultrasound pulses are analyzed, they should be completely identical, provided that the reflections originate from non-moving tissue. Reflections from moving tissue structures such as from flowing erythrocytes, however, lead to slight differences (Fig. 4.7), since the reflecting structures are already in a slightly different location at the time of the second sound pulse. If both signals are subtracted from each other, stationary structures lead to mutual cancellation, whereas echo pulses of moving structures can be selectively filtered out in this way.

The subtraction signals caused by moving blood can be made visible in the B-mode image by means of brightness coding (**B-flow** = **Brightness Flow**) of (Fig. 4.8). Stationary tissue echoes can either be completely masked or displayed in the background for better anatomical orientation.

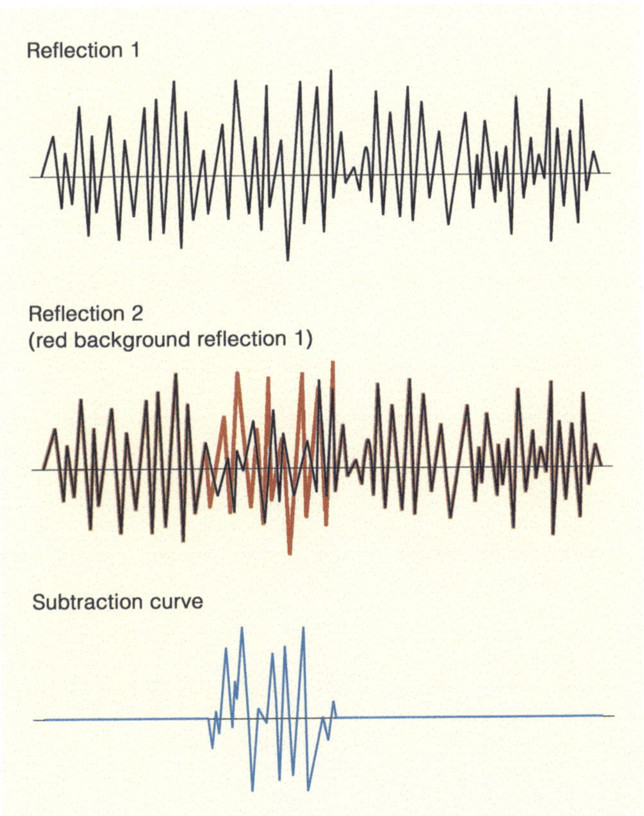

Fig. 4.7 Principle of B-flow technique. Successive ultrasound signals only lead to identical reflection signals if the ultrasound structures remain stationary (red curve in reflection 2). A blood flow localized in the sound field results in circumscribed changes of the signal pattern, which can be filtered out by subtracting the reflected signals

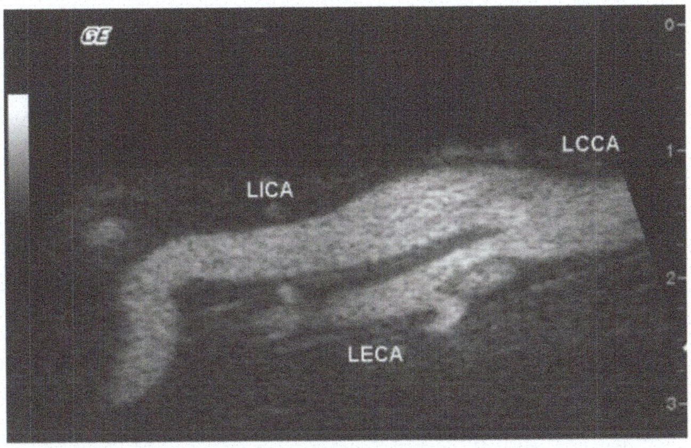

Fig. 4.8 Normal carotid bifurcation using B-flow technique. (Dr. H.-P. Weskott, Hannover)

4.2.2 Possible Applications of B-flow Technique

Compared to "conventional" color coded duplex sonography, B-flow technique has the advantage of a much better resolution in imaging blood perfused areas, since it is based on B-mode imaging with its high resolution and not on a Doppler-based color window with a limited number of sample volumes. In addition, the flow imaging is almost not dependent on the angle between the Doppler beam and the vessel, so that even curved vessel courses can be reliably displayed (overview).

Advantages and Disadvantages of the B-flow Technique on the Arteries Supplying the Brain

- Advantages
  - High spatial resolution of the flow representation
  - Only minimal dependence on the "insonation angle" of the sound
- Disadvantages
  - Can only be used for superficial vessels
  - No reliable detection of flow direction
  - No quantitative measurement of blood flow velocity
  - Cannot be used on intracranial vessels.

However, B-flow technique also has several disadvantages that limit its use. The main disadvantage is the strong dependence of display quality on a low-noise reflection signal. However, as already described in Sect. 3.2, the signal-to-noise ratio decreases exponentially with increasing penetration depth. Accordingly, extracranial B-flow technique gives usable results only in relatively slim patients with optimal examination conditions, while the imaging of the vertebral arteries, which are regularly located somewhat deeper, already leads to problems. Intracranially the technique is not useful.

Table 4.2 Valence of different ultrasound methods in the evaluation of flow information

	Pin probe	Duplex sonography		
	Doppler spectrum	Doppler spectrum	Color coding	B-flow
Flow localization	–	–	+	+
Flow direction	+	+	(+)	(+)
Flow velocity	–	+	(+)	–
Flow volume	–	+	+	–
Flow disturbances	+	+	(+)	–
Flow characteristics	+	+	–	–

Summary
B-flow technique is currently the only method used in clinical practice for assessing blood flow that is not based on Doppler principle. In the B-mode ultrasound image, moving blood is shown in a brightly coded form. The method has a very high spatial resolution, but is currently only suitable for superficially located vessels.

4.3 Diagnostically Relevant Flow Parameters

In summary, the Doppler sonographic evaluation of cerebral blood vessels is confined to six hemodynamic criteria. In addition to the detection of the flow direction and the localization of blood flow, these include flow velocity as the most important parameter for the detection of stenoses, but also flow disturbances and pulsatile characteristics as well as the determination of the flow volume as an indirect indication of changes in cerebral hemodynamics. Details on this can be found in the Chaps. 5 and 6 as well as in the clinical Chapters. Table 4.2 gives an overview of the diagnostic value of the different ultrasound techniques.

5 Flow Assessment Using the Doppler Spectrum

Bernhard Widder and Gerhard F. Hamann

5.1 Methodology of Spectrum Analysis

After the so-called demodulation of the ultrasonic waves reflected back to the transducer, the low Doppler frequency 1–20 kHz shift mentioned in Sect. 4.1 remain. These frequencies are converted into digital signals with the aid of an analog-digital (AD) converter and can then be further processed in any standard PC.

The detection of the frequency components of the Doppler spectrum is usually done by the method of **Fast Fourier Transformation** (FFT). As already mentioned in Sect. 4. 1.4 above, the frequency-time spectrum, that is, the representation of the individual frequency components on the y-axis over time (x-axis), has become the standard in medicine. The incidence of the individual frequency components ("power") can be "coded" in color or brightness levels.

5.1.1 Fast Fourier Transformation (FFT)

As shown in Fig. 3.7, any complex curve function can be decomposed into numerous sinusoidal oscillations and thus analyzed in its frequency components. This finding is connected with the name of the French mathematician Jean Baptiste Fourier (1768–1830). The "FFT" is merely a special calculation rule for the rapid decomposition of the individual frequency components. The frequency resolution is usually given in "points." A 128-point FFT means nothing else than that, for example, a Doppler spectrum with a maximum frequency of ±3.2 kHz can be decomposed into 2 × 64 individual frequency components with a resolution of 50 Hz each. The FFT point values of 64, 128, 256, 512, etc. have a compelling mathematical background, which needs not be discussed in detail here.

Summary

Doppler signals can be analyzed in their individual frequency components using spectrum analysis and displayed graphically over time (frequency time spectrum). The Fast Fourier Transformation (FFT) is used mathematically for this purpose.

5.2 Diagnostic Parameters of the Doppler Spectrum

Starting from Sect. 4.3, this chapter provides a detailed description of the various parameters of the Doppler frequency time spectrum ("Doppler spectrum"), as it can be detected with the single pencil probe as well as with duplex devices.

5.2.1 Detection of Flow Direction

All Doppler and duplex devices available today automatically detect the direction of flow toward or away from the Doppler sound beam and display it on the monitor above or below the zero line. Usually there is a graphic symbol (icon) at the edge of the screen, which indicates which direction of flow is displayed above and below the zero line. Problems with directional differentiation only occur if the Doppler frequencies are higher than the pulse repetition frequency in pulsed Doppler applications (**Alias effect** Sect. 5.3.4).

B. Widder (✉)
Expert Opinion Institute, District Hospital, Guenzburg, Germany
e-mail: bernhard.widder@bkh-guenzburg.de

G. F. Hamann
Clinic of Neurology and Neurological Rehabilitation, District Hospital, Guenzburg, Germany

B. Widder, G. F. Hamann (eds.), *Duplex sonography of the brain-supplying arteries*, https://doi.org/10.1007/978-3-662-65566-5_5

Practical Tips

If the sound beam is directed largely perpendicular to the vessel, amplitudes in the frequency spectrum can be derived in both directions of flow, almost equal to each other on both sides (Mirroring). "This is due to the fact that the Doppler sound beam is, physically speaking, not a narrowly defined line," but also has a lateral extension, as explained in the Sect. 3.1.1. Similar artifacts (cross talk) can also be found if the amplification of the Doppler or duplex device (gain) is set too high (Fig. 5.1).

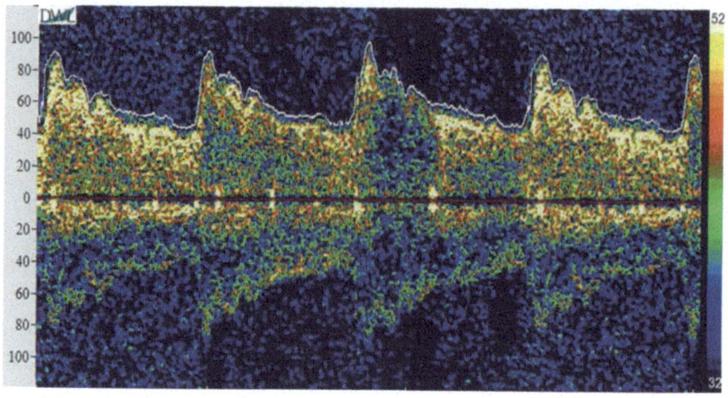

Fig. 5.1 Artifacts caused by "crosstalk" to the other channel of the Doppler device when the gain is set too high

5.2.2 Detection of Flow Velocity

First of all, it should be noted that the Doppler spectrum alone permits only **statements** about flow velocities, but no **measurement** in the narrow sense. The measurement of flow velocities always requires additionally the presence of imaging techniques that can be used to determine the angle between the sound beam and the vessel (insonation angle). For details see Sect. 5.3.2.

Background Information

When using the "simple" Doppler pin probe without the possibility of assessing the insonation angle between the sound beam and the vessel, it must always be remembered that changes in the position of the sound probe as well as curved vessels can simulate changes in flow velocity (Fig. 5.2). If, for example, a maximum systolic frequency of 4 kHz is used at the extracranial carotid artery as the limit between "normal" and "pathological," which usually leads to correct results at a transmission frequency of 4 MHz and at the usual insonation angle of 60°, completely different Doppler frequencies can be measured if the vessel passes in the medial or lateral direction (Fig. 1.8). When using standard values, these angle problems must therefore always be taken into account by using Doppler probes without additional B-mode imaging.

Assessment Parameters

The description of the Doppler spectrum is generally based on three parameters (Fig. 5.3).

Systolic Maximum Frequency

It is measured at the apex of the systole and represents the maximum flow velocity occurring in a vessel. ◀

End Diastolic Maximum Frequency

It is measured in the cardiac cycle immediately before the start of the next systole. It is a complex measure of the elasticity of the vascular system and of the peripheral resistance. ◀

Mean Value

The mean value describes the intensity-weighted average of the Doppler frequencies at any point in the spectrum. It correlates best with the actual amount of blood flow volume through the vessel. ◀

Diagnostic Significance

Systolic Maximum Frequency

Due to physiological circumstances (continuity law, Sect. 2.3), there is a quadratic relationship between the degree of stenosis and the systolic maximum frequency, which can usually be detected without major problems in the Doppler spectrum (Fig. 5.4). However, the increase in flow velocity is additionally determined by the length of the stenosis (Fig. 13.7). Of particular practical importance is the fact that the systolic (and enddiastolic) maximum frequency decreases again in subtotal stenoses. There are two reasons for this:

- According to the law of Hagen-Poiseuille (Sect. 2.3), the flow resistance increases drastically for very high grade stenoses and leads to a decrease in flow velocity.
- With increasing degree of stenosis, the proportion of the remaining high flow components becomes increasingly smaller due to turbulence effects. Their backscattered intensity is then no longer sufficient to be detected.

◀

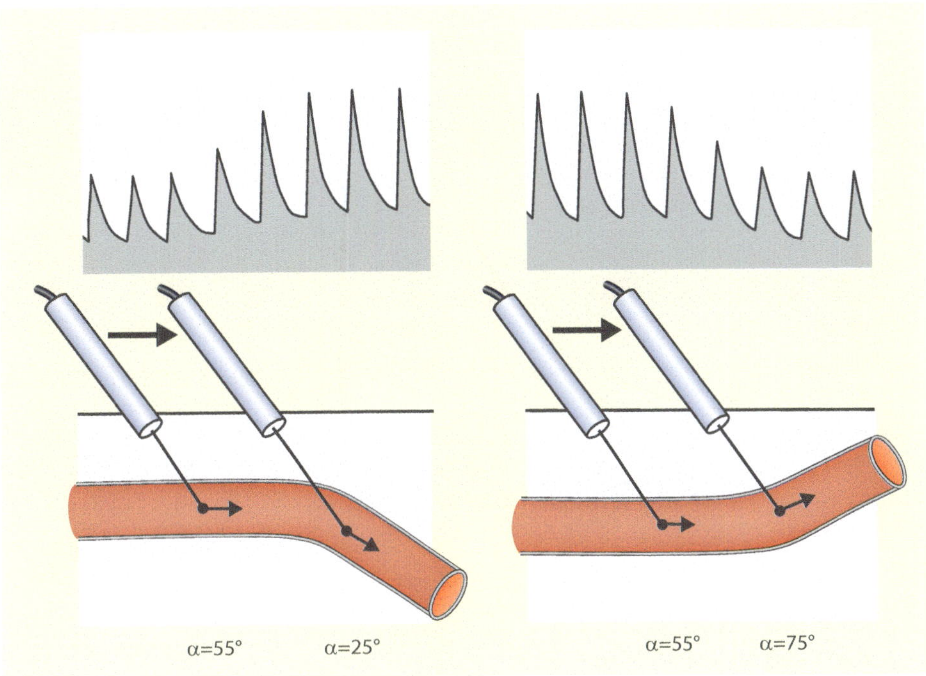

Fig. 5.2 Changes in Doppler frequencies induced by vessel bending at constant vessel diameter. Medial bends (left) lead to an apparent "flow acceleration," a lateral bend (right) results in an apparent "flow reduction"

End Diastolic Maximum Frequency

A similar relationship to the degree of stenosis exists for the end-diastolic maximum frequency. However, due to its greater variability, it has never gained importance for the diagnosis of stenosis. However, this value is indispensable for the measurement of pulsatility (Sect. 5.2.4). ◀

Mean Value

Due to its close relationship with the total amount of blood flowing through a vessel, it is particularly important for determining flow volume (Sect. 5.3.3). ◀

Possible Errors

The detection of systolic maximum frequency can lead to misinterpretations if the sound transmission power and/or the Doppler gain are set too high or too low (Fig. 5.5). If the setting is too high, device artifacts (**crosstalk**) are displayed faking a flow signal; if the setting is too low, less powerful frequency components no longer reach the threshold value of the spectrum display and are "cut off." In case of doubt, an attempt should be made to adjust the spectrum display optimally by slowly increasing or decreasing the Doppler gain. This requires a certain "sure instinct," fixed rules cannot be given.

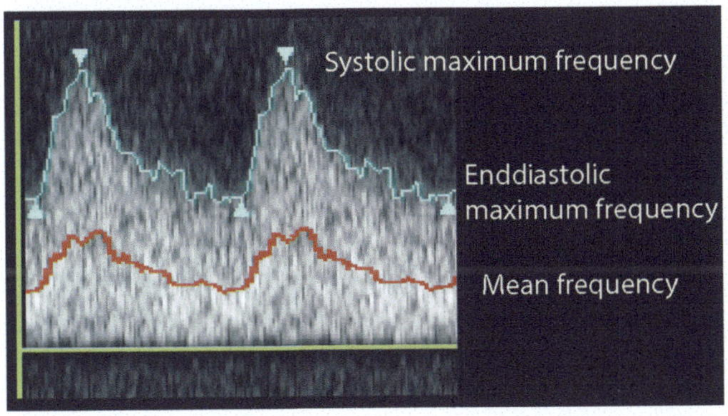

Fig. 5.3 Measurement parameters of the Doppler frequency time spectrum

> **Practical Tips**
> For optimal power or Doppler gain adjustment, in non-pathological cases the observation of the systolic window is recommended (Fig. 5.7). If this is just visible, the signal adjustment is usually correct.

5.2.3 Flow Disturbances

Acoustically, flow disturbances in the loudspeaker of the Doppler and duplex device impress as hissing or rather bubbling noises reaching into the diastole. They are often compared with "steps in the gravel" or "snowball crunching."

Assessment Parameters

Spectrum analysis enables a differentiated assessment of the degree of flow disturbances on the basis of typical changes in the Doppler spectrum (Fig. 5.6). A distinction is made between three forms of manifestation and one special case:

1. **Minor flow disturbances** can be recognized by the disappearance of the so-called systolic window. This is the

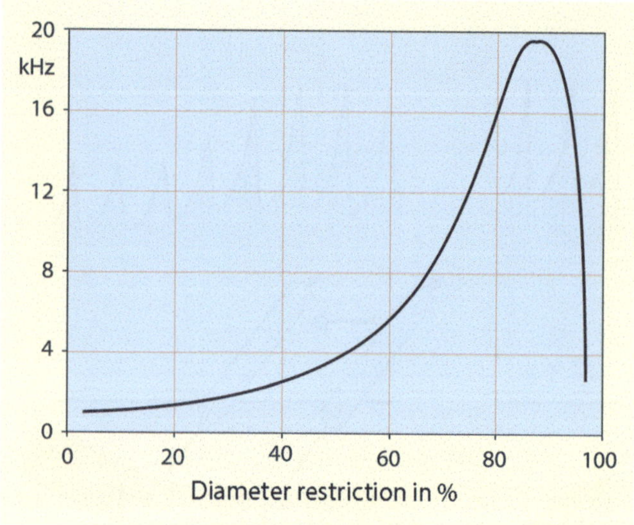

Fig. 5.4 Quadratic relationship between the degree of stenosis and the maximum systolic Doppler frequency (peak frequency) with respect to an ultrasonic transmission frequency of 5 MHz in a flow model. (According to Spencer and Reid 1979)

"empty" area below the systolic peak caused by the predominance of higher-frequency flow components in the laminar flow profile. The disappearance of this window is caused by the occurrence of low-frequency Doppler frequencies. In this case one also speaks of spectral broadening (Fig. 5.7).

2. **Moderate flow disturbances** show a predominance of low-frequency components during systole.
3. **High-grade flow disturbances** also show flow components running retrograde to the flow direction. In extreme cases, only the portion of the flow disturbance and no longer the undisturbed high-frequency "jet flow" can be detected in the Doppler spectrum.

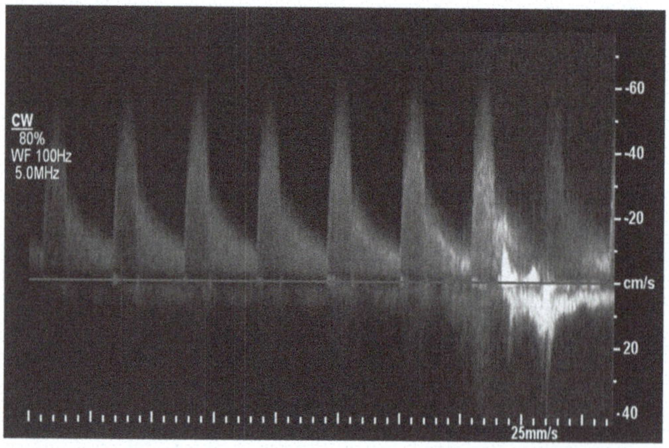

Fig. 5.5 Problems in assessing the systolic maximum frequency due to different settings of the Doppler gain. Example with continuously increased gain from left to right. In addition, at the end of the curve a swallowing artifact

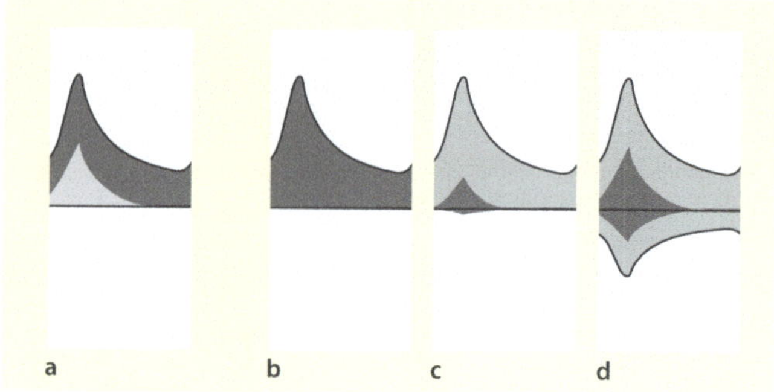

Fig. 5.6 (**a**–**d**) Characteristics of flow disturbances in the Doppler spectrum. Normal pulse curve (**a**), minor flow disturbance with disappearance of the "systolic window" (**b**), moderate flow disturbance with predominance of low frequency components (**c**), high-grade flow disturbance with additionally apparent retrograde flow components (**d**)

4. **Seagull crying:** A special form of high-grade flow disturbances are harmonic frequencies, which are recognizable in the Doppler spectrum as band-shaped stripes with (approximately) uniform frequency during systole (Fig. 5.8). In the loudspeaker of the Doppler device they impress as "whistling" or "squeaking" signals, which are often vividly compared with the cries of seagulls. This noise is probably caused – similar to the transverse flute or panpipe – by a rapid flow of blood "whistling" over a cavity (e.g., vessel outlet). Experience has shown that such signals are more frequent in stenoses of the external carotid artery, which has numerous branches.

Diagnostic Significance

As already mentioned in Sect. 2.4, flow disturbances are basically non-specific and can occur physiologically in the case of vessel bends, branches and dilatations (e.g., carotid bulb) as well as in the pathological case of stenoses, hyperperfusion or aneurysms. The non-specificity, however, only applies to minor and moderate flow disturbances, while pronounced flow disturbances occur almost exclusively in the vicinity of high-grade stenoses. Thus, they are to be used as an essential diagnostic criterion if the diagnostically more significant flow velocity in the maximum of the stenosis cannot be detected reliably.

This situation is given in three constellations:

1. **Insufficient sound window:** Transcranial Doppler/duplex sonography often is limited by an inadequate sound window, which does not allow low-energy, higher Doppler frequencies due to a high-grade stenosis to pass through sufficiently (Fig. 5.9).
2. **Perpendicular insonation angle:** If, as for example in the area of the carotid siphon, the insonation angle is regularly more than 70° for anatomical reasons, the systolic

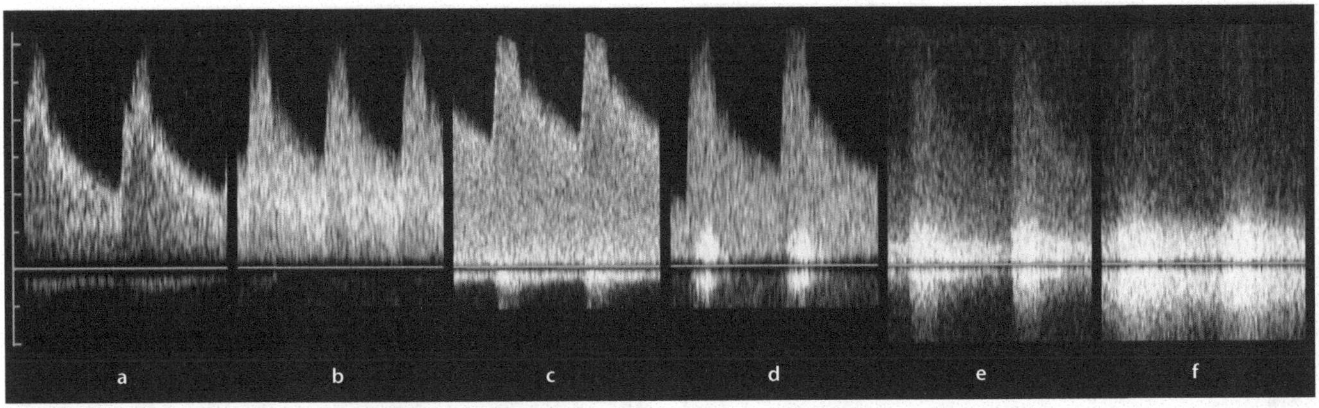

Fig. 5.7 (**a**–**f**) Examples of flow disturbances. Normal Doppler frequency time spectrum with recognizable "systolic window" (**a**); minor flow disturbance with loss of the "systolic window" (**b**); transition to medium flow disturbance with increasing low-frequency components (**c**, **d**); high-grade flow disturbance with still recognizable maximum frequencies (**e**); maximum frequencies can no longer be reliably detected (**f**)

maximum frequency can no longer be used as a valid parameter for the detection of stenoses. In this case the diagnosis must be based on the occurrence of flow disturbances (Fig. 5.10).

3. **Non-assessable stenosis maximum:** If the stenosis is located in an area that is inaccessible by sonography (e.g., when the internal carotid artery passes through the base of the skull) or if the maximum stenosis is obscured by calcification (Fig. 5.11), stenosis detection must be indirectly based on the occurrence of poststenostic flow disturbances.

> Note
> **Severe flow disturbances in a vessel must always be considered pathological.**

Possible Errors

False-negative results in stenoses only occur if for some reason the flow velocity in the stenosis is lower than expected (e.g., tandem stenoses, Sect. 13.1.6). False-positive misinterpretations are more frequent and are possible in the following cases:

1. **Vascular superpositions** can lead to an apparent broadening of the frequency density spectrum. This is particularly important in transcranial Doppler sonography, where several vessel sections are often derived due to the relatively large sample volume (Fig. 5.12).
2. **Vessel branches and bends** physiologically lead to locally circumscribed flow disorders (Fig. 5.12) and should not be misinterpreted as stenoses. The decisive factor for differentiation from stenoses is the fact that physiological flow disturbances immediately distal to a vessel junction or bend are detectable over a distance of at most twice the vessel diameter and then disappear, whereas flow disturbances distal to higher-grade stenoses regularly persist over a longer distance.
3. **Hyperperfusion** is often associated with the characteristics of a slight flow disturbance. The long-distance involvement of the entire vessel is indicative of this.
4. **Anemia** lead to turbulence due to their influence on the Reynolds number (Sect. 2.4). Typically, however, they affect all the vessels investigated, but are increasingly found in the area of vessel branches and bends.

5.2.4 Flow Characteristics (Pulsatility)

As already described in the previous Sect. 2.5, skin and muscle arteries with high peripheral resistance (e.g., subclavian and external carotid arteries) show low diastolic blood flow, while vessels supplying the brain and those leading to parenchymatous organs (e.g., thyroid) also show considerable diastolic blood flow due to their low peripheral resistance.

> Practical Tips
> The relationship between systolic and end-diastolic flow velocity is not only important for the differentiation of vessels, but also represents a quantitative criterion suitable for side comparison.

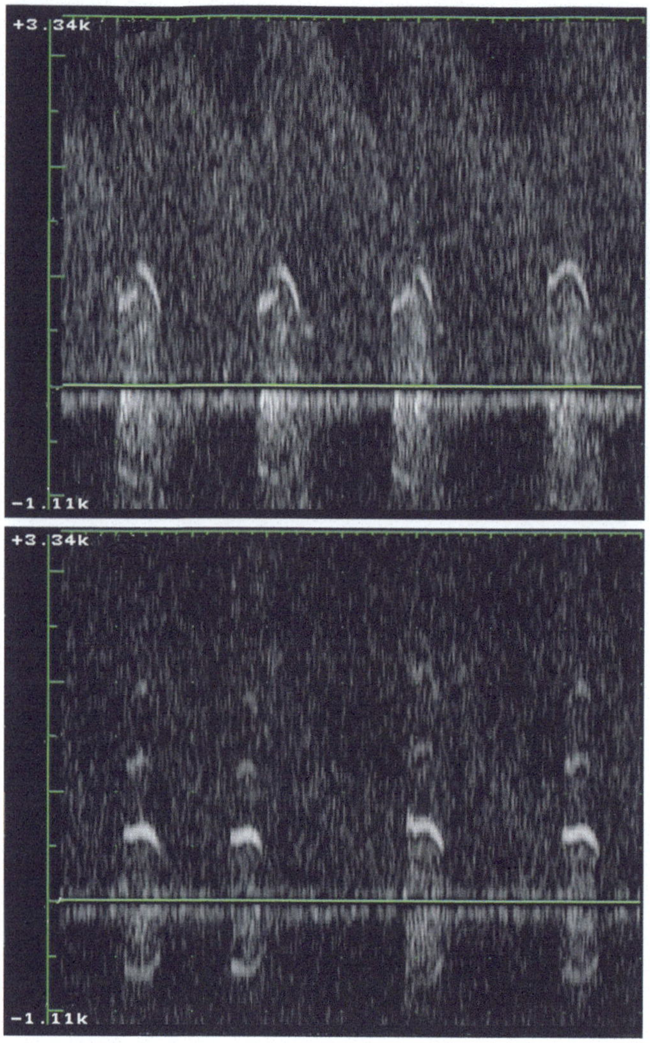

Fig. 5.8 Examples of harmonic "seagull crying" in the Doppler spectrum of the middle cerebral artery in 2 patients with high-grade stenosis in the main stem of the middle cerebral artery. In the upper picture "Seagull crying" subordinated to the just visible flow signal of a high-grade stenosis. Below as a special feature multiple harmonics (in addition irregularity of the pulse curve caused by cardiac arrhythmia)

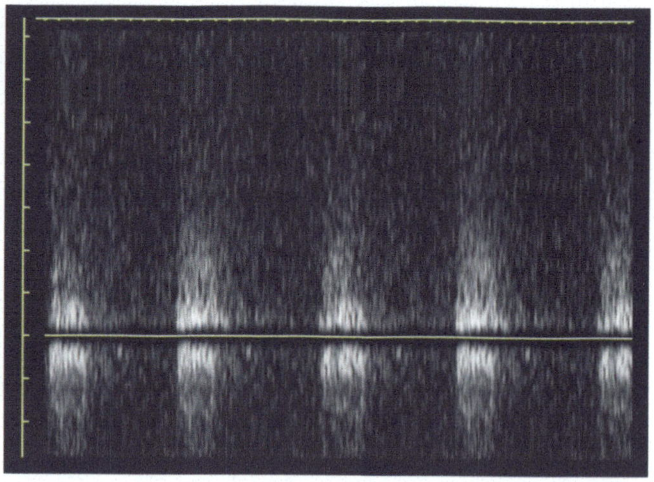

Fig. 5.9 High-grade stenosis of the middle cerebral artery. Since the temporal sound window is insufficient, the maximum systolic flow velocity cannot be defined and the stenosis can only be recognized by the pronounced flow disturbance

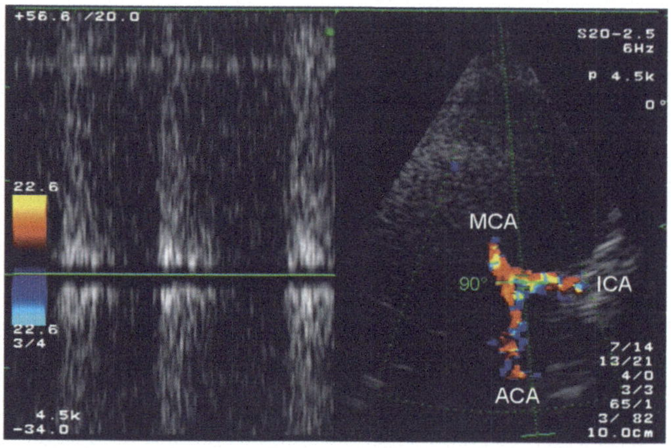

Fig. 5.10 Due to the almost 90° insonation angle, a high-grade stenosis in the distal course of the internal carotid artery (ICA) can only be verified on the basis of the pronounced flow disturbance immediately before division into the cerebral media (MCA) and anterior (ACA)

Assessment Parameters

For the acquisition of pulsatile flow characteristics, usually abbreviated as **pulsatility**, there are three approaches described in the literature (Table 5.1).

Resistance Index (RI)

The pulsatility index described by Pourcelot (1974) and therefore also called Pourcelot index is calculated as the difference between the systolic and end-diastolic maximum divided by the systolic maximum (Fig. 5.3). ◀

Pulsatility Index (PI)

The index introduced by Gosling and King (1974), which can be used as an alternative, requires knowledge of the mean frequency by which the difference between systole and diastole is divided. ◀

Diastolic Ratio

For daily use, qualitative assessment of the relative proportion of diastole in the systolic amplitude ("diastolic ratio") appears to be the easyest reference for pulsatility. If the systole is assumed to be 100%, diastolic flow fraction is less than 1/3 of the systole for skin- and muscle-supplying vessels and more than 1/3 of the systole for brain-supplying arteries. ◀

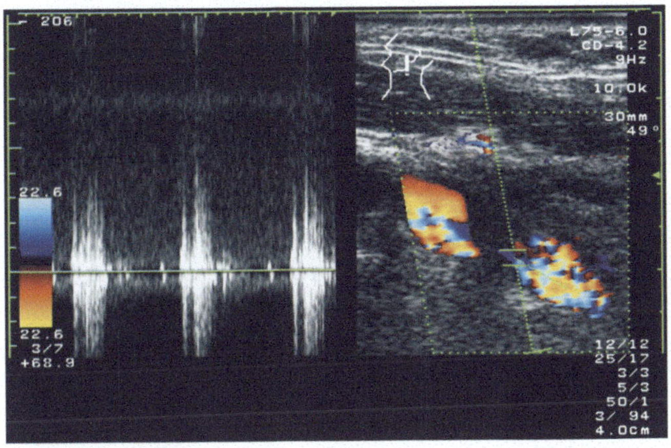

Fig. 5.11 Maximum of a higher degree carotid stenosis hidden by "sound shadow" due to a calcification. The pronounced poststenotic flow disturbance, however, indicates the stenosis

> **Practical Tips**
> Unfortunately, the Resistance (RI) and Pulsatility Index (PI) are often used synonymously in studies without more detailed information, which can lead to misunderstandings.

Diagnostic Significance

The assessment of pulsatility not only allows statements about possibly pathologically altered peripheral vascular resistance (e.g., with increased intracranial pressure), but also provides important indirect indications of occlusive cerebrovascular diseases. Thus, pulsatility typically increases proximal to a high-grade stenosis augmenting the peripheral resistance (Fig. 5.13). Conversely, distal to high-grade stenoses, pulsatility is characteristically reduced, since in this case the peripheral resistance vessels are dilated and thus the peripheral resistance is reduced in order to maintain blood supply. Together with an increased flow velocity, however, abnormally reduced pulsatility can also indicate a cerebral arteriovenous malformation (Table 5.2).

Possible Errors

Misinterpretations of pulsatility can occur if the wall filter of the device at low Doppler frequencies is more than approx. 10% of the detected maximum systolic frequency (Fig. 5.14). The task of the wall filter is to suppress artifact signals due to radial pulsations of the vessel wall. An electronic high-pass filter is used for this purpose, which eliminates low frequency components in the Doppler spectrum and is usually set to 50–200 Hz.

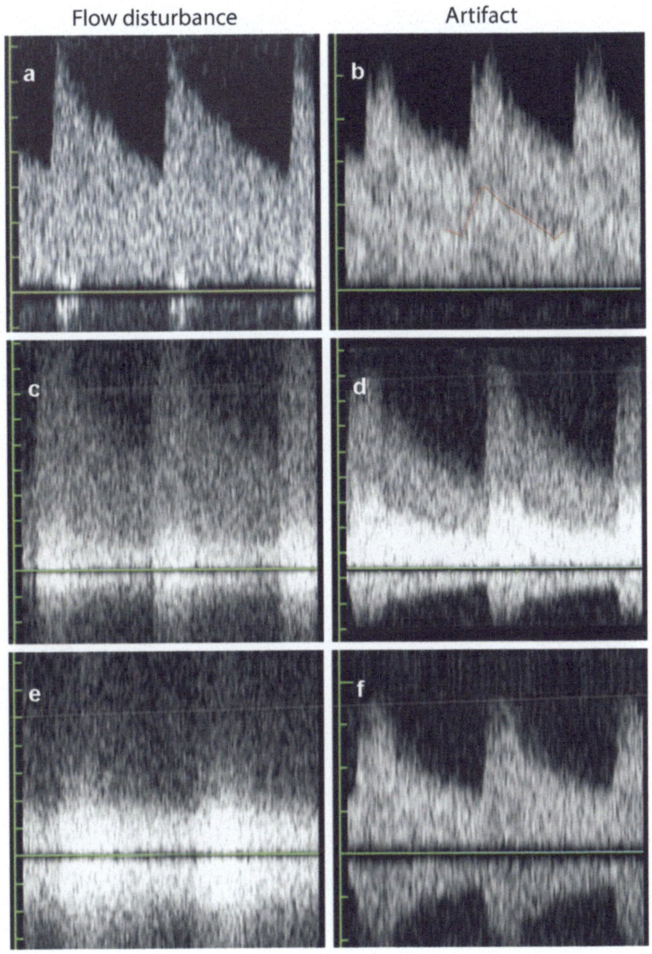

Fig. 5.12 (**a**–**f**) Real (left) and false (right) flow disturbances in the Doppler spectrum. Superposition of 2 vessels flowed through in the same direction (**b**, **d**) deceives a missing "systolic window" (**a**) or a pronounced flow disturbance (**c**, **e**); simultaneous representation of two vessels with opposite flows (**f**)

> **Practical Tips**
> When detecting low Doppler frequencies <1 kHz, care should be taken to set the wall filter as low as possible (<100 Hz) to avoid misinterpretation of pulsatility.

Special Case "flattened systolic increase"

A further flow characteristic that is important in individual cases is the systolic increase in the pulse curve. Due to the rapid contraction of the left ventricle, the pulse curve reaches its (largely) maximum after only about 0.1 s in healthy individuals. Behind very high grade stenoses there is a flattened systolic rise, which in extreme cases can lead to the image of a **delta signal** with an almost identical rise and fall

Table 5.1 Possibilities to describe the pulsatility of Doppler flow curves

Parameters	Calculation	Normal values	
		Brain supplying vessel	Muscle vessel
Resistance index (RI)	(systole – diastole)/systole	<0.75	>0.75
Pulsatility index (PI)	(systole – diastole)/mean	<1	>1
Diastolic ratio	Diastole/systole	>1/3	<1/3

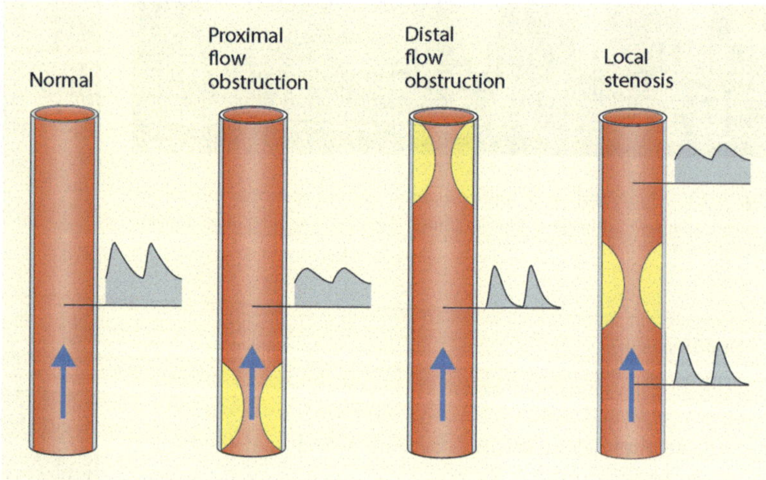

Fig. 5.13 Changes in pulsatility in proximal and distal to a high-grade vascular stenosis of the brain supplying arteries

Table 5.2 Significance of pathologically altered pulsatility values in the brain supplying arteries

Pulsatility compared to normal values	Cause
Diminished pulsatility	Upstream high level flow obstruction Arteriovenous malformation at further vascular course Hyperperfusion through other causes (e.g., to ischemia) Aortic stenosis
Increased pulsatility	Downstream high level flow obstruction Increased intracranial pressure Cerebral microangiopathy Aortic insufficiency

of the systole (Fig. 13.22). However, a flattened systolic increase is also to be expected with reduced heart contractility and aortic stenosis. Accordingly, side comparison is of importance here.

Summary
The diagnostic assessment of the Doppler spectrum is based on few parameters: The measured Doppler shift is proportional to blood flow velocity and shows a quadratic relationship to the degree of stenosis. Although flow disturbances are an unspecific phenomenon, pronounced flow disturbances characteristically only occur with higher degrees of stenosis and can then be used diagnostically. The pulsatility of the Doppler spectrum over the systolic-diastolic cycle is chances in the case of upstream and downstream stenoses. Various pulsatility indices are available for quantification.

5.3 Special Features of Pulsed Doppler Technology

Compared to CW technique, pulsed Doppler and duplex applications have some special features, which mainly have an advantageous effect on the diagnostic possibilities, but also have a typical disadvantage (**Aliasing effect**).

5.3.1 Flow Assessment at Defined Tissue Depths

As already described in the previous Sect. 3.1.2, the use of pulse-echo technique in Doppler sonography makes it possible to search for the presence of blood flow at tissue depths

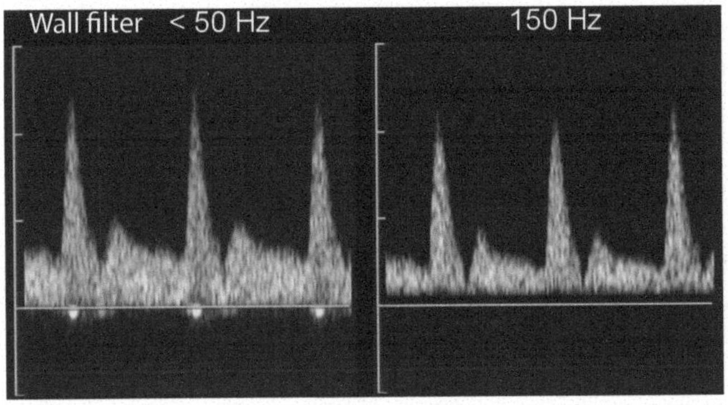

Fig. 5.14 Possible misinterpretation of pulsatility with wall filter set high (right)

defined by the examiner. This possibility is defined by two parameters that can be set on the device.

Depth

The **depth** of the Doppler measurement can either be selected directly for Doppler devices without imaging, or, for duplex sonography, it can defined using "trackball".

Sample Volume

The **sample volume** characterizes the distance along the Doppler sound beam within which a Doppler sonographic flow measurement is to be performed. Knowledge of two physical principles is important for the optimum setting of the measuring volume.

Size of the Sample Volume

As the size of the sample volume decreases, the "total quantity" of ultrasound signals available for Doppler spectrum analysis also decreases (Fig. 5.15), so that a sufficient Doppler signal may no longer be detected, especially in deeper-lying vessels or in cases of transmission difficulties through the skull. In addition, the probability of "dropping out" of the vessel increases even with small movements of the ultrasound probe or the patient. Accordingly, larger measurement volumes should be preferred when examining deep-lying vessels and in restless patients (Table 5.3). ◄

Practical Tips
If it is not possible to recognize a vessel either in B-mode or color-coded imaging, a "blind" attempt can be made to obtain a flow signal in the examined area setting the sample volume to a maximum value. By gradually reducing the size of the sample volume, it can then be localized step by step.

3D-Extension of the Sample Volume

Due to the clear-cut limits on the device screen, the sample volume is often considered to comprise a sharply defined area. For physical reasons, however, the sensitivity of the measurement volume does not break off sharply along the sound axis, but shows a relatively slow decrease toward both sides (Fig. 5.16). In addition, the sample **volume,** as the name suggests, has a three-dimensional shape and

Fig. 5.15 Influence of different sample volumes on the Doppler spectrum in transtemporal Doppler insonation of the middle cerebral artery

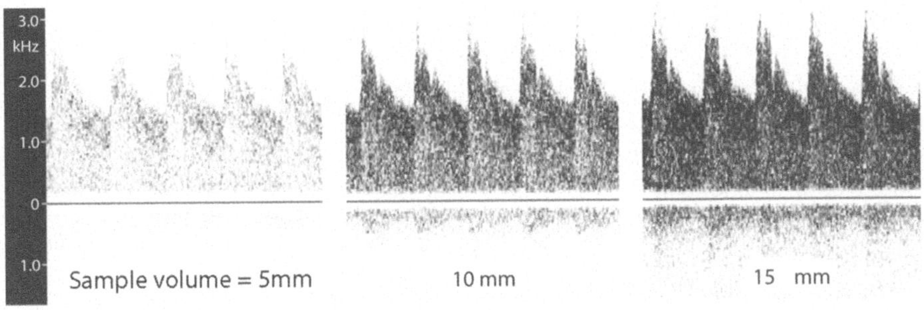

Table 5.3 Basic principles for setting the sample volume in pulsed Doppler and duplex sonography

Sample volume compared to the examined vessel diameter		
Larger	Comparable size	Smaller
Deep lying vessels Insufficient temporal window in the transcranial Doppler/duplex sonography "Blind" search for blood flow with the duplex device Restless patient	Standard setting	Distinguishing vessels lying close together

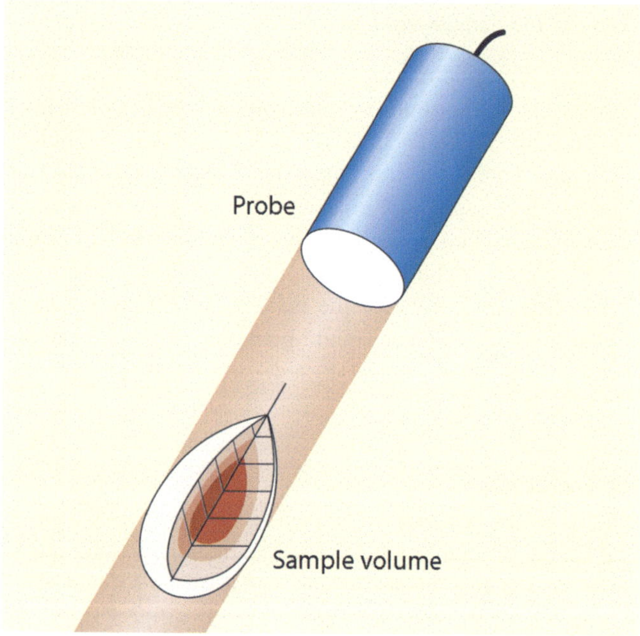

Fig. 5.16 Three-dimensional expansion of the sample volume in pulsed Doppler and duplex sonography. (After von Reutern et al. 2000)

therefore also has a certain lateral extension. If the Doppler gain is set very high, it is therefore possible that vessels lying next to the actual sample volume are also recorded and can cause confusion, especially when differentiating between an occlusion and a still open vessel. ◀

5.3.2 Measurement of Flow Velocity

In contrast to the simple Doppler pin probe, where only frequencies can be assessed, the combination of B-mode image and Doppler sound beam used in duplex sonography allows concrete measurements of flow velocity in cm/s or m/s. A prerequisite for this is the determination of the angle between the Doppler sound beam and the vessel axis (so-called insonation angle). Every duplex device offers the possibility performing such an angle correction by means of a rotatable bar (Fig. 5.17). After setting the angle, the velocity can usually be read directly on the monitor in cm/s or m/s.

Diagnostic Significance

In addition to the possibility of recording a physiological parameter instead of the purely technical criterion of Doppler frequency shift, the angle-corrected measurement of flow velocity offers further significant diagnostic advantages:

1. In the case of a medial or lateral bend of the vessel, false negative and false positive results can occur without knowledge of the insonation angle (Fig. 5.2).
2. If a sufficiently reproducible setting of the angle correction is technically possible (see below), the determination of the flow velocity leads to a more reliable assessment of the degree of stenosis.

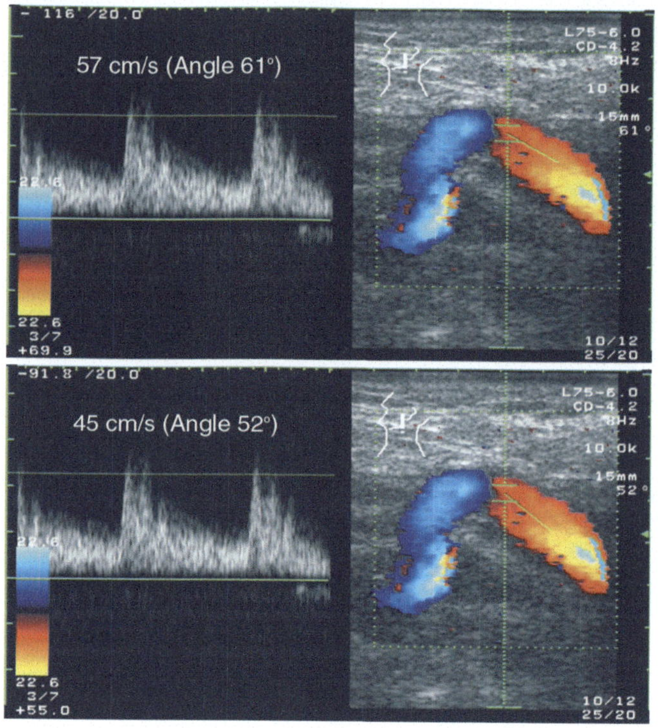

Fig. 5.17 Determination of the flow velocity in the internal carotid artery at different settings of the insonation angle. Note the different measured values even with relatively small fluctuations of the angle setting

> Note
>
> **When duplex sonography is used, an angular correction of the angle between the Doppler beam and the vessel axis should always (!) be performed.**

Possible Errors

Various sources of error must be taken into account in angle-corrected measurements of flow velocity.

"Unfavorable" Insonation Angle

Due to unavoidable inaccuracies in the setting of the angular correction insonation angles of 70° and more should be avoided, otherwise unacceptable measurement errors may occur (Fig. 5.18). This is due to the already mentioned cosine function in the Doppler equation (Sect. 4.1.2). ◀

Vessel Displayed Too "short"

A measurement error which is not obvious at first glance can occur if the correct angle is set in the insonated plane but the vessel runs across this plane, resulting in an angular error in the plane perpendicular to the B-mode section

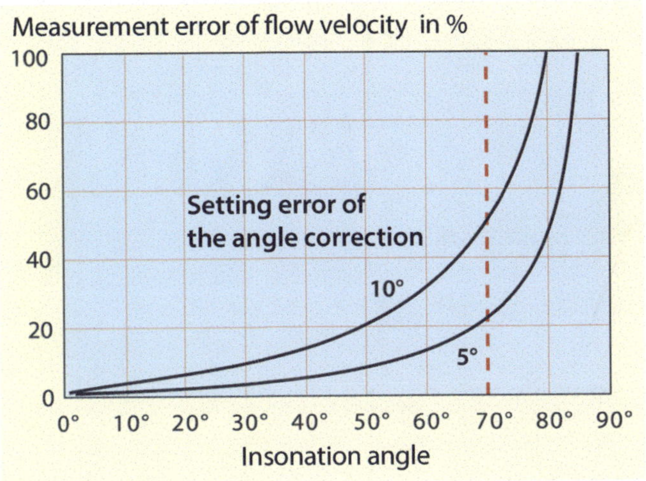

Fig. 5.18 Disproportionate increase of the measurement error when determining flow velocity due to the cosine function in the Doppler relationship. Unavoidable inaccuracies in the adjustment of the insonation angle in the order of 5–10° are only moderately relevant at small angles between the Doppler sound beam and the vessel <60°, whereas pronounced incorrect measurements are obtained from an insonation angle of 60–70°

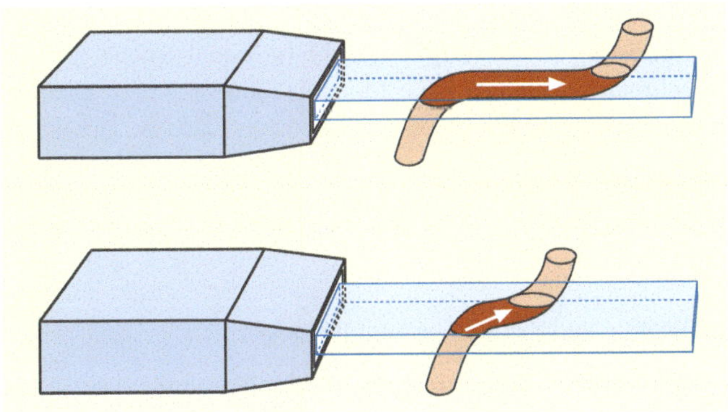

Fig. 5.19 Possible measurement errors when determining the flow velocity through a vessel running across the sectional image plane. If the vessel can only be traced briefly in the sectional image, this can result in an unpredictable angle between the axis of the sound beam and the vessel axis (bottom)

(Fig. 5.19). Such an angle error is to be avoided if the vessel can be represented "band-shaped" from the area of the measuring at least over a distance corresponding to twice the diameter of the vessel on both sides (e.g., in the case of internal carotid artery ± 1 cm) with clearly distinguishable vessel walls. ◀

Note

The reliable determination of blood flow velocity requires an insonation angle of < 70° and a "band-shaped" display of the vessel course over a length of ± 1 cm proximally and distally to the measuring point.

Poststenotic Flow Disturbances

Immediately behind higher grade stenoses, considerable flow disturbances are regularly found, in the case of short-distance stenoses not infrequently combined with a helically twisted blood flow (**helix flow**, Fig. 13.13). Poststenotic determination of flow velocity should therefore always be carried out as far as possible distal to the stenosis to avoid incorrect measurements. ◀

Note

Measurements of the poststenotic flow velocity should not be taken immediately behind a stenosis, but as far as possible away from it.

Elongations and Kinkings

In cases of with elongations and kinkings problems can occur, since the setting of the angle correction leaves variation possibilities, which may result in considerably different measured velocities (Fig. 5.20). ◀

Eccentrically Running Stenoses

Problems with the adjustment of the insonation angle cannot be avoided either in the case of eccentric residual lumina in stenoses (Fig. 5.21). ◀

Practical Tips

If measurement errors cannot be avoided in the case of elongations and eccentric stenoses, the examiner should at least know the "bandwidth" of the measurement error. This can be done by measuring flow velocity at various insonation angles.

5.3.3 Measurement of Flow Volume

If the mean flow velocity and the vessel cross section are known, duplex sonography is also a suitable method for determining flow volume. The calculation is based on the formula

$$I = F \cdot v_m$$

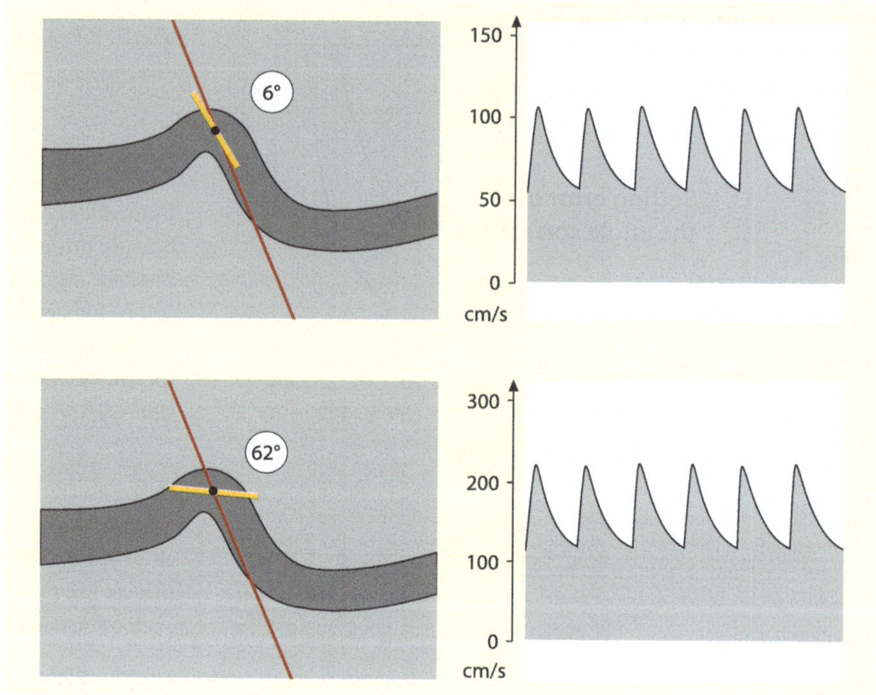

Fig. 5.20 Problem of angle-corrected measurement of flow velocities in kinking. In this case, there are considerable variation possibilities in the setting of the angle correction with considerably variable flow velocity values. In the schematic example shown, maximum systolic velocity has a range from 105 cm/s (angle 6°) to 220 cm/s (angle 62°)

I Flow volume
F Cross-sectional area (= $\pi/4\ d^2$)
v_m Intensity weighted average flow velocity (mean)

As a measure of flow velocity, the intensity-weighted average **mean velocity** correlates best with the total number of "flow threads" in the vessel. A prerequisite for correct determination, however, is a sufficiently large sample volume over the entire cross section of the vessel (Fig. 5.22).

Background Information
As far as the mean velocity is not automatically output by the device, the arithmetically averaged flow velocity can be used as an alternative after angle-corrected conversion of the Doppler frequencies according to the formula.

$$v_m = 1/3\ (v_s + 2v_d),$$

where v_s is the maximum systolic velocity and v_d represents the enddiastolic velocity. Taking the vessel diameter d in mm and the flow velocity v_m in cm/s flow volume I is calculated as

$$I = 0{,}47 \cdot d^2 \cdot v_m [ml/\min]$$

In clinical routine it is sufficient to estimate the average flow velocity by optical interpolation of the Doppler spectrum on the screen. The area above the movable measuring bar (systole) should be equal to the area below the measuring bar (diastole) (Fig. 5.23).

Diagnostic Significance
The determination of flow volume is particularly important in two situations.

Alternative to rCBF Measurements

Sonographic determination of blood volume is a cost-effective, non-invasive alternative to other methods, for example, nuclear medical measurements of cerebral blood flow (CBF). Indications for this are, for example, the estimation of the cardiac load due to the shunt flow in the case of an arteriovenous malformation, but also the assessment of flow volume after extra-intracranial bypass surgery. ◀

"Abnormal" Vessel Diameters

Sonographic vascular diagnostics is generally based on the comparison of measured flow velocities with reference values and/or with the conditions on the contralateral side. However, this only makes sense in "normal" vessel diameters on both sides. This is not the case with congenital hypoplasia or acquired constrictions of individual vessels (e.g., "normal" flow velocity in a highly constricted vessel in the case of a long-distance dissection). ◀

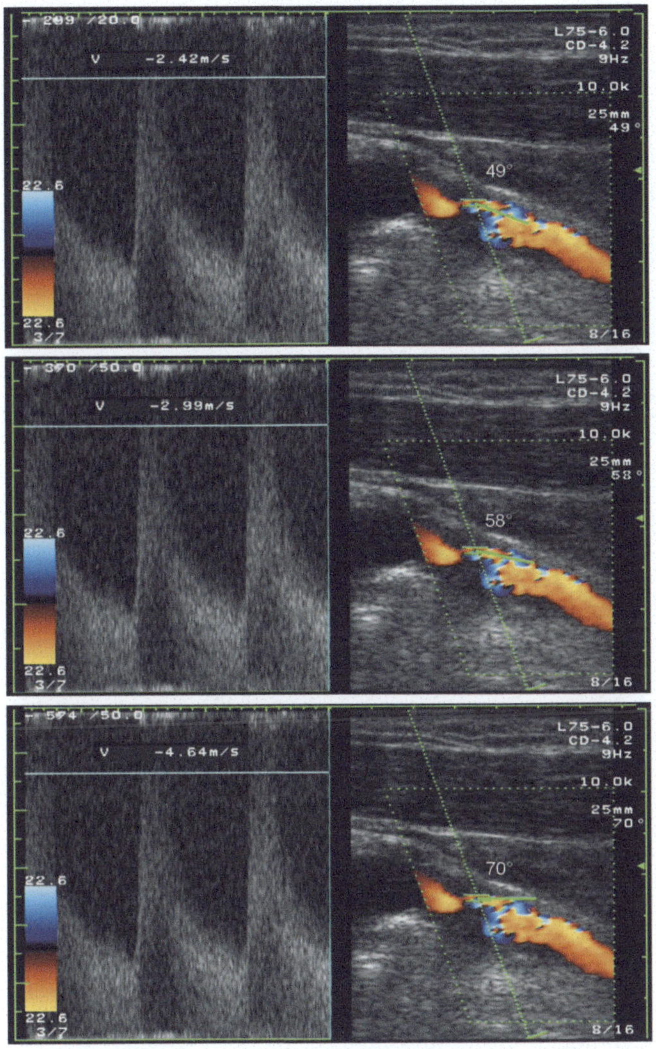

Fig. 5.21 Measurement of flow velocity at the maximum of a short-distance, eccentric stenosis of the internal carotid artery at different settings of the angle correction. Depending on the positioning of the insonation angle, systolic flow velocities between 240 and 460 cm/s result!

> Note
>
> **In all cases of "abnormal" vessel diameter in B-mode imaging, a determination of flow volume should be carried out, as the determination of flow velocity does not allow reliable statements in this case.**

Possible Errors

The main source of error when assessing flow volume concerns the determination of the vessel diameter. Since this is entered quadratically into the calculation formula of flow volume, even small inaccuracies become considerably noticeable (Fig. 5.24). These can occur in several ways (see following overview):

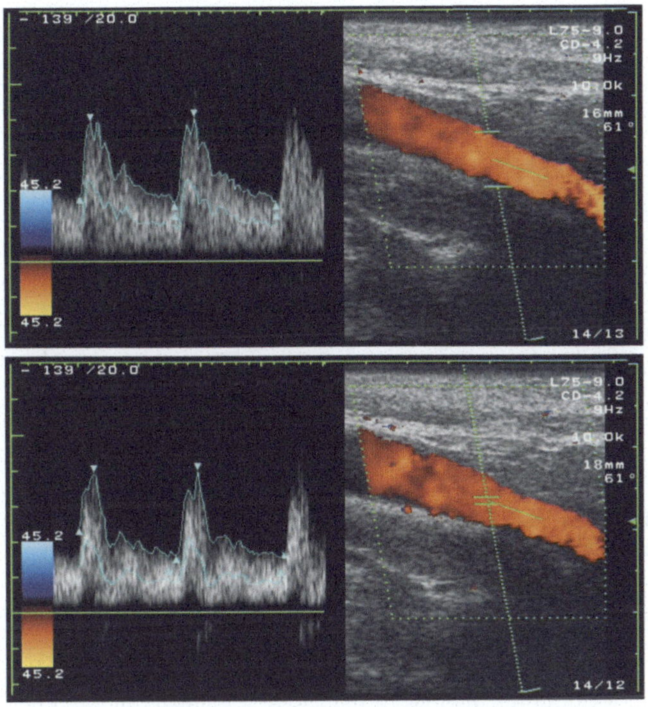

Fig. 5.22 The recording of the flow spectrum in a vessel cross section requires a sample volume that covers the entire lumen (top) otherwise the derived "mean velocity" is incorrect (bottom)

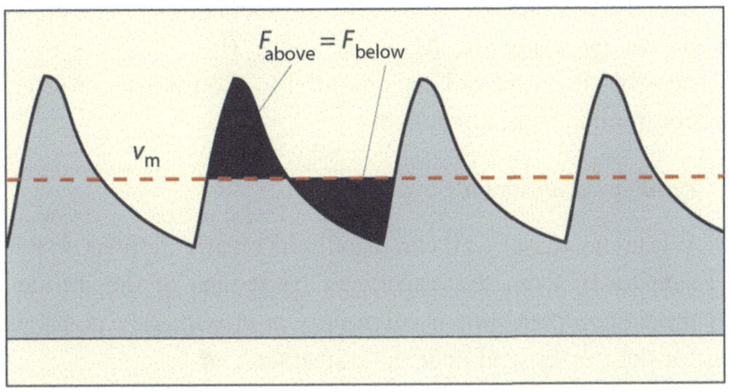

Fig. 5.23 Estimation of average flow velocity on the screen. Further explanations in text

Sources of error in the sonographic determination of flow volume

1. Measurement error of the vessel diameter
   1. Systolic-diastolic diameter fluctuations
   2. Vessel borders not clearly recognizable in B-mode imaging
   3. Vessel has no ideal circular cross section
   4. Determination of the vessel diameter only by means of the color coded display
2. Measurement error of the average flow velocity
   1. Sample volume smaller than the vessel diameter
   2. Angle between the sound beam and the vessel ≥70°
   3. Presence of flow disturbances in the measuring range

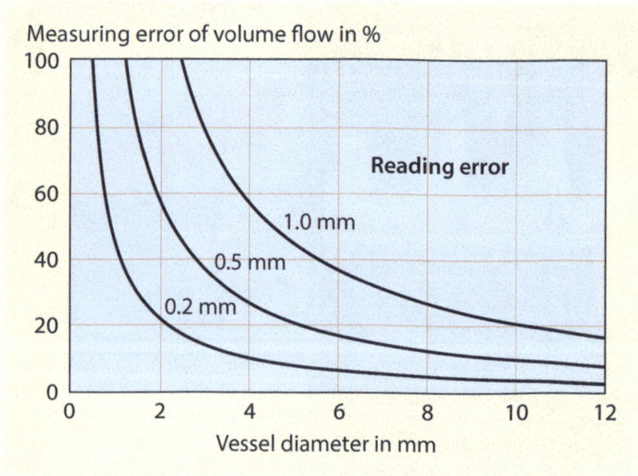

Fig. 5.24 Possible measuring errors in the determination of flow volume as a function of vessel diameter and its measuring (in)accuracy

Problem of Vascular Pulsations

In the systolic-diastolic cycle, radial vascular pulsations result in fluctuations of the vascular diameter in the order of usually about 10%. There is no consensus in the literature on the point in time in the cardiac cycle at which the diameter should be determined. The most correct method would be ECG-triggered averaging, but this has not become established for reasons of practicability. The alternative by using the M-mode image (Fig. 5.25) is only possible if the vessel runs parallel to the transducer (e.g., common carotid artery). ◀

Problem of Vascular Borders

While the vessel wall can usually be clearly defined on the side away from the transducer by means of the intima-media complex, this is often only approximately possible for the vessel wall near the transducer. ◀

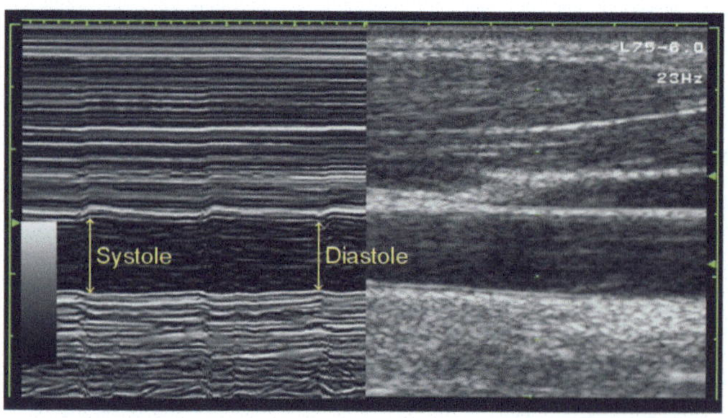

Fig. 5.25 Evaluation of systolic-diastolic vessel pulsations by M-mode imaging

Problem of Cross Section Calculation

The calculation of the area based on the diameter of the vessel requires a circular cross section. Outside the carotid bulb, this situation in arteries is normally present with sufficient accuracy. However, problems arise when eccentric changes in the vessel wall are present. In this case, the cross section may have to be calculated on the basis of the transverse cross-sectional image. ◀

Problem of the Resolution

Compared to B-mode imaging, the resolution of the color coded image is significantly worse. This must be taken into account if, as is often the case in the internal carotid artery, the course of the vessel cannot be adequately defined in the B-mode image and the diameter must be determined using color coded representation. Intracranially, the resolution of color coded duplex sonography is completely inadequate anyway, so that flow volume determinations are not possible here. ◀

> Note
> **As far as technically possible, B-mode (or B-flow) imaging rather than the color coded image should be used to determine the vessel diameter when determining flow volume.**

In addition to the above mentioned problems in determining the vessel diameter, there are further sources of error resulting from the measurement of flow velocity. If there are more pronounced flow disturbances in the area of the measuring point, the averaging of flow velocity is only roughly appropriate due to the no longer laminar and rotationally symmetrical flow conditions in the vessel. Other avoidable sources of error are a 70° or more angle between the sound beam and the vessel as well as a too small measuring volume.

> Note
> **In and immediately behind stenoses with flow disturbances no determination of flow volume should be performed.**

Due to the inaccuracies mentioned, it goes without saying that flow volume determinations are only relatively rough estimates. Especially when measuring smaller vessel diameters, considerable errors must be expected, which can

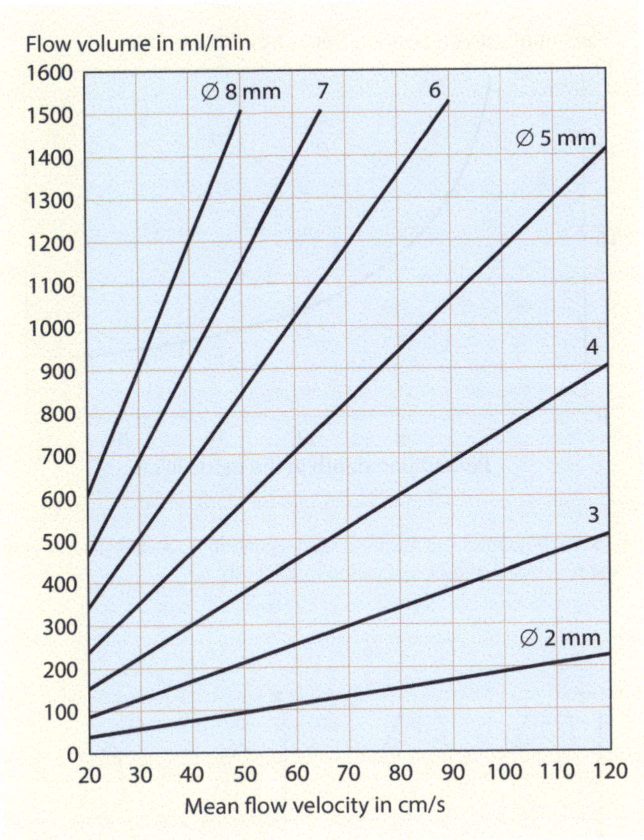

Fig. 5.26 Nomogram for determining flow volume in vessels from mean flow velocity and vessel diameter

reach 50–100%(!) (Fig. 5.24). In the common and internal carotid artery, however, the flow volume can usually be estimated with an accuracy of ±20–30%, which corresponds to the measurement accuracy of other methods (e.g., MRI, SPECT). As far as the existing duplex device does not include the possibility of flow volume determination, the nomogram in the Fig. 5.26 can be used to quickly estimate flow volume.

Practical Tips

Due to the unavoidable inaccuracies in the determination of flow volume, it should be avoided to simulate an apparent accuracy by giving exact calculation values. Rather, relatively coarse subdivisions, for example, 250, 300, 350 ml/min, appear to be more appropriate.

5.3.4 Problems with the Aliasing Effect

The advantages of the selective flow investigation in pulsed Doppler sonography are bought by a physically caused

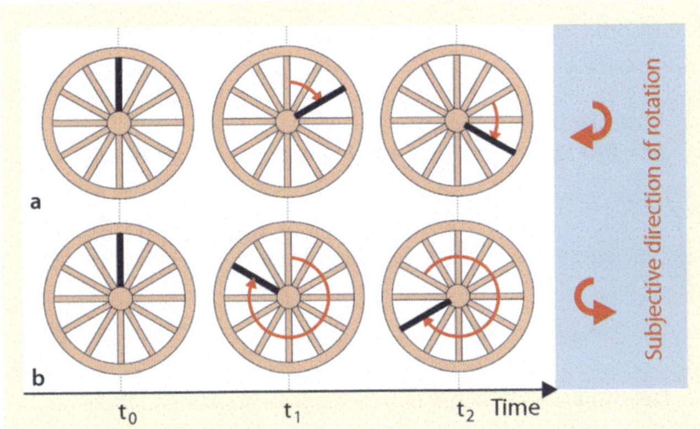

Fig. 5.27 Aliasing effect using the example of spoked wheels rotating clockwise at different speeds in a TV or cinema film with the display. Individual images shown at times t_0, t_1 and t_2. While at slow rotational speed (**a**) the direction of rotation of the wheel appears to be correct, a faster movement results in the subjective impression of a wheel turning in the opposite direction (**b**)

disadvantage called **Aliasing**. This effect is well known from cinema films, for example, when the spoked wheels of moving carriages seem to turn in the wrong direction. The reason is that film recordings consist of individual frames that are recorded and played back at a "frame rate" above the limit of 16 Hz, which is characteristic of the temporal resolving power of the eye. Correspondingly, rotational movements are equally divided into individual images (Fig. 5.27). At a certain speed of rotation, the wheels seem to stand still, and as they increase further, the impression of a wheel turning in the opposite direction is created.

A similar situation exists in pulsed Doppler sonography. Here, the relatively low-frequency Doppler shift in the range of a few kHz with oscillation durations of around 1 ms must be developed from very short consecutive ultrasonic pulses whose oscillation period is 1000 times shorter (Fig. 5.28). This requires very frequent ultrasonic pulses enabling the electronic device to correctly detect the Doppler shift. The measure for this is the so-called **Pulse repetition frequency** (PRF) (Sect. 3.3.1). According to the so-called **Nyquist Theorem** however, only Doppler frequencies that do not exceed half of the PRF can be displayed correctly (**Aliasing threshold**). If Doppler frequencies greater than PRF/2 are to be displayed, the aliasing effect described above will occur.

In Doppler spectrum analysis, aliasing is characterized by the fact that frequency peaks are cut off and reappear on the screen with apparently opposite flow direction (Fig. 5.29). If the Doppler frequency to be derived is above the pulse repetition frequency, the pulsatility of both the acoustically audible Doppler signal and the spectrum image may be lost, or a flow signal may be produced that can no longer be interpreted.

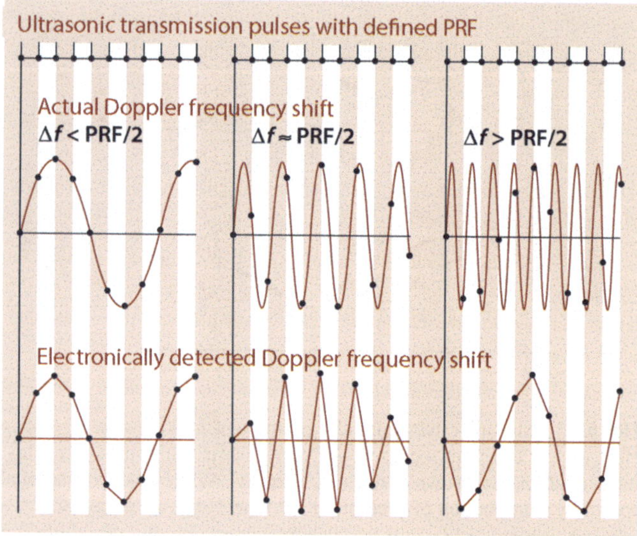

Fig. 5.28 Reconstruction of sinusoidal oscillations of different frequencies (Doppler shift) from single ultrasonic pulses with a defined pulse repetition frequency (PRF). If the Doppler frequency shift Δf to be displayed exceeds half of the PRF (right), a misinterpretation of the measured Doppler frequency (aliasing effect) occurs with an apparently slower frequency, which seems to go in the other direction due to phase inversion

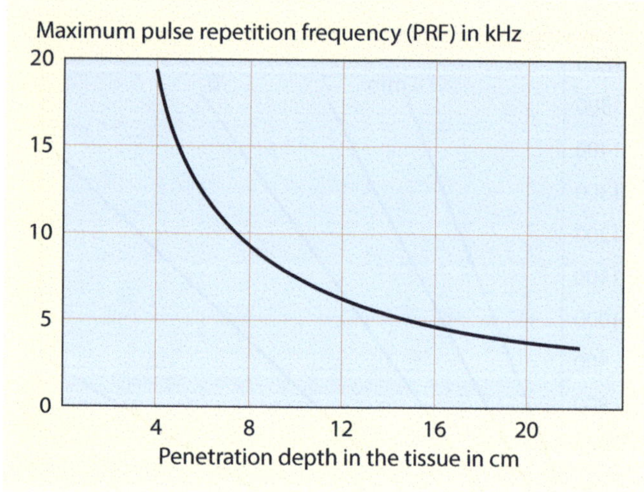

Fig. 5.30 Maximum achievable pulse repetition frequencies depending on the required depth of insonation in the body

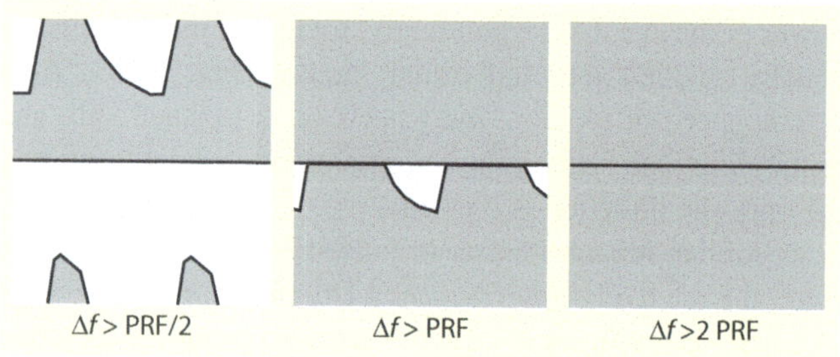

Fig. 5.29 Display of a Doppler spectrum with frequency shift Δf for different pulse repetition frequencies (PRF)

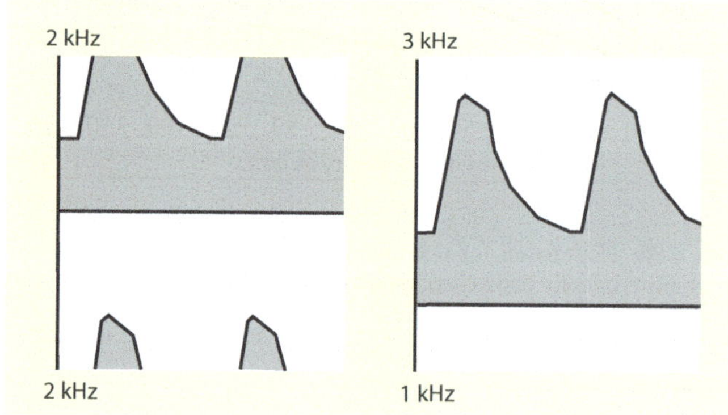

Fig. 5.31 Improved display of higher Doppler frequencies using pulsed Doppler technique by shifting the zero line

> **Note**
> **"Aliasing" means a physically induced phenomenon where the displayed Doppler frequency shift may be misrepresented in the opposite direction of flow.**

Maximum PRF Versus Penetration Depth

The desire to increase the pulse repetition frequency is limited by the fact that the emission of a new sound pulse must be waited until the echoes from the maximum tissue depth to be examined have reached the transducer (Fig. 5.30). This can lead to problems, especially when examining intracranial vessels, since in this case an insonation depth of 8–10 cm is regularly required. The only way to increase the imaging quality is to shift the zero line of the device (Fig. 5.31).

High-PRF Mode

The limitations of the Nyquist theorem on the representability of Doppler frequencies can be partially overcome in most duplex devices by the so-called **High-PRF mode**. Here, the emission of a new ultrasonic pulse does not wait until all reflections have reached the transducer again, but halfway through the time a new pulse is already emitted. Thus a doubling of the displayable Doppler frequency up to the level of the pulse repetition frequency can be achieved. However, this is bought by setting up another sample volume in the middle between the transducer and the measuring volume set on the screen. If a vessel "randomly" runs in this further sample volume, its flow signal is also displayed. Accordingly, the High-PRF mode should not be used, for example, in the diagnostics of vessel occlusions.

Summary
The pulsed Doppler technique enables blood flows to be selectively detected at freely selectable tissue depths by positioning a defined sample volume. If the Doppler examination is carried out in combination with B-mode imaging (duplex sonography), flow velocities and flow volumes can be measured quantitatively after determining the angle between the sound beam and the vessel (insonation angle) and, if necessary, also the vessel diameter. A disadvantage of pulsed Doppler and duplex sonography is the occurrence of the aliasing effect with apparently reversed flow direction if the Doppler frequencies to be displayed exceed half the frequency at which ultrasonic pulses are emitted (pulse repetition frequency).

References

Gosling RC, King DH (1974) Arterial assessment by Doppler shift ultrasound. Proc R Soc Med 67:447–449

Pourcelot L (1974) Applications cliniques de l'examen Doppler transcutane. Inserm 34:213–240

Spencer MP, Reid JM (1979) Quantitation of carotid stenosis with continuous-wave Doppler ultrasound. Stroke 10:326–330

Von Reutern GM, Kaps M, Büdingen HJ von (2000) Ultraschall-diagnostik der hirnversorgenden Arterien, 3rd edn. Thieme, Stuttgart New York

Flow Assessment Using Color Coding

6

Bernhard Widder and Gerhard F. Hamann

6.1 Technical Principles of Color Coded Imaging

6.1.1 Color Coded Flow Detection

Despite its designation as "Fast Fourier Transformation," FFT (Sect. 5.1) is far too slow for physical reasons to be used for color coded imaging of arterial flow with its numerous scan lines. Since, however, the requirements for frequency resolution are not very high and color coded imaging serves much more to localize flow than to measure flow parameters in detail, other techniques – especially the so-called **autocorrelation method** – can be used to obtain at least approximate information about the intensity-weighted mean Doppler shift frequency. The exact knowledge of the principle behind is unnecessary for the ultrasound user.

6.1.2 Parameters of the "color window"

As already mentioned in Sect. 4.1.3, color coded flow imaging is basically a pulsed Doppler device with numerous small sample volumes along a larger number of "virtual" Doppler sound beams which are successively electronically controlled. This results in a two-dimensional field of distinct measuring points whose flow information is displayed in different colors ("color coded"). This field is characterized by the following parameters.

Color Window
This is a box within the B-mode image, in which flow information is displayed in color coded form. Depending on the transducer used, the color window is displayed as a (tilted) rectangle or as a circle sector (Fig. 6.1). Together with the number of scan lines (see below), the width of the color window selected by the examiner, is responsible for the frame rate (Sect. 6.2.4).

Tilted Angle of Color Window
With linear array transducers, the rectangular color window can usually be tilted with its lower part several steps to the right or left to achieve a more favorable insonation angle (Sect. 6.2.1)

Scan Lines
The position of the "virtual" Doppler sound beams can only be recognized indirectly by the shape of the color window. The number of scan lines can usually be adjusted by the examiner in several steps and influences both the resolution of the color coded image (Sect. 6.1.4) and the frame rate (Sect. 6.2.4). In order not to reduce the latter too much, the flow signal is usually only analyzed for each 3rd – 4th sound beam of the B-mode image, and the color representation of the scan lines between is interpolated.

6.1.3 Methods of Color Coded Presentation

The already shown frequency density spectrum at any point of time of the systolic-diastolic cycle can be color coded by different methods. The most important ones for vascular diagnostics are listed below (Fig. 6.2).

Frequency-Dependent Display (Velocity Mode)
The so-called "velocity mode" gives information about the magnitude of the intensity weighted Doppler frequency shift (mean frequency). There is consensus among equipment

B. Widder (✉)
Expert Opinion Institute, District Hospital, Guenzburg, Germany
e-mail: bernhard.widder@bkh-guenzburg.de

G. F. Hamann
Clinic of Neurology and Neurological Rehabilitation, District Hospital, Guenzburg, Germany

B. Widder, G. F. Hamann (eds.), *Duplex sonography of the brain-supplying arteries*, https://doi.org/10.1007/978-3-662-65566-5_6

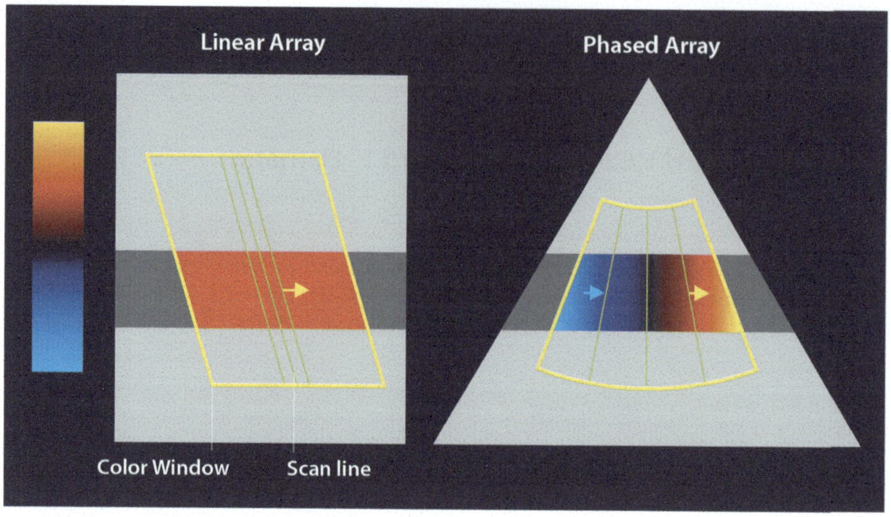

Fig. 6.1 Shape and position of the color window of a linear array (left) and a phased array transducer (right). The position of the "virtual" sound beams (scan lines) can only be recognized by the shape of the color window. Using a linear array transducer, the color window and thus the scan lines can be tilted to the left or right within certain limits. This allows an improvement of the "color filling" of vessels that are almost parallel to the transducer surface by reducing the insonation angle, which is otherwise near 90°. Using phased array transducers, the changing relative direction of flow toward and away from the scan lines causes a color change in transvers running vessels. In addition, when crossing the 90° insonation angle, color extinction must be expected

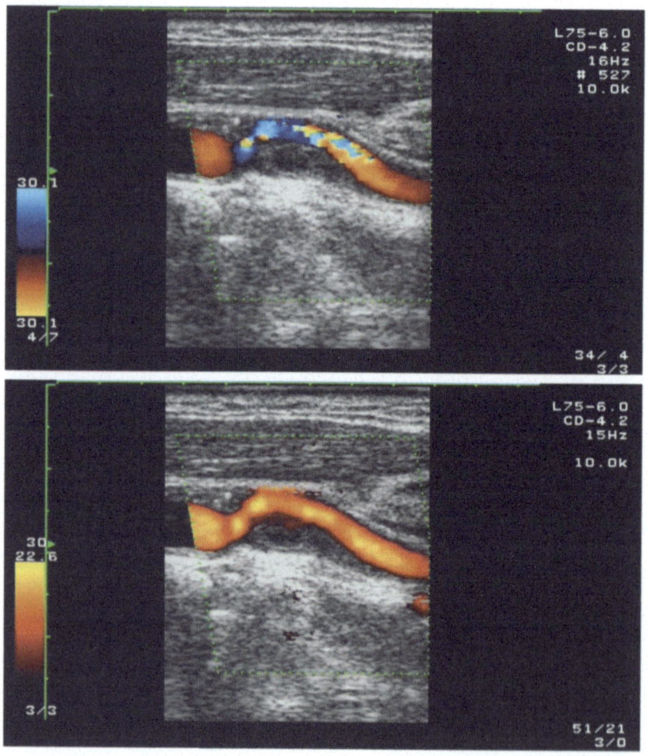

Fig. 6.2 Color coded presentation of the internal carotid artery in velocity mode (top) and power mode (bottom) using the example of a moderate stenosis at the origin of the internal carotid artery. Note the better presentation of the contours of the vessel lumen in the power mode, while the velocity mode provides information on the maximum stenosis based on the local increase in flow velocity

manufacturers that the higher the Doppler frequency shift, the brighter or more intense the color coding becomes (Fig. 6.3). The red-blue coding of the two directions of blood flow to and from the transducer is the most common, but it should not be confused with the red-blue representation of arteries and veins that is common in anatomy textbooks due to possible misinterpretations caused by aliasing effects (Sect. 6.2.2).

Usually color coded duplex scanners show at the side of the screen a bar or wheel, in which the colors selected for color coding of the two flow directions and Doppler frequencies are displayed (color map). The value usually displayed at the top and bottom corresponds to the maximum mean frequency until the alias threshold is reached (Sect. 6.2.2), but most manufacturers indicate this in cm/s or m/s. Since an angle correction is not possible fro color coded imaging, the indication of velocity appears methodically nonsensical and is misleading, but for some inexplicable reasons it has become widely accepted. This also concerns the term "velocity mode" for this technique. The velocity indicated refers to an angle of 0° and can therefore be easily converted to kHz (Table 6.1).

Power-Dependent Display (Power Mode)
Using this method, color coding is based on the intensity (power) of the backscattered frequency components and is thus proportional to the diameter of the investigated vessel within certain limits. Since this method is rather insensitive to artifacts and is only slightly dependent on the insonation angle, any vessel in which blood flows – at whatever

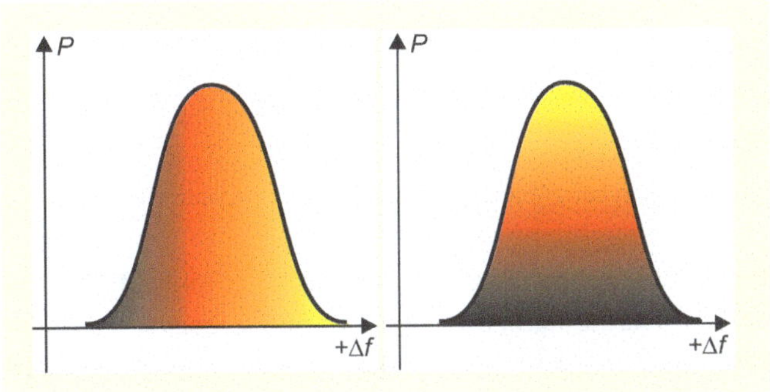

Fig. 6.3 Principle of the different color coded representations of blood flow. While higher Doppler frequencies Δf lead to brighter color values in frequency-dependent methods (velocity mode, left), the energy P of the reflected Doppler spectrum is used for color coding in power-dependent methods (power mode, right)

speed – can be represented in this way when the threshold is set low. Statements about flow velocity, however, are not possible, and – at least with older devices – the direction of flow cannot be determined either. Table 6.2 gives an overview of the advantages and disadvantages of both methods.

6.1.4 Resolution of Color Coded Imaging

Spatial Resolution
As with B-mode imaging, the axial and lateral resolution must be considered separately for the color coded imaging.

Axial Resolution

In contrast to B-mode imaging, where ultrasound pulses as short as possible are selected, (Fig. 3.6), pulse duration in Doppler applications must be considerably longer in order to enable a sufficient Doppler frequency determination. Correspondingly, color coded imaging has a worse axial resolution by a factor of 5–10 as compared to B-mode imaging. ◀

Lateral Resolution

Due to the considerably smaller number of scan lines compared to B-mode imaging, comparable limitations also result with regard to the lateral resolution. If one assumes about 20–30 scan lines as "usual", an extracranial lateral resolution of at most 1–2 mm can be achieved. In the transcranial examination of intracerebral vessels, the situation is even worse in the range of 2–3 mm due to the low ultrasound frequency and possible distortions when penetrating the bony skull. Since the diameter of the major cerebral arteries is also only in this range, it goes without saying that it is not possible to make statements about the width of theses vessels. ◀

Note
Resolution of color coded display:

- **Extracranial**
  - **Axial 0.5–1 mm**
  - **Lateral 1–2 mm**
- **Transcranial**
  - **Axial 1–2 mm**
  - **Lateral 2–3 mm**

Temporal Resolution
The temporal resolution of color coded imaging represents a compromise between the desire for a flow representation that is as pulsatile as possible ("high temporal resolution") on the one hand and the highest possible spatial and detail resolution on the other. The frame rate of color codes decreases:

- By increasing the scan line density in the color window
- By widening the "Color Window"
- By increasing the number of scan lines.

If one assumes a common frame rate of 5 Hz and takes into account a heart rate of for example, 70/min, the color coded image is recreated just 4 times over the heart cycle. Accordingly, color coding is only suitable to a very limited extent for statements on flow pulsatility.

6.1.5 Special Methods of Color Coded Image Processing

Today, ultrasound devices are no longer conceivable without extensive digital image post-processing, although the line between relevant processing of the ultrasound information and pure "image embellishment" with possible loss of information is fluid. This applies in particular to color coded imaging, where the image is generated from a very limited number of scan lines with likewise limited axial resolution. In order to achiveve a sufficient "color filling" auf the vessels

Table 6.1 Conversion of displayed velocity values in mean frequencies with respect to the Doppler transmission frequency

Velocity value [cm/s]	Doppler transmission frequency			
	2.5	5.0	7.5	MHz
10	0.3	0.7	1.0	kHz
20	0.6	1.3	2.0	kHz
50	1.6	3.3	5.0	kHz

Table 6.2 Comparison of velocity and power dependent color coded display methods

Display method	Advantages	Disadvantages
Frequency dependent presentation *(Velocity mode)*	Information about flow velocity	Flow display dependent from insonation angle
Intensity dependent presentation *(Power mode)*	"Color filling," relatively independent of angle, "angiography-like" imaging	Missing information about flow velocity, at slow flow velocities (e.g., poststenotic) "color filling" of vessels not optimal

investigated, averaging techniques plays a role here, Two techniques are mainly used for this aim.

Persistence Index

By continuous interpolation of several consecutive images, artifacts can be suppressed and the image appears "smoother." However, this is bought by a reduction of the temporal resolution. The number of interpolated images can be controlled by the user by means of the so-called persistence index.

Color Capture

Continuous summation of the color information of successively taken images with subsequent "freezing" of the summed image is particularly helpful when vessels cannot be displayed in one plane. Such a situation is found almost regularly in kinkings, but also in the area of the circle of Willis. By slightly tilting the transducer back and forth, a spatial segment with all the vessels in this segment can be recorded and displayed on the screen (Fig. 6.4). In CT and MR angiography this method is known as "maximum intensity projection" (MIP).

Summary

In color coded duplex sonography, blood flow can be displayed within a defined color window as colored structures. Standard methods of color coding are frequency-dependent (velocity mode) and power-dependent (power mode) display. Compared to B-mode imaging, the resolution of color coded imagingis lower by a factor of 5–10. Special techniques of image processing (persistence index, color capture) result in a more homogeneous color presentation in individual cases.

6.2 Influencing Variables on Color Coded Flow Imaging

6.2.1 The Insonation Angle

As mentioned above, the angle between the sound beam and the vessel under investigation is essential for all Doppler applications. Of course, this also applies to color coded flow imaging. However, what makes this more difficult is the fact that the numerous "virtual" sound beams (**color- or scan lines**) are visible only indirectly by means of the shape and position of the **color window** (Fig. 6.1).

In the case of sector or curved transducers, the insonation angle changes across the screen, so that in a straight vessel there may be flow both toward and away from the probe. An angle approaching 90° can lead to the incorrect diagnosis of a vessel occlusion. A vessel detected with an increasing insonation angle can give rise to the misdiagnosis of a stenosis due to the increasing Doppler frequencies.

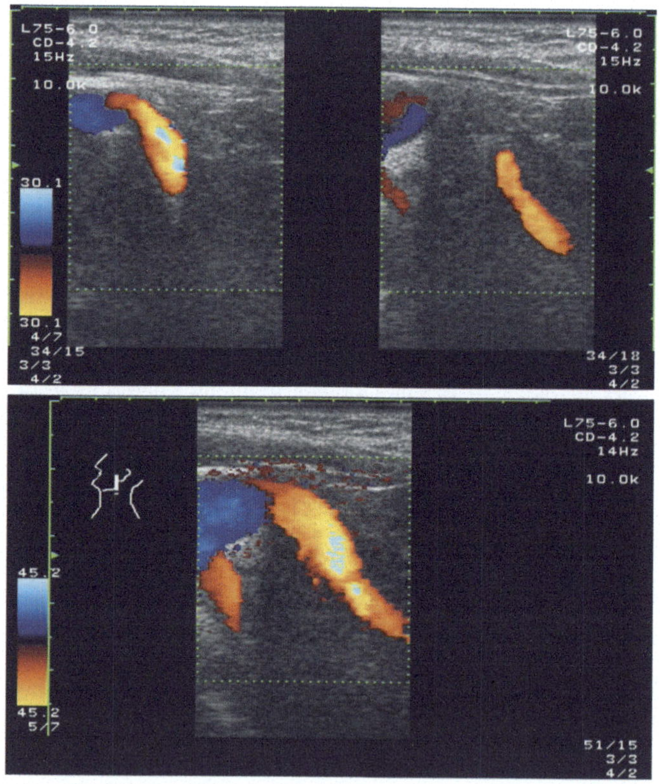

Fig. 6.4 Color coded representation of an elongation of the internal carotid artery without (top) and with (bottom) use of color capture. Due to the fact that the course of the vessel does not lie in a single sectional plane, either the proximal or the distal section of the extracranial internal carotid artery can normally be displayed

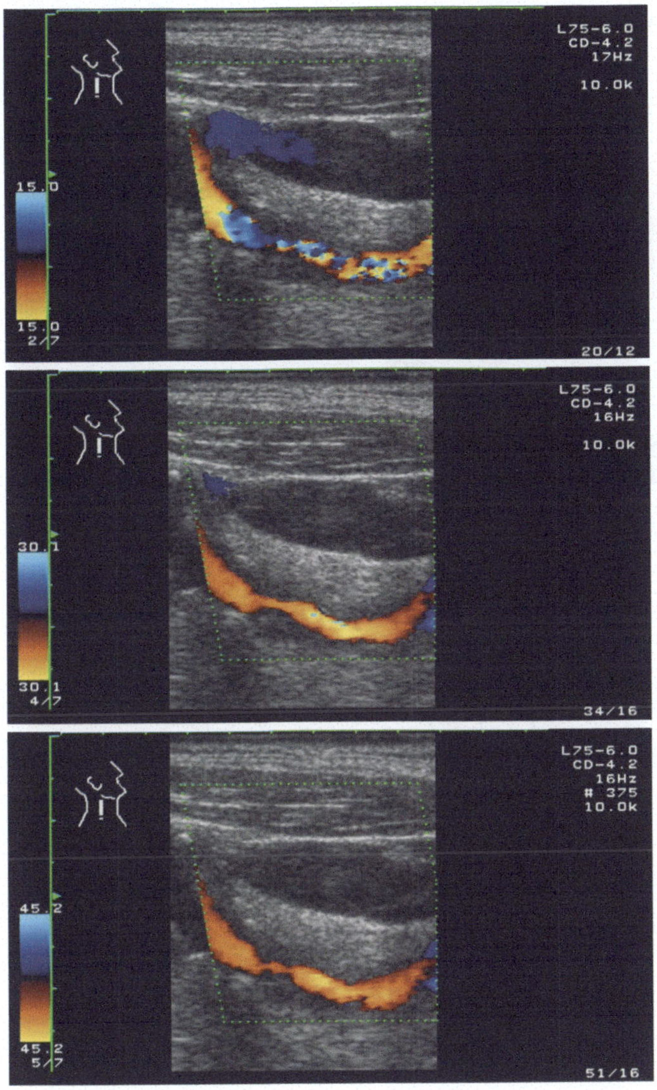

Fig. 6.5 Color coded representation of a long-stretched stenosis at the origin of the internal carotid artery with an alias threshold increasing from top to bottom

6.2.2 Aliasing

Since color coded duplex sonography is a pulsed Doppler application, the aliasing effect also plays an important role. Therefore Doppler frequencies exceeding the **alias threshold** (Sect. 5.3.4) are displayed with apparently reversed flow direction.

Color Map

As already mentioned, the color map visible at the side of the screen provides information about the maximum mean frequency that can currently be displayed without aliasing. Most manufacturers prefer a vertical **color bar** (Fig. 6.5), with some devices there is also a **color wheel**. The latter is particularly suitable for illustrating the principle of the alias effect, according to which the opposite colorsbegins when the "alias threshold" is exceeded (Fig. 6.6).

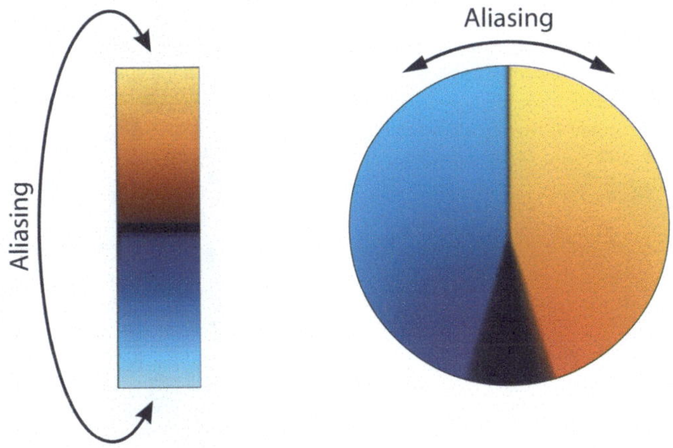

Fig. 6.6 Color map in the most frequently used form as a vertical bar (left) as a color wheel (right). If the alias threshold is exceeded due to higher Doppler frequencies, the opposite coloration is achieved

Differentiation Aliasing: Retrograde flow

Showing similar color coding, Doppler frequencies that exceed the alias threshold cannot be easily distinguished from retrograde flow in a vessel. However, a reliable aid is provided by the fact that the crossing of the alias threshold runs across lighter colors, so that a light boundary layer is formed between regions of different colors (Fig. 6.7). Retrograde flow components, on the other hand, typically show a dark border (Fig. 6.8).

> Note
> **Differentiation between aliasing effect and backflow:**
> - **Aliasing effect: color transition with light hem**
> - **Backflow: Color transition with dark hem.**

> Practical Tips
> As a rule of thumb for the setting of the alias threshold, a value of 10–20 cm/s should normally be set initially, both extra- and intracranially, in order to first detect the vessels. To exclude stenosis respectively to detect a local aliasing phenomenon, the aliasing threshold is then gradually increased by increasing the PRF. If there is a stenosis, there remains a distinct aliasing area indicating the stenosis (Sect. 6.3.2).

6.2.3 Lower Cut-Off Frequency (Wall Filter)

In color coded duplex sonography, it is necessary to differentiate unmoved from moving structures in order to display them either gray shaded or in color. For this purpose – in

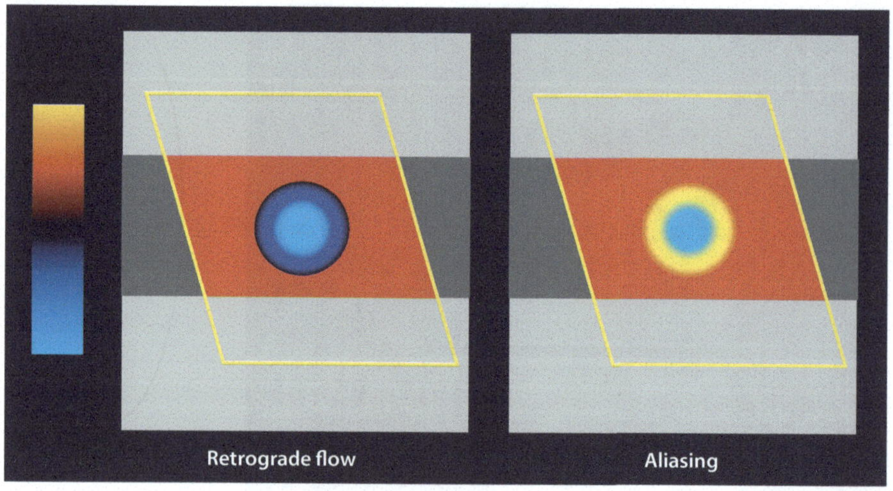

Fig. 6.7 Differentiation between aliasing and retrograde flow based on the coloration in the border area of the color change (retrograde flow = dark border zone; aliasing = light border zone)

simplified form – a high-pass filter is used, which excludes low Doppler frequency shifts from the color display, as they also occur with (mostly) unmoved structures (Fig. 6.9). Since such a separation is also necessary in the "conventional" Doppler sonography in order to suppress the low but highly reflective lateral pulsations of the vessel walls from the Doppler spectrum, the term "**wall filter**" has been derived from this application. However, it should be noted that the filter used does not represent a sharp dividing line for

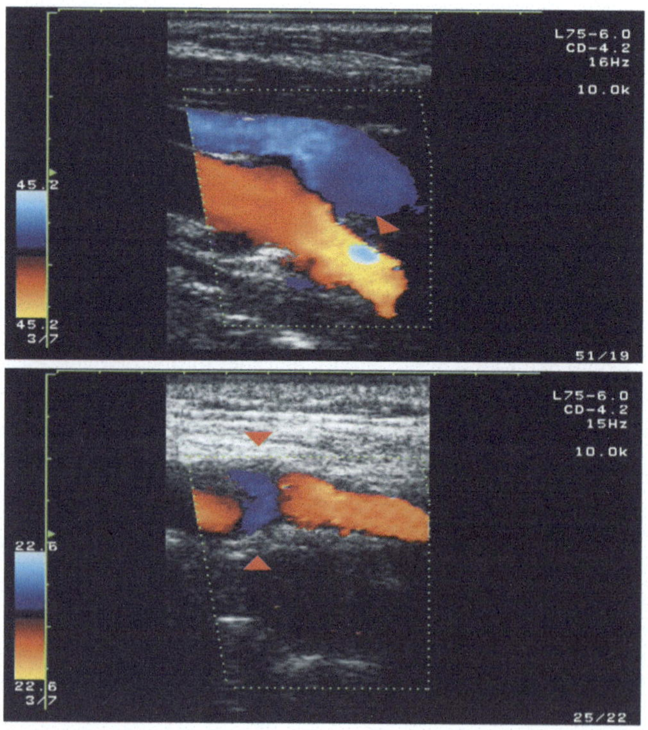

Fig. 6.8 Circumscribed aliasing effect approx. 2 cm distal to the origin of the internal carotid artery as an indication of a stenosis located there (above). Retrograde flow components in the region of the carotid bulb caused by helically twisted flow ("helix flow") (bottom)

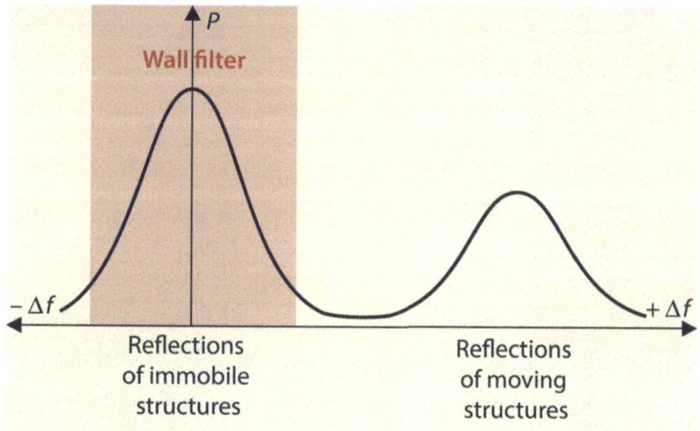

Fig. 6.9 Separation of unmoved echoes ($\Delta f \approx 0$) from Doppler frequency shifts by means of a wall filter (ideally sharp-edged in the figure)

technical reasons. Accordingly, strong stationary echoes can overcome the filtering and appear as color dots when the wall filter is set low.

Minimum Detectable Blood Flow

In practice, the lower cut-off frequency represents only a relatively minor problem, since even behind most severe stenoses, flow velocities in the order of 1–2 cm/s can be expected in the poststenotic lumen. Flow velocities below that obviously lead to thrombosis in larger arteries. Thus, for example, at a transmission frequency of 5 MHz and an angle of 60° between the sound beam and the vessel, a wall filter or a minimum resolution in the order of 50 Hz should be sufficient to be able to detect the remaining blood flow even behind a high-grade stenosis (Fig. 6.10). Due to the problem of angle dependence, however, higher insonation angles should be avoided, since otherwise a sufficient detection of low flow velocities can no longer be expected.

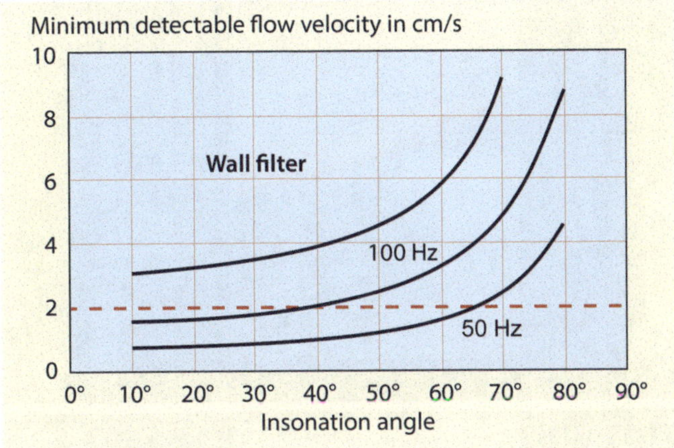

Fig. 6.10 Dependence of the minimum detectable flow velocity on the insonation angle and the wall filter set (for example using an ultrasonic transmission frequency of 5 MHz). To be able to detect a velocity of 2 cm/s, the insonation angle should not exceed 60–70° (with 50 Hz wall filter)

6.2.4 Frame Rate

Without influence on the diagnostic accuracy, but disturbing the ultrasound investigation, slow frame rates can be a problem in color coded imaging. While the build-up of a B-mode image takes place in almost negligible time, image build-up times for color coding in the range of 100–200 ms are not uncommon, resulting in frame rates of 5–10 Hz. In individual cases, a compromise is required between the minimum still derivable Doppler frequency on the one hand and the width of the color window and the number of color lines on the other hand (Table 6.3). Other influencing variables are the required imaging depth, which limits the maximum achievable pulse repetition frequency, and the number of desired focal points.

Background Information
As in B-mode sonography the use of several focus points would be desirable in order to achieve optimum resolution not only at a certain depth in the tissue, but over the entire scanning range. While this is not critical for B-mode imaging due to the fast image build-up, the use of several focus points in color coded imaging leads to a hardly acceptable slowdown of the frame rate, since a separate color image must be built up for each focus point. Most device manufacturers therefore use only one focus zone for color display.

Table 6.3 Factors influencing the frame rate

Technical parameter	Frame rate higher	Frame rate lower
Width of color window	Smaller	Larger
Quantity of the scan lines	Less	More
Pulse repetition frequency	Higher	Lower
Lower cut-off frequency	Higher	Lower

6.2.5 Color Gain and Color Balance

In contrast to B-mode sonography, which requires only a single gain control, color coded duplex sonography has separate controls for B-mode and color gain as well as a control for the ratio of the two to each other ("color balance") (Fig. 6.11).

Too little color gain causes the color coded flow information to disappear, too much gain leads to dotted color artifacts in the area of non-moving structures. The latter should not be confounded with the **confetti effect** which can occur behind high-grade stenoses (Fig. 13.12).

The relationship between the color coded and B-mode imaging is determined by the **color balance**. If the balance is adjusted too much in favor of the gray-scale image, the colored flow image disappears. If the balance is set too much in the direction of the color coding, the edges of the vessel are overwritten in color. It takes some experience to achieve a reasonable compromise between a still sufficient B-mode representation and a good "color filling" of the examined vessels.

Summary
The angle dependency known from Doppler sonography can be observed in the same way in color coded imaging, that is, the color coding fails if the angle between the "virtual" sound beam and the vessel is approximately 90°. The aliasing effect is also of importance, which leads to an apparent backflow at flow velocities that exceed the aliasing threshold. A prerequisite for a reliable color coded vessel display is sufficient color gain and an adapted color balance.

6.3 Basic Techniques of Color Coded Duplex Examination

In the practice of color coded duplex examination, there are two fundamentally different forms of approaching the goal: on one hand the best possible pathoanatomic vascular

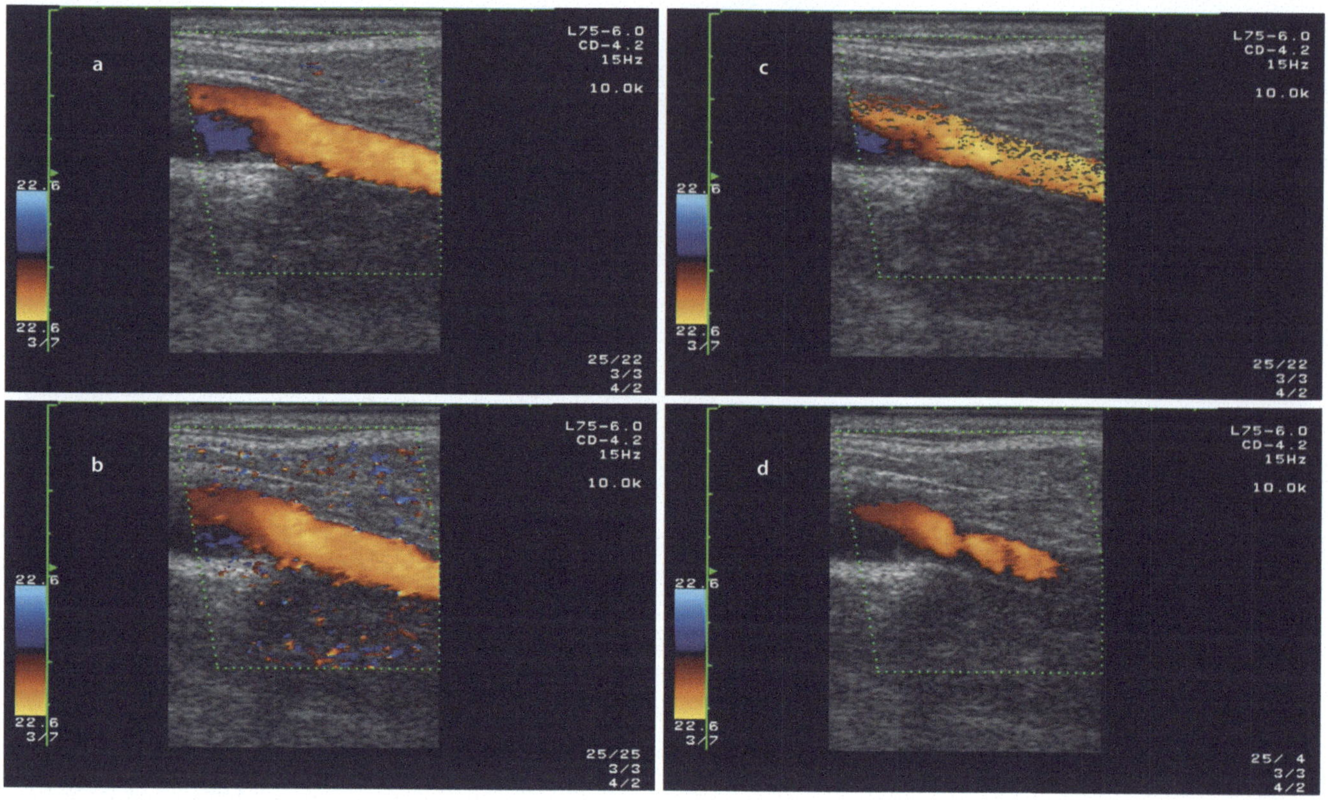

Fig. 6.11 (**a**–**d**) Appearance of a normal extracranial internal carotid artery at different settings of color gain and balance. "Normal" appearance with isolated color spots outside the vascular lumen (**a**), color gain set too high (**b**), balance set to the disadvantage of the color coding (**c**), color gain set too low (**d**)

presentation, on the other hand the best possible assessment of flow characteristics (Table 6.4). It is not realistic to fulfil both requirements together, which is why a selection has to be made depending on the question.

6.3.1 Optimized Vessel Imaging ("Low-flow setting")

Probably the most important significance of color coded technique is the possibility of localizing flow in vessels. This makes the best possible "color filling" important, while statements about the Doppler frequency and the pulsatile course are subordinate and are the domain of "conventional" duplex technique with a singular ultrasound beam. The best possible representation of vessels can be achieved by considering several factors (see overview below).

Possibilities for Improving the "color filling" of Vessels ("Low-Flow Setting")

- Low Doppler transmission frequency (if adjustable on the device side)
- Low pulse repetition frequency PRF (alias threshold ≤10 cm/s)
- Low wall filter (≤50 Hz)
- Optimization of the angle between sound beam and vessel
- Increase of the color gain
- Use of digital image processing (persistence, color capture)
- Use of the "power mode."

Practical Tips

The combination of low PRF, low wall filter, optimized insonation angle and high color gain up to the occurrence of single color dots in soft tissue is called low-flow setting and is used to detect slow flow velocities when differentiating from vascular occlusions.

Low Doppler Transmission Frequency

If color coded flow investigation is the main focus of a particular diagnostic problem, a transducer with a lower transmission frequency should be selected despite the

Table 6.4 Basic techniques of color coded duplex examination in the area of the extracranial arteries supplying the brain

Technology	Objective	Field of application
Optimized vessel imaging	Reaching a good "color filling" of the examined vessel	Assessing the course and the continuity of the vessels investigated
Optimized flow assessment	Step by step increasing an initial low pulse repetition frequency PRF until almost all alias phenomena largely disappear	Localizing stenoses und their maximum narrowing

possibly poorer image resolution. This can be expected to significantly increase the penetration depth in individual cases, while the already limited color resolution is only marginally affected.

Low "wall filter"

Since flow velocity in vessels only shows higher velocities in the middle and decreases toward the vessel wall due to the typical parabolic flow profile, the setting of a relatively low cut-off frequency (wall filter) with the possibility of detecting even low flow velocities is a prerequisite for a on optimal color filling of the whole vessel. This can be achieved by selecting a low pulse repetition frequency in combination with a suitable wall filter.

Optimized Insonation Angle

In addition, there is a requirement for a lowest possible angle between the virtual sound beam and the vessel. However, this is countered by the fact that, if the color window is tilted strongly, the distance to reach the vessel can increase considerably, which leads to a reduced penetration depth (Fig. 6.12). When sonicating deep-seated vessels, it is therefore necessary to find a compromise between the two opposing effects.

Increasing the Color Gain

The setting of a sufficient color gain is one of the most important measures to achieve optimal color filling of a vessel. As a rule, color enhancement is correctly adjusted when some color dots also appear in motionless structures.

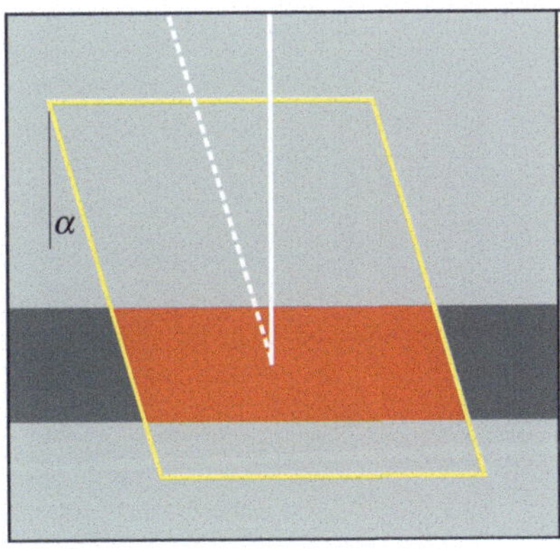

Tilt angle	Time extension
0°	0 %
10°	4 %
20°	13 %
30°	31 %

Fig. 6.12 Enlargement of the distance between transducer and vessel by increased tilting of the color window

Digital Image Processing

The various techniques of image processing have already been mentioned. It seems to make sense to use these measures, because although information about the pulsatile course of flow is lost, this information is of little importance anyway for the reasons mentioned and priority should be given to an optimal "color filling."

Using Power Mode

As already mentioned in Sect. 6.1.3, **Power mode** results in a better "color filling" with the possibility to display even very slow flows. The price for this, however, is the loss of flow velocity information (in older devices also of direction information), so that this method can only serve as a supplement to the velocity mode.

6.3.2 Optimized Flow Imaging

This technique is used to make local flow accelerations in stenoses visible (Fig. 6.13). Starting from a low PRF value (or a low aliasing threshold of 10–20 cm/s), the PRF is gradually increased until aliasing phenomena in the vessel course have largely disappeared. If a local aliasing is still present and cannot be explained by changes in the insonation angle, this indicates a stenosis. In this way, it is also easy to detect the maximum of a stenosis and then to place the Doppler beam in this area specifically for measuring maximum flow velocity.

Summary

Depending on the diagnostic objective, two different device settings can be considered for color coded duplex sonography:

- The aim of "optimized vessel imaging" by achieving the best possible "color filling" of vessels, which may be managed by using various "low-flow parameters."
- The aim of "optimized flow imaging" for recognizing circumscribed flow accelerations as an indication of the presence of a stenosis, which is possible by varying the PRF.

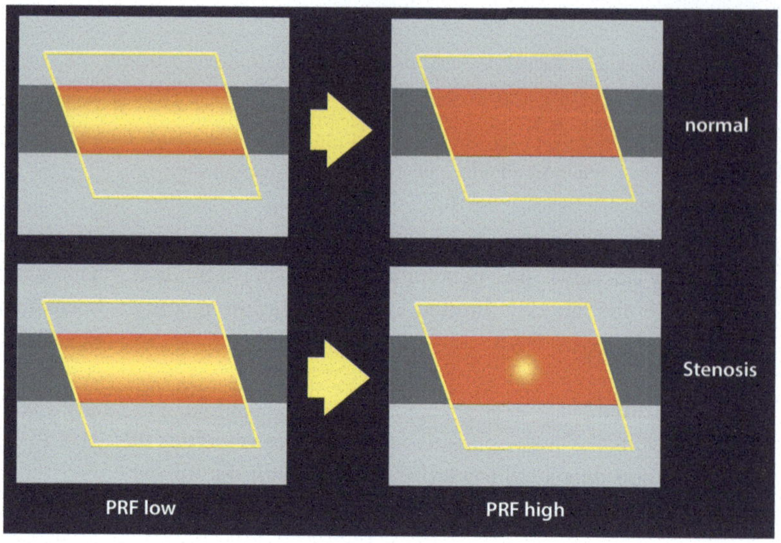

Fig. 6.13 Principle of optimized flow imaging by slowly increasing the PRF. In the case of a straight vessel, a band-like elongated aliasing only occurs in the centre of the vessel when PRF is low. If a circumscribed stenosis is present, this can be easily recognized by a localized aliasing effect in the stenosis area when PRF is increased

Part II

Investigation Techniques

Extracranial Doppler Sonography

7

Bernhard Widder and Gerhard F. Hamann

7.1 Indications

CW Doppler sonography with the "simple" pen probe is the oldest ultrasound method for detecting stenoses and occlusions of the arteries supplying the brain. Initially, only the ultrasound of the end branches of the ophthalmic artery was known as an "indirect" method. However, it was soon shown that carotid bifurcation, the branches leaving the aortic arch and the vertebral arteries could also be examined "directly." In view of color coded duplex sonography which is now widely used, CW Doppler sonography is still of significance for a few indications (see overview below).

Screening for Higher Grade Carotid Stenoses
CW Doppler sonography is a cost-effective and reliable screening method for detection or exclusion of higher grade stenoses of the extracranial internal carotid artery in symptomatic patients with hemiplegic symptoms, amaurosis fugax, aphasia and/or asymptomatic patients with auscultable bruits of the neck. Systolic maximum frequencies above 7–8 kHz indicate higher grade stenoses with high certainty. Errors occur only in the usually avoidable confusion with vascular processes of the external carotid artery (Sect. 13.4). Conversely, a high-grade stenosis can be reliably excluded if the transition from the common to the internal carotid artery is inconspicuously traceable. Last but not least, the Doppler sonographic determination of systolic maximum frequency is also suitable for monitoring the course of high-grade carotid stenosis in order not to overlook a possible progression.

Supplement to Color Coded Duplex Sonography
Despite of advanced duplex device technology, unclear situations in the area of carotid bifurcation, for example, with deep lying and/or strongly calcified vessels, cannot be excluded. In this case, the Doppler assessment of the end branches of the ophtalmic arteries ("periorbital arteries") represents an important additional criterion for sonographic carotid diagnostics (Sect. 7.3).

Detecting Subclavian Steal Effects
Together with the upper arm compression test, CW Doppler sonography is suitable for excluding or detecting a vertebro-vertebral overflow (subclavian steal effect) in the case of larger blood pressure differences in the arms. However, its practical significance is limited, since even in the case of a complete subclavian steal effect, typical clinical symptoms only rarely interferes with everyday life, which is the indication for an interventional procedure or a carotid-subclavian bypass. Moreover, experience has shown that these patients do not suffer from embolic brainstem infarctions, since emboli from a subclavian stenosis do not spread cranially due to the blood flow leading to the arm.

Indications for CW Doppler Sonography of the Extracranial Arteries Supplying the Brain

- Screening procedure to exclude and, if necessary, to monitor the progress of higher-grade stenoses of the extracranial internal carotid artery
- Complementary method to color coded duplex sonography by examining the periorbital arteries
- Clarification of a subclavian steal effect in the case of larger blood pressure differences in the arms.

In **acute stroke**, however, CW Doppler sonography does not possess any significance. The method is not reliable enough to draw immediate therapeutic consequences, and

B. Widder (✉)
Expert Opinion Institute, District Hospital, Guenzburg, Germany
e-mail: bernhard.widder@bkh-guenzburg.de

G. F. Hamann
Clinic of Neurology and Neurological Rehabilitation, District Hospital, Guenzburg, Germany

B. Widder, G. F. Hamann (eds.), *Duplex sonography of the brain-supplying arteries*, https://doi.org/10.1007/978-3-662-65566-5_7

thus only costs unnecessary time, which is needed for more important measures (Chap. 21). In addition, CW Doppler sonography of the **vertebral arteries** is considered obsolete. A sufficiently reliable assessment of the vertebral artery is not possible by Doppler sonography without knowledge of the diameter and the course of the vertebral arteries. Thus, the method is also dispensable for the clarification of vertigo. The only exception is the abovementioned proof or exclusion of a subclavian steal effect in the case of a corresponding clinical suspicion.

7.2 Technical Settings

The setting of CW Doppler devices is generally uncritical, as only a few parameters are relevant. In order to be able to work as quickly as possible, it is advisable to set the device in such a way that normally as few knobs or buttons as possible have to be operated during the examination procedure.

Flow Direction
The flow direction setting should be selected in such a way that it points upward in non-pathological cases (e.g., periorbital arteries toward the probe, carotid branches away from the probe).

Zero Line
If the direction of flow is fixed, it is advisable to leave the zero line also fixed in the middle of the screen. If the direction of flow is set to change, it seems more sensible to move the zero line to about 1/3 of the screen height.

Frequency Range
If the maximum displayable frequency is set to 4 kHz (in both directions of flow), this is sufficient in the non-pathological case to adequately display the frequency spectrum of all investigated neck vessels.

Power (Sound Transmission Energy)
It is recommended to set the maximum value as standard, since thermal stress is not to be expected in CW Doppler sonography.

Gain
The signal amplification is optimally adjusted if there are isolated artifact points outside of the displayed flows on the screen.

Sweep
The display speed should be set so that the compression maneuvers listed below can be recorded on the screen without the need to press any further keys (5–6 s/screen width).

7.3 Examination of the Periorbital Arteries

Although Doppler sonography of the end branches of the ophthalmic artery appears obsolete at first glance as a merely "indirect method", it is still important – even in combination with color coded duplex sonography. On the one hand, it increases the "redundancy" of the ultrasound examination and thus its reliability, and on the other hand, together with the assessment of the common carotid artery, it can at least provide rough information about the vascular situation in case of unclear conditions at the carotid bifurcation (Sect. 13.1.3). Finally, it indicates the localization of intracranial occlusive processes of the internal carotid artery before or after the ophthalmic artery.

7.3.1 Physiological Principles

The ophthalmic artery is the only branch of the internal carotid artery that leaves the skull. It runs outward on the medial side of the eye socket and gives off the ethmoidal artery medially and the supraorbital artery laterally. Via its end branch, the supratrochlear artery, it anastomosizes with branches of the external carotid artery (Fig. 1.5). Since the blood pressure at eye level in the internal carotid artery is normally significantly higher than in the thin branches of the external carotid artery, the branches of the ophthalmic artery are normally perfused from the inside to the outside (so-called **antegrade flow** in Doppler terminology). As a result, the medial, supraorbital part of the forehead skin is usually supplied with blood from the internal carotid artery.

If the pressure in the proximal internal carotid artery decreases due to a high-grade stenosis or occlusion, the flow in the ophthalmic artery and its end branches also decreases. When there is an equilibrium between the external and internal pressure, the anastomosis is not supplied with blood and represent a kind of watershed between the internal and external carotid arteries. If the pressure drop in the internal carotid artery is even greater, a retrograde flow from the outside to the inside can occur. In this case, the **ophthalmic collaterals** contributes to cerebral perfusion (Fig. 7.1).

7.3.2 Examination Procedure

Due to their better spatial resolution in the superficial area, a pencil probe with a nominal frequency of 8–10 MHz should preferably be used, but low-frequency probes of 4–5 MHz also lead to useful results.

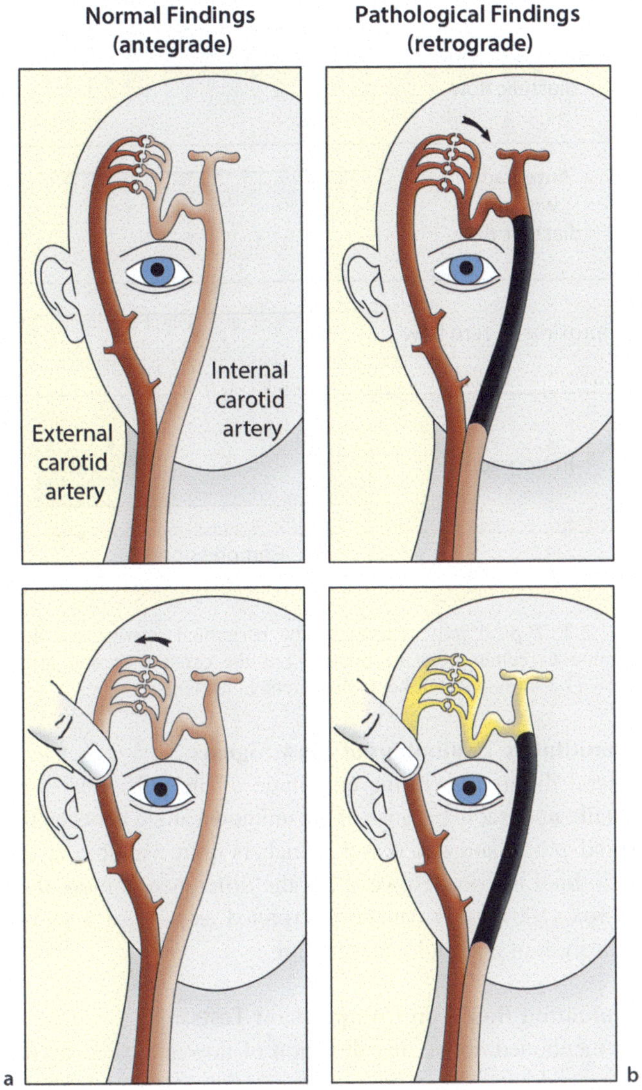

Fig. 7.1 (**a**, **b**) Schematic representation of the flow relation between internal and external carotid arteries with and without compression of external branches. Normal findings with antegrade flow (**a**), pathological findings with retrograde flow (**b**). Further explanations in the text

Doppler Examination

The largest branch of the ophthalmic artery, the supratrochlear artery, is examined by placing the Doppler probe without pressure in the medial corner of the eye in a slightly medial and parietal position (Fig. 7.2). Since the anatomical variations in the orbital cavity are very numerous, they are summarized as **periorbital arteries**.

> **Practical Tips**
> An optimal low contact pressure with the probe can be achieved by holding the probe cable with your hand instead of the probe. Irritation of the eyes by the usually formalin-containing ultrasound contact gel is avoided if the gel is not placed directly in the medial corner of the eye but slightly above it under the eyebrows.

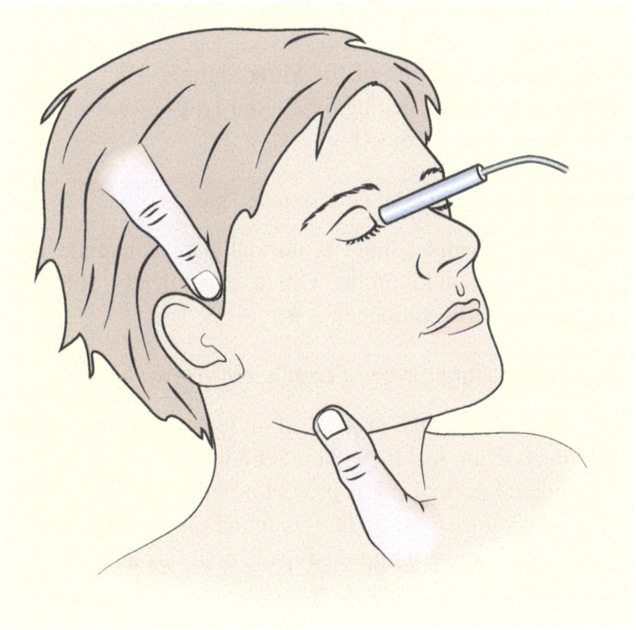

Fig. 7.2 Assessment of the periorbital arteries in the medial corner of the eye. Note the compression points of the superficial temporal and the facial artery

Under acoustic control, the angle and position of the probe are changed until a sufficient signal amplitude is reached. In individual cases it is possible that several vessels with different signals and – in pathological cases – also different flow directions are diverted. The signal with the most "pathological" finding is decisive for the assessment (Sect. 7.3.3).

Compression Maneuvers

Since the anatomical vascular conditions in the area of the medial angle of the eye are very variable and vascular loops are also common, the direction of flow indicated by the Doppler device cannot be considered reliable. Compression maneuvers should therefore be performed routinely to confirm the findings (Sect. 7.3.3).

> **Practical Tips**
> The main problem with compression maneuvers is to perform them without changing the transducer position. In case of doubt, it is advisable to apply compression at another point (e.g., in the area of the zygomatic arch) and to observe the reaction of the Doppler spectrum. A further possibility for error is if the vessel is not reliably compressed. Compression should therefore always be applied only when the vessel in question could be palpated.

7.3.3 Criteria for the Evaluation of Findings

Qualitative Evaluation of the Flow Signals

Doppler sonography distinguishes four types of pulse curves of the periorbital arteries (Fig. 7.3).

Antegrade Signal with Enddiastolic Flow

In healthy people, there is normally an antegrade flow toward the sound probe with a diastolically still well detectable flow component. ◀

Antegrade Signal Without Enddiastolic Flow

In the elderly and at cool skin temperature, a signal directed from inside without enddiastolic flow is also considered normal if it is present on both sides. However, if a detectable diastolic flow is found on the contralateral side, this is to be interpreted ipsilaterally as an indication of a pathological process. ◀

(Approximate) Zero Flow

Almost always pathological is a complete or approximate blood stasis in the periorbital arteries, which is secured by compression tests and confirms a pressure equilibrium between the outside and the inside. ◀

Practical Tips

To distinguish a suspected zero flow from an examination artifact, it is recommended to search for a flow signal from the periorbital arteries during continuous compression of external branches. If such a signal is found, it will typically (largely) disappear in pathological cases when the compression is released.

Retrograde Signal

A retrograde flow away from the sound probe is also regarded as pathological and indicates a high-grade flow obstruction or occlusion in the underlying internal carotid artery. ◀

Practical Tips

Since the periorbital arteries only reflect the pressure equilibrium between the external and internal carotid arteries, it is not possible to distinguish whether there ist an ipsilateral flow obstruction in the ipsilateral internal carotid artery or in the contralateral external carotid artery leading to an increased antegrade blood flow in the periorbital arteries in the latter case. Therefore, the palpation of the superficial temporal artery may be helpful in order to exclude an external carotid artery obstruction.

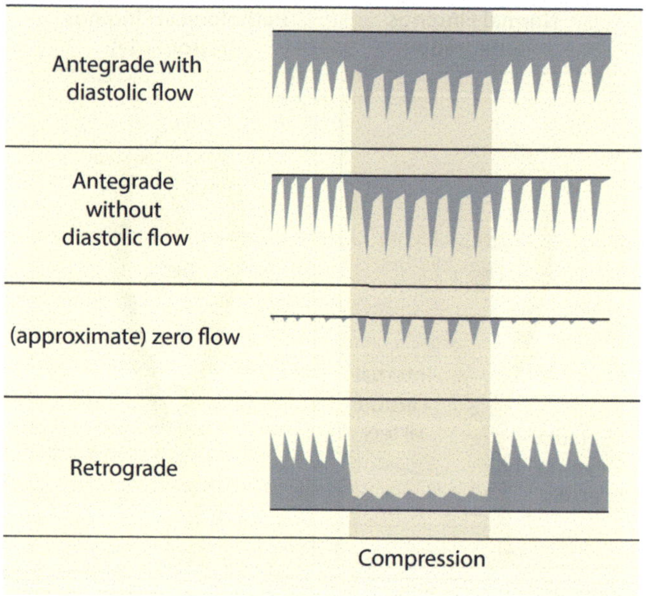

Fig. 7.3 Typical pulse curves of the periorbital arteries and their reaction to compression of branches of the external carotid artery (brown background). Further explanations in the text

Quantitative Evaluation of Flow Signals

Lateral differences in the amplitude of the pulse curve are usually not usable because of the unknown angle between the sound probe and the vessel, which is quite variable at the periorbital arteries. However, if the difference is more than approx. 100%, this can be interpreted as at least a strong indication of a pathological finding.

Evaluation Based on Compression Tests

As mentioned above, the direction of flow indicated by the Doppler device cannot be considered of an ante- or retrograde flow without any doubt. This proof can only be provided by short-term compression maneuvers in which the internal-external pressure equilibrium is artificially reduced on the side of the external carotid artery. Here, a distinction must be made between two basic reactions (Fig. 7.3).

Increase in Flow

An increase in the flow velocity when compressing the superficial temporal and/or facial artery proves an antegrade flow, because when the counterpressure in the external carotid artery is reduced, the pressure difference and thus the flow velocity directed from the inside to the outside increases. ◀

Decrease in Flow

A reduction in the flow velocity or even a change in the other direction of flow prove a retrograde flow in the sense of an ophthalmic collateral flow, which runs over branches of the external carotid artery through the eye to the internal carotid artery. ◀

Procedure in the Absence of Compression Effect
If neither compression of the superficial temporal artery nor the facial artery shows a usable flow effect, no reliable statement can be made about the direction of flow. In this case, two possibilities should be considered for differential diagnosis:

- There is no pathological situation, since there are no significant anastomoses between the compressible external branches and the ophthalmic artery due to the anatomical conditions.
- A pathological situation is present in which the ophthalmic artery is supplied retrogradely via the maxillary artery, which is not compressible from the outside and also may contribute to cerebral collateral supply.

For differentiation, flat compression of the medial, supraorbital forehead region, which in non-pathological cases is supplied by the internal carotid artery, helps further. If this region is compressed with several fingers, the physiological flow velocity in the supplying periorbital arteries drops significantly. If, on the other hand, the ipsilateral internal carotid artery is occluded by an ophthalmic collateral via the maxillary artery, the forehead is not supplied via the ophthalmic artery in view of the existing cerebral blood requirement, so that no (noteworthy) reaction to the compression maneuver can be detected.

Background Information
A relatively rare case of ophthalmic collaterals is an anastomosis running across the bridge of the nose between the periorbital arteries on both sides. It can occur in hypoplastic anterior communicating artery. The decrease in the flow velocity in both periorbital vessels during compression of the nasal dorsal artery proves such an "extracranial communicating artery".

7.3.4 Possible Errors

False Negative Findings
Indirect assessment of the periorbital arteries fails if, in addition to a higher degree of stenosis of the internal carotid artery, there is also a stenosis of the external carotid artery. In this case, the pressure gradient between the internal and external arteries may be normal again. The same applies to stenoses and occlusions of the common carotid artery, which, as expected, do not influence the pressure gradient.

In rare cases, Doppler drainage of the periorbital arteries in the corner of the eye can lead to confusing results if a reliably antegrade flow signal is present at one site and a demonstrably retrograde flow signal at another site. This is due to the anatomical variations already mentioned above. Different flow directions can be explained by the fact that sometimes not all of these branches anastomose with the external carotid artery. For the Doppler sonographic assessment, the derived vascular branch with the most "pathological" findings is decisive.

False-Positive Findings
A retrograde signal can be faked if the flow velocity in the periorbital arteries appears to decrease due to moving the probe position during compression. Typically, however, in this case there is a continuous reduction of the pulse curve amplitude and a continuous increase after the end of compression. In contrast, in the case of an actual retrograde flow, it is to be expected that both the flow decrease and increase will occur abruptly (Fig. 7.4).

Summary
Doppler sonographic examination of the periorbital arteries (especially the supratrochlear artery) provides important information about the presence of flow obstructions in the ipsilateral internal carotid artery. If the vessel, which normally is perfused from the inside to the outside, shows a retrograde flow, this can be considered pathological. The same applies to a significantly increased pulsatility compared to both sides. The direction of flow in the periorbital arteries must be secured in each case by compression tests of the palpable branches of the external carotid artery and the skin of the forehead.

7.4 Examination of the Carotid Bifurcation

7.4.1 Sound Distribution Levels

The insonation of the carotid bifurcation at the neck can be performed in three different planes, each with a different transducer position:

- **Anterior position** from the front with the probe inserted between the sternocleidomastoid muscle and the larynx.
- **Lateral position** from the side with the probe vertically positioned on the sternocleidomastoid muscle. The ultrasound passes through the muscle. The head position is straight and slightly reclined in order to keep the muscle as flat as possible.
- **Posterior position** from the back with a sound probe behind the sternocleidomastoid muscle and radiating forward. The head is slightly turned to the opposite side.

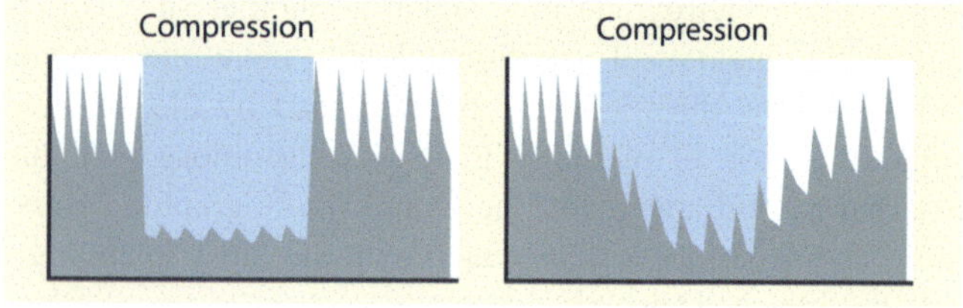

Fig. 7.4 Retrograde flow in the supratrochlear artery with abrupt change in flow velocity at the beginning and end of compression (left) and artifact due to change of probe position during compression of external branches (right)

Since the branches of the carotid bifurcation often lie in one plane behind each other and therefore cannot be reliably differentiated, the most favorable plane must be determined by trial in each individual case.

7.4.2 Examination Procedure

Carotid Artery

The examination using a 4 to 5 MHz probe begins with the derivation of the common carotid artery as far as possible proximally with the probe directed 50–60° cranially. An angle that is too steeply directed toward the cranial makes little sense, since in this case the penetration depth is no longer sufficient, especially in obese patients (Fig. 7.5).

The common carotid artery is the easiest to identify, since no other major arterial vessels run in the lower third of the neck.

Practical Tips

If the Doppler probe is placed flat on the upper thoracic aperture, side comparison examinations of the common carotid artery can be performed, since the angle of incidence is largely identical in this case.

Differentiation of the Carotid Branches

The common carotid artery can now be followed cranially to its two branches, the internal and external carotid artery. The internal carotid artery is usually best found when the sound probe is positioned about 2 cm below the jaw angle. The external carotid artery can usually be reached by slowly moving the probe frontal in direction of the chin.

The differentiation of the two vascular branches can be performed with varying degrees of reliability according to three methods.

Location

The internal carotid artery is usually located dorsally to the external carotid artery. In about 10% of cases, however, the vessels overlap, and rarely does the internal carotid artery also run frontally to the external carotid artery (Fig. 1.6). ◀

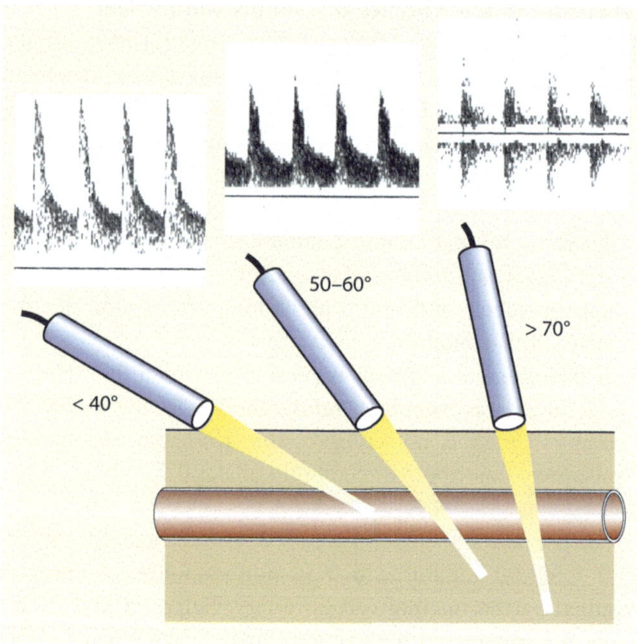

Fig. 7.5 Doppler spectra at different sound probe positions. If the probe is too steeply directed cranially, the vessel lies outside the sensible penetration depth of the ultrasound beam (left); optimum probe position with an angle of 50–60° between the sound beam and the vessel (center); too vertical position with resulting mirror artifacts and an only marginal flow curve (right)

Pulsatility

At least in the non-pathological case the vessels can be identified by their different pulsatility (Fig. 7.6). In the pathological case, however, variable findings can occur in both vascular branches. ◀

Compression Maneuvers

In case of doubt, oscillating compression of the superficial temporal artery is helpful, which – even when using duplex sonography – is the only reliable criterion for the external carotid artery. During this oscillating compression (preferably with only one finger), the simultaneously derived pulse curve of the external carotid artery shows a kind of rebound effect, which becomes clear both acoustically in the loudspeaker and by observing the curve on the monitor (Fig. 7.7). ◀

Practical Tips

In order to ensure that the rebound effect is not caused by movement of the head but actually by short-term

(continued)

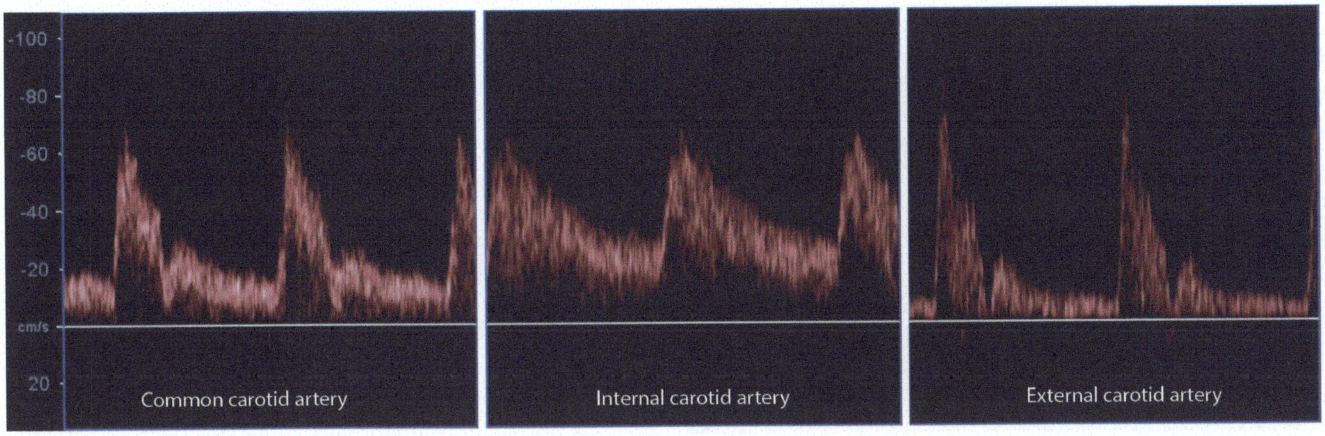

Fig. 7.6 Typical pulse curves of the carotid branches. High end diastolic flow (acoustic: soft, full-sounding signal) in the internal carotid artery, low end diastolic flow in the external carotid artery (acoustic: sharp, whipping signal), common carotid artery as a "mixture" of both signals

compression of the temporalis superficialis, it is recommended to apply oscillating compression to the adjacent zygomatic bone as a "crosscheck." If the effect in the Doppler signal is maintained, a movement artifact is present.

Examination Procedure

Since stenoses are most frequently found directly in the area of the carotid bifurcation, the initial sections of the internal and external carotid arteries are particularly important. Continuous tracking of the common carotid artery into the internal carotid artery by slowly moving the Doppler probe cranially with a sufficient amount of ultrasound gel has proven to be the most reliable method. The probe guide is flexibly adapted to the course of the vessel by slightly swinging it back and forth and the vessel is followed cranially as far as possible (Fig. 7.8).

7.4.3 Diagnostic Criteria

Systolic Maximum Frequency

As already explained in the previous Sect. 5.2.2, the Doppler sonographic assessment is based primarily on the evaluation of the maximum systolic frequency. In all three vessel sections of the carotid artery, the site with the highest occurring maximum systolic frequency in the Doppler spectrum must therefore be located and documented accordingly. In the case of a conspicuous maximum frequency (>4 kHz at 4–5 MHz transmission frequency), an attempt should always be made to derive the vessel again as far as possible cranially from the suspected stenosis in order to obtain information about the post-stenotic signal.

Further Flow Criteria

In addition, flow disturbances (Sect. 5.2.3) as well as the pulsatility (Sect. 5.2.4) should be recorded. In particular, the comparison of both sides should be taken into account.

Fig. 7.7 Rebound effect on the pulse curve of the external carotid artery during oscillating compression of the superficial temporal artery

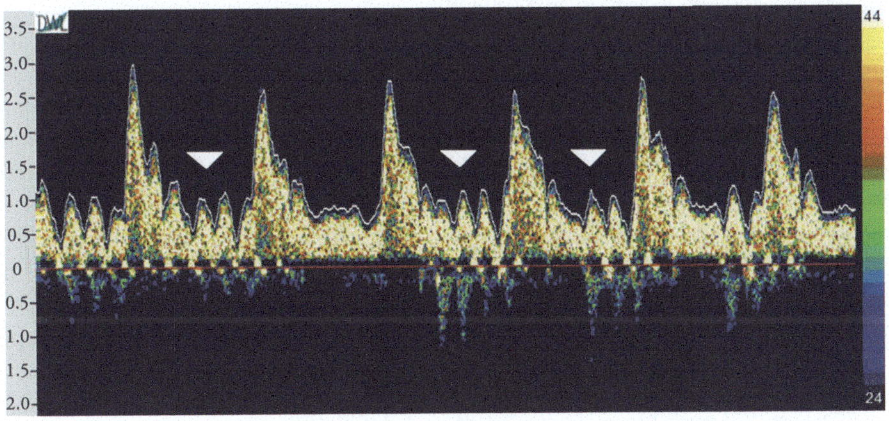

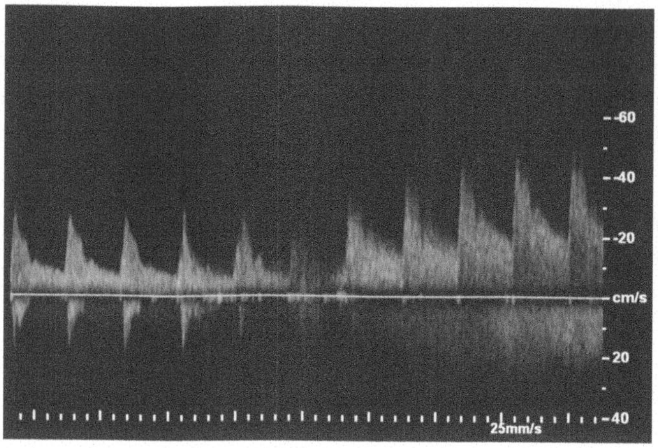

Fig. 7.8 Continuous assessment of the common carotid artery up to the internal carotid artery by slowly moving the Doppler probe. Notice the typical drop in Doppler frequencies in the carotid bulb

7.4.4 Possible Errors

The three most important sources of error result from the given technical limitations of CW Doppler sonography.

No Knowledge of the Insonation Angle
Since the angle between the sound beam and the vessel is not known, all kinds of curved vessel courses can lead to misinterpretations: For example, a vessel running medially results in increased Doppler frequencies and thus in the false-positive findings of a stenosis. In contrast, a vessel that runs laterally causes a moderate stenosis to be overlooked. The accuracy of the method is therefore limited to high-grade stenoses if the systolic maximum frequency exceeds 7–8 kHz and/or pronounced flow disturbances are recognizable.

No Knowledge of the Vessel Course
Since the Doppler examination ist performed without additional imaging, irregular vascular courses complicate the assessment and can lead to misinterpretations.

No Depth Information
Vessels overlapping in the direction of sound cannot be distinguished from each other by CW Doppler sonography. If the external carotid artery lies medially and covers the internal carotid artery, the latter can be misinterpreted as occluded or a stenosis can be overlooked.

Summary
The carotid bifurcation can be insonated with the CW Doppler probe in three planes (from the front, from the side and from behind). The most favorable examination position must be determined by trial and error. The internal carotid artery is usually located dorsally to the external carotid artery and normally shows a significantly lower pulsatility than the external carotid artery. A reliable differentiation of the two vessels can be achieved by means of the "rebound effect" in the external carotid artery by oscillated compression of the superficial temporal artery.

7.5 Examination of the Vertebral Artery

Although the Doppler sonographic recording of the vertebral artery is no longer of importance in the diagnosis of cerebrovascular disorders (Sect. 7.1), the examination technique is described briefly below.

7.5.1 Examination Procedure

With the CW Doppler probe, the vertebral artery can be detected both in the area of ist origin and the atlas loop (Fig. 7.9).

Origin
The examination is performed with a medially and caudally directed Doppler probe approx. two transverse fingers above the clavicle. The vertebral artery can be distinguished from other vessels by the fact that oscillating compression of the atlas loop results in a similar rebound effect as described above for the external carotid artery (Fig. 7.10).

Atlas Loop
In order to assess the atlas loop, the head is turned slightly to the opposite side and the Doppler probe points approximately in the direction of the contralateral zygomatic arch. Due to the close proximity, confusion with the internal carotid artery or the occipital artery must be excluded:

- The **internal carotid artery** has the same signal character as the vertebral artery, but usually has slightly higher Doppler frequencies. Typically, it can be followed proximally, which is not the case with the vertebral artery.
- The **occipital artery** has a much higher pulsatility than the vertebral artery. In addition, its pulse curve decreases or even disappears by digital compression of the occipital scale above the mastoid.

Upper Arm Compression Test
In case of different radial pulse and/or supraclavicular bruits, the so-called upper arm compression test can be performed while simultaneously recording the vertebral artery in the area of the atlas loop. It serves to assess the influence of subclavian artery stenoses and occlusions on the blood flow in the vertebral artery. This concerns in particular the proof of

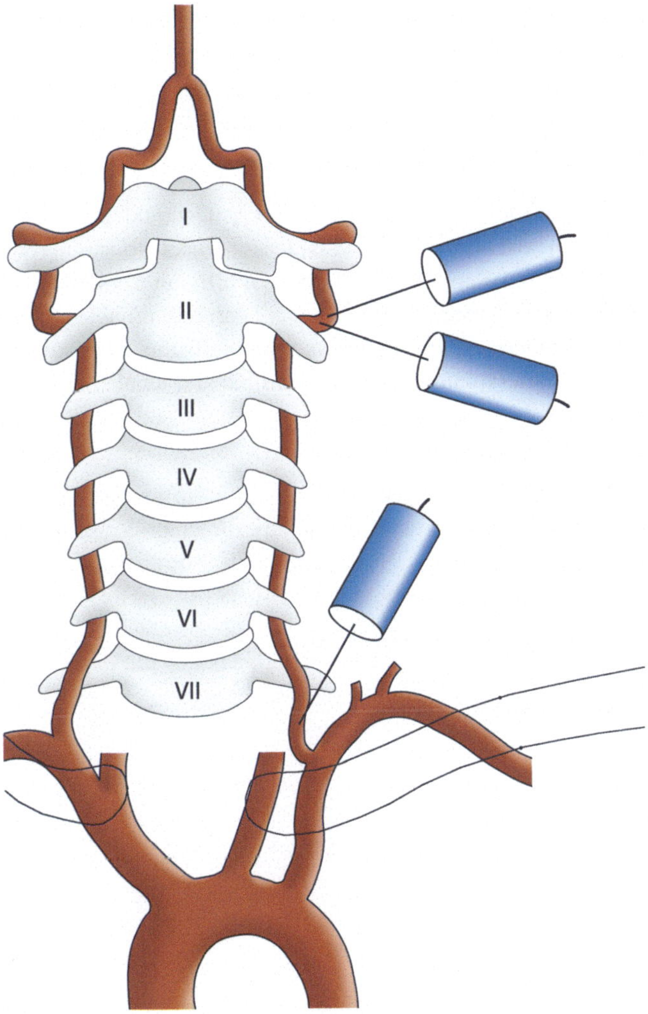

Fig. 7.9 Doppler sonographic examination positions for the assessment of the vertebral artery in the area of the atlas loop and at ist origin

a so-called vertebro-vertebral overflow or **subclavian steal effect** with retrograde flow in the ipsilateral vertebral artery. Since the direction of flow in the vertebral artery cannot be clearly defined by CW Doppler sonography either at the atlas loop or at its origin due to the numerous possible course variations, this is done on the basis of the reaction in the upper arm compression test.

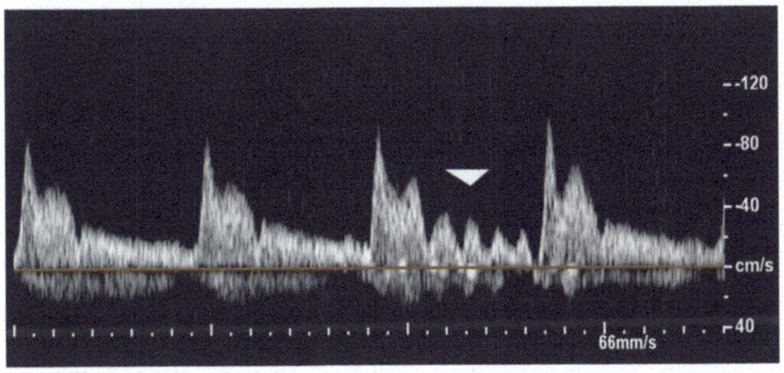

Fig. 7.10 Doppler spectrum of the vertebral artery when assessed at its origin from the subclavian artery. The reboud effect by oscillated compression of the vertebral artery in the area of the atlas loop helps to differentiate it from other vessels in this area

For this purpose, the affected upper arm is oversystolically compressed with the blood pressure cuff for approx. 20 s. The resulting ischemia leads to a dilatation of the arm vessels and, accordingly, to an increased blood demand in the arm when the cuff pressure is released quickly. The reaction is observed in the Doppler curve of the ipsilateral vertebral artery. If a proximal obstruction of flow is found in the subclavian artery, an increase in pathological phenomena in the vertebral artery occurs during the reactive phase of hyperemia. For further details see Sect. 15.1.3.

7.5.2 Diagnostic Criteria

Without knowledge of the vessel diameter, the possibilities of assessing the Doppler signal of the vertebral artery are very limited. The assessment of signal strength as a measure of vessel diameter, which was previously used in the absence of color coded duplex sonography, appears obsolete. Thus, CW Doppler sonography of the vertebral artery is limited to the reaction in the upper arm compression test.

Summary
The vertebral artery can be derived by Doppler sonography in the area of the atlas loop as well as at its origin with a caudally directed probe. Since no information on the vessel diameter is possible, the procedure is only of some significance in conjunction with the upper arm compression test in clarifying a subclavian steal effect.

7.6 Examination of the Subclavian Artery

The diagnostic significance of Doppler sonography of the subclavian artery is significantly lower than that of clinical examination with auscultation and side-comparison radial pulse palpation or blood pressure measurement. However, since duplex sonography often fails in this area, the "simple" Doppler examination is important in individual cases for clarifying diseases in this vessel.

7.6.1 Examination Procedure

The probe position for the examination of the subclavian artery is the same as for the assessment of the origin of the vertebral artery. As a skin- and muscle-supplying vessel, the subclavian artery typically shows high pulsatility with an early diastolic backflow (Sect. 2.5), which makes it easy to detect in non-pathological cases. In pathological cases the curve may be deformed. In this case it is recommended to examine the vessel on the basis of the already known **rebound effect** during oscillating compression of the brachial artery.

Differentiation between the proximal and distal leg of the subclavian artery is possible on the basis of the direction of the pulse curve. If the flow is in the direction of the probe, it is probably the proximal section of the vessel before the vertebral artery branches off. In the distal section of the vessel, on the other hand, a flow directed away from the probe can be obtained.

7.6.2 Diagnostic Criteria

Due to frequent overlaps and the unknown angle between the ultrasound beam and the vessel, the systolic maximum frequency as well as the shape of the pulse curve is of little importance. The findings of flow disturbances are therefore the most important criterion. If these – correlating to auscultation findings – are present in a pronounced form and can be clearly assigned to the subclavian artery, a subclavian artery stenosis can be considered certain.

7.6.3 Possible Errors

When deriving the subclavian artery, it should always be borne in mind that the vessel is subject to numerous variations in its course, which make it difficult to distinguish between the "proximal" and "distal" parts. A reliable differentiation therefore only appears possible if the origin of the vertebral artery can be clearly identified and localized.

Summary
The subclavian artery can be assessed in its proximal and distal section with a caudally directed ultrasound probe. The flow curve normally shows a high pulsatility with early diastolic backflow. The most important diagnostic criterion is the occurrence of pronounced flow disturbances, which ensures the diagnosis of a subclavian artery stenosis.

8 Extracranial Duplex Sonography

Bernhard Widder and Gerhard F. Hamann

8.1 Indications

> **Practical Tips**
> The examination of the extra- (and intracranial) cerebral vessels is best carried out in a semi-recumbent position of the patient with slightly overextended head. According to the experience of the authors, examination chairs that fold backward have proven to be the best for this purpose, as they are used, for example, for electroencephalogram (EEG) recordings or for the transport of handicapped, non-bed-ridden patients in the clinic ("seat trolley"). When purchasing such a chair, care should be taken to ensure that the head section can be folded away to allow trans-nuchal examinations. Sitting behind the patient's head has proven to be the best position for the examiner. Sitting next to the patient leads to a considerably cramped examination posture for a long time.

Duplex sonography – if necessary together with MRA and CTA – is the method of choice for individual assessment of the indication and risk of vascular surgery and interventional procedures on the supra-aortic arteries (following overview). If the sectional image of the carotid artery shows multiple arteriosclerotic changes extending into the aortic arch, the benefit of such an intervention will have to be estimated more critically than in the case of a circumscribed stenosis at the origin of the internal carotid artery. Particularly in the case of low and moderate stenoses, statements on the stenosis morphology are often possible. However, the reliability of the method in detecting morphological features such as ulcerations is unsatisfactory.

> **Indications for Extracranial Duplex Examination**
> - Further clarification of abnormal Doppler sonographic findings
> - Clarification of therapeutic consequences in carotid artery stenoses and occlusions (extension of arteriosclerotic changes, morphology)
> - Contribution to the differential diagnosis in transient and permanent cerebral ischemia
> - Assessment of circulatory disorders in the vertebrobasilar system
> - Clarification of pulsating neck tumors
> - Exclusion of extracranial vasculitis
> - Controls after reconstructive surgery of the carotid artery.

Duplex sonography is also the method of choice for the clarification of pulsating neck tumors, and the same applies to the exclusion of extracranial vasculitis. At least once duplex sonographic examination should applied after surgical or interventional procedures on the brain-supplying arteries.

8.2 Device Settings

> **Practical Tips**
> Ultrasonic probes are subject to premature aging if they are not switched off when not in use and "run dry." Since in this case they cannot transfer their sound

(continued)

B. Widder (✉)
Expert Opinion Institute, District Hospital, Guenzburg, Germany
e-mail: bernhard.widder@bkh-guenzburg.de

G. F. Hamann
Clinic of Neurology and Neurological Rehabilitation, District Hospital, Guenzburg, Germany

B. Widder, G. F. Hamann (eds.), *Duplex sonography of the brain-supplying arteries*, https://doi.org/10.1007/978-3-662-65566-5_8

energy to tissue, heating of the transducer and the adhesive layers inside the transducer, which are essential for sound transmission, occurs. Between the individual examinations the sound probes should therefore always be switched off by “freezing” the image. Although it is technically easy to switch off the sound probe automatically when not in use, this is not established in most devices.

8.2.1 Ultrasound Transducers

For the examination of the extracranial brain-supplying arteries, **Linear array transducers** with a transmission frequency of 5–10 MHz ar best suited. The image width of 3–4 cm is ideal for displaying the cervical vessels in a longitudinal section over a sufficiently long distance.

In obese patients with vessels deep in the tissue, abdominal **Curved-array transducers** (also known as convex transducers) with transmission frequencies around 3.5 MHz may be used. In the case of multi-frequency transducers, the transmission frequency should be set as high as possible to improve the otherwise poor resolution (see Sect. 3.3.2). Such transducers also have advantages in assessing the distal course of the internal carotid artery, which can be regularly followed cranially by another 2–3 cm compared to the linear probe.

8.2.2 B-mode Imaging

Apart from the ultrasound transmission frequency, there are only few parameters to consider when setting the gray-scale B-mode imaging (Fig. 8.1).

Display Depth

As standard, a display depth of 3–4 cm has proven to be a good choice. This means that all relevant structures can be depicted for most patients. Only in individual cases, for example, in slender patients or for imaging the superficial temporal artery, shorter imaging depths appear to be useful. Also only in individual cases, especially for imaging deep-lying vertebral arteries, an imaging depth of 5 cm must be selected.

Focus Points

Due to the existing dynamic focusing of the device, one or more focus points can be set at variable depths. For the visualization of carotid and vertebral arteries, it is generally sufficient to use one focus point at a depth of 2–2.5 cm.

Time Gain Compensation (TGC)

The runtime-dependent gain (Fig. 3.8) must be set so that even deeper structures are still clearly displayed, while the intensity in the area close to the transducer must usually be reduced. Depending on the device used, an S-shaped curve of the gain control must be set manually, whereby experience shows that the start of the rise is at a depth of approx. 1 cm, the end at 2–3 cm (Fig. 8.2). With other devices this is already fixed in the so-called **preset** so that a further setting of the gain controls is not necessary.

B-mode Gain

In order not to overlook low-echo structures, the overall amplification of the B-mode display should be selected in such a way that the (unstenosed) vessel lumen does not appear completely echo-free, but that isolated “echo points” are visible in it.

Image Processing

Depending on the manufacturer, numerous image processing parameters such as dynamics, contrast, contour enhancement, persistence as well as various gray curves can be selected in almost any combination. Fixed rules for setting the **Pre-** and **Postprocessing** cannot be specified, and the most appealing image must be determined by trial and error.

8.2.3 Color Coded Imaging

Power

The signal amplification is usually set to the maximum. Due to the good blood circulation of the soft tissue in the neck, thermal problems are not to be feared. A slight warming at the interface to the cervical spine is possible, but practically without significance. Since these structures are located relatively deep in the tissue, a pronounced weakening of sound energy (power) has already occurred by passing the tissue until the cervical spine is reached.

Display Modes

At the start of the examination, the use of the **Velocity mode** useful for quick orientation ist recommended. If required, the user can then – especially for documentation puposes – switch to the **Power mode** or – if available – to **B-flow technology**.

Size of the Color Window

A color window width of 2–2.5 cm appears to be necessary in order to display the neck vessels in longitudinal section in color coded form over a sufficient length (Fig. 8.3). Only then is it possible to determine the angle-corrected flow velocity (Sect. 5.3.2). The depth of the color window should also be in the same order of magnitude so that it does not have to be

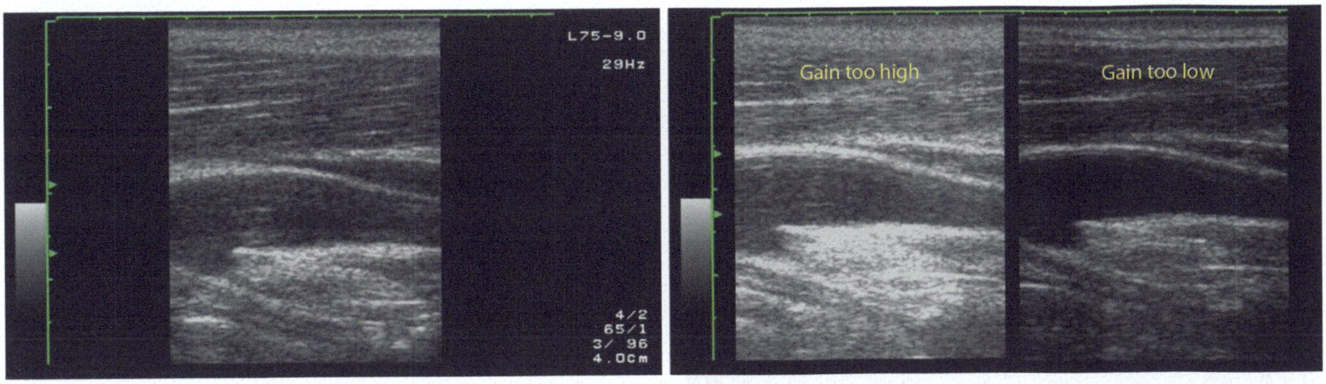

Fig. 8.1 "Standard settings" for B-mode imaging of the extracranial arteries with a display depth of 4 cm and focus zones at 2–3 cm depth. Correct setting of the gain with individual "echo points" in the vessel lumen (left); gain set too high/too low (right)

moved continuously during the examination. However, these requirements reach their limits, especially with low-cost devices, when either the frame rate drops below 6–7 Hz, which considerably worsens the examination conditions (see Sect. 6.2.4), or the scan line density must be reduced to such an extent that ultimately no meaningful color coded imaging is possible. A compromise will have to be made here.

Tilting the Color Window

Although a maximum tilting of the color window seems to make sense as a standard for theoretical considerations, in order to realize the smallest possible angle between the "virtual" sound beams in the color window and the vessels insonated. However, as already shown in Fig. 6.12, this also increases the transit time of the ultrasound with a resulting reduction in penetration depth. Correspondingly, only a slight tilting with an angle of 10–15° appears to be reasonable as standard.

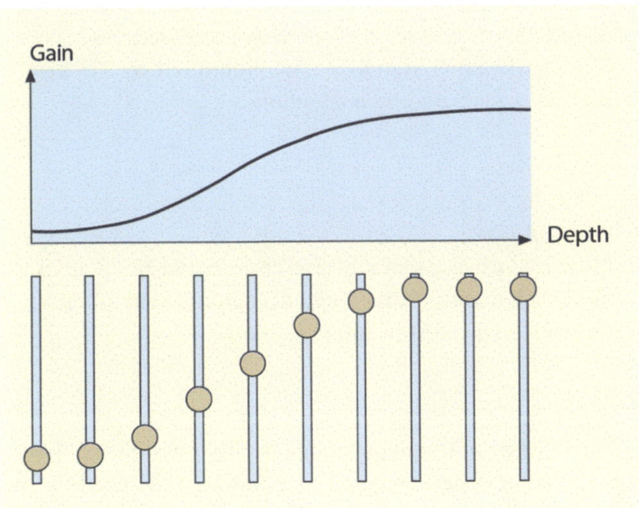

Fig. 8.2 S-shaped adjustment of time gain compensation (TGC) for imaging of superficial vessels, only required for some types of devices

The question of whether the color window should be tilted to the right or left cannot be answered in general. The tilting direction depends mainly on whether the course of the vessels runs from caudal to cranial on the screen or vice versa. Although there have been repeated attempts in the past to define this in a standardized way, this has not been accepted. In the opinion of the authors, this also represents overregulation, and every examiner should be free to choose the screen orientation depending on the position of the ultrasound device by the patient.

Color Gain

In order to achieve the most complete "color filling" of vessels, the color gain should be set so high that individual color dots are still visible in the surrounding soft tissue (Fig. 6.11).

> **Note**
> The presence of individual color dots in the soft tissue serves on image documentation as proof that the color gain of the duplex device was set sufficiently high in the examined vessel.

Color and B-mode Balance

By default, the balance should be set strongly to a predominance of color coding. Otherwise, the vessel will not be sufficiently filled with color (Fig. 6.11). It should be noted, however, that this can cause the edges of the vessel to be "overfilled" with color, which must be taken into account when determining the vessel diameter using the color coded image.

Aliasing Threshold

In the first step of each examination, the vessels to be examined must be located. For this purpose the sensitivity of the

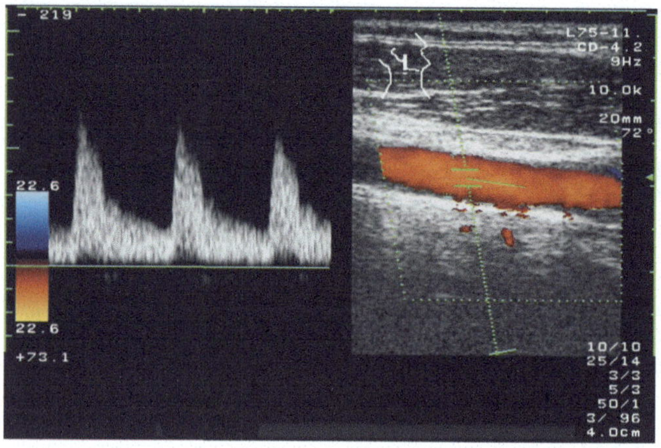

Fig. 8.3 "Standard settings" for color coded imaging of the extracranial arteries. Color coded image: Color window tilted 10–15° cranially, alias threshold ±20–25 cm/s. Also note the individual color dots in the tissue not perfused as an indication of a sufficiently adjusted gain. Doppler spectrum: angle between sound beam and vessels at 50–70°, sample volume approx. 3 mm, adjusted angle correction. Flow away from the sound beam runs upward

color coded flow detection must be high. Accordingly, the aliasing threshold should initially be set to approx. ±20 cm/s. An even lower aliasing threshold does not seem to be helpful because of increasing artifacts. Maximum low aliasing thresholds are generally only useful when differentiating vascular occlusions (see Sect. 13.3.1).

Wall Filter

With regard to the wall filter a compromise must be found between a setting as low as possible in order to still be able to display slow flows, and an artifact sensitivity that is not too high. If the wall filter is not already coupled to the aliasing threshold of the unit, which is the case with some units, a value in the order of 100 Hz is recommended.

8.2.4 Doppler Spectrum

For most parameters of the Doppler spectrum, the rules already described for extracranial CW Doppler sonography apply. However, the use of Doppler sonography "within" the color coded vessel imaging needs some further considerations.

Doppler Sound Beam

In most devices, the Doppler sound beam is coupled to the tilting of the color window, so that there is no possibility of specific presetting. If the color window and the Doppler beam can be controlled separately, an angle of 20–30° should be set as standard in order to detect vessels running horizontally across the screen with an insonation angle of less than 70°.

Sample Volume

The smaller the sample volume selected for Doppler recording, the more accurate the measurement, but the lower the reflected ultrasound energy (Fig. 5.15) and the more susceptible the recording is to patient movements. A sample volume of 3–4 mm, which is slightly less than the "normal" diameter of the internal carotid artery, should be regarded as a sensible compromise.

> **Practical Tips**
> In individual cases, a large sample volume has the advantage that the duplex transducer can be "used" as a Doppler probe. This is of interest, for example, if it is not possible to assign a pathological finding previously found with the CW Doppler probe by duplex imaging (e.g., retroauricular arteriovenous fistula). In this case, "blind" searching with a large sample volume until the vessels of interest are found again is helpful.

Frequency Range

Particularly in the **Triplex mode**, that is, the combined "online" display of color coded image and Doppler spectrum, only very low Doppler frequencies can be displayed without occurrence of aliasing phenomena. This is due to the fact that, while the frame repetition rate of the color coded display is still acceptable, there is simply not enough time to provide a sufficiently high PRF for the Doppler spectrum.

> **Practical Tips**
> In order to at least slightly increase the displayed frequency range, it is recommended in duplex sonography to always shift the zero line from the center (Fig. 5.31). Also the "quality" of the Doppler spectrum is not very satisfactory in "triplex mode." This means that flow disturbances cannot be correctly assessed and the acoustic Doppler signal sounds is muffled by the low PRF as if mediated by a telephone.

> **Practical Tips**
> Flow disturbances should not be assessed in "Triplex mode," but only with "frozen" color coded images, otherwise false results are possible.

An increase in frequency range is only possible by "freezing" the color coded image. This eliminates the need for the repeated build-up of the time-consuming color coded flow image, and the computer time is available for detecting Doppler signals.

Additional Information

With a "frozen" color image, the maximum displayed frequency can also be further increased by increasing the PRF of the device, so that even high flow speeds can be displayed and, above all, can be measured without aliasing. However, with increasing increase in frequency range, the depth of blood flow detecting is decreasing. In most devices this is evident from the fact that a mark on the Doppler sound beam moves upward toward the sample volume. The increase of the frequency range comes to its natural end when the sample volume shown on the screen is reached.

Recommended "default settings" of the Duplex Device for the Examination of Extracranial brain Arteries

1. Traansducer
   - Linear-array transducer
   - Nominal frequency 5–7.5 MHz
2. B-mode imaging
   - Display depth 4 cm
   - Focus range 2–2.5 cm
   - B-mode gain as high as necessary with single artifact points in the vessel lumen
3. Color coded imaging
   - Power set to the maximum
   - Color window 2–2.5 cm wide and high
   - Scan line density adapted to a frame rate of at least 6 Hz
   - Tilting of the color window cranially by 10–15°
   - Aliasing threshold at approx. ±20 cm/s
   - Wall filter approx. 100 Hz
   - Color gain increased until single artifact points are visible in the non-perfused tissue
   - Color and B-mode balance "color lasting"
4. Doppler spectrum
   - Doppler beam (if not coupled to color window) tilted to 20–30° cranially
   - Sample volume 3–4 mm

8.3 Examination of the Carotid Bifurcation

The duplex sonographic examination of the carotid bifurcation is of course always carried out in combination of B-mode imaging, color coded vessel imaging and Doppler spectrum analysis. For didactic reasons, the individual procedures are presented separately in the following.

8.3.1 Diagnostic Sections

Longitudinal Section

Analogous to the probe positions mentioned for extracranial Doppler sonography (Sect. 7.4.1), longitudinal sections through the carotid bifurcation can be made from the front, lateral and dorsal plane. The most favorable position in each case must be determined by trial and error.

Transversal Section

As a further examination criterion, B-mode and color coded imaging with the probe held transversely to the neck and tilted slightly cranially or caudally can be used (Fig. 8.4). Transversal images are also particularly suitable for taking a look at the surrounding structures of the neck. Directly next to the common carotid artery, the **internal jugular vein** is found. In addition to its flow direction from cranial to caudal, it is usually easy to recognize because, in contrast to the common carotid artery, it does not have a circular shape, no delimitable vascular walls, and can be compressed with the ultrasound probe. In case of doubt, a Valsalva maneuver can also be used in which the jugular vein regularly "inflates." Other structures shown are the thyroid gland and possibly also lymph nodes, which are round or oval and normally low echogenic.

8.3.2 Examination Procedure

Carotid Bifurcation in Longitudinal Section

The examination begins with a longitudinal section of the common carotid artery. The vessel should be followed as far proximally as possible in order not to overlook any vascular changes present here. Since the common carotid artery can generally be reliably displayed in B-mode imaging and the intima-media thickness in particular can be assessed here (Sect. 8.3.3), this part of the examination should be performed without switching on color coding.

In the next step, a slow cranial movement of the transducer head is performed – usually with color coding switched on – until the bifurcation becomes visible or – much more frequently – a slight widening (**carotid bulb**) with subsequent narrowing of the vessel diameter is apparent and the internal carotid artery is reached. Because the internal and external carotid arteries are usually not in one plane, it is only in relatively rare cases that they can imaged both as a fork (Fig. 8.5).

By slightly rotating the transducer dorsally, one usually reaches the internal carotid artery, by rotating it ventrally one reaches the external carotid artery. In order not to lose orientation, it is important to ensure that the "pivot point" of the transducer in the common carotid artery remains unchanged.

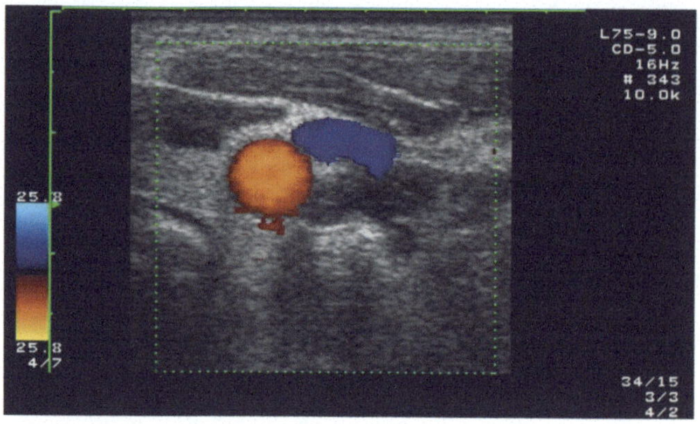

Fig. 8.4 Transversal section through the common carotid artery (red) with preceding jugular vein (blue)

Even when "falling out" of the vessel, it is advisable to always start again in the easily visualized common carotid artery.

> **Practical Tips**
> Confusion may be caused by the findings of pronounced retrograde flow components in the color coded image of the carotid bulb. However, this is not a backward directed blood flow, but a spiral flow that is regularly found at vessel outlets (helix flow; Fig. 8.6).

Both for reasons of identification (see below) and for the assessment of the various flow parameters not detectable by color coded imaging, the Doppler sound beam should be switched on in all three vessel sections and the respective Doppler spectrum assessed and documented.

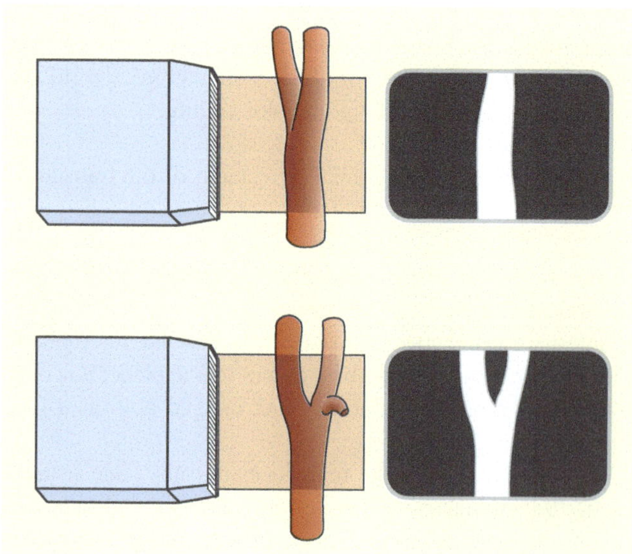

Fig. 8.5 Longitudinal view of the carotid bifurcation as a fork (bottom) or – much more frequently – with only the internal or external carotid artery (top)

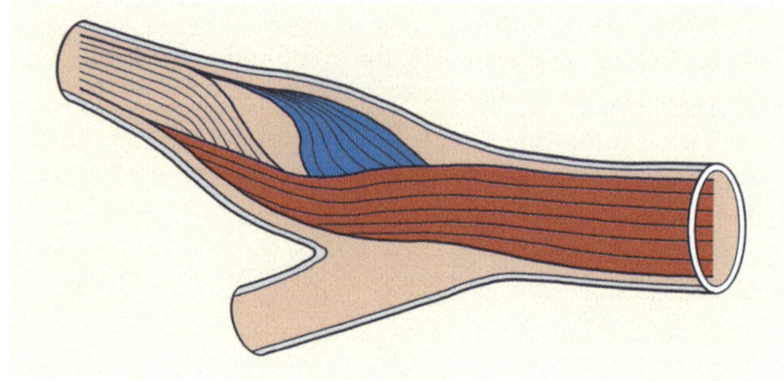

Fig. 8.6 Twisted blood flow in the carotid bulb (helix flow) impressing as retrograde flow components visible in color coded imaging

You should always try to follow the carotid branches as far as possible to below the angle of the jaw. While the B-mode image usually fails early on, the color coded examination helps here and enables in particular the display of kinkings and coilings located below the skull base. In case of doubt, the use of the 3.5 MHz convex probe can also help here.

Identification of the Carotid Branches

In general, the external carotid artery can be identified by the presence of vascular branches in the color coded image. However, since in individual cases a branch of the internal carotid artery may also be present (Case Study 18.5), this criterion can only be regarded as certain if several (!) vascular branches are visible (Fig. 8.7). According to all experience, such conditions are only found in the external carotid artery. Otherwise the differentiation is made according to the criteria of the Doppler spectrum already mentioned in CW Doppler sonography. These include different pulsatilities and the reaction to oscillating compression of the superficial temporal artery (Fig. 7.7).

Image Quality Assessment

The formal assessment of the image quality is an essential part of the duplex sonographic examination, as it provides information afterward on how reliably the sonographic findings can be assessed. Since stenoses may be inadequately represented in both B-mode and color coded images, the estimation of image quality is not based on the detectability of vascular changes, but on the ability to delimit the vessel walls. Since the color coded technique is usually superior to B-mode imaging in the presentation of vascular processes, the color coded image is the standard for evaluation.

A sufficient image quality is always given if the vessel lumen can be separated from the surrounding tissue structures without disturbing artifacts (Table 8.1). In addition, in non-pathological cases, the internal carotid artery should be traceable in a longitudinal section of at least 2 cm. But also in pathological cases the unstenosed lumen should be clearly delimited proximally and distally to the stenosis at least over a length of 0.5–1 cm.

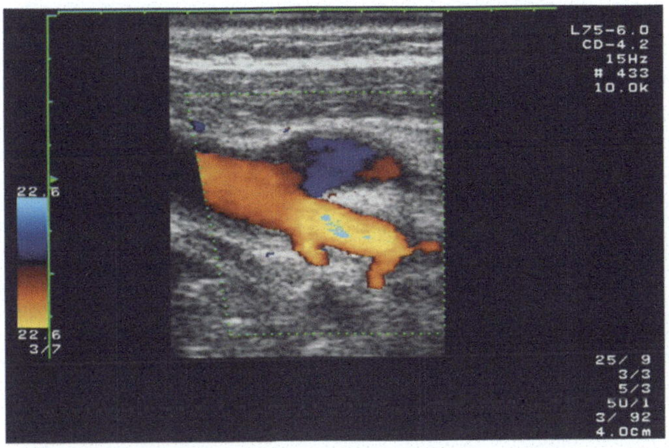

Fig. 8.7 Identification of the external carotid artery by two or more recognizable branches. Only one branch is not sufficient for reliable detection

Carotid Bifurcation in Transversal Section

In addition to the longitudinal section, color coded cross-sectional images of the carotid artery should be used if one of the following situations exists.

Unclear Findings in Longitudinal Section

In the case of overlapping and/or strongly elongated vascular branches, a clear assignment in longitudinal section is often not possible. The slow back and forth movement of the cross-sectional image gives a three-dimensional impression, which often makes it easier to make a clear assignment. ◀

Quantification of Stenoses

Especially low and moderate stenoses can be assessed well in transversal section if the open residual lumen (color coded) is shown and at the same time the unstenosed vessel lumen is recognizable as a low-echo structure (Fig. 8.8). ◀

Practical Tips
When attempting an exact quantification of stenoses, it should always be taken into account that color coded imaging – for methodological reasons – is associated with only low resolution and that the representation of the perfused lumen is strongly dependent on the setting of the color gain.

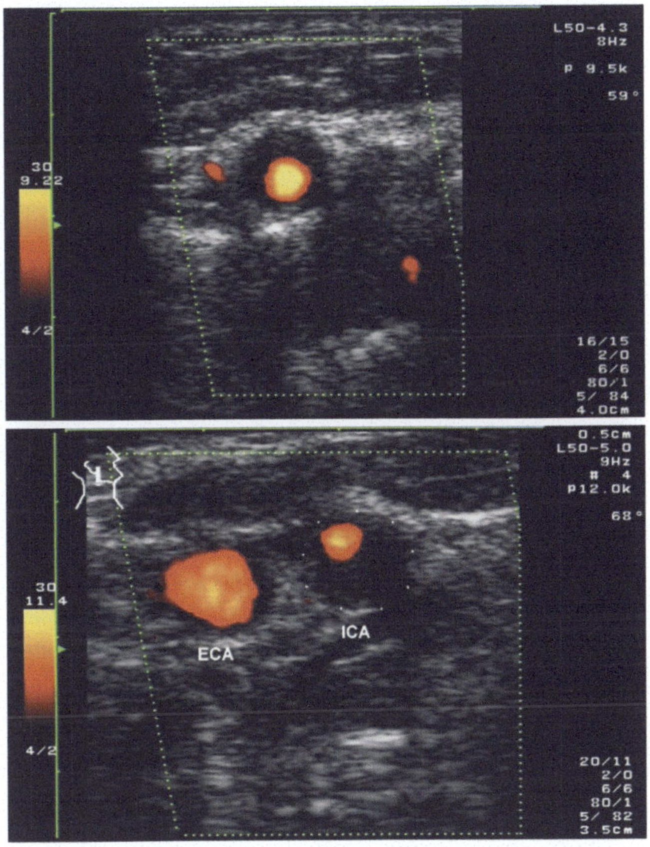

Fig. 8.8 Transversal section through the carotid bulb in medium to high grade stenoses of the internal carotid artery. Concentric stenosis (top), eccentric stenosis (bottom)

8.3.3 Diagnostic Criteria Using B-mode Imaging

Using B-Mode imaging, three aspects can be assessed.

Intima-Media Thickness (IMT)

B-mode imaging (without color coding!) is of essential importance for the assessment of the intima-media thickness

Table 8.1 Assessment of the image quality of duplex sonograms of carotid bifurcation

Evaluation	Criteria
Well	Vascular lumen delimitable without relevant artifacts from surrounding tissue structures, internal carotid artery traceable at more than 2 cm length. In the pathological case vessel length proximal and distal the stenosis at least 0.5–1 cm clearly delimitable
Moderate	Vascular lumen sufficient delimitable, internal carotid artery at least 2 cm length traceable. In the pathological case vessel proximal and distal the stenosis still visible
Bad	Vascular lumen bad delimitable *or* internal carotid artery not at 2 cm traceable *or* vessel in particular distal a stenosis not delimitable

(IMT) and possible generalized vascular wall changes (Sect. 16.1.1). To assess IMT, the vessel should run as parallel as possible to the surface auf the ultrasound transducer (Fig. 8.9). Only in this case will reflection occur (see Sect. 3.2), which is a prerequisite for optimal imaging of the vessel wall layers. By slightly moving the transducer back and forth between the vessel walls, the sectional plane can usually be placed exactly through the middle of the vessel.

Note
The intima-media thickness should only be assessed if the vessel is approximately parallel to the transducer surface.

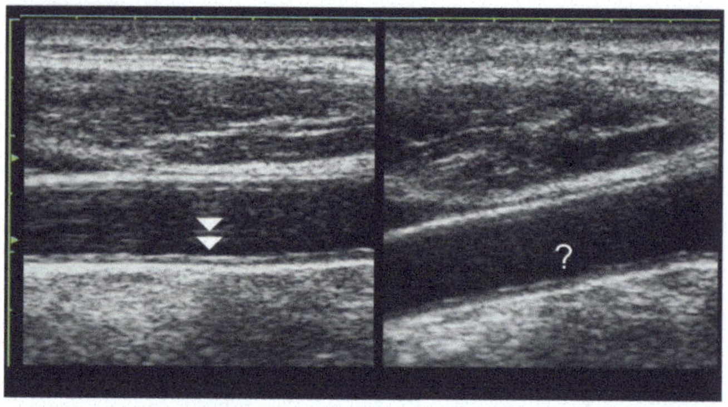

Fig. 8.9 Imgaing of the wall layers of the common carotid artery with different tilting of the transducer. Clear representation of the intima-media layer when the vessel runs parallel to the transducer surface (left); insufficient representation when the vessel runs at an angle (right)

The intima-media thickness is usually best assessed on the vessel wall far from the transducer, since this is where the most favorable reflection conditions exist. The measurement is performed according to the so-called **leading-edge method**. The first measurement line is the transition ("leading edge") between the low-echo lumen and the first, more echo rich band, the second measurement line is the transition between the low-echo intermediate layer and the thicker, more echo rich outer seam (Fig. 8.10).

The rule according to which the intima-media thickness should be assessed 2 cm below the bifurcation may be useful for follow-up examinations under study conditions. However, since atherosclerotic changes can occur in different focal areas, it is recommended in clinical routine to always examine the entire common carotid artery with the exception of the bifurcation and to use the site with the maximum extent of vascular changes for assessment.

Practical Tips
The determination of the intima-media thickness should be performed at the site in the common carotid artery where the thickness of the vessel wall is most pronounced. Plaques in the immediate vicinity of the carotid bifurcation (up to approx. 1 cm proximal to the bifurcation) should be considered separately.

Vascular Morphology
Although sonomorphological criteria in arteriosclerotic and inflammatory disease have an only limited reliability, they contribute to the estimation of etiology and risk in individual cases. Further details can be found in Sect. 16.2.3.

Vascular Pulsations
Particularly in the clarification of vascular occlusions, attention should also be paid to vascular pulsations. In this case, a distinction is made between two main types:

1. **Transversal pulsations** are found physiologically in every (major) artery. Their disappearance can be interpreted as an indication of an occlusion or at least low perfusion.
2. **Longitudinal pulsations** occur mainly when the pulse wave hits a structure lying in the flow axis. This can be a high-grade stenosis or occlusion, but also a kinking or coiling of the vessel. Longitudinal pulsations present on both sides are also found in pronounced hypertension.

8.3.4 Diagnostic Criteria Using Color Coded Imaging

In addition to the localization of the vascular branches of the carotid artery, color coded imaging contributes to the following purposes:

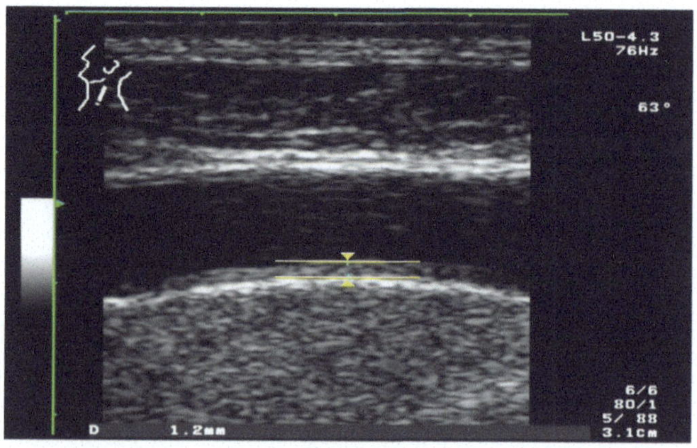

Fig. 8.10 Determination of intima-media thickness according to the leading-edge method

Detection of Vessel Occlusion

Color coded imaging in the longitudinal section under low-flow conditions (Sect. 6.3.1) is the method of choice for detecting carotid artery occlusion (Sect. 13.3).

Localization of the Stenosis Maximum

According to the principle of optimized flow imaging (Sect. 6.3.2), the maximum of a stenosis can be localized (Fig. 8.11) for exact positioning of the Doppler beam.

Detection of Caliber Fluctuations

In addition to the detection of circumscribed stenoses, it is important – especially in combination with flow volume measurement – to recognize abnormal changes in the vessel diameter in comparison to the contralateral side with and to standard values.

> **Practical Tips**
> Abnormal vessel diameters of the carotid artery are often caused by a vessel dissection, but can also occur before and after high-grade stenoses.

Detection of Abnormal Vessel Patterns

Color coded imaging is the method of choice for assessing elongations and kinkings in the internal carotid artery (Sect. 20.1).

8.3.5 Diagnostic Criteria Using the Doppler Spectrum

As already mentioned above, Doppler spectra of the common carotid artery, internal and external should also be routinely derived in non-pathological cases. In addition, Doppler spectra from the maximum stenosis and the poststenotic area should be assessed after prior color coded localization of the stenosis. The evaluation of the Doppler spectrum is based on the following parameters.

Angle Corrected Flow Velocity

The maximum **systolic flow velocity** is the most important criterion for the quantification of stenoses. In comparison to the maximum systolic frequency in CW Doppler sonography, the angle correction results in significantly fewer error possibilities, especially in stenoses that are not yet very severe.

> **Practical Tips**
> When using duplex sonography, the angle-corrected flow velocity should always be measured, as it offers considerable diagnostic advantages over the "blind" determination of the Doppler frequency shift. However, insonation angles of 70° and more should be strictly avoided. Possible errors with eccentric stenoses and kinked stenoses (Sect. 20.1.1) can be reduced if the examiner obtains an impression of the "bandwidth" of the flow velocities to be measured by adjusting the angle correction differently (Fig. 13.15).

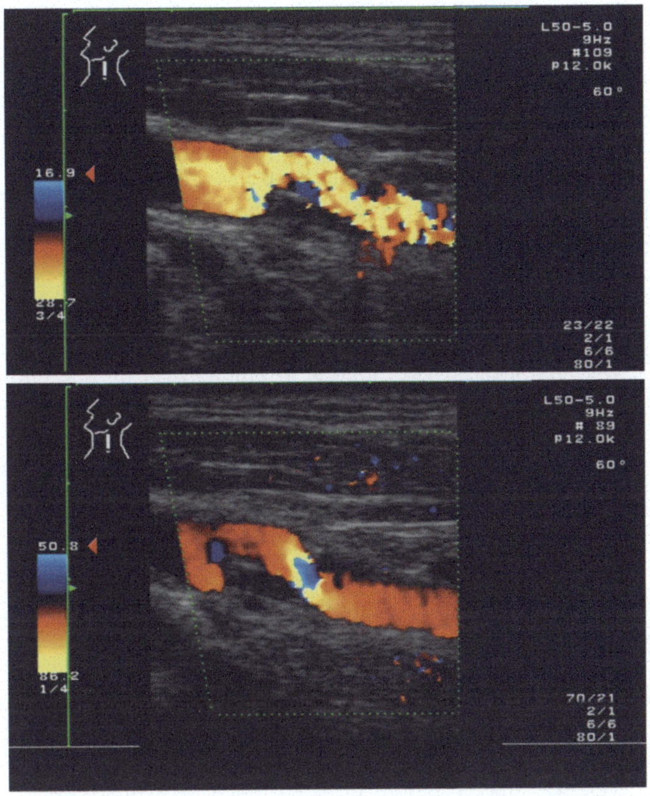

Fig. 8.11 Localization of the maximum stenosis of the internal carotid artery by (gradually) increasing the alias threshold (in the example from 17 to 51 cm/s) until only at a circumscribed aliasing phenomenon remains ("optimized flow imaging")

The maximum **end diastolic flow velocity** is only of minor importance and is only an "auxiliary criterion" if a measurement of the systolic value fails. The main reason for this are very high Doppler frequencies, which exceed the PRF even when the image is "frozen" and the zero line is set downward and can no longer be detected. This situation occurs mainly in low-cost duplex devices, which have only a relatively low maximum PRF.

The **mean value**, that is, the intensity-weighted mean flow velocity, is only important for flow volume measurement, but not for the quantification of stenoses.

Determination of Flow Volume
Determinations of the absolute flow volume in ml/min are recommended in two cases:

1. **Unusually high or low flow velocities** in a carotid branch that cannot be explained by local vascular processes. On the one hand this could be due to hyperperfusion in a vessel leading to an arteriovenous fistula (Sect. 20.4), on the other hand to an intracranial flow obstruction (Sect. 13.2).
2. **Unusually large or small vessel diameters** compared to the contralateral side and/or in comparison to standard values. In the first case, a pathological hyperperfusion should be considered even with "normal" flow velocity detected, since flow volume increases quadratically with the vessel diameter. The second case is regularly found in front of higher grade intracranial stenoses, for example, in the context of dissections, in which the flow volume measurement is the method of choice for observing the course of the disease (Chap. 18).

Practical Tips
As far as possible, for flow volume measurement the vessel diameter should be determined by B-imaging, since the error possibilities in the color coded image are much greater due to the low resolution of color coding.

Flow Disturbances
As shown in Sect. 5.2.3, the evaluation of flow disturbances is important when the detection of the flow velocity fails. In the area of the extracranial carotid arteries this situation is given in two cases:

1. **Maximum stenosis not assessable** due to an acoustic shadow (Fig. 13.10)
2. **Uncertain insonation angle** especially for kink formations, but also for eccentric stenoses (Fig. 13.15).

Pulsatility
Deviations in pulsatility from the normally expected findings can occur on one or both sides and then give indications of the following findings (Table 8.2):

1. **Unilateral increased pulsatility** if the flow obstacle is further cranial
2. **Increased pulsatility on both sides** in the case of microangiopathy, increased intracranial pressure values or in aortic insufficiency
3. **Unilateral reduced pulsatility** especially in the common carotid artery in case of high grade obstruction at the origin of the vessel
4. **Reduced pulsatility on both sides** in case of pronounced aortic stenosis in combination with a corresponding auscultation result.

Summary
Duplex sonographic examination of the carotid bifurcation starts with a longitudinal sectional image of the common carotid artery to make statements about the intima-media thickness. Then color coding should switched on and the branches of the carotid bifurcation are located. The differentiation between internal and external carotid artery as well as the specific search for flow irregularities is carried out on the basis of the Doppler spectrum by positioning the Doppler sound beam at different points of the vessels. The domain of color coding is the detection of vessel occlusions. In addition, "optimized vessel display" in color coded imaging helps in the targeted search for circumscribed stenoses.

8.4 Examination of the Vertebral Artery

8.4.1 Examination Procedure

Intervertebral Course (V2 Segment)
Duplex sonographic longitudinal imaging of the vertebral artery in its intertransverse course between the sixth and second cervical vertebra is almost always successful without major difficulties. Accordingly, this access route is routinely the first to be mentioned. Sound irradiation is always from the front, since in lateral and dorsal irradiation, especially in older people, bony attachments to the transverse processes obstruct the view of the vessel (Fig. 8.12).

The color coded technique makes it much easier to locate the vertebral artery, which is why the examination should always be performed in color mode. Since the vessel is usually located relatively deep in the tissue, the color window should be tilted only slightly by 10–15°, the aliasing threshold should be set sufficiently low and, in particular, the color gain should be turned up as high as possible in order to achieve sufficient "color filling" in the depth.

Practical Tips
In individual cases, it may be possible that the vertebral artery can be identified in the B-mode image, but a

(continued)

Table 8.2 Pathological changes in pulsatility in the extracranial internal carotid artery and their causes

Pulsatility		
Ipsilateral	Contralateral	Cause
Increased	Normal	Downstream flow obstruction
Increased	Increased	Cerebral microangiopathy, increased intracranial pressure, aortic insufficiency
Diminished	Normal	Upstream flow abstruction
Diminished	Diminished	Aortic stenosis

sufficient "color filling" of the vessel cannot be achieved. In such situations, however, it is usually possible to detect a Doppler spectrum by positioning the Doppler sound beam in the visible vessel.

Guiding structures are the transverse processes of the cervical spine, which can be easily recognized in longitudinal section by their acoustic shadow (Fig. 8.13). The vertebral artery runs between them, together with the associated vertebral vein (Fig. 8.14). Compared to the vein, the artery often shows a slightly more echogenic wall structure, but transverse arterial pulsations are often not sufficiently visible. Differentiation is easily possible, provided there is no subclavian steal effect, on the basis of the different flow direction in color coded imaging.

Practical Tips

Problems may arise in color coded imaging of hypoplastic vertebral arteries. Especially in the case of deep-seated vessels, all available **"low-flow parameters"**(Sect. 6.3.1) should be used (Fig. 8.15). In the presence of osteochondrotic changes with barely visible space between the transverse processes, an attempt should always be made to depict the vessel not only in one segment but along the entire cervical spine. In most cases, the vertebral artery can also be visualized in the V1 segment (see below).

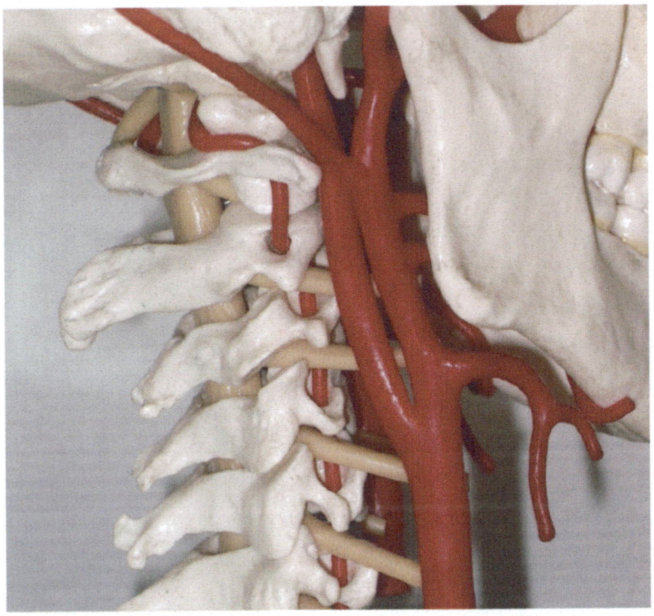

Fig. 8.12 Sonographic access to the vertebral artery in the V2 section from the front. Photo vascular model

Non-routine Examinations

In addition to the imaging of the V2 segment, examinations in the caudal and cranial segments are generally only necessary if the V2 findings are unclear or abnormal.

Prevertebral Course (V1 Segment)

If the vertebral artery cannot be clearly visualized in the V2 segment or if there are conspicuous findings, the next step is to derive the prevertebral course. As already mentioned in Sect. 1.3.1, the entry of the vertebral artery into the transverse foramina is quite variable. Accordingly, it is not uncommon to find a rather long prevertebral course of the proximal vertebral artery (Fig. 8.16). It is also not uncommon, especially in elderly people with pronounced osteochondrosis, for the vertebral artery to be displayed only in this area. In this case, the guiding structure for reliable identification of the vessel is the transverse process at which the vertebral artery enters the V2 segment. ◄

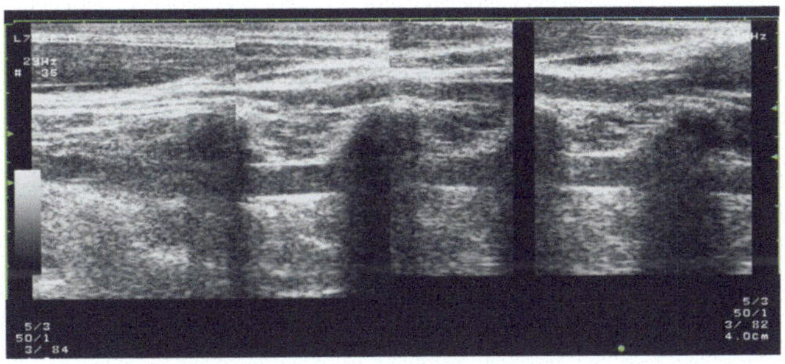

Fig. 8.13 Representation of the vertebral artery in its course between the transverse processes of the cervical spine in B-mode imaging

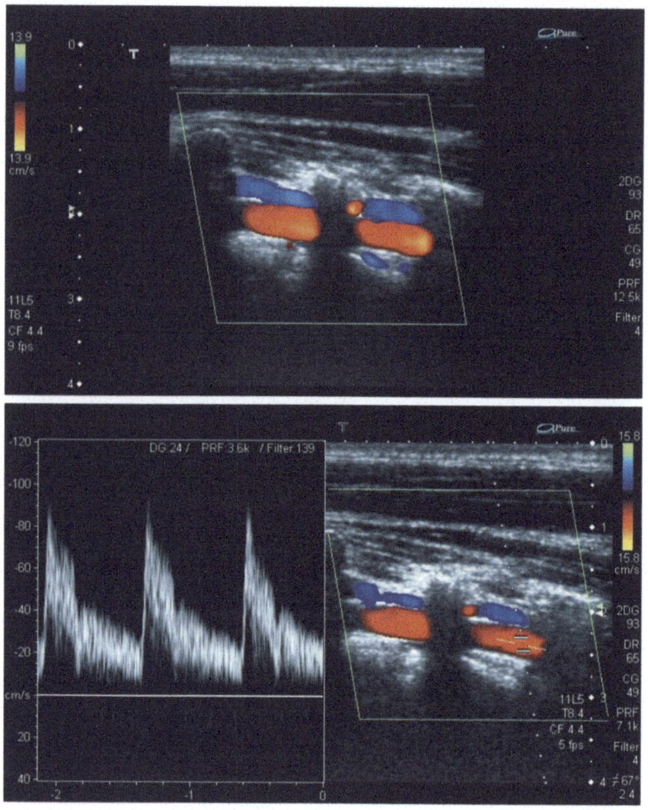

Fig. 8.14 Color coded representation of the vertebral artery (red) and vertebral vein (blue) in the intertransversal V2 section

Vertebral Origin (V0 Segment)

In contrast to the segments mentioned above, the origin of the vertebral artery is not always to be presented reliably. In the ideal case, the vertebral artery can be followed in an almost stretched course, starting from the V1 segment, until it exits the subclavian artery (Fig. 8.17). However, loop formations are often found in the area, which make imaging difficult (Fig. 1.12). As expected, the method often fails in obese patients with short necks. ◀

Atlas Loop (V3 Segment)

Especially in the case of clinically suspected vertebral dissection (Sect. 18.3), the atlas loop should be investigated. The lower, proximal part of the atlas loop between the axis and the atlas is generally easy to visualize and, in contrast to the other intervertebral sections, shows a curve toward the transducer which resembles the handle of a coffee cup (Fig. 8.18). ◀

8.4.2 Diagnostic Criteria

Vessel Diameter

The main advantage of sectional imaging of the vertebral artery compared to CW Doppler derivation is the possibility to determine the diameter of the vessel with high reliability. This measurement can contribute significantly to differentiating between congenital hypoplasia and proximal or distal occlusion. Measuring the diameter should therefore be a routine part of the examination. In clinical suspicion of a dissection, the diameter should also be observed continuously over all sections of the vertebral artery that can be examined.

> **Practical Tips**
> As far as possible, after identification of vertebral artery the color coding should be switched off and the diameter determination should be carried out in gray-scale B-mode imaging, as this allows more accurate measurements.

Flow Velocity

The determination of the angle-corrected flow velocity at the vertebral arteries is only of importance if a circumscribed stenosis can be detected in a section that can be examined. Otherwise the qualitative assessment of the flow signal is sufficient.

> **Practical Tips**
> The determination of the flow velocity in the vertebral artery is not without problems, since the angle between the Doppler sound beam and the vessel is usually in the range of 80° and therefore considerable measuring errors must be taken into account. In this case, an attempt must be made to achieve an "acceptable" insonation angle of less than 70° by further tilting the sound beam and, if necessary, tilting the sound probe.

Flow Volume

Although the determination of flow volume is of some importance in the area of the vertebral arteries for pathophysiological reasons (Sect. 20.3), the method has not yet become established. Nevertheless, there are standard values available which can serve as a reference (Chap. 28).

> **Flow Disturbances**
> Similar to the carotid artery, flow disturbances are always an important parameter when the maximum stenosis is not visible and/or there are unclear relationships. In the area of the vertebral arteries these situations are found in the following cases:
>
> 1. **Maximum stenosis not assessable** within transverse processes
> 2. **Uncertain insonation angle** caused by elongations and kink formations of the vertebral artery.

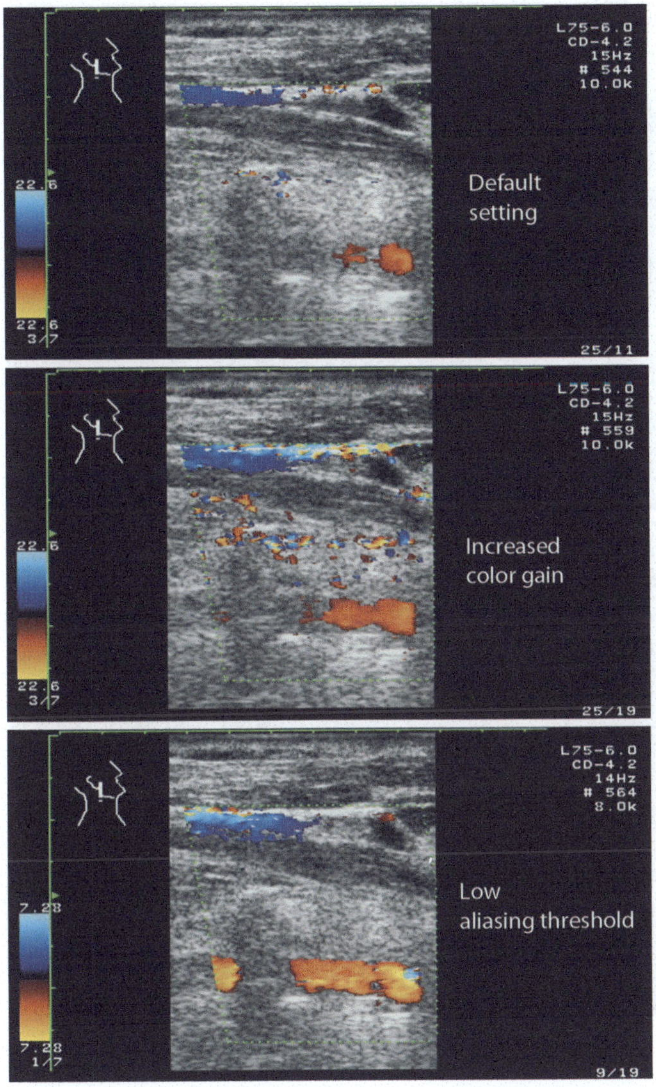

Fig. 8.15 Possibilities to improve the color coded imaging of a deep lying vertebral artery (approx. 3 cm depth) by increasing the color gain (middle) and/or decreasing the aliasing threshold to values <10 cm/s (below)

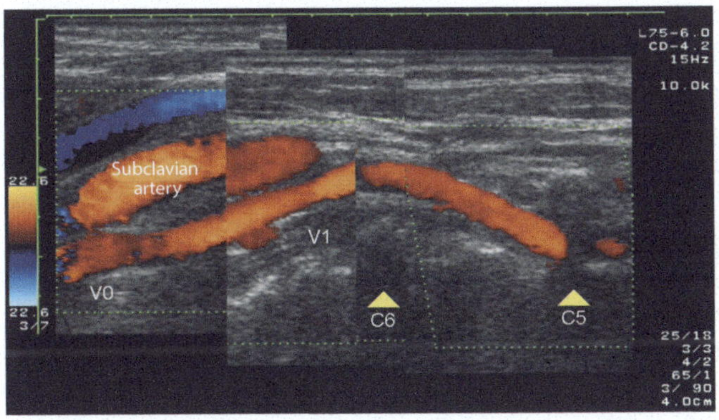

Fig. 8.16 Origin of the vertebral artery from the subclavian artery and course of the vessel in the prevertebral V1 segment with "high" entry into the transverse foramen C5

Pulsatility

Pulsatility is an essential parameter of the diagnosis at the vertebral arteries with a broad differential diagnosis. An increased pulsatility compared to the contralateral side is found in the following cases:

1. **Hypoplasia of the vertebral artery.** With an asymmetry of the vertebral arteries of 1:2 and more or a diameter < 2.5 mm, the hypoplastic vessel regularly shows an increased pulsatility. In this case, the vertebral artery supplies (mainly) neck muscles, often the vessel has no connection to the basilar artery (Sect. 1.3.1).
2. **Distal occlusive process.** As expected, high-grade flow obstructions in the distal course of the vessel are associated with increased pulsatility in Doppler sonographic recording of the extracranial section.
3. **Proximal occlusive process.** At first glance, the finding of increased pulsatility distal to a flow obstruction contradicts the information given in the basics (Sect. 2.5), according to which reduced (!) pulsatility is to be expected in this case. However, the vertebral artery is a vessel with numerous spinal branches, which in the case of an occlusion at the origin of the vertebral artery "jump off" as collaterals, but usually only produce a "muscular flow signal."
4. **Unfavorable insonation angle.** Not to be forgotten is an apparently increased pulsatility at low Doppler frequencies due to an angle of almost 90° between the Doppler beam and the course of the vessel when diastolic flow components are cut off due to the wall filter (Fig. 5.14).

Practical Tips

The main difference between "only" hypoplasia and a distal occlusion of the vertebral artery is the finding that the end-diastolic flow velocity never reaches the zero line in hypoplasia.

Summary

The method of choice for the assessment of vertebral artery is color coded duplex sonography, with which the vessel diameter and usually the entire course from its origin to the atlas loop can be recorded. Problems arise in obese patients with a short neck if the vessel is very deep or osteochondrotic changes block the "sonographic view" to the vertebral artery. The minimum requirement is the recording at one point (V2 section); if constrictions (especially dissections) are suspected, the entire course of the vessel should be displayed.

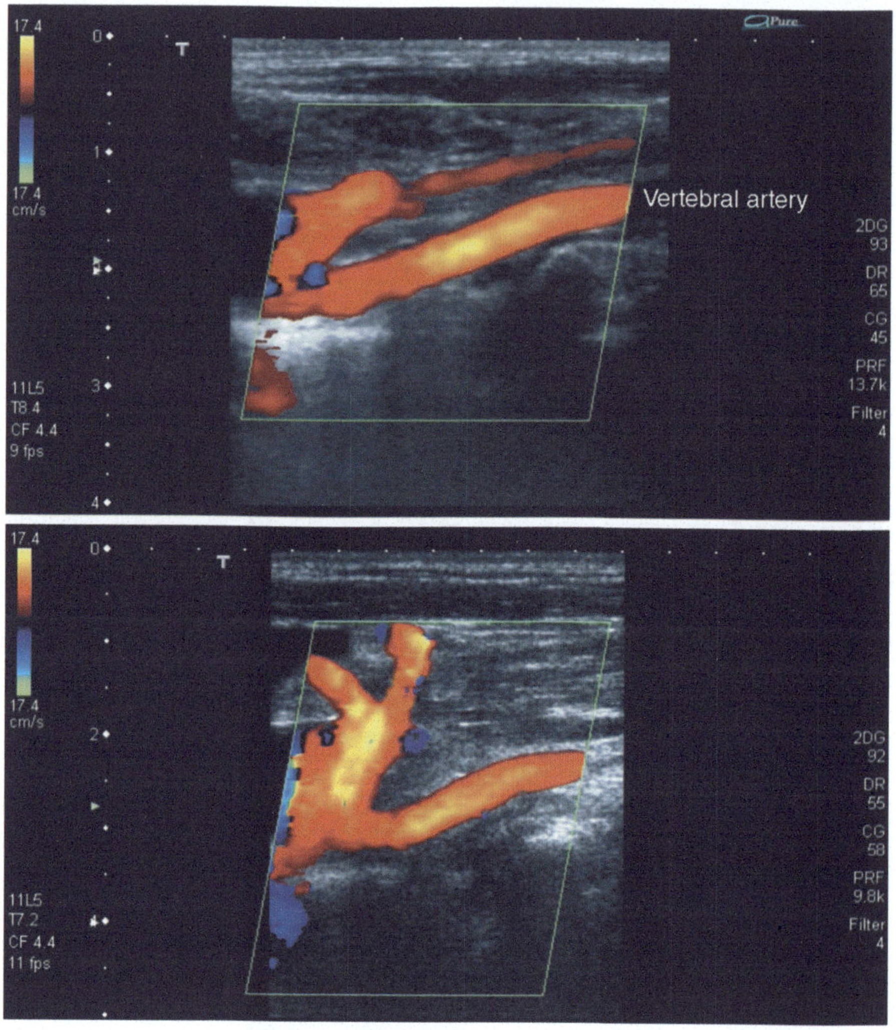

Fig. 8.17 Exit of the vertebral artery from the subclavian artery. Note the numerous other branches of subclavian artery in this area

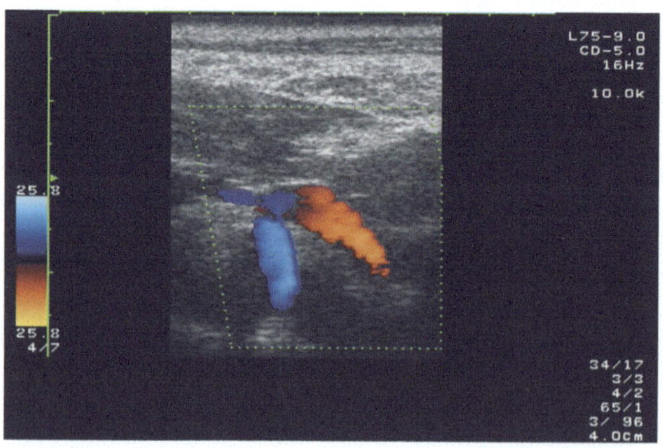

Fig. 8.18 Color coded representation of the 'atlas loop' of vertebral artery with its characteristic handle-shaped appearance

8.5 Error Sources

8.5.1 B-mode Imaging

In B-mode imaging of extracranial vessels, various biologically and physically caused sources of error must be taken into account (Fig. 8.19), which also affect the color coded display.

Reverberations

Reverberation occur when two strong reflectors are facing each other in parallel. In such a case a "ping-pong effect" results, in which the ultrasonic pulse is thrown back and forth. Since part of the energy penetrates the reflector each time it hits it, the back and forth thrown part usually weakens within a short time, but it can cause considerably artifacts on the screen.

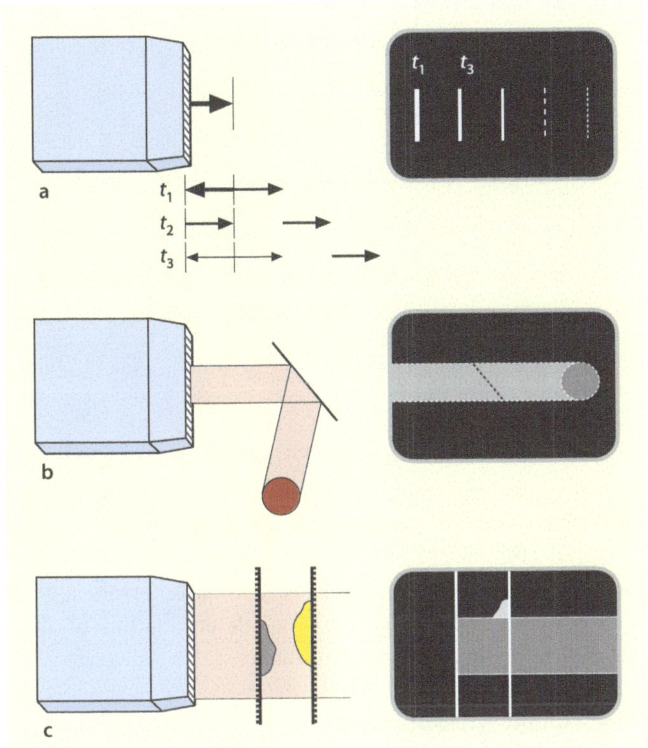

Fig. 8.19 (a–c) Physically caused artifacts in B-mode imaging. Reverberation echoes due to "ping-pong effect" between 2 parallelly located strong reflectors (**a**). Mirror artifact caused by reflection of a reflector inclined to the sound beam displaying by a structure lying outside the acoustic irradiation plane (**b**). Acoustic shadow due to echogenic, sound-impermeable wall sections with extinction of the structures behind them (**c**)

Practical Tips

The differentiation of plaques from artifacts can be performed in daily routine mainly based on two effects: In plaques the "normal" intima-media interface is missing, whereas in artifacts the interface is "underlaid" (Fig. 8.20). In addition, artifacts change their position and appearance by tilting or moving the transducer (see below).

Mirror Artifacts

They occur with reflectors lying in the sound axis, which act as a mirror and image structures not located in the sectional plane (Fig. 8.19). Experienced examiners recognize reverberations and mirror artifacts in the vascular lumen by the fact that such structures do not pulsate or pulsate atypically (e.g., in the wrong direction) and disappear or at least change their location when the transducer is tilted (Fig. 8.21).

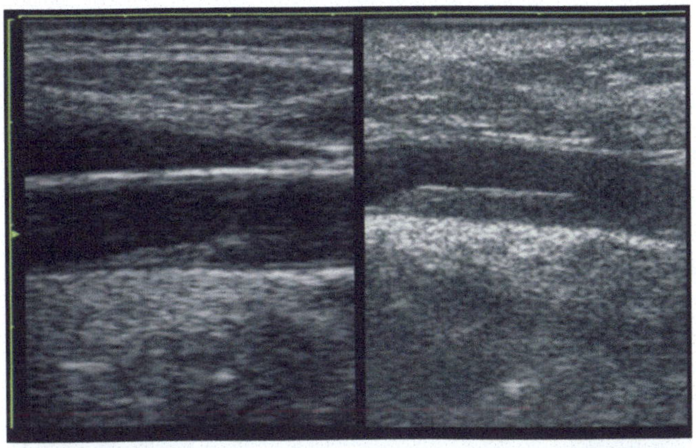

Fig. 8.20 In the case of artifact echoes, the intima-media boundary layer remains "underlaid" continuously visible (left), whereas it is interrupted in this area in the case of plaques in the vessel wall (right)

Acoustic Shadow

A frequent problem in the diagnosis of vascular stenosis are echogenic, usually calcified structures in the vessel wall, which are more or less impermeable to ultrasound and prevent or at least make it more difficult to assess the structures behind them in the direction of sound propagation (Fig. 13.10).

Eccentric Stenoses

If the insonation plane lies not exactly in the middle of the vessel, eccentrically located stenoses can be over- or underestimated (Fig. 8.22). Careful adjustment of the transducer by "oscillating" between the walls of the vessel as well as the validation of findings by using as many insonation planes as possible regularly help here.

Blooming Artifacts

Echogenic structures on the lateral vessel wall (e.g., plaques) can project into the vessel lumen due to the limited lateral resolution of the transducers (Fig. 8.23). Again, this can only be solved by combining as many imaging planes as possible, including transverse sections.

8.5.2 Doppler Spectrum

In addition to unavoidable sources of error due to an acoustic shadow or a not clearly recognizable course of the vessel, further avoidable errors have to be considered.

Flow Velocity Measurement

The main sources of error are insonation angles of 70° or more between the sound beam and the vessel course as well as a forgotten (!) or incorrectly set angle correction (see overview below).

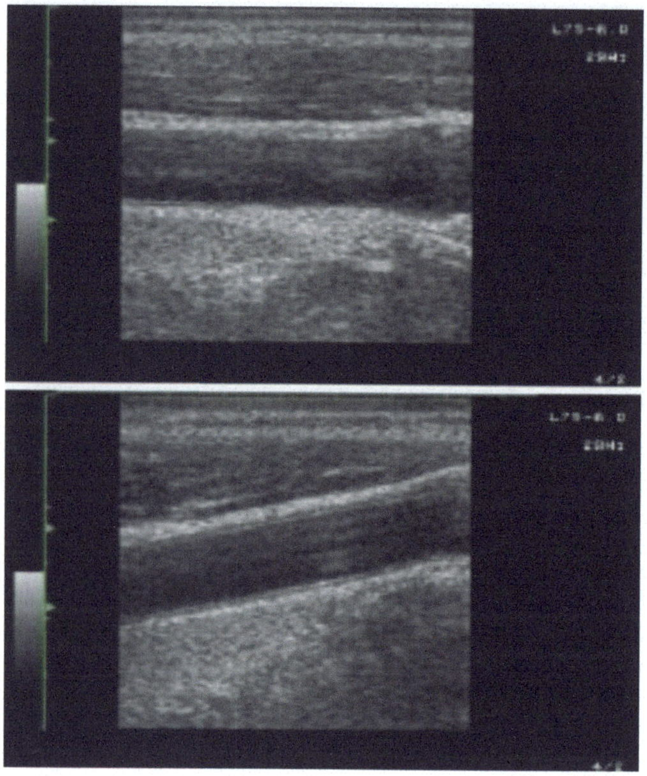

Fig. 8.21 Artifact echoes in the area of the lateral vessel wall (top), which cannot be distinguished from a low echogenic stenosis or a vasculitis at first, but they disappear when the sound probe is tilted slightly (bottom)

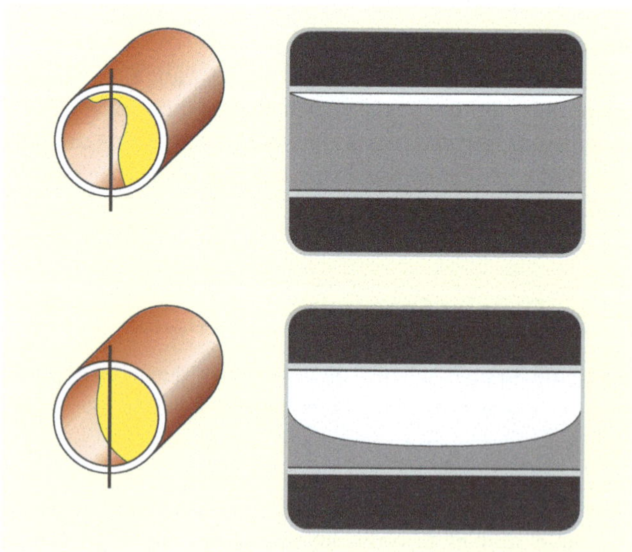

Fig. 8.22 Under- and overestimation of an eccentrically located stenosis in the longitudinal image depending on the insonation plane

The Most Important Sources of Error When Determining Angle-Corrected Flow Velocity

1. Power or gain set too high/too low
2. Insonation angle ≥70°
3. Incorrectly set angle correction
4. Insufficiently depicted vessel course in longitudinal section
5. Velocity measurement in the area of flow disturbances.

If the latter cannot be clearly defined, for example, for reasons of eccentric stenosis, the investigator should at least know the range of variation of the flow velocities to be measured (Fig. 5.21) and consult "secondary criteria" for the exact stenosis grading. Other avoidable errors are an incorrectly set gain (Fig. 5.5) and determination of flow velocity in the area of flow disturbances.

Flow Volume Measurement

In addition to the above mentioned errors in the determination of flow velocity, an incorrect assessment of the vessel diameter must be regarded as the main source of error due to the quadratic influence (Fig. 5.24). As far as possible, the determination should therefore always be carried out in gray-scale B-mode imaging. An evaluation based on color coding represents only a bad compromise due to the lower resolution. Furthermore, it must be ensured that the – usually smaller set – sample volume is at least as large as the vessel lumen for flow volume measurement.

8.5.3 Color Coded Imaging

In addition to the problems already mentioned in Sect. 8.5.1, errors in color-coded imaging are usually due to two avoidable negligences.

Color Gain Set Too Low

If the color gain is set too low, it cannot be expected that vessels will be adequately represented. A sufficient color gain can be recognized by the appearance of singel "color dots" outside the vessels (Fig. 6.11).

90° Insonation Angle

Due to the mentioned specifications in the Doppler equation, no meaningful color coded flow representation can be expected for an insonation angle of approximately 90°. However, a relatively high angle of incidence of 70–80° usually seems to be reasonable, especially for deep-lying vessels (e.g., vertebral artery), in order not to cause too much attenuation in the tissue by prolonging the transit time of the ultrasound (Fig. 6.12).

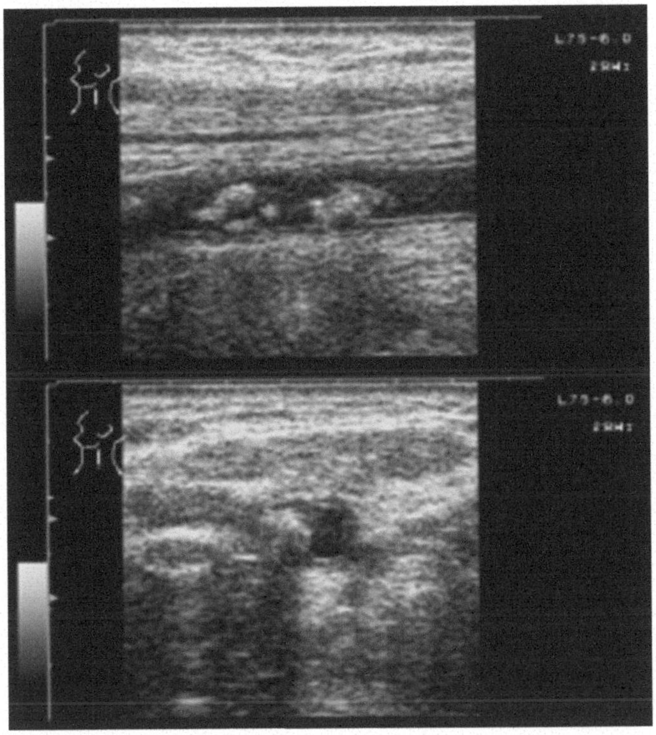

Fig. 8.23 An echogenic plaque localized on the lateral vessel wall as demonstrated in transverse section (bottom) leads to an apparently high-grade stenosis in longitudinal section (top)

Summary
Biologically and physically caused sources of error in B-mode and duplex sonography are reverberation echoes from strong reflectors, mirror artifacts due to reflections and acoustic shadows caused by soundproof structures. Strongly reflecting structures on the lateral vessel wall can lead to blooming artifacts and be overestimated as relevant stenoses. Errors in Doppler flow measurement and color coded imaging can usually be avoided if the instrument settings are carefully observed.

9 Transcranial Doppler Sonography

Bernhard Widder and Gerhard F. Hamann

9.1 Indications

While extracranial CW Doppler sonography is only of minor importance today in view of the considerably more valid duplex examination, transcranial Doppler sonography does not significantly lag behind transcranial duplex sonography with regard to its diagnostic significance in quite a large number of applications (Table 9.1). Furthermore, due to the smaller contact surface of the pin probe and the usually significantly higher sound transmission energy, the single beam Doppler sonography has advantages in transmitting the temporal bone window (Fig. 9.2).

The main indications for transcranial Doppler sonography are

- Recognition and monitoring of **high-grade intracranial stenoses** in the presence of transient or permanent hemiplegic symptoms and/or speech disorders.
- Assessment of the **cerebrovascular reserve capacity** in the case of known high-grade stenoses or occlusions of the cerebral arteries to evaluate their hemodynamic significance for cerebral blood flow (Chap. 12).
- Detection of **right-left cardiac shunts** (patent foramen ovale PFO) after intravenous administration of contrast agents as part of the investigation of the causes of cerebral ischemia (Chap. 26).
- Detection and monitoring **increased intracranial pressure**. Slightly elevated intracranial pressure values cannot be reliably detected, however, which limits the clinical usefulness of the method (see Chap. 23).

B. Widder (✉)
Expert Opinion Institute, District Hospital, Guenzburg, Germany
e-mail: bernhard.widder@bkh-guenzburg.de

G. F. Hamann
Clinic of Neurology and Neurological Rehabilitation, District Hospital, Guenzburg, Germany

9.2 Device Settings

9.2.1 Standard Setting

Due to the problem of having to tranmit the bony skull, transcranial Doppler sonography necessarily requires the use of low-frequency sound probes (usually 2 MHz). Another basic requirement is the use of pulsed Doppler technique in order to be able to differentiate sufficiently between the different intracranial vessels.

Flow Direction
Since the main vessels of the skull base run toward the probe (middle and posterior cerebral artery), it has become generally accepted that flow toward the probe is displayed on the screen above the zero line.

Zero Line
It is recommended to leave the zero line fixed in the middle of the screen. In this way, in non-pathological cases, all large intracranial vessels can be displayed without manipulation of the device.

Frequency Range
If the maximum displayable frequency is set to about 3 kHz (in both directions of flow), this is sufficient in the non-pathological case to display the frequency spectrum of all intracranial arteries sufficiently.

Power
By default, a maximum sound transmission energy (power) can be used to obtain quick examination results. However, if the examination takes longer, the sound energy should be reduced. In particular, the orbital vessels should only be dissipated with low transmitted sound energy to avoid any danger (see Sect. 3.5).

B. Widder, G. F. Hamann (eds.), *Duplex sonography of the brain-supplying arteries*, https://doi.org/10.1007/978-3-662-65566-5_9

Table 9.1 Differences in diagnostic significance between transcranial Doppler and duplex sonography

	Doppler sonography	Duplex sonography
Detection and monitoring of intracranial stenoses	++	++
Detection of intracranial vascular occlusions in acute stroke	(+)	++
Assessment of intracranial collaterals	(+)	++
Assessment of cerebrovascular reserve capacity	++	++
Assessment of cardiac right-left shunts (foramen ovale)	++	(+)
Detection and monitoring of vasospasms	+	++
Detection and monitoring of intracranial pressure	+	+
Detection of cerebral circulatory arrest (brain death)	+	++

Gain
The gain is optimally adjusted if there are single artifact points outside of the displayed Doppler spectrum on the screen.

Sample Volume
The use of a medium size sample volume (8–10 mm) is recommended as standard. If this is set smaller, the spatial resolution is improved, but at the same time the already problematic derivability of the vessels is reduced.

Depth
For the beginning of the transtemporal examination, an examination depth of 55–60 mm is most suitable, since the probability of hitting a vessel is highest here. For further examination, however, a variation of the examination depth of 40–80 mm is usually required.

9.2.2 Insufficient Temporal Bone Window

In the case of an insufficient temporal bone the detectability of the vessels can – to a limited extent – be increased by the following measures.

Maximum Power
For some devices the specified power limit of 100 mW/cm^2 can be exceeded after confirmation of the knowledge about the use of the high sound energy.

Maximum Sample Volume
In this way, the "quantity" of reflections available for the determination of the Doppler frequency shift can be significantly increased.

Increasing the Frequency Range
By increasing the maximum frequency that can be displayed, the PRF is increased, which leads to a (further) increase in sound transmission energy. However, this measure is limited by the fact that the maximum possible examination depth is reduced.

9.3 Examination Procedure

9.3.1 Transtemporal Access

The temporal bone is the only area of the skull that regularly shows a reduced bone thickness and can therefore be penetrated by ultrasound. There are three "sound windows" to distinguish (Fig. 9.1):

- The anterior window near the lateral orbital rim
- The middle window directly before the upper base of the auricle
- The posterior window above the external auditory canal.

Since the middle "sound window" has proven to be the most favorable location in the majority of cases, it is recommended to start with this one.

> **Practical Tips**
> In older patients it is not uncommon to find only a rear "sound window" above the ear, which is the preferred location for posterior cerebral artery detection. With plenty of contact gel and by tilting the probe forward it is often possible to obtain Doppler signals even from the middle and anterior cerebral arteries.

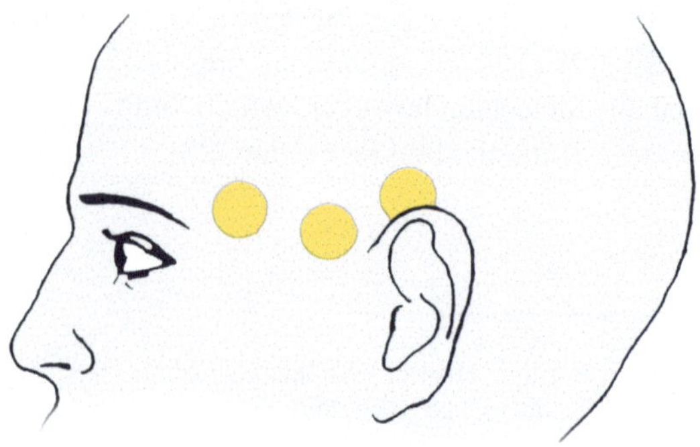

Fig. 9.1 Sound windows for transtemporal insonation of the basal cerebral arteries

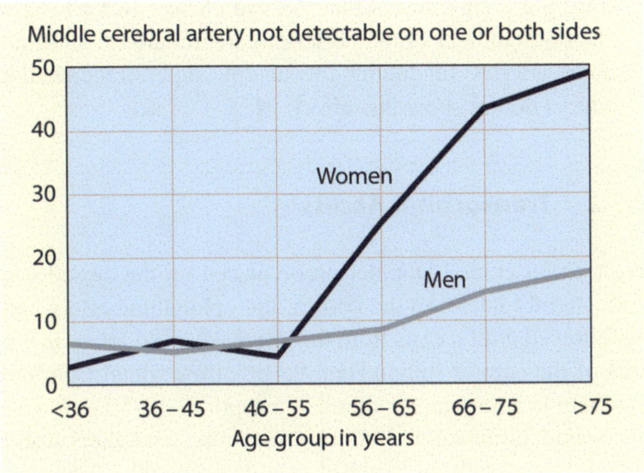

Fig. 9.2 Insufficient feasibility of transtemporal Doppler examinations in 1740 patients depending on age and sex

The necessity of transmitting the bony skull represents the most essential problem of transcranial Doppler sonography in practice. Especially in older women, it must be expected that almost half of them cannot be sufficiently examined. But also in men and younger women, 5–10% of cases reveal no sufficient temporal window, whereby single sided problems are not uncommon (Fig. 9.2). Accordingly, information on the signal quality should always be provided in transcranial Doppler examinations (Table 9.2).

> **Practical Tips**
> In order to improve the examination conditions, it must always be ensured that the ultrasound probe is optimally coupled by using sufficient ultrasound gel. It is also recommended to start the examination with maximum transmission power and a large sample volume. Once the vessels have been found, the sample volume can be reduced to achieve good localization resolution (Fig. 5.16).

Middle and Anterior Cerebral Arteries

The anterior arteries of the brain are usually reached by slightly tilting the probe forward, directing the sound beam to the contralateral zygomatic bone. In individual cases, however, the position of the vessels can vary considerably. The main stem of the middle cerebral artery is regularly found at a depth of 50–55 mm (M1 segment; Table 9.3). In some cases, the vessel can also be followed further laterally to its branches in the sylvian fissure (M2 segment), which is usually reached at a depth of 40–45 mm. When the probe is shifted medially and slightly tilted caudally, the distal part of the internal carotid artery is recorded at a depth of 60–65 mm, but the transition between the two vessels cannot be reliably identified on the basis of the Doppler signal without additional color coded imaging.

By augmenting the depth of the sample there occurs usually a downward component – away from the probe – in addition to the pulse curve which has always been directed upward. This is assigned to the anterior cerebral artery (A1 segment), which can normally be followed up to the midline (depending on the width of the skull at 75–80 mm). In younger patients with a well-developed sound window, it is not uncommon that also vessels of the contralateral hemisphere can be recorded at greater depths.

Posterior Cerebral Artery

The initial section of the posterior cerebral artery (P1 segment) is reached at a depth of 70–75 mm with the sound probe turned slightly dorsally and caudally. Often, a signal from the contralateral cerebral posterior artery is also seen at this depth, which is directed away from the probe.

The transition from the P1 to the P2 segment is usually derived at a depth of 60–65 mm. However, since the posterior cerebral artery emerges from the anterior cerebral circulation in about 20% and numerous mixed constellations occur (Sect. 1.7.2), the classification is unreliable.

Differentiation of the Cerebral Arteries

Due to the close topographical relationships and numerous variants, the assignment of the cerebral arteries based on the three criteria of flow direction, probe position and depth of the sample volume are not sufficiently reliable. In order to achieve a clear vascular differentiation, various short-term compression maneuvers of the common carotid artery were suggested. Although the cerebral can indeed be differentiated in this way based on their reaction to the compression maneuver, the carotid compression test is an invasive method and involves an unavoidable risk of stroke. Since differentiation

Table 9.2 Evaluation of the temporal bone window in transcranial Doppler sonography

Assessment	Conditions
Well	Doppler spectrum all 3 cerebral arteries clearly derivable
Moderate	Doppler spectrum restricted derivable, but still of diagnostic value
Bad	Doppler spectrum from only single vessels detectable
Missing	No Doppler signal derivable

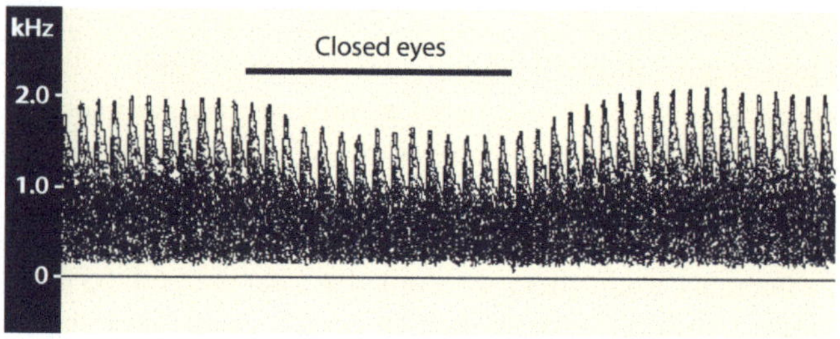

Fig. 9.3 Eye closure test to identify the posterior cerebral artery. Closing the eyes and then looking at a brightly illuminated, high-contrast object leads to a significant increase in blood flow velocity in the posterior cerebral artery within a few seconds

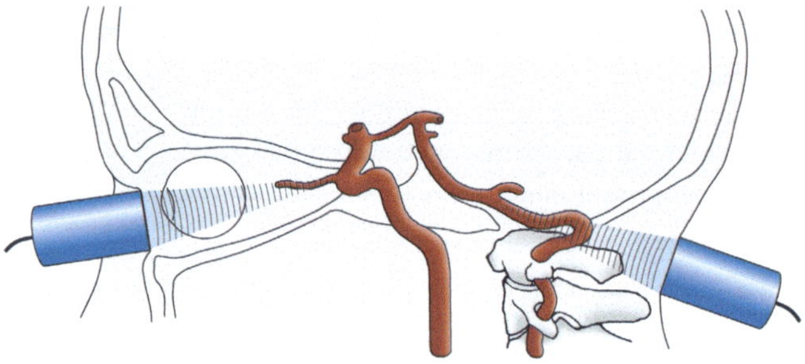

Fig. 9.4 Transorbital and transnuchal examination

of the brain basal arteries is possible using color coded duplex sonography, the carotid compression test must therefore be regarded as obsolete. Therefore, only 2 vessels can be clearly assigned by Doppler sonography.

Middle Cerebral Artery

A vessel that can be found transtemporally at a depth of 40–45 mm is almost certainly the middle cerebral artery or one of its branches. In particular, the posterior cerebral artery is no longer to be expected at this depth of examination, as it very soon after its origin runs dorsally around the midbrain. ◀

Posterior Cerebral Artery

Opening the eyes and looking at a brightly illuminated, high-contrast object leads to a 20 to 30% increase in the flow velocity in the posterior cerebral artery within a few seconds compared to the situation with closed eyes (Fig. 9.3). This means that the eye closure test allows a clear assignment of the posterior cerebral artery, since all other arteries (including the nearby superior cerebellar artery) do not show this effect. ◀

9.3.2 Transorbital Access

With a transcranial Doppler probe placed on the closed eye bulb slightly lateral to the cornea, the ophthalmic artery can be followed until it exits from the internal carotid artery in the area of the carotid siphon (Fig. 9.4). A flow signal from the ophthalmic artery can be found at a depth of 40–50 mm with the sound probe turned slightly medially, and the carotid siphon can usually be reached at a depth of 60–70 mm. A flow toward the probe indicates that it is the caudal section. By slightly tilting the transducer cranially, the cranial section can also be assessed in many cases.

An overview of the depths of examination of transorbital ultrasound vessels is given in Table 9.4.

Practical Tips

Although damage to the lens of the eye has only been observed at much higher ultrasound powers, it is recommended to reduce the transmission energy in transorbital Doppler sonography as much as possible and to avoid direct ultrasound exposure of the lens.

9.3.3 Transnuchal Access

The Foramen magnum offers a further access route. Here the examination is best performed in a sitting position and the patient is asked to lower his chin as far as possible to the chest with his neck stretched. The sound probe is placed in the midline of the neck approximately 2–3 cm below the occipital bone cusp and directed slightly cranially. The vertebral arteries are located at a depth of 60–80 mm. Under normal anatomical conditions, they can be differentiated by slightly tilting the probe and serve as a "guide" to the basilar artery (Table 9.5).

Depending on the thickness of the neck and anatomical variations, the basilar artery begins at a rather variable depth

Table 9.3 Examination depths for transtemporal sonication and vessels normally expected in this area

Depth [mm]	Direction of probe tilting	Flow direction	Vessel
40–45	Frontal	Toward probe	Middle cerebral artery (M2 segment)
50–55	Frontal	Toward probe	Middle cerebral artery (M1 segment)
60–65	Frontal	Toward probe	Carotid T-area
70–75	Frontal	Away from the probe	Anterior cerebral artery (A1 segment)
60–65	Dorsal	Changing	Posterior cerebral artery (P1/P2 segment)
70–75	Dorsal	Toward probe	Posterior cerebral artery (P1 segment)

Table 9.4 Depths of examination of transorbital insonated vessels

Depth [mm]	Vessel
40–50	Ophthalmic artery
60–70	Carotid siphon

Table 9.5 Depth of examination in transnuchal Doppler sonography

Depth [mm]	Vessel
60–80	Vertebral artery
70–110	Basilar artery

between 70 and 110 mm. If no additional color coding is available, it can be assumed with sufficient certainty that the basilar artery is reached at a depth of approx. 100 mm. Both the vertebral and basilar arteries show a flow direction away from the probe. A vessel running along the vertebral artery toward the sound probe is often found at variable depths. This is usually the posterior inferior cerebral artery (PICA), but in individual cases it may also be the anterior spinal artery.

Summary
When the sound probe is placed in the area of the temporal bone (transtemporal examination), the middle, anterior and posterior arteries as well as the distal internal carotid artery can be derived. The main problem of the examination is the often insufficient temporal bone window (in about 10% of all patients, in up to 50% of older patients). In addition, the transorbital examination allows the carotid siphon to be derived. When the sound probe is placed in the neck (transnuchal examination), the transition from the vertebral artery to the basilar artery can be followed by varying the depth of the examination. Due to the existing variability, a reliable identification of the basilar artery is only possible at an examination depth of 100 mm.

9.4 Diagnostic Criteria

9.4.1 Doppler Frequencies

Since the angle between the sound beam and the vessel is not known in transcranial Doppler sonography, Doppler frequencies should be specified in kHz and not in cm/s – comparable to extracranial Doppler sonography. As in other vascular regions, the determination of the maximum systolic Doppler frequency is of primary importance. For the assessment of the cerebrovascular reserve capacity (Chap. 12), the intensity-weighted mean Doppler frequency (mean) is also of significance.

In the area of the middle cerebral artery, side comparisons are possible within narrow limits, since this vessel is usually very symmetrical and problems with the angle of incidence are therefore of little consequence. The intraindividual side differences of the Doppler frequencies have a maximum of ±10%. The intraindividual differences are in the same order in repetitive examinations, which is important for follow-up examinations.

Additional Information
In transcranial Doppler sonography, flow velocities are sometimes given instead of frequency values. This seems legitimate for the middle cerebral artery, since the angle of incidence in the M1 segment is almost always less than 30° when the vessel is irradiated transtemporally (Table 9.6). Since the cosine at angles below 30° by definition shows only slight deviations from the maximum value 1 (cos 30° = 0.87), there are correspondingly only small measurement errors compared to angle-corrected velocity measurement. The conversion can be done according to the simple formula.

$$\text{Flow rate}\ [\text{cm/s}] = 40 \times \text{Doppler frequency}\ [\text{kHz}]$$

Table 9.6 Angle between the Doppler beam and the cerebral arteries by using transtemporal ultrasound. In addition, indication of the measurement error caused by this when using a one-dimensional probe in comparison to angle-corrected measurement with color coded duplex sonography

	Frequency of different insonation angles [%]		
Vessel	≤30°	31–40°	>40°
Middle cerebral artery	78	22	–
Anterior cerebral artery	73	17	10
Posterior cerebral artery	61	33	6
Measurement error [%]	**<14**	**14–23**	**>23**

According to Fujioka et al. (1994)

However, the situation is different for the other cerebral arteries, especially for the distal internal carotid artery, so that this procedure is not recommended.

9.4.2 Flow Disturbances

As in the case of extracranial vessels, assessment of flow disturbances is also of importance when the detection of the flow velocity fails in the area of the intracranial vessels. This situation is given in two cases.

Assessment of the Distal Internal Carotid Artery
The distal internal carotid artery runs almost perpendicular to the sound beam of the Doppler probe up to its branching at the so-called carotid T, so that the maximum systolic Doppler frequencies are in no way meaningful, even in the case of high-grade stenoses. Correspondingly, only indirect evidence can be obtained from the occurrence of pronounced flow disturbances.

Problems with the Temporal Sound Window
Due to turbulent flow occurring distal to high-grade stenoses, the laminar fast flow components become less and less (Fig. 2.7). For transcranial Doppler sonography, this means that if the temporal bone window is insufficiently developed, the high-frequency but low-energy frequency components are no longer reliably displayed, while the high-energy, low-frequency turbulence may still be visible in the Doppler spectrum and can be used as an indirect criterion for a high-grade stenosis.

9.4.3 Pulsatility

Deviations in pulsatility indicate the following situations:

- **Increased pulsatility** in the main stem of the middle cerebral artery indicates an occlusion of a main branch of the middle cerebral artery.
- **Increased pulsatility** in the cerebral arteries of both sides indicated either an increased intracranial pressure ord a cerebral microangiopathy.
- **Reduced pulsatility** in the cerebral arteries can bei found in the case of occlusion or severe stenosis of the supplying extracranial arteries, especially in connection with reduced collateral supply.

Summary
The Doppler sonographic evaluation of the cerebral arteries is based on three criteria: Determination of the maximum systolic Doppler frequencies, occurrence of flow disturbances and assessment of pulsatility. In the area of the middle cerebral artery, the side differences of the Doppler frequencies are in the order of only 10%. The same applies to repetitive examinations. Due to the many variations in the course of the vessels, these conditions are not present in the other cerebral arteries.

Reference

Fujioka KA, Gates DT, Spencer MP (1994) A comparison of transcranial color Doppler imaging and standard static pulsed wave Doppler in the assessment of intracranial hemodynamics. J Vasc Tech 18:29–35

10 Transcranial Duplex Sonography

Bernhard Widder and Gerhard F. Hamann

10.1 Indications

Today, transcranial color coded duplex examination is the standard method for sonographic evaluation of the intracranial vessels. There are several clinically important indications for the performance of this technique.

Acute Cerebral Infarction
The sonographic detection and localization of occlusions of the middle cerebral artery in acute cerebral infarction is still a viable alternative, even in view of the fact that CTA and MRA are available almost everywhere (Chap. 21). In addition, ultrasound examinations are suitable for monitoring the course of a thrombolytic therapy. In the posterior circulation, however, the informative value appears limited.

Intracranial Stenoses or Occlusions
The transcranial color coded duplex examination is suitable to detect stenoses or occlusions of the intracranial vessels supplying the brain. There is very good agreement with CTA, which is the gold standard in the acute situation (Demchuk et al. 2016).

Intracranial Collateral Supply
Not least in addition to CTA and/or MRA examinations, transcranial duplex sonography can provide valid information on the quality and quantity of the intracranial collateral supply in occlusions of the extracranial brain-supplying arteries due to the possibility of recording hemodynamic parameters.

B. Widder (✉)
Expert Opinion Institute, District Hospital, Guenzburg, Germany
e-mail: bernhard.widder@bkh-guenzburg.de

G. F. Hamann
Clinic of Neurology and Neurological Rehabilitation, District Hospital, Guenzburg, Germany

Vasospasms
It is true that vasospasms can in principle also be detected by "simple" transcranial Doppler sonography. Color coded duplex sonography, however, has significant advantages, since it allows reproducible detection of even smaller vessels and angle-corrected measurements of flow velocity are possible (Chap. 22).

"Brain Death Diagnostics"
Cerebral circulatory arrest can also be detected with "simple" transcranial Doppler sonography. However, in the absence of a flow signal, imaging can be used to differentiate between a problem due to an insufficient temporal bone window and a cerebral blood flow that actually no longer exists. In addition, extracranial duplex examination can reliably differentiate between the various arteries supplying the brain, so that the diagnosis may already be limited to these vessels.

Further indications have been described for the assessment of intracranial structures, for example in connection with Parkinson's disease (Berg et al. 2011). In addition, numerous studies on the detection of cerebral aneurysms, angiomas, and tumors can be found in the literature. However, in view of the high accuracy and much higher resolution of the competing CT and MRI procedures, the authors believe that ultrasound has no relevant practical use here.

10.2 Device Settings

> **Practical Tips**
> What is true for extracranial linear array transducers, is even more true for the much smaller phased array transducers used in transcranial duplex sonography: If they are not switched off when not in use and "run

(continued)

B. Widder, G. F. Hamann (eds.), *Duplex sonography of the brain-supplying arteries*, https://doi.org/10.1007/978-3-662-65566-5_10

empty", excessive heating of the transducer may occur resulting in continuous deterioration of image quality. Between the individual examinations, the transducers should therefore always be switched off by "freezing" the image, especially if the color or Doppler mode is switched on.

10.2.1 Transducers

Transducer Type
For the examination of the intracranial brain-supplying arteries, only phased-array transducers with the smallest possible contact surface are considered, in order to be able to make use of the often very small temporal bone window.

Ultrasound Transmission Frequency
Due to the problems with the transmission of ultrasound through the bony skull, the ultrasound frequency should be as low as possible. Nominal frequencies of more than 2.5 MHz are generally (in adults) not suitable. If it is a multi-frequency transducer, the lowest nominal frequency should be set as standard. Under good examination conditions, the frequency can still be switched higher to improve the resolution of the B-mode image.

10.2.2 B-mode Imaging

Depth Settings
There is no uniform standard for this. For the transtemporal examination, two variants with different advantages and disadvantages come into consideration (Fig. 10.1):

- **15 cm depth setting:** In this setting, the contralateral skull bone including the ventricular system is regularly displayed. Especially for the less experienced as well as for B-mode examinations of the cerebral parenchyma (Fig. 10.3), this has the advantage of easier orientation in the image. In addition, due to the representability of the contralateral skull, it can be seen at first glance whether the examination can be performed successfully (Fig. 10.5). On the other hand, the color coded image shows the cerebral arteries very small.
- **10 cm depth setting:** Here the vessels of the circle of Willis are shown in an acceptable size so that this setting is particularly suitable for standard color coded examination.

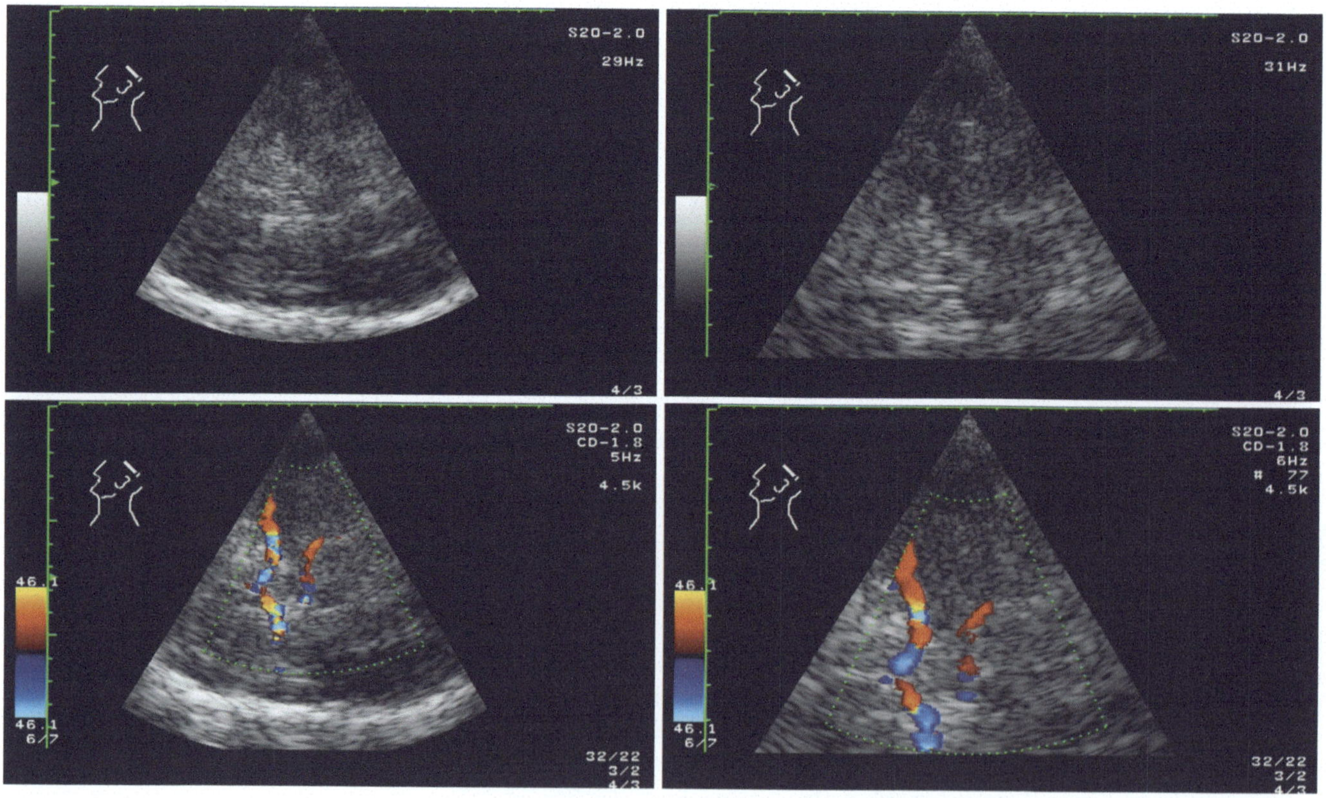

Fig. 10.1 Appearance of intracranial structures in the axial B-mode and color coded image at different display depths (left 15 cm, right 10 cm)

For the transnuchal study, a standard depth of 12 cm is recommended in order to cover the entire vertebrobasilar system.

Focus

Since the diagnostically "most interesting" vessels are located at a depth of about 6 cm, it is recommended to set the focus in this region. If the assessment of the ventricular system in the B-mode image is the main focus, a deeper focus may have to be selected.

B-mode Gain

The adjustment of the signal amplification including the time gain compensation (Fig. 8.2) should be oriented toward the clearest possible representation of the lead structures important for the examination (especially the midbrain and the third ventricle, possibly also the thalamus).

Signal Dynamics

The dynamic range of the B-mode image should be set to 40–50 dB in order to ensure sufficient soft tissue resolution on the one hand and to achieve a high-contrast image with good representation of the contours of the brain parenchyma on the other.

Image Processing

Depending on the manufacturer, numerous image processing parameters such as contrast, contour enhancement, persistence index as well as various gray scales can be changed in almost any combination. Fixed rules for setting the **pre-** and **postprocessing** cannot be specified, and the best interpretable picture must be determined by trial and error.

10.2.3 Color Coded Imaging

Power

The signal power should be set to a maximum as standard in order to obtain sufficient reflections from the inside of the skull. A quite considerable warming of the skull bone has been described (Sect. 3.5), but no damage to patients caused by this is known. Due to the pronounced ultrasound absorption at the skull bone, no significant thermal effects are to be expected intracranially. However, a reduction of ultrasound transmission energy should be carried out in two cases:

- **Examination in case of bone defects.** If there is no sound absorption by the cranial bone (e.g., after extra-intracranial bypass operations), the entire ultrasound energy reaches the brain, which can lead to significant heating both on the surface and – in the case of Doppler recordings – in the focal area.
- **Examination of the orbital cavity.** Comparable to the examination with the transcranial Doppler probe, a significant reduction of transmission power should be made here in order not to damage the eye lens.

Display Mode

At the start of the examination, the use of the **Velocity mode** is useful for quick orientation. If required, the user can then – especially for the image documentation of findings – switch over to the **Power mode**.

Size of the Color Window

General rules cannot be given here. Though the largest possible color window is desirable, not least for documentation reasons, due to the long transit times of the ultrasound in the skull, the size of the color window is limited by the frame rate, which – especially when the Doppler sound beam is switched on in **Triplex mode** – can become very low and thus impair the examination procedure. Particularly low-cost devices quickly reach the limits of their capabilities. In the best case, the angle of the color window should be 30–40°, which is slightly more than half of the total image angle of 60° usually used, in order to be able to document both the anterior and posterior basal brain arteries in one image.

Color Gain

In order to achieve a most complete **color filling** of vessels, the color gain should be set so high that single color points are also visible in the surrounding soft tissue.

> **Practical Tips**
> The presence of single color dots in the soft tissue serves on image documentation as proof that the color gain of the duplex device was correctly adjusted in the examined vessel.

Color/B-mode Balance

The balance should be set to maximum color representation by default. Since the cerebral arteries cannot be reliably delineated in B-mode imaging, color coded vascular imaging is of major importance.

Aliasing Threshold

In the first step of each examination, the vessels to be examined must be located. For this purpose the sensitivity of the color coded flow detection must be high. Accordingly, the aliasing threshold should be adjusted to a lower range by about ±20 cm/s or 0.2 m/s. An even lower aliasing threshold usually appears to be of little help, since then the frequency of artifacts also increases, while the sensitivity for imaging the cerebral arteries no longer increases significantly.

Wall Filter
If the wall filter is not already coupled to the aliasing threshold in the device, a value in the order of 50 Hz appears to be recommended.

10.2.4 Doppler Spectrum

Sample Volume
In order to be able to clearly differentiate the vessels, the smallest possible sample volume should be selected. Enlarging the sample volume – as extracranially useful – is of no importance for transcranial examinations, since the Doppler sound beam is only used to "scan" the color coded visible vessels.

Frequency Range
As with the extracranial examination, especially in **Triplex mode** as the combined "online display" of color coded image and Doppler spectrum, only very low Doppler frequencies can be displayed without occurrence of aliasing effects.

> **Practical Tips**
> In order to at least slightly increase the displayed frequency range, it is recommended to shift the zero line of the Doppler spectrum from the center down or up in duplex sonography.

Also, the "quality" of the Doppler spectrum in **Triplex mode** is not very satisfactory. For example, flow disturbances cannot be correctly assessed and the acoustic Doppler signal sounds dull due to the low PRF and often gives the wrong impression of a flow disturbance.

> **Practical Tips**
> Flow disturbances should not be evaluated in Triplex mode, but only be judged with "frozen" color coded images, otherwise misinterpretations are possible.

An increase of the frequency range is only possible by "freezing" the color coded image. This eliminates the need for the repeated build-up of the time-consuming color coded flow image and the analysis time is available for Doppler sprectrum analysis.

With a "frozen" color image, the maximum displayed frequency can also be further increased by increasing the PRF of the device, so that even high flow speeds can be displayed and, above all, measured without aliasing. However, as the frequency range is increased, the depth of blood flow is also reduced. In most devices this is evident from the fact that a mark on the Doppler sound beam moves upward toward the sample volume. The increase of the frequency range comes to an end when the sample volume shown on the screen is reached.

> **Recommended "default settings" of the Duplex Device on the Intracranial Arteries Supplying the Brain**
> - Sound probe
>   - Phased-array sound probe
>   - Nominal frequency < 2.5 MHz (optimal 1.5–2 MHz)
> - Black and white image
>   - Display depth transtemporal 10 or 15 cm, transnuchal 12 cm
>   - Focus range 6 cm
>   - Adapt black and white amplification to the representation of the midbrain as a guiding structure
> - Color coded image
>   - Sound transmission power (Power) maximum
>   - Color window as large as possible (optimal 30–40° = half angle of the overall image)
>   - Alias threshold at approx. ±20 cm/s
>   - Wall filter approx. 50 Hz
>   - Color gain until individual artifact points are visible in the fabric
>   - Color B-mode balance maximum "color blasted"
> - Doppler spectrum
>   - Measuring volume as small as possible

10.3 B-mode Sonography of the Brain

Before the main topic of transcranial color coded duplex examination of the intracranial vessels is addressed, the following section provides some information on B-mode imaging of brain structures. At first glance, this may seem strange to the neurovascular ultrasound examiner. However, B-mode sonography of the brain provides the lead structures for the examination of the cerebral arteries, which should therefore be known.

10.3.1 Ultrasonic Anatomy of the Brain

The temporal ultrasound window is used for the representation of brain structures, the penetration depth is primarily set to 15–16 cm. Of the sectional planes through the brain

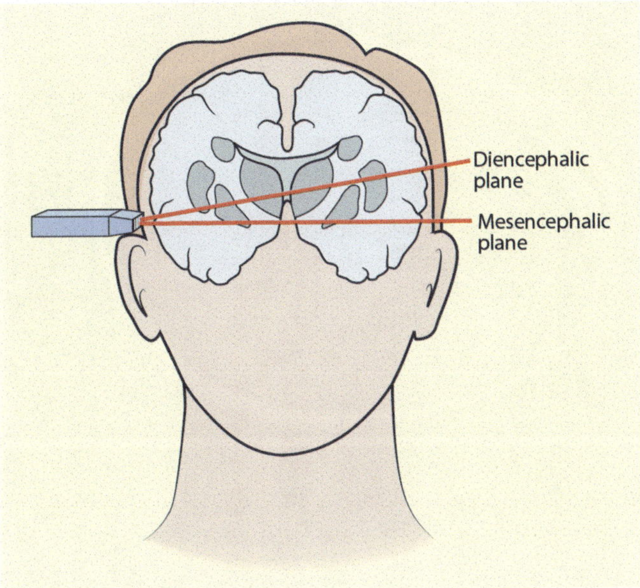

Fig. 10.2 Most important sectional planes in transtemporal insonation of the brain

described in the literature, two are of particular importance (Fig. 10.2), which will be described in more detail below.

Mesencephalic Plane

The examination always begins with a horizontal axial section through the brain parallel to the orbitomeatal line. The guiding structure here is the butterfly-shaped, low-echo mesencephalic brain stem (Fig. 10.3). The two pedunculi cerebri can be defined as the "wings" of the butterfly, the roundish, echogenic aqueduct can be seen in the midline of the dorsal posterior margin. Directly in front of it lies the moderately echogenic brainstem raphe as a longitudinal structure.

The mesencephalon is surrounded by the strongly echogenic basal cisterns and is thus almost always clearly distinguishable. Towards frontolateral, the basal cisterns continue into the lateral sulcus, where the middle cerebral artery is visible as a pulsating line. On the side of the basal cisterns structures of the temporal lobe are visible. Dorsal of the mesencephalon is the upper worm of the cerebellum.

Diencephalic Plane

The so-called diencephalic plane is reached with a slight cranial tilt of 10–20°. The guiding structure here is the low-echo third ventricle in the midline at a depth of approx. 75 mm, which is bordered on both sides by two echogenic lines. Laterally, the thalamus, which is not very echogenic, is visible as a rounded structure. Dorsolaterally, the choroideal plexus of the trigonum is found as an echogenic structure. Dorsal of the third ventricle the mostly strongly echogenic pineal gland is visible in the midline. Frontally, the third ventricle continues into the "comma-shaped," low-echo anterior horns of the lateral ventricle, which are bordered by an echogenic seam. Toward the middle, the two anterior horns are separated by the echogenic septum pellucidum.

10.3.2 Ventricle Width Measurements

The determination of the third ventricle and its deviation from the midline were the first diagnostic applications of ultrasound already in the 1960s before the beginning of the CT era in the form of the so-called **echoencephalography.** Even then, midline shifts were reliably detectable, which of course also applies to the much better technical possibilities of color coded duplex sonography today. Midline shifts can also be easily and quickly detected in the ultrasound B-mode image and followed closely over time, which is an advantage over CT examinations, since ultrasound controls are easy to perform, especially in unstable patients who are hard to be transported (Blanco et al. 2015).

Similarly, the width of the third ventricle can generally be determined without difficulty as the distance between the two echogenic lines of the ventricular walls (Fig. 10.4). According to comparative studies, there is a close correlation between the determination of ventricular width with B-mode sonography and CT examinations (Table 10.1) (Seidel et al. 1995), which may be important for follow-up controls. Due to resolution problems, the width of the lateral ventricle, which is defined as the maximum distance between the lateral edge of the ventricle on the opposite side (!) and the midline (**septum pellucidum**) is more difficult to measure.

Summary

With transtemporal insonation, various brain structures can be assessed by axial B-mode imaging. The most important planes are the mesencephalic plane, in which the midbrain and adjacent structures become visible, and the diencephalic plane, which, in addition to the basal ganglia, mainly shows the third ventricle and the lateral ventricles. The position and width of the ventricles are suitable as parameters for the assessment of increased cerebral pressure.

10.4 Color Coded Examination

Similar to transcranial Doppler sonography, color coded duplex sonography also focuses on the examination through the temporal bone, followed by the transnuchal insonation of the vertebrobasilar junction. In contrast, examination through

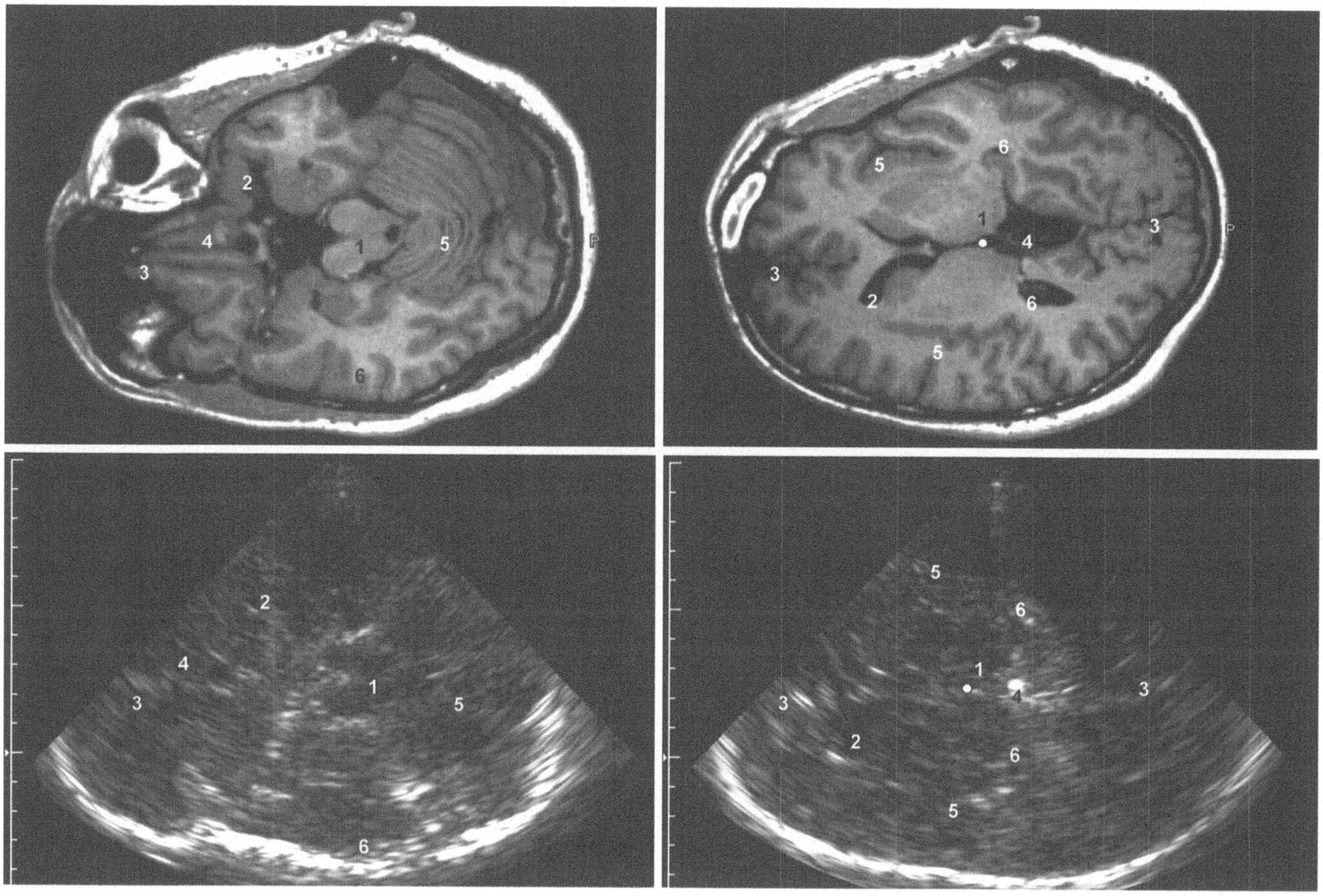

Fig. 10.3 Sonographic imaging of brain structures in transverse section (Prof. Dr. M. Mäurer, Würzburg). Mesencephalic plane (left): 1 mesencephalic brain stem, 2 lateral sulcus with middle cerebral artery, 3 falx cerebri, 4 cerebellar vermis, 5 temporal lobes, 6 contralateral skull. Diencephalic plane (right): 1 thalamus with adjacent third ventricle (dot), 2 anterior horns of the lateral ventricles, 3 cerebral falx, 4 pineal gland, 5 sylvian fissure, 6 retrothalamic cistern

the orbital cavity has no practical significance in duplex sonography.

Transcranial Duplex Examination in Non-Pathological Cases

- Transtemporal – axial plane
  - Locating and optimizing the temporal bone window in the B-mode image
  - Localization of the leading structures (midbrain, sphenoid bone wing, lateral fissure)
  - Color coded assessment of the middle, anterior and posterior cerebral artery
  - "Optimized flow detection" to exclude local flow acceleration
  - Assessment maximum flow velocity in the different vessels
- Transtemporal – coronary plane
  - Color coded examination of the carotid T
  - Assessment of the Doppler spectrum (flow disturbances) in the carotid T region
  - Optional display of the top of basilar artery
- Transnuchal
  - Assessment of the vertebrobasilar junction
  - Assessment of the maximum flow velocity in the different vessel sections

10.4.1 Transtemporal Access

Temporal Bone Window

For the special features of the temporal bone window see Sects. 9.2.2 and 9.3.1. As with transcranial Doppler examination, a valuation of the examination conditions seems to be reasonable when using duplex sonography. This is based on the color coded display of the cerebral arteries (Table 10.2).

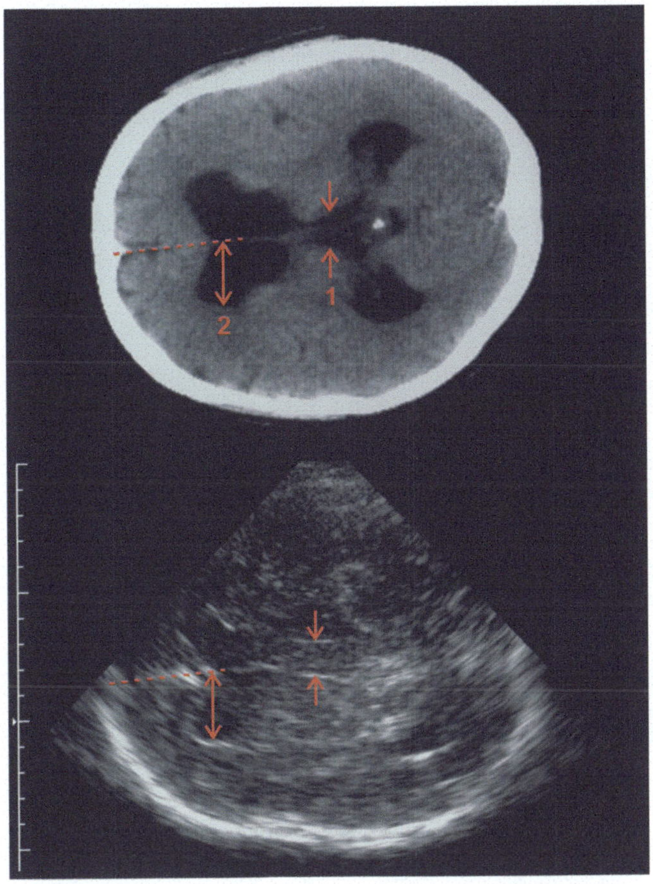

Fig. 10.4 Determination of the width of the third ventricle and the lateral ventricle in an axial B-mode imaging (Prof. Dr. M. Mäurer, Würzburg)

Axial Section

The examination always starts with an axial B-mode image in the mesencephalic plane (Sect. 10.3.1). A penetration depth of 15–16 cm, which includes the contralateral skull, allows a quick overview of all important brain structures. For more detailed examinations of a hemisphere, an imaging depth of 10–12 cm seems to be more favorable, since the ipsilateral vessels including the circle of Willis are shown in sufficient size.

Practical Tips

When starting the examination in B-mode imaging, it is usually possible to predict at first glance whether the color coded examination will be successful or not. If the B-mode image shows clearly distinguishable brain structures and the contralateral skull can also be displayed, it can be assumed that the intracranial vessels can also be displayed in color coded form. If, on the other hand, a diffuse, (largely) unstructured image is found, the bone window appears insufficient, at least at the current position of the transducer (Fig. 10.5). Thus the time of the "blind" search for a temporal bone window, as required in transcranial Doppler sonography, can be shortened considerably.

As in the sonographic parenchyma assessment, the color coded identification of the cerebral arteries is based on the butterfly-shaped guiding structure of the mesencephalon, around which the posterior cerebral artery wraps itself (Fig. 10.6). In the frontolateral structure of the lateral sulcus, the middle cerebral artery is expected. The anterior cerebral artery runs from the main stem of the middle cerebral artery at a variable height toward the midline and is easy to identify by its direction of flow away from the probe, at least in non-pathological cases. Under good insonation conditions, the contralateral vascular system is also revealed, comparable to the examination with the one-dimensional Doppler probe. Only in rare cases, however, is it possible to display the entire circle of Willis in a color coded manner "in accordance with the anatomy book."

Coronary Section

The axial sections are supplemented by the coronary section with the transducer rotated by 90° and tilted slightly forward toward the contralateral zygomatic bone. The sonoanatomical guiding structure here is the echogenic sella region, on whose lateral wall a double contour is regularly recognizable, which can be assigned to the sinus cavernosus respectively to the distal end of the internal carotid artery (Fig. 10.7). Based on this guiding structure, two vessels can be examined here.

Carotid T

The coronary section is the method of choice for assessing the transition of the internal carotid artery into the middle cerebral and anterior artery (**Carotid T**). In addition, it is not uncommon to follow the carotid artery proximally until immediately before the origin of the ophthalmic artery. ◀

Table 10.1 Age-dependent standard values of ventricle width

Age (years)	40 ± 13	68 ± 8
Third ventricle (mm)	5 ± 2	8 ± 2
Lateral ventricle (mm)	17 ± 2	19 ± 3

According to Seidel et al. (1995)

Table 10.2 Valuation of the temporal bone window in transcranial duplex sonography

Valuation	Conditions
Well	All 3 cerebral arteries without difficulties visible
Moderate	All 3 cerebral arteries still visible
Bad	Only single cerebral arteries visible
Missing	Intracranial vessels not visible

Practical Tips
In most cases, the internal carotid artery is relatively straight and elongated in the sellar section. In some cases, however, there are also pronounced vascular arches and loops, which are difficult to classify.

Top of Basilar Artery

Only after (!) reliable identification of the carotid T should an attempt be made to reach the head of the basilar artery by slightly tilting the transducer dorsally. This is typically also a T-shaped vessel structure (Fig. 10.8). However, the basilar artery is significantly deeper than the carotid T in the midline at about 75 mm and there is no close anatomical relationship to an echogenic structure behind the vessel in the direction of sound propagation as for the internal carotid artery. In addition, the basilar artery can usually only be traced over a relatively short distance. ◀

Practical Tips
In order to avoid confusion with the carotid T, it is recommended to mark the expected localization at a depth of 75 mm with a cursor on the screen of the duplex device to locate the head of the basilar artery.

10.4.2 Transnuchal Access

The examination is best carried out from behind with the patient sitting, lowering the chin as far as possible to the

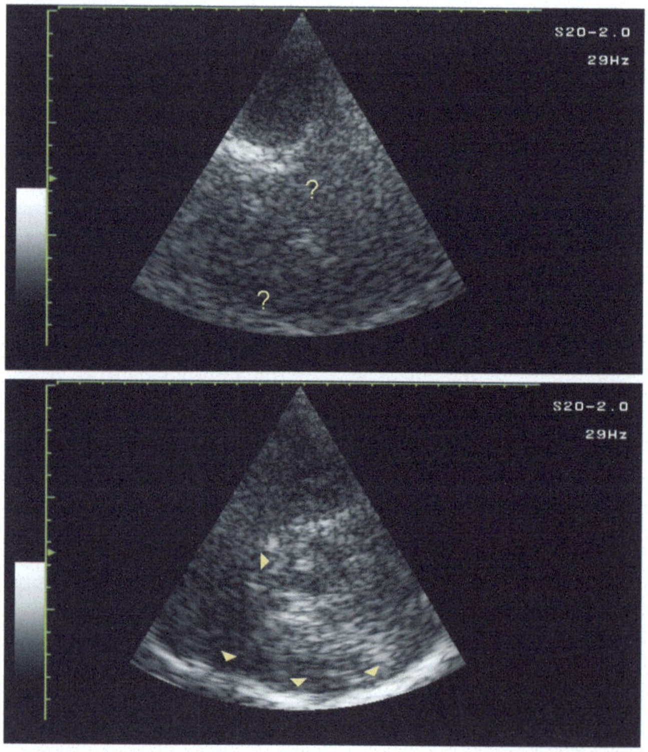

Fig. 10.5 "Prima vista assessment" of the temporal bone window in the B-mode image. Clearly discernible echo structures with a clearly defined midbrain and a continuously visible contralateral skull (bottom) indicate a well-developed bone window, while otherwise (top) color coded searching for a vessel is usually unnecessary

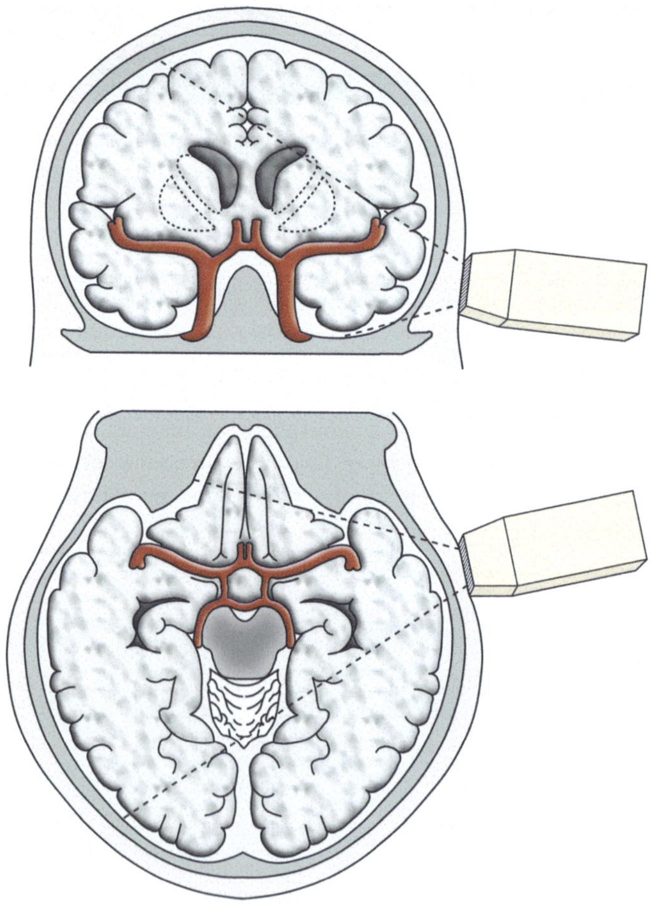

Fig. 10.6 Schematic representation of intracranial vascular structures in axial (bottom) and coronary (top) sectional view

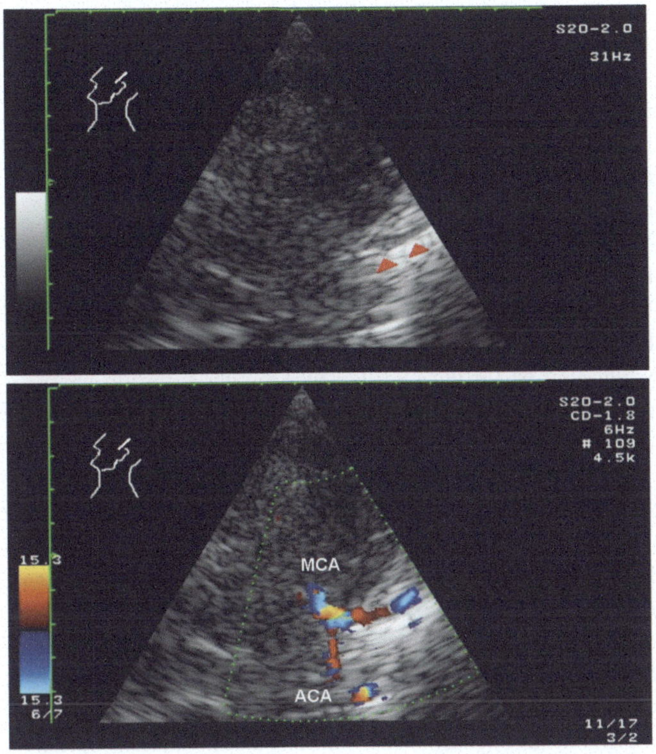

Fig. 10.7 Representation of the distal course of the internal carotid artery within a low-echo "channel" (red arrows) in front of the echogenic sella structure

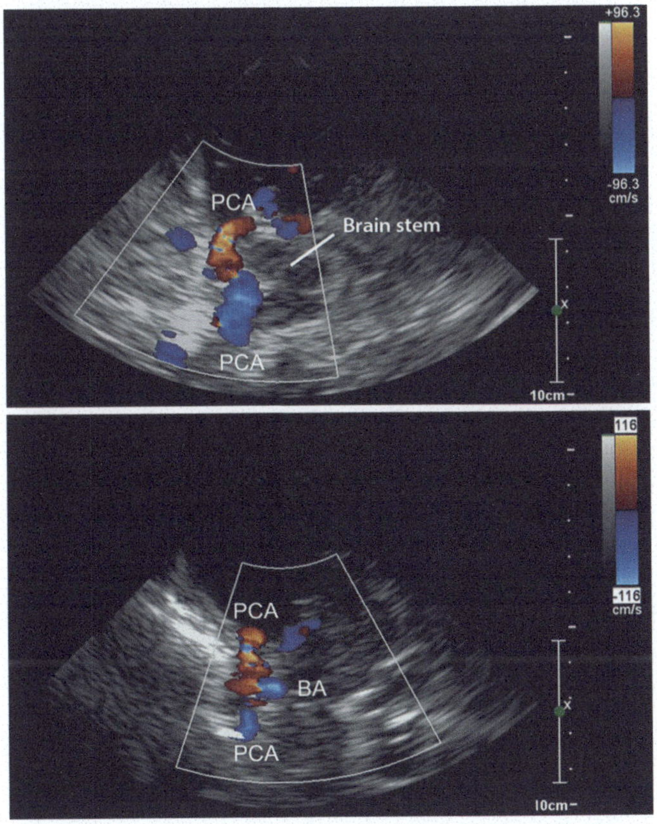

Fig. 10.8 Color coded representation of the head of the basilar artery in the axial (top) and coronary (bottom) section

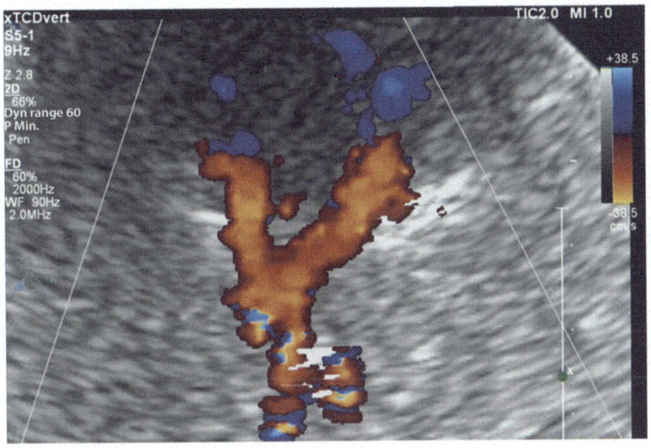

Fig. 10.9 Vertebrobasilar artery Y in transnuchal color coded duplex examination

chest. In contrast to the examination with the Doppler probe, the vertebrobasilar junction when using color coded imaging is usually best shown when the sound probe is placed underneath the skull bone slightly offset from the center line and directed slightly cranially. In contrast to transtemporal recording, only the axial section is important for the transnuchal examination; the depth of representation should be approx. 12 cm. The guiding structure in the B-mode image is the roundish Foramen magnum, which is found at a depth of approx. 6 cm and can be recognized by a walnut-sized low-echo recess.

After switching on the color mode, the vertebrobasilar junction is ideally visible distal to the foramen magnum in the form of a Y (Fig. 10.9). The blood flow is directed away from the sound probe – that is, opposite to the middle cerebral artery – which must be observed. The confluence of the vertebral arteries is usually found at a depth of approx. 7–8 cm, but in individual cases in patients with a strong neck it can be much deeper. The first 2/3 of the course of the basilar artery can be followed regularly by duplex sonography. The distal third of the vessel to the **top of basilar artery**, however, is often not reliably assessable and can only be presented under good examination conditions.

Practical Tips

Since the vertebrobasilar junction is often not sufficiently visible when the transducer is held in the middle, it should be positioned slightly laterally offset from the midline. The smaller vascular branches leaving the distal vertebral artery are also only inconstant and unreliable visible. A vessel that branches off laterally is usually the posterior inferior cerebral artery (PICA), whereas vessels located medial to the vertebral artery (probably) are to be interpreted as spinal arteries.

Possible Errors
Transcranial duplex sonographic examinations of the vertebrobasilar arteries contain several problems which can only be solved in part.

Curved Vessel Course

Especially in hypoplasia of a vertebral artery, the vertebral arteries and the basilar artery show a strongly curved course, which can lead to interpretation difficulties. ◀

Vessel Course Outside the Insonation Plane

It is not uncommon for the basilar artery not to lie in an axial plane, so that the vessel can be detected punctiform when traced cranially and may give rise to confusion with other vessels due to the lack of continuity. ◀

Summary
Transtemporal examination using color coded duplex sonography allows to display all major cerebral arteries in their initial sections. The leading structure in the axial image is primarily the upper brain stem, around which the posterior cerebral artery wraps. In the coronary image, the distal internal carotid artery can also be assessed with the carotid T, and with somewhat less reliability also the top of the basilar artery.

10.5 Diagnostic Criteria

10.5.1 B-mode Imaging

Although determining the width of the ventricle is not part of the standard examination of the cerebral arteries, measuring the distance between the two horizontal borderlines of the third ventricle provides quick and easy evidence of an existing dilatation of the internal CSF spaces. In individual cases, the assessment of the lateral ventricles can also help here.

10.5.2 Color Coded Imaging

Since the resolution of the color coded representation of the intracranial arteries is not sufficient to make statements about the vessel diameter and thus also about constrictions of the vessel lumen, the value of color coding is limited to two assessment criteria.

Localization of the Brain-Based Arteries
Compared to the "blind" vascular assessment with the simple Doppler probe, the visualization of the vascular course represents a significant gain in information. This applies in particular to anatomical variants, which are frequently present in the area of the major cerebral arteries, but also to the clarification of collateral pathways.

Localization of Stenoses
With the help of an **optimized flow display** (Sect. 6.3.2), locally increased Doppler frequencies can be identified, which can be further clarified by Doppler sprctrum analysis (Fig. 14.6).

10.5.3 Dopppler Spectrum Analysis

By examining the main stem of the middle cerebral artery the results of the simple pen probe do not differ significantly to angle corrected Doppler measurements by color coded duplex sonography due to the small insonation angle. In all other cerebral vessels, however, angle correction for measuring maximum systolic flow velocity is of major importance for the graduation of stenoses.

Practical Tips
Incorrect findings can occur if the vessel to be examined cannot be clearly visualized over a distance of at least approx. 1 cm. In this case, a bending of the vessel leading out of the sounding plane cannot be ruled out (Fig. 5.19), which can then lead to inaccuracies in the assessment of the flow velocity due to the angle error.

10.5.4 MCA/ICA Index (Lindegaard Index)

The ratio value described by Lindegaard et al. (1989) and often referred to in the literature as the "Lindegaard index" between the flow velocities in the middle cerebral artery and the extracranial internal carotid artery helps to differentiate increased flow velocities in the middle cerebral artery. In the case of hyperperfusion, a simultaneous increase in flow velocity in both the extracranial and cerebral arteries is to be expected, while stenoses of the middle cerebral artery lead to an isolated increase in the flow velocity in the affected vessel.

MCA/ICA Index	
Normal/hyperperfusion	MCA/ICA Index 1.0–2.5
Stenosis/vasospasm	MCA/ICA Index ≥3

10.5.5 Asymmetry Index (Zanette Index)

Zanette et al. (1989) proposed an asymmetry index (AI) to quantify differences in flow velocity of the middle cerebral artery between both sides, especially with regard to the localization and extent of vascular occlusions in acute stroke. The somewhat cumbersome calculation in the original version becomes more manageable in the case of a modification (AI_{mod}). Thus, an ipsilateral occlusion of the middle cerebral artery ($MCA_{ipsi} = 0$) results in an AI_{mod} of 100%; AI is considered pathological – provided that the vascular situation is unremarkable at the contralateral side – if the AI_{mod} exceeds 10–20%.

Modified Asymmetry Index (AI_{mod})

$$AI_{mod} = \frac{MCA_{contra} - MCA_{ipsi}}{MCA_{contra} + MCA_{psi}} \times 100\ [\%]$$

Standard value	$AI_{mod} < 10\%$
Occlusion of a MCA branchs	$AI_{mod} > 20\%$
Occlusion od the MCA main stem	$AI_{mod} = 100\%$

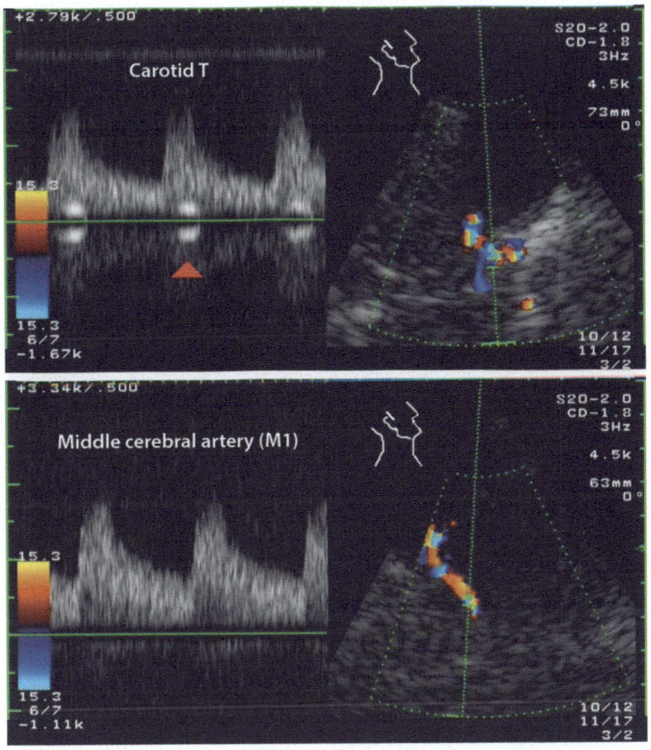

Fig. 10.10 A moderate flow disturbance in the distal internal carotid artery, which is only found in the immediate carotid T-region (above) and which can no longer be detected in the main stem of the middle cerebral artery (below), is to be considered physiological

10.5.6 Flow Disturbances

The distal internal carotid artery is a "problem zone" for intracranial duplex sonographic examination, since the insonation angle in coronary imaging is approximately 90° and thus reliable measurements of flow velocity are not possible. Thus, the predominant part of the sonographic assessment in the carotid T region is based on the detection of flow disturbances.

This is aggravated by the fact that in this area, due to bendings of the internal carotid artery, flow disturbances already occur in the normal case, which must not then be assessed as pathological. "Physiological" flow disturbances in the carotid T are to be distinguished from "pathological" flow disturbances by the following criteria.

Degree of Flow Disturbance

Low-grade and, in the case of vessel branches and bends, also medium-grade flow disturbances (Fig. 10.10) are usually the expression of a physiological situation in the area of the carotid T. However, the occurrence of severe flow disturbances with additional flow components running retrograde to the direction of flow must be considered pathological as an expression of a more severe stenosis.

Expansion of the Flow Disturbance

Physiological flow disturbances are found locally in the area of a bifurcation and/or vessel bending. A few mm further along the distal course of the vessel, however, they have disappeared again. If flow disturbances are therefore still detectable more than 1 cm distal to the suspected site, they must be considered pathological as an expression of a higher grade stenosis.

> **Practical Tips**
> Incorrect findings can occur if flow disturbance is an expression of hyperperfusion, for example, in the anterior cerebral artery, due to a collateral supply of the contralateral hemisphere via the anterior communicating artery (Fig. 10.11). A reliable differentiation is not possible in such case and it can only be argued against the presence of a stenosis "with probability" on the basis of the overall situation (e.g., contralateral vessel occlusion, flow disturbance also in the anterior communicating artery, high flow velocity in the entire A1 segment).

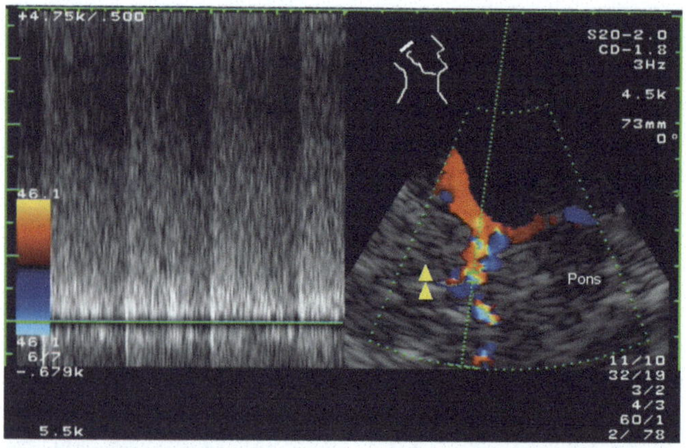

Fig. 10.11 Flow disturbance in the A! segment of the anterior cerebral artery due to collateral supply (cross flow) to the contralateral hemisphere

10.5.7 Pulsatility

Deviations in pulsatility from the normally expected results indicate the following situations:

- **Increased pulsatility** in the main stem of the middle cerebral artery indicates an occlusion of a main branch of the middle cerebral artery.
- **Increased pulsatility** in the cerebral arteries of both sides indicated either an increased intracranial pressure ord a cerebral microangiopathy.
- **Reduced pulsatility** in the cerebral arteries can bei found in the case of occlusion or severe stenosis of the supplying extracranial arteries, especially in connection with reduced collateral supply.

Summary
Since vessel diameters cannot be determined in the ultrasound image of intracranial vessels, the color coded vessel imaging serves primarily to localize the vessels and as a "guide rail" for the evaluation of the Doppler spectrum. The main diagnostic criteria are the angle-corrected flow velocity, the occurrence of flow disturbances and changes in pulsatility.

10.6 Duplex Sonography of the Intracranial Veins

In addition to the arteries, transcranial color coded duplex examination sometimes reveals intracranial veins. A distinguishing feature is the missing or at least low pulsatility. Figure 10.12 gives an overview of the veins that can be detected in individual cases. In view of the diagnostic possibilities of CTA and MRA, sonographic imaging of the intracranial veins is of no practical importance.

Fig. 10.12 Intracranial veins and sinus that can be displayed by duplex sonography

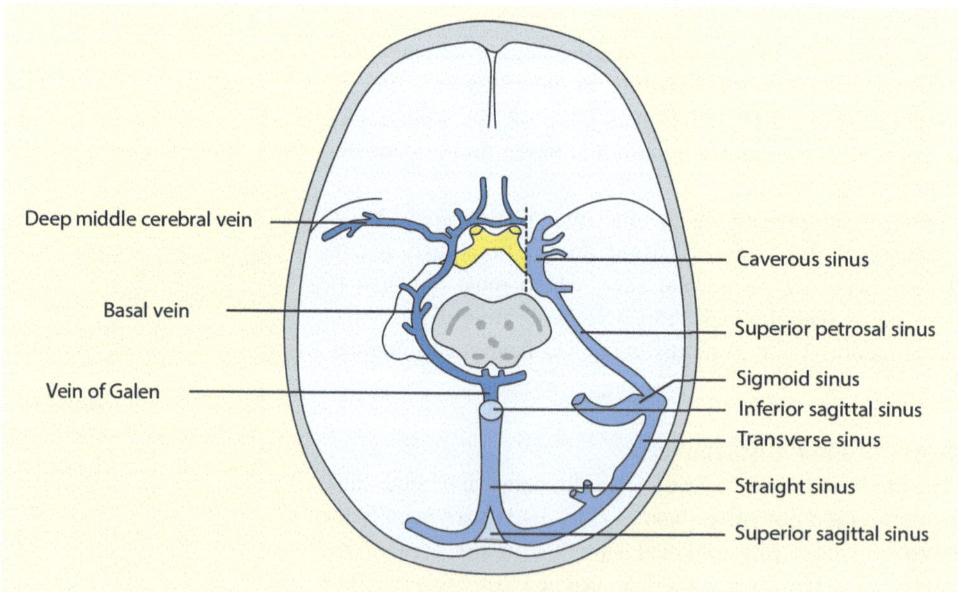

References

Berg D, Seppi K, Behnke S, Liepelt I, Schweitzer K, Stockner JG et al (2011) Enlarged substantia nigra hyperechogenicity and risk for Parkinson disease. A 37-month 3-center study of 1847 older persons. Arch Neurol 68:932–937

Blanco P, Do Pico JL, Matteoda M (2015) Intracranial hematoma and midline shift detected by transcranial color-coded duplex sonography. Am J Emerg Med 33:1715.e5–1715.e7

Demchuk AM, Menon BK, Goyal M (2016) Comparing vessel imaging: noncontrast computed tomography/computed tomographic angiography should be the new minimum standard in acute disabling stroke. Stroke 47:273–281

Lindegaard KF, Nornes H, Bakke SJ, Sorteberg W, Nakstaad P (1989) Cerebral vasospasm. Acta Neurochir 100:12–24

Seidel G, Kaps M, Gerriets T, Hutzelmann A (1995) Evaluation of the ventricular system in adults by transcranial duplex sonography. J Neuroimaging 5:105–108

Zanette EM, Fieschi C, Bozzao L, Roberti C, Toni D, Argentino C, Lenzi GL (1989) Comparison of cerebral angiography and transcranial Doppler sonography in acute stroke. Stroke 20:899–903

Assessment of Intracranial Collateral Pathways 11

Bernhard Widder and Gerhard F. Hamann

Especially in connection with multiple vascular stenoses and occlusions of the brain-supplying arteries or a progression of stenoses, the question of already existing or in future possible intracranial collateral pathways arises. As already described in Sect. 1.8, there are essentially three major collateral pathways (Fig. 11.1), which can be very differently designed for each individual:

- **Extra-intracranial collateral.** Here, the ophthalmic artery should be mentioned in the first place, which is almost regularly supplied retrogradely in the case of high-grade stenotic processes of the proximal internal carotid artery (Sect. 1.5.1).
- **Collaterals of the circle of Willis.** The anterior communicating artery and the posterior communicating artery represent the main intracranial collateral pathways, whereby the anterior connection is usually much better developed (Table 11.1).
- **Leptomeningeal anastomoses**. The anastomoses running over the cerebral convexity maintain a "basic blood supply" to a variable extent when the large cerebral vessels are blocked and are particularly important for the "time window" of thrombolysis and interventional therapies in acute cerebral infarction.

11.1 Indications

Examinations of the intracranial collateral vessels are not part of the routine program of ultrasound examinations of the brain-supplying arteries and are bound to a few concrete questions (see overview below).

B. Widder (✉)
Expert Opinion Institute, District Hospital, Guenzburg, Germany
e-mail: bernhard.widder@bkh-guenzburg.de

G. F. Hamann
Clinic of Neurology and Neurological Rehabilitation, District Hospital, Guenzburg, Germany

Indications for Assessment of Intracranial Collateral Pathways

- Estimation of the risk of hemodynamically induced cerebral infarction in the case of occlusion of the internal carotid artery
- Diagnostic aid for the clarification of occlusive diseases of the brain-supplying arteries
- Risk assessment before ligation of the internal carotid artery
- Contribution to the indication of surgical and interventional procedures in carotid stenoses.

11.1.1 Assessment of Existing Collateral Channels

An occlusion of the extra- and intracranial arteries supplying the brain regularly leads to the formation of anastomoses, which attempt to maintain blood flow in the area of the brain that is no longer directly supplied. The indication for the sonographic recording of these collaterals is mainly due to two reasons.

Assessment of the Hemodynamic Risk
Especially in the case of the relatively frequent carotid occlusions, the question arises whether the collateral supply is sufficient. Inadequate collateral relationships are remarkably rare (Fig. 1.20), but are then associated with a high risk of hemodynamically induced border zone infarction. The method of choice for quantifying collateralization is the determination of cerebrovascular reserve capacity (Chap. 12).

Use as a Diagnostic Aid
The detection of intracranial collaterals is an important diagnostic criterion for detecting occlusive disease in the brain-supplying arteries (Sect. 13.3.2). If a clear assessment of the

B. Widder, G. F. Hamann (eds.), *Duplex sonography of the brain-supplying arteries*, https://doi.org/10.1007/978-3-662-65566-5_11

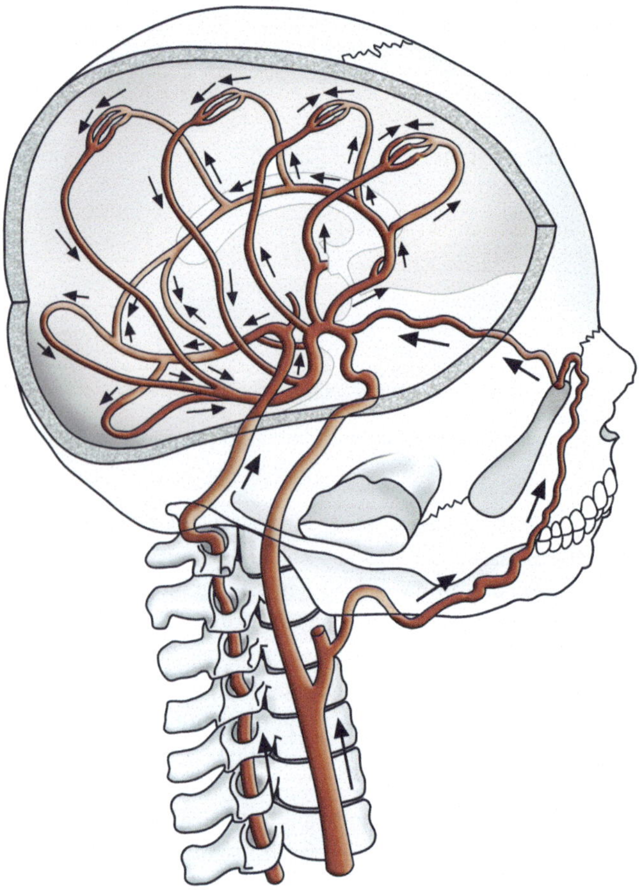

Fig. 11.1 Most important collateral pathways in addition to the circle of Willis in occlusive disease of the brain-supplying arteries

findings is not possible and other methods such as CTA and MRA fail, in rare individual cases there is still an indication to perform carotid compression tests.

11.1.2 Assessment of Future Collateral Pathways

The situation is somewhat more complex for predicting future possible collateral pathways, including their importance for brain perfusion. This question arises in the indication for surgical or interventional procedures in three cases:

- Ligature of the internal carotid artery in tumors or aneurysms
- Ipsilateral internal carotid artery occlusion with contralateral stenosis
- High-grade carotid artery stenosis in asymptomatic patients.

By definition, a vascular occlusion to be expected in the future cannot be clarified on the basis of the currently existing vascular situation, but in this case requires the "simulation" of the occlusion by short-term compression of the common carotid artery (carotid compression test). Due to the risk of plaque detachment or local vascular dissection, which cannot be ruled out, a decision will only be made to do this if no clarification can be achieved by other procedures. According to older studies with large numbers of patients (Zoltay et al. 1987), the risk is, however, considered extremely low, especially since relevant plaques in the area of the common carotid artery can be easily excluded sonographically.

11.2 Examination Procedure and Criteria

11.2.1 Localization of Collateral Vessels

The method of choice for localizing collateral vessels is transcranial color coded duplex sonography. With the help of this technique, both the "usual" anastomoses via the anterior and posterior communicating artery as well as the other collateral connections in the area of the large cerebral arteries, which are impressively variable in individual cases, can be reliably displayed. Figure 11.2 shows typical examples of the anterior and posterior communicating artery in unilateral and bilateral occlusion of the internal carotid arteries.

Other methods appear to be of practical importance only in two exceptions:

- **Transcranial Doppler sonography** without imaging is able to detect with a high degree of reliability a collateralization via the anterior common artery if high Doppler frequencies and/or pronounced flow disturbances are observed in the anterior region at an examination depth of 75–80 mm.
- **CW Doppler sonography of the periorbital vessels** enables reliable clarification of a possible collateral supply via the ophthalmic artery (Sect. 7.3). A retrograde flow ensures the findings of such anastomosis.

> **Practical Tips**
> If Doppler sonography of the periorbital arteries remains unclear, the ophthalmic artery can also be detected directly through the ocular bulb with both the 4-MHz CW probe and the pulsed 2-MHz probe

(continued)

Table 11.1 Blood flow volumes in the main collateral pathways (in normoplasia)

Ophthalmic artery	50–100 ml/min
Anterior communicating artery	150–200 ml/min
Posterior communicating artery	100–150 ml/min

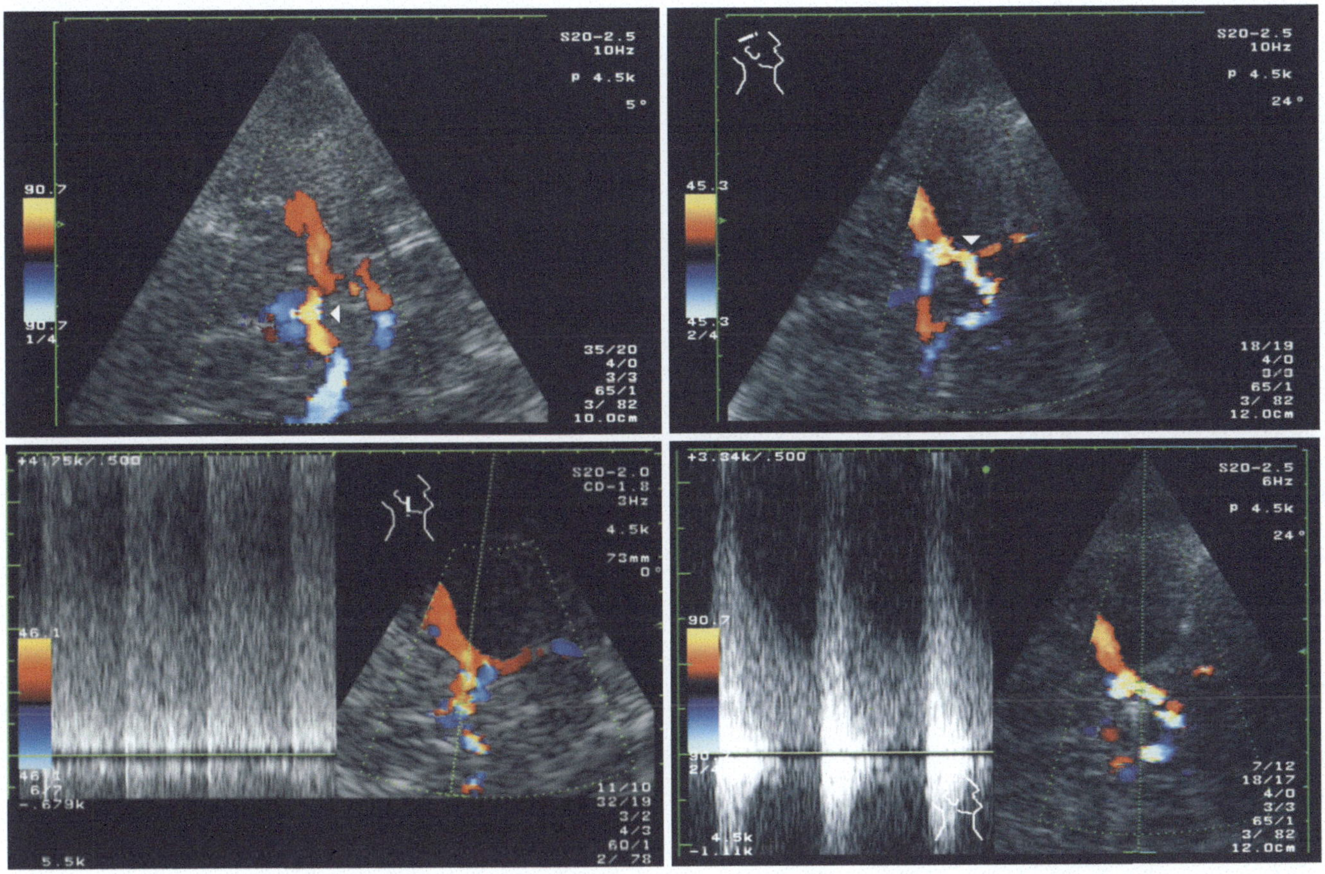

Fig. 11.2 Color coded representation of the circle of Willis in occlusions of the internal carotid artery. Collateralization via the anterior communicating artery in ipsilateral occlusion auf the internal carotid artery (left); collateral supply via both posterior communicating arteries in bilateral occlusion of the internal carotid artery (right)

(cave biological effects due to the high sound transmission energy).

11.2.2 Functional Assessment of Collateral Pathways

Determination of the Flow Volume

Although obvious from a pathophysiological point of view, the determination of flow volumes (Sect. 5.3.3) in the extracranial arteries has so far gained surprisingly little importance for the functional assessment of collaterals in the associated literature. An intracranial flow volume determination is not yet possible for technical reasons.

Practical Tips

According to studies by Eicke et al. (1998), the increase of ipsilateral flow volume in the case of an occlusion of the contralateral internal carotid artery is 30–150 ml/min (normal flow volume in the order of 250 ml/min). Ho et al. (2002) state a flow volume in the common carotid artery of more than 370 ml/min and/or in the vertebral artery of more than 120 ml/min as predictive for the presence of collateral flow.

Cerebrovascular Reserve Capacity

The determination of cerebrovascular reserve capacity gives a quantitative impression of the "quality" of the collateral supply in a vascular supply area. For further details see Chap. 12.

Summary

With transcranial color coded duplex sonography, the collateral pathways in extracranial occlusive disease can usually be clarified without difficulty. In order to be able to quantitatively estimate the contribution of the various collateral pathways prior to a planned

(continued)

operation or intervention in the area of the brain-supplying arteries, compression maneuvers of the common carotid artery are required in individual cases.

11.3 Findings in Different Collateral Pathways

11.3.1 Extra-Intracranial Collaterals

As already mentioned above, the most important collateral through the ophthalmic artery can be secured by the Doppler findings of a retrograde flow through the periorbital arteries. A quantitative estimation could also be made by duplex sonographic flow volume determination of the ophthalmic artery, but there is no experience or standard value available.

11.3.2 Circle of Willis

Anterior Communicating Artery

The majority of unilateral occlusions of the internal carotid artery are collateralized mainly by the anterior common artery (Fig. 11.2). Characteristic findings are:

- Retrograde A1 section of the ipsilateral anterior cerebral artery
- Hyperperfusion and frequently pronounced flow disturbances in the area of the anterior communicating artery (Hensel and Müller 2014)
- Hyperperfusion in the A1 section of the contralateral middle cerebral artery.

However, it should be noted that no quantitative statements on the "quality" of collateral care can be derived from the presence of all these findings. The reason for this is that intracranially there is no possibility to determine vessel diameter. Thus, no conclusions can be drawn about the flow volume from an increased flow velocity. The determination of the flow volume in the extracranial internal carotid artery is more important here.

Note

The detection of hyperperfusion and flow disturbances in the anterior section of the circle of Willis allows qualitative, but not quantitative statements about the existing collateral supply.

Posterior Communicating Artery

Compared to the anterior part of the circle of Willis, the posterior communicating artery regularly shows smaller caliber and cannot be displayed under normal circumstances. A reliable assessment is only possible by color coded examination, as otherwise, due to the numerous anatomical variations in this area, considerable false statements can occur. The embryonic variant of the circle of Willis with an posterior cerebral artery originating from the internal carotid artery (Case Study 18.5) must also be considered.

11.3.3 Leptomeningeal Anastomoses

A direct sonographic presentation is not possible here. Only indirect evidence for the presence of leptomeningeal anastomoses is given if the contralateral middle cerebral artery shows an increased flow velocity in the case of ipsilateral occlusion.

Sonographic Evidence of Collateral Pathways in the Closure of the Extracranial Internal Carotid Artery

- Collaterals via the ophthalmic artery
  - Retrograde supratrochlear (and ophthalmic) artery
  - Evidence of an orthograde flow in the distal internal carotid artery by color coded imaging
- Collaterals over the anterior communicating artery
  - Retrograde A1 section of the ipsilateral anterior cerebral artery
  - Increased flow in the contralateral anterior cerebral artery
  - Hyperperfusion in the anterior communicating artery
- Collaterals over the posterior communicating artery
  - Detectability of the vessel by color coded imaging
  - Increased flow in the initial section of the ipsilateral cerebral posterior artery
- Collaterals about brain convexity (leptomeningeal anastomoses)
  - Increased flow in the contralateral middle cerebral artery.

Summary

The Doppler recording of the ophthalmic and periorbital arteries allows qualitative statements about the most important extra-intracranial collaterals. The

(continued)

collateral pathways of the circle of Willis can be visualized using transcranial color coded duplex sonography.

References

Eicke BM, Meckes S, Tettenborn B, Ringel K, Keyhan K (1998) Indirect assessmant of distal high grade carotid stenoses – superiority of extracranial volume flow rate determination. Electroenceph Clin Neurophysiol 107:P56–P57

Hensel O, Müller T (2014) Strömungsstörungen bei Verschluss der A. carotis interna. Klin Neurophysiol 45:P22

Ho SS, Metreweli C, Yu CH (2002) Color velocity imaging quantification in the detection of intracranial collateral flow. Stroke 33:1795–1798

Zoltay G, Czopf J, Szirmai I (1987) Der Wert des Karotis-Kompressions-Tests für die Diagnose zerebraler Durchblutungsstörungen. EEG EMG Z 18:207–213

Cerebrovascular Reserve Capacity 12

Bernhard Widder and Gerhard F. Hamann

12.1 Indications

The cerebrovascular reserve capacity (synonymous: **autoregulation reserve, vasomotor reserve, cerebrovascular reactivity**) is a measure of the ability of the intracerebral arterioles to dilate further (and to constrict). Since the autoregulation of the cerebral vessels is the main mechanism for maintaining cerebral blood flow even in the event of a severe drop in blood pressure (Sect. 2.2.2), quantitative statements on the function of cerebral hemodynamics can be derived from it.

> **Practical Tips**
> First hints for the presence of disturbed cerebral hemodynamics can be found by observing the pulse curve. Only in the case of reduced pulsatility with a diastolic flow fraction of approximately 50% and more (Sect. 5.2.4) is it to be expected that there is a relevant impairment of cerebrovascular reserve capacity. The pulse curve should be assessed as far as possible distal to an existing vascular occlusion (e.g., in the M2 segment of the middle cerebral media).

Cerebral autoregulation can be disturbed or altered by several underlying causes (Table 12.1). Based on the expected abnormalities in dilatation and/or constriction, four cases can be distinguished.

Reduced Dilatation Ability
In the case of an upstream flow obstruction reducing cerebral perfusion pressure, the cerebral autoregulation attempts to maintain the cerebral blood flow by widening the intracerebral arterioles. However, it can no longer react to a drop in blood pressure by additional dilatation, so that a further reduction in blood pressure leads to a drop in cerebral perfusion (Fig. 2.2). Numerous prospective studies have shown that patients with carotid occlusion and exhausted cerebrovascular reserve capacity have a significantly increased risk of stroke. The assessment of hemodynamic limitations in high-grade stenoses and occlusions of the brain-supplying arteries is therefore the most important indication for the investigation of cerebrovascular reserve capacity (see overview below; Douvas et al. 2016).

> **Indications for the examination of the cerebrovascular reserve capacity**
> - Indications of proven clinical significance
>   - Assessment of hemodynamic impairment in high-grade stenosis and occlusion of the brain-supplying arteries
> - Indications with a rather scientific character
>   - Assessment of neural decoupling in traumatic brain injury and cerebral ischemia
>   - Follow-up of cerebral microangiopathies
>   - Examinations for migraine.

In contrast, minor disturbances of the cerebrovascular reserve capacity are only of minor importance and are not associated with an increased risk of brain infarction. The reason for this is that the brain possesses a further protective mechanism against ischemia due to the possibility of increasing the oxygen extraction rate (Fig. 2.2). If the flow obstruction

B. Widder (✉)
Expert Opinion Institute, District Hospital, Guenzburg, Germany
e-mail: bernhard.widder@bkh-guenzburg.de

G. F. Hamann
Clinic of Neurology and Neurological Rehabilitation, District Hospital, Guenzburg, Germany

B. Widder, G. F. Hamann (eds.), *Duplex sonography of the brain-supplying arteries*, https://doi.org/10.1007/978-3-662-65566-5_12

Table 12.1 Regulation disorders of the width of intracerebral arterioles and their causes

Clinical picture	Cause	Capability to dilate	Capability to constrict
Upstream vascular occlusion	Reactive dilatation	Signifcantly diminished	Maintained
Severe traumatic brain injury, cerebral ischemia	Neural decoupling	Maximally dilated	(Largely) repealed
Hyperperfusion syndrome	Unknown	Maximally dilated	(Largely) repealed
Cerebral Microangiopathy	Hyalinosis	Moderately diminished	Moderately diminished
Migraine	Unknown	Increased	Increased

is removed, for example, as a result of carotid surgery, the cerebrovascular reserve capacity regularly normalizes.

Reduced Constriction Ability

In acute cerebral ischemia and/or severe traumatic brain injury, the control mechanisms of the intracerebral arterioles may become uncoupled. In this case, the resistance vessels are maximally dilated and do not react with adequate constriction when blood pressure is raised or when other stimuli are applied (e.g., hyperventilation). There is a correlation here between reduced dilatation capacity and prognosis, that is, if the dilatative reserve capacity has disappeared, the risk of stroke is increased (Douvas et al. 2016). Due to the associated tendency to develop brain edema, the determination of the cerebral reserve capacity in acute cerebral trauma probably has prognostic significance. An at least similar mechanism is also found in the so-called **hyperperfusion syndrome** after carotid surgery, where a dilatation of the intracerebral arterioles occurs in the first hours to days after the operation (Sect. 24.1.4).

Reduced Dilatation and Constriction Ability

In contrast to the mechanisms mentioned above, disturbances of the cerebrovascular reserve capacity result from primary damage to the intracerebral arterioles. This is the case in pronounced cerebral microangiopathies with hyalinosis of the vessel walls. The reduction of the cerebral reserve capacity is significantly less pronounced in microangiopathies than in the cases mentioned above (Nazzaro et al. 2013).

Increased Dilatation and Constriction Ability

In migraine patients, an increased ("overshooting") cerebrovascular reserve capacity compared to normal values mentioned above is often found in the interval even at low stimulus levels. However, it is not known whether this finding is related to the pathomechanism of migraine or whether it is merely an epiphenomenon.

12.2 Examination Procedure and Criteria

The Doppler or duplex sonographic determination of the cerebrovascular reserve capacity is one of several available technical methods for the quantitative assessment of cerebral hemodynamics. Here, stimulation of the intracerebral arterioles is necessary in order to be able to make indirect statements about the ability of the arterioles to dilate or constrict.

The strongest influence on the width of the intracerebral arterioles is the CO_2-partial pressure of the blood. Thus hypercapnia leads to a pronounced dilatation of the vessels, while hypocapnia leads to a constriction. This results in an S-shaped relationship between pCO_2 and cerebral blood flow (CBF; Fig. 12.1).

If the cerebral perfusion pressure drops due to an upstream flow obstruction, the cerebral blood flow can be maintained over a certain area by dilating the intracerebral resistance vessels. In this case, however, there is a left-shift of the pCO_2-CBF curve, until finally the absence of a change in cerebral blood flow in pCO_2-changes indicates maximum dilated arterioles and thus an exhausted cerebrovascular reserve capacity.

Background Information

A natural prerequisite for the determination of cerebrovascular reserve capacity using transcranial Doppler or duplex sonography is the assumption that the diameter of the cerebral arteries remains largely constant when

(continued)

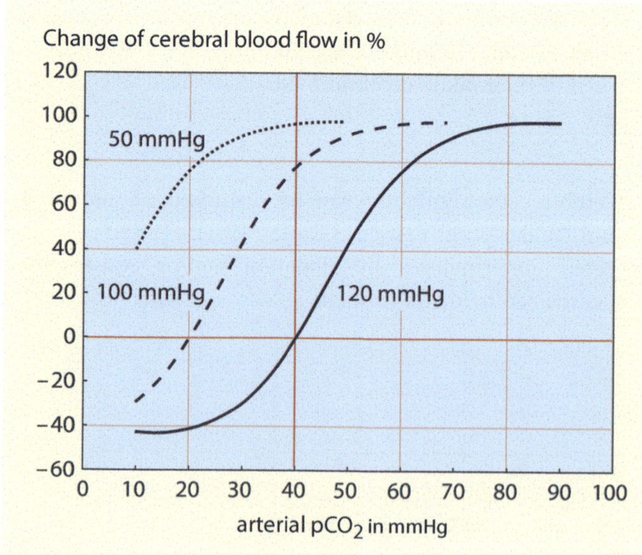

Fig. 12.1 Relationship between pCO_2 and cerebral blood flow at different values of cerebral perfusion pressure in mm Hg

the cerebral arterioles are stimulated. Only then a proportionality between flow velocity in these vessels and cerebral blood flow can be expected. Otherwise a over- or underestimation would occur by Doppler examination in comparison to measurements of cerebral perfusion. However, various investigations were able to exclude significant caliber variations.

Practical Tips

The Doppler findings of the periorbital arteries can also provide important informations about the cerebral hemodynamic situation. If zero flow or retrograde flow can be reliably ruled out (including a collateral flow via the maxillary artery) (Sect. 7.3), there is a high probability that there is *no* severely reduced cerebrovascular reserve capacity (Krapf and Widder 1998). However, the reverse conclusion is not possible, since only a small percentage of patients with pathological findings in the periorbital arteries show a significant disturbance of cerebral hemodynamics. A reduced reserve capacity contralateral to a stenosis or occlusion can be an expression of collateralization with a corresponding impairment of the possibility of dilatation on the supposedly healthy side of cerebral blood flow (Sam et al. 2014). It is thus a genuine "Robin Hood phenomenon," that is, the "poor" hemisphere with a poor blood supply receives so much support from the "rich" hemisphere with a supposed normal blood supply that the cerebrovascular reserve capacity is exhausted.

The determination of cerebrovascular reserve capacity can in principle be carried out on all cerebral arteries by Doppler sonography. Whereas in earlier years complex tests with CO_2-insufflation and i.v. administration of acetazolamide (Diamox®) were performed, today only apnea and hyperventilation tests are usually used, after it has been shown in practise that these are comparably reliable.

These procedures take advantage of the fact that in the majority of cooperative patients it is possible to achieve a relevant increase or decrease in pCO_2 by simple breath holding or hyperventilation. Accordingly, this test does not require any additional equipment other than the Doppler or Duplex device. Two different measuring methods are described in the literature.

Breath-Holding Index (BH Index)

With this method the patient is asked to hold his breath as long as possible (at least 30 s) (Fig. 12.2). The relative increase in blood flow velocity divided by the time of holding breath results in the so-called **BH Index**. The standard value was determined to be 1.2 ± 0.6 (Markus and Harrison 1992):

$$\text{BH Index} = \frac{v_{Apnea} - v_{Rest}}{v_{Rest} \times t_{Apnea}} \times 100$$

v_{Rest} Average flow velocity at rest,
v_{Apnea} Average flow velocity after breath holding $\geq$30 s,
t_{Apnea} Time of holding breath (at least 30 s).

Practical Tips

The start of the apnea phase should preferably be from the middle of the breath. Due to possible feelings of suffocation, breath holding after maximum exhalation is unpleasant for the patient. Holding breath from deep inspiration regularly leads to a Valsalva maneuver with an increase in intracranial pressure. In order to exclude a too low increase in flow velocity due to intracranial pressure augmentation, it is recommended to always wait

(continued)

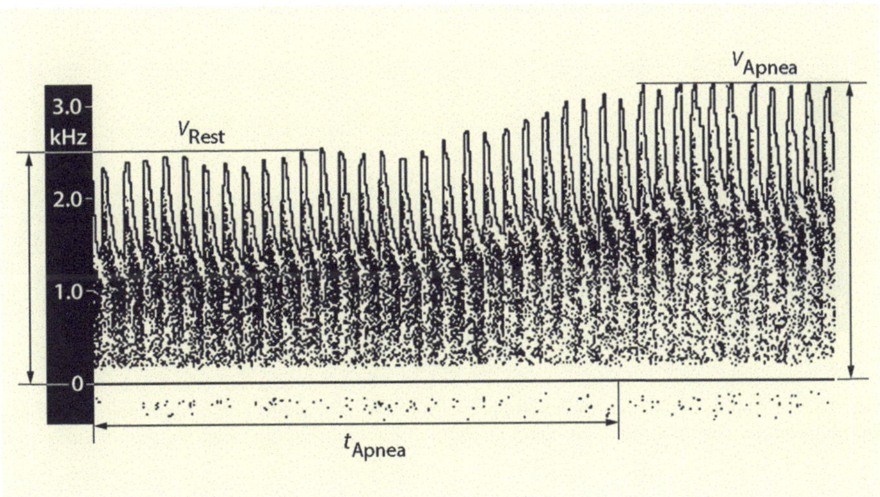

Fig. 12.2 Example of an apnea test in a healthy volunteer. With $v_{Apnea} = 3.2$ kHz, $v_{Rest} = 2.4$ kHz and an apnea time of 30 s the resulting BH index amounts to 1.1

for the maximum increase in flow velocity, which regularly is reached 5–10 s after the end of the apnea phase.

Hyperventilation-Apnea Test

The combination of hyperventilation and subsequent breath holding has significant advantages over breath holding alone (Fig. 12.3) 2:

- **Better compliance.** Some patients are barely able to hold their breath for long periods of time. Hyperventilation is more reproducible and its efficiency can easily be observed by the examiner.
- **Clinically clearer statement.** The reaction during hyperventilation provides better information about whether the cerebrovascular reactivity is completely exhausted or still borderline. According to the S-shaped curve shown in the Fig. 12.1, hyperventilation leads to a measurable decrease in flow velocity in the cerebral arteries in borderline cases, whereas in apnea there is no reaction in both cases.

In the combined test, the patient is first asked to breathe in and out rapidly at one-second intervals or at the rhythm of the heartbeat heard from the Doppler device (see overview below). Rapid breathing has proven to be more advantageous than forced breathing because it causes less intracranial pressure fluctuations, puts less strain on the patient and also makes him less inclined to shake the head and thus change the position of the probe. After about 30–40 s, he is asked to hold his breath as long as possible according to the protocol for the apnea test shown below. When performing the test with transcranial duplex sonography, the three situations normocapnia, hyperventilation and apnea can be recorded by freezing the corresponding images (Fig. 12.4).

In healthy persons the drop in flow velocity during hyperventilation is at least 15% with respect to the initial base value (Widder 1992). During the subsequent breath holding a pronounced increase in flow velocity is to be expected with a delay of 10–20 s, which increases further after the end of breath holding for a few seconds.

In moderate pathologic cases the increase in flow velocity is diminished during the subsequent apnea phase, while the decrease is still maintained during initial hyperventilation. If this falls below 10% of the baseline or even **inverse reaction** with an increase in flow velocity during hyperventilation and subsequent decrease during the apnea phase can be detected, evidence of a highly impaired cerebrovascular reserve capacity is provided. The reason for this "worst case" with inverse reaction is that during hyperventilation, due to vasoconstriction of the arterioles on the contralateral side, more blood is available ipsilaterally via the remaining collateral, while conversely, contralateral vasodilatation leads to reduced ipsilateral collateral supply.

Hyperventilation-Apnea Test
- Measurement of the base value of maximum Doppler frequency or mean frequency
- 30–40 s hyperventilation by rapid breathing (for example in rhythm with the own heartbeat from the loudspeaker of the Doppler device)
- Measurement of the hypocapnia value of Doppler frequency
- Hold the breath as long as possible (minimum approx. 30 s), then continue breathing normally
- Measurement of the hypercapnia value of Doppler frequency 5–10 s later.

Practical Tips

Hyperventilation first and subsequent breath holding has practical advantages over the reverse procedure,

(continued)

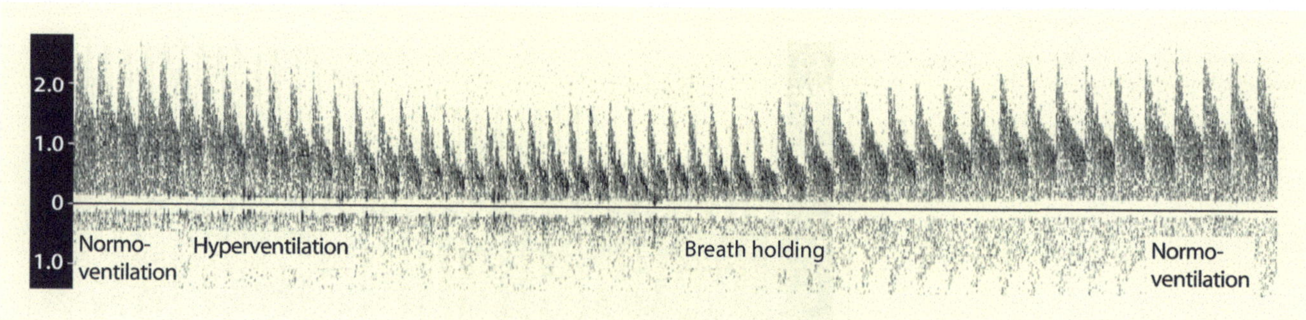

Fig. 12.3 Example of a hyperventilation-apnea test in a healthy subject with continuous registration of the Doppler spectrum of the middle cerebral artery

since it is easier to keep the probe still during the air-holding phase, so that there is greater certainty regarding possible fluctuations in the position of the probe and thus smaller changes in flow velocity can be detected.

Practical Tips
The reaction speed of the brain vessels to changes in pCO_2 plays a significant role in the assessment of the cerebrovascular reserve capacity. For example, after recent ischemia (especially border zone infarctions), a considerable delay of the reaction time of 10–20 s to double or more is often observed, which is probably an expression of metabolically disturbed autoregulation. However, no systematic studies on this are available.

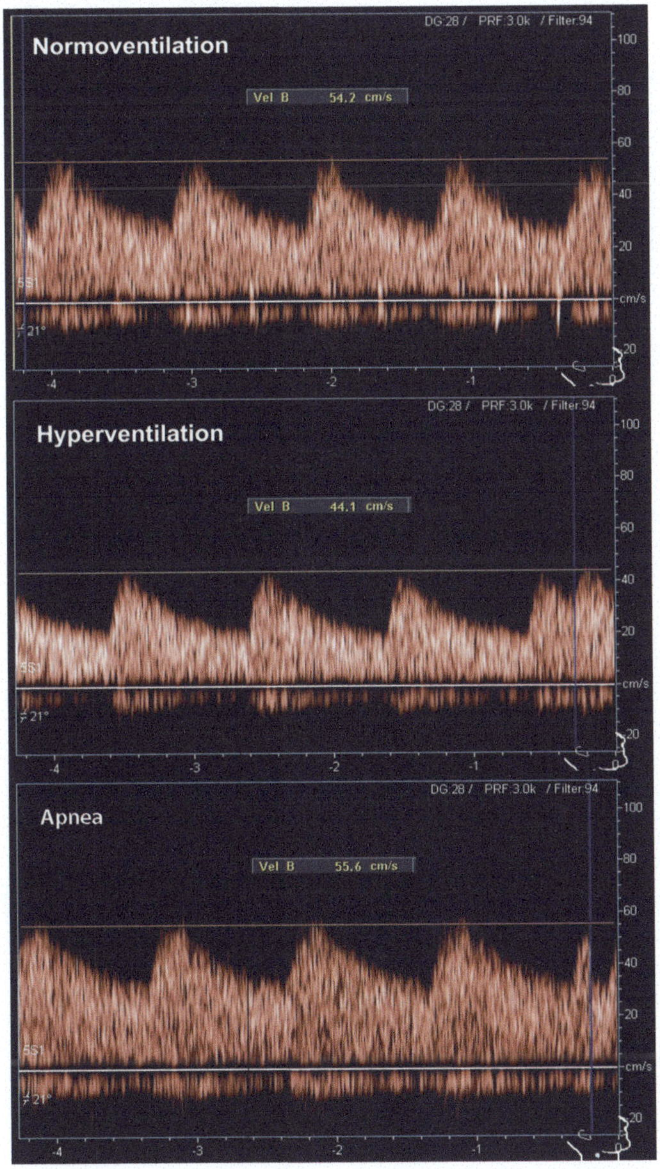

Fig. 12.4 Example of a hyperventilation-apnea test performed by transcranial duplex sonography in a healthy person

Possible Errors

The main source of error in Doppler or duplex determination of cerebrovascular reserve capacity is unintentional changes in the position of the probe. In addition, the assessment of cerebrovascular reserve capacity may become impossible if cardiac arrhythmia is present which cause considerable fluctuations in flow velocity.

Caution is also advised in the first weeks after a stroke. In the case of large infarcts, false-positive values can occur during this time due to the disturbed cerebral metabolism.

Summary
Doppler sonographic assessment of the cerebrovascular reserve capacity requires stimulation of the intracerebral arterioles to change their width. This can be done by hyper- and hypoventilation (breath holding).

References

Douvas I, Moris D, Karaolanis G, Bakoyiannis C, Georgopoulos S (2016) Evaluation of cerebrovascular reserve capacity in symptomatic and asymptomatic internal carotid stenosis with transcranial Doppler. Physiol Res 65:917–925

Krapf H, Widder B (1998) Die A. supratrochlearis als Indikator für die zerebrale Hämodynamik bei Karotisverschlüssen. Ultraschall Med 19:114–119

Markus HS, Harrison MJG (1992) Estimation of cerebrovascular reactivity using transcranial Doppler, including the use of breath-holding as the vasodilatory stimulus. Stroke 23:668–673

Nazzaro P, Schirosi G, Mezzapesa D, Petruzzellis M, Pascazio L, Serio G et al (2013) Effect of clustering of metabolic syndrome factors on capillary and cerebrovascular impairment. Eur J Intern Med 24:183–188

Sam K, Small E, Poublanc J, Han JS, Mandell DM, Fisher JA et al (2014) Reduced contralateral cerebrovascular reserve in patients with unilateral steno-occlusive disease. Cerebrovasc Dis 38:94–100

Widder B (1992) Use of breath holding for evaluating cerebrovascular reserve capacity. Stroke 23:1680–1681

Part III

Findings in Stenoses and Occlusions

13 Stenoses and Occlusions of the Extracranial Carotid Artery

Dirk Sander and Bernhard Widder

The prevalence of asymptomatic carotid stenosis >50% is 2–8%, that of asymptomatic carotid stenosis >80% is 1–2% (Hill 1998). The prevalence increases with age. In a systematic review of 40 population-based studies, a total prevalence of 4.2% was found. The prevalence was 4.8% in men under 70 and 2.2% in women under 70. From the age of 70 onward, the prevalence was 12.5% in men and 6.9% in women. The overall prevalence of high-grade carotid stenosis (>70%) was 1.7% (de Weerd et al. 2009, 2010).

13.1 Stenoses of the Internal Carotid Artery

Since the introduction of color coded duplex sonography, it has become common practice in many places to determine the local findings of carotid bifurcation solely on the basis of color coded information. However, since the internal carotid artery is not an isolated vessel, but rather the cerebral arteries are part of a network and upstream and downstream occlusion processes are also important, this procedure involves considerable risks.

The criteria for stenosis grading were updated in 2010 (Arning et al. 2010), in particular with the aim of enabling conversion from local (ECST) to distal stenosis grade (NASCET) (Sect. 13.1.1). In accordance with the German S3 guideline for carotid stenosis (Ringleb et al. 2012), it is recommended to indicate the degree of stenosis according to NASCET criteria. The current criteria for stenosis quantification are summarized in Table 13.1; an overview of the four most important steps is given in Fig. 13.1.

The numerical values given are for orientation only and may vary upward or downward in individual cases. Relevant deviations are to be expected in particular in the case of contralateral carotid occlusions, very short or excessively long vascular constrictions and tandem stenoses (for details see text).

13.1.1 Definition of the Degree of Stenosis

Although the origin of the internal carotid artery is by far the most common localization of stenosis in the brain-supplying arteries, the definition of degree of stenosis of the internal carotid artery is not uniform in the literature. The main reason for this is that the initial section of the internal carotid artery regularly shows a considerable dilatation compared to the rest of the vessel (**Carotid bulb**). Accordingly, there are two fundamentally different possibilities for assessing the degree of stenosis (Table 13.1) (Fig. 13.2).

Local Degree of Stenosis (ECST Criteria)
This is calculated from the ratio between the minimum residual diameter and the local unstenosed lumen and provides the best information about the actual extent of the stenosis. From the CTA/MRA image, it can usually only be determined approximately by interpolation between the immediately pre- and post-stenotic lumen, since, unlike duplex sonography, the original vessel diameter cannot be detected. The local degree of stenosis was also included in the European study on the surgical treatment of symptomatic carotid stenosis (European Carotid Surgery Trialists' Collaborative Group 1991). This is the basis for the term "ECST criteria."

Distal Stenosis Degree (NASCET Criteria)
In contrast, this is oriented to the distal, non-stenosed vessel diameter as a reference. Since the vascular lumen of the distal internal carotid artery remains largely constant up to the base of the skull, this definition allows better statements to be made about the hemodynamic effects of a stenosis. On the other hand, moderate stenoses in the area of the carotid bulb

D. Sander
Department of Neurology, Benedictus Hospital, Tutzing, Germany

B. Widder (✉)
Expert Opinion Institute, District Hospital, Guenzburg, Germany
e-mail: bernhard.widder@bkh-guenzburg.de

B. Widder, G. F. Hamann (eds.), *Duplex sonography of the brain-supplying arteries*, https://doi.org/10.1007/978-3-662-65566-5_13

Table 13.1 Stenosis graduation of the internal carotid artery (mod. according to Arning et al. 2010)

Degree of stenosis (NASCET definition) %	10	20–40	50	60	70	80	90	Closure
Degree of stenosis, old (ECST definition) %.	45	50–60	70	75	80	90	95	Closure
Main criteria								
1) B-mode imaging	++ +							
2) Color coded imaging[a]	+	+++	+	+	+	+	+	+++
3) Systolic peak velocity at the maximum of the stenosis (cm/s) approx.[b]			200	250	300	350–400	100–500	
4) Systolic peak velocity poststenotic (cm/s) approx.[c]					> 50	<50	<30	
5) Collaterals (periorbital arteries / anterior communicating artery)[d]					(+)	++	+++	+++
Additional criteria								
6) Diastolic prestenotic flow deceleration in the common carotid artery		–			(+)	++	+++	+++
7) Poststenotic flow disturbances			+	+	++	+++	(+)	
8) End diastolic flow velocity at the stenosis maximum (cm/s)			Up to 100	Up to 100	Over 100	Over 100		
9) Confetti sign[e]				(+)	++	++		
10) ICA/CCA stenosis index[f]			≥ 2	≥ 2	≥ 4	≥ 4		

Degree of stenosis according to NASCET [%]: The figures are for a 10% range (±5%)
[a]Detection of low-grade stenosis (local, alias effect) in contrast to non-stenosing plaque, visualization of the direction of flow in medium and high-grade stenoses, and detection of vascular occlusion
[b]Criteria apply to stenoses with a length of 1–2 cm and only to a limited extent to multi-vessel processes
[c]Measurement as far distal as possible, outside the zone with jet flow and flow disturbances
[d]Possibly only one of the collaterals affected: If extracranial examination alone is performed, the findings are less reliable
[e]Confetti sign is only visible when PRF is set low
[f]CCA common carotid artery, ICA internal carotid artery

are either ignored in this procedure or would even have to be assigned negative stenosis degrees. As this was used in the North American Symptomatic Carotid Endarterectomy Trial (NASCET) (Eliasziw et al. 1995), it is also referred to as "NASCET criteria." When comparing study results, the different approaches must be taken into account. Since the relationship between the carotid bulb and the distal internal carotid artery is relatively constant, an approximate conversion can be made (Table 13.1).

Note

In this book, all informations on stenoses refer exclusively to the "distal degree of stenosis" according to the NASCET definition (Table 13.1).

Practical Tips

Following the radiological practice of graduating degrees of stenosis as precisely as possible, the sonographic assessment of internal carotid stenoses has become widely accepted in the German-speaking world in recent years. This assessment is based on 10 divisible percentages including intermediate steps (70–80%). In view of the various possibilities for error, this may not always make sense and implies the problem of "pseudo accuracy." However, if all criteria are carefully considered, differentiated and reproducible process observations are possible in this way. The definitions used in this book can be found in Table 13.1.

Background Information

Occasionally – especially when using the CTA – the cross-sectional constriction is also used as a measure for stenoses. The relation to the surface could be regarded as advantageous in principle, since stenoses are rarely concentric but usually eccentric, so that a too low degree of constriction may be assumed in one plane, but too high a degree of constriction in the other plane (Fig. 13.3). However, this method has not become generally accepted.

13.1.2 Main Criteria for Stenosis Grading

The detection and graduation of stenoses of the extracranial internal carotid artery is essentially based on the use of four

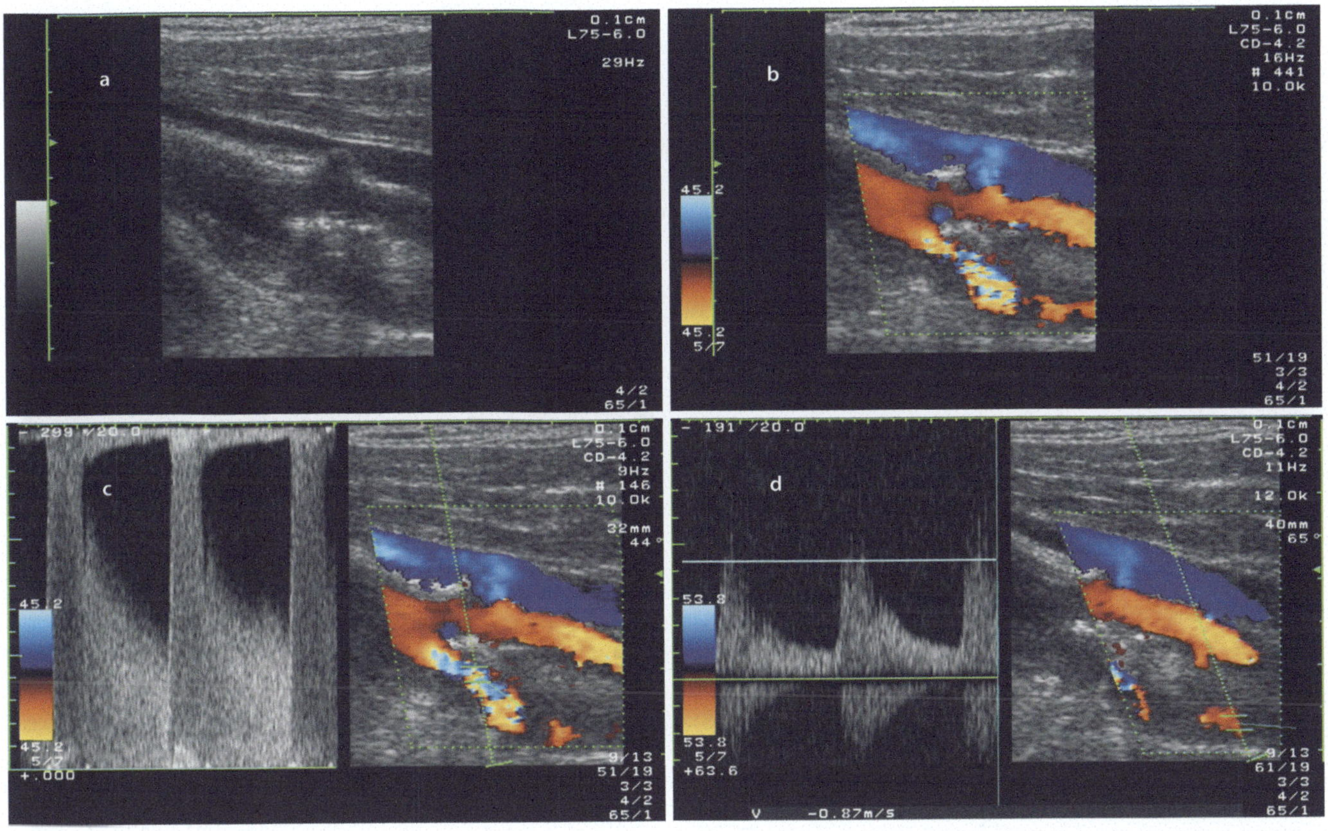

Fig. 13.1 (**a–d**) Steps for graduation of an stenosis of the internal carotid artery. B-mode (**a**) and color-coded (**b**) cross-sectional images show evidence of a stenosis, but a more precise assessment is not possible. The Doppler spectrum at the maximum of the stenosis (**c**) shows a maximum systolic flow velocity of around 300 cm/s. Note the not exactly definable maximum due to the limited frequency resolution of the device and the "co-presentation" of retrograde flow components at the upper edge of the image due to the aliasing effect, which, however, does not significantly affect the diagnostic statement. Together with the maximum poststenotic flow velocity of about 85 cm/s (**d**) a stenosis degree of 70% according to NASCET can be defined. The additional criteria of retrograde flow in the periorbital arteries and an ICA/CCA index of 300/60 = 5 (maximum flow velocity in the common carotid artery 60 cm/s, not shown) confirm the findings of a circumscribed, high-grade – but not yet highest – degree stenosis of the internal carotid artery

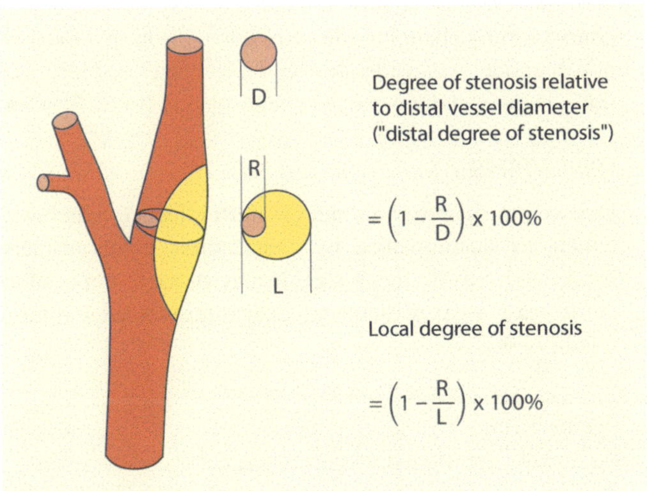

Fig. 13.2 Calculation of the local degree of stenosis and the degree of stenosis relative to the distal vessel diameter (distal stenosis degree)

criteria, which complement each other in their sensitivity and specificity (Fig. 13.4).

Color Coded Display of the Stenosis Maximum

Slight to moderate vascular stenoses can be regularly recognized in the color coded longitudinal image by the constriction of the "ribbon" and – based on the comparison with the non-stenosed vessel wall shown in B-mode imaging – the degree of stenosis can also be determined quite accurately. The same applies to cross sections through the stenosis maximum, which can be used to visualize and grade eccentric constrictions in particular. Difficulties generally only occur when a sound cancellation artifact (**Acoustic Shadow**) prevents the view of the stenosis maximum (Fig. 13.10).

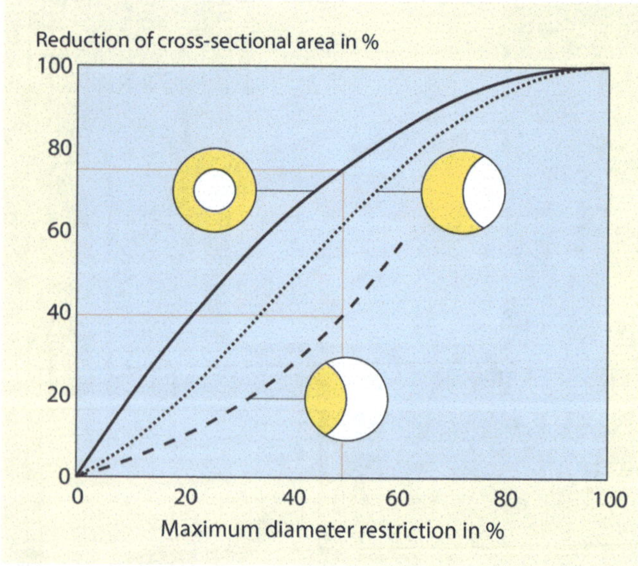

Fig. 13.3 Relationships between cross-sectional and diameter narrowing in concentric and eccentric stenoses

> **Practical Tips**
> For the graduation of eccentric stenoses in the cross section of the vessel, the plane in which the largest diameter restriction is visible is decisive.

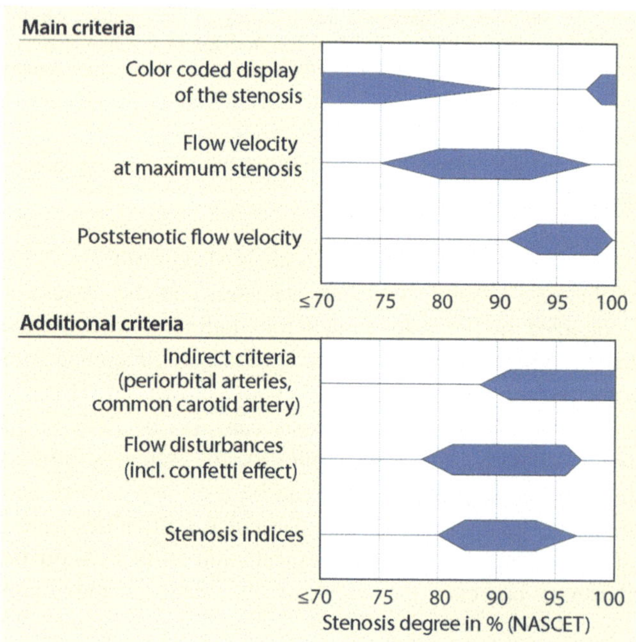

Fig. 13.4 Diagnostic domains of the various sonographic criteria, differentiated into the three main criteria color display, intra and poststenotic flow velocity and additional criteria, which serve primarily to check the plausibility of the findings determined on the basis of the main criteria

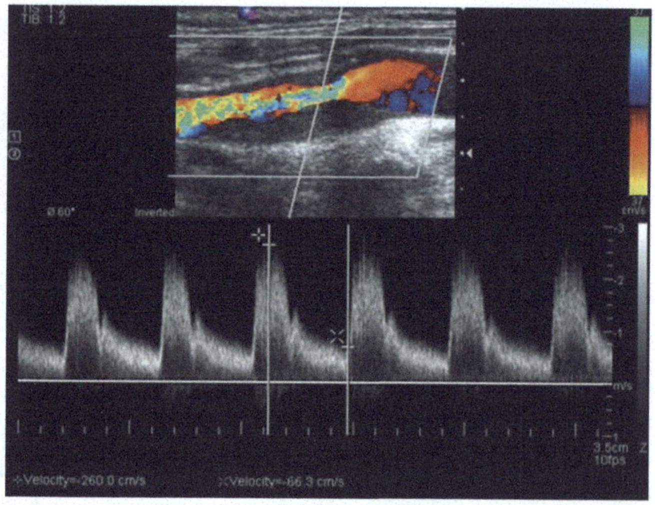

Fig. 13.5 Graduation of stenoses of the internal carotid artery in a color coded duplex image. In the color coded image, the circumscribed flow acceleration can be recognized by the color reversal ("Alias phenomenon"). Poststenotically, a "colorful" color spectrum is found as an expression of a flow disturbance. The Doppler spectrum at the maximum of the stenosis shows systolic peak velocities of 260 cm/s and thus corresponds to an almost 70% stenosis according to NASCET

However, the more severe the stenosis is, the more uncertain the stenosis grading based on the color coded image becomes. The main reasons for this are:

Resolution Problems of Color Coding

As already described in Chap. 6, the resolution of the color coded display is in the mm range. In view of the fact that the residual diameter of a 70% carotid stenosis is approx. 1 mm and the difference to a stenosis of 80–90% is only 0.5 mm, it is clear why the method is overtaxed here. In addition, there is the problem that in the systolic-diastolic course and by changing the color intensification – even in power mode – considerably variable vessel borders and thus also vessel diameters can be displayed (Fig. 13.5). ◀

Color Artifacts

Due to flow disturbances and **Confetti effects** (see below), which are accompanied by considerable color artifacts inside and outside the vessel, it may become impossible or at least very difficult to detect the residual lumen reliably. ◀

> **Practical Tips**
> As already mentioned several times, color coded vessel imaging is able to localize the maximum of the stenosis in higher grade stenoses, if a local alias phenomenon can be detected at a specific location in the vessel within the scope of "optimized flow imaging."

Flow Velocity at Maximum Stenosis

Due to the relationship between the degree of stenosis and Doppler frequency shift, which has already been mentioned several times, the angle-corrected measured flow velocity has proven to be the most reliable parameter for the detection of stenoses of the internal carotid artery. However, stenoses in the area of the exit of the internal carotid artery lead to a significant increase in the flow velocity at a local stenosis level of 50–60% at the earliest. The main reason for this is that, due to the regularly widening "carotid bulb," hemodynamic effects of stenoses only occur at higher degrees of constriction.

Background Information

The equation of Doppler frequency and flow velocity made here is always based on the assumption that the angle between the sound beam and the vessel is in the order of 60°. In this case, a flow velocity of for example, 120 cm/s results in a Doppler frequency of 4 kHz (at 4–5 MHz transmission frequency). Although this "normal" angle is surprisingly often achieved by the experienced examiner when using the simple Doppler probe, the angle-corrected determination of the flow velocity with duplex sonography leads to significantly more reliable results in view of the relatively frequent bending of the vessels.

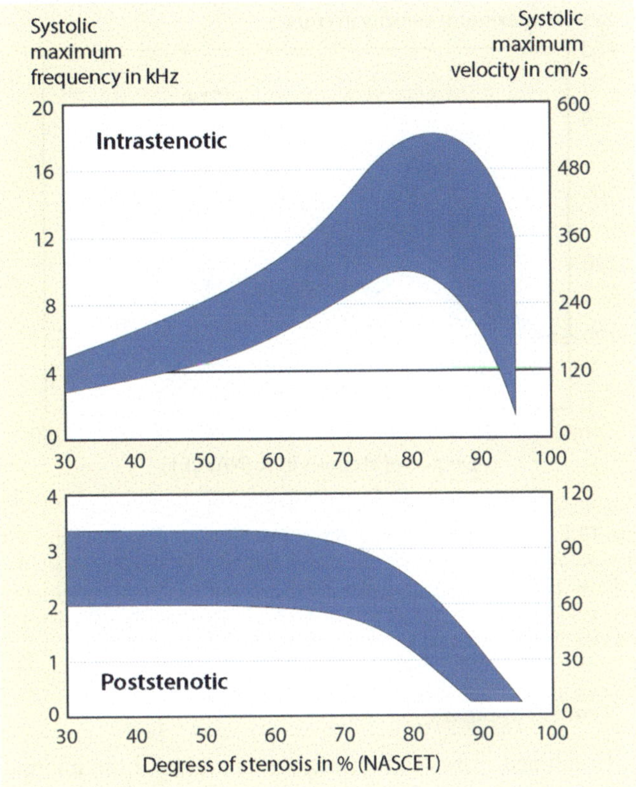

Fig. 13.6 Relationship between the degree of stenosis of internal carotid artery and the systolic maximum velocity (or frequency) at the maximum of the stenosis (top) and poststenotic (bottom). The frequency specifications refer to a transmission frequency of 4–5 MHz. Blue area: Usual tolerance range caused by differences in stenosis length, angular artifacts, physiological expansion of the carotid bulb and changing cerebral blood flow

When spectrum analysis is used, a maximum systolic flow velocity of 120 cm/s or a Doppler frequency of about 4 kHz (related to a transmission frequency of 4 MHz) is considered to be the limit between normal and pathological (Fig. 13.6). Diameter restrictions of 50% according to NASCET criteria result – with a "normal" length of the stenosis of 1–2 cm – in velocities of approx. 200 cm/s (or 7 kHz Doppler frequency), high-grade stenoses of 70% and more lead to velocities of 300 cm/s and above (or Doppler frequencies of 10 kHz).

Deviations from the above values are to be expected in 5 cases:

Filiform Stenoses

Highest-grade stenoses, in which only a minimal blood flow is forced through the stenosis, lead to variable flow phenomena at the stenosis maximum (Fig. 13.6). In this area, therefore, the poststenotic flow velocity gains in importance (see below). ◄

Contralateral Carotid Occlusions

Contralateral carotid occlusions (or very severe stenoses), in which the affected hemisphere of the brain is supplied via the ipsilateral, stenosed internal carotid artery, lead to increased flow velocities, which are 25–35% higher due to compensatory multi-perfusion (Busutill et al. 1996; Henderson et al. 2000). This situation must be taken into account when graduating such stenoses, otherwise a higher degree of stenosis will be described. ◄

Short-/Long-Distance Stenoses

The length of stenosis has a significant impact on flow velocity. According to the law of Hagen-Poiseuille explained in Sect. 2.3, the flow resistance of a stenosis is determined by its length. The above mentioned information on typical flow velocities at different degrees of stenosis is always based on the assumption of a "usual" stenosis length of 1–2 cm. However, very short, high-grade stenoses lead to significantly higher flow velocities, while long-distance stenoses, for example, in dissections, can be associated with considerably slower flow velocities (Fig. 13.7). However, there are no systematic studies in the literature. ◄

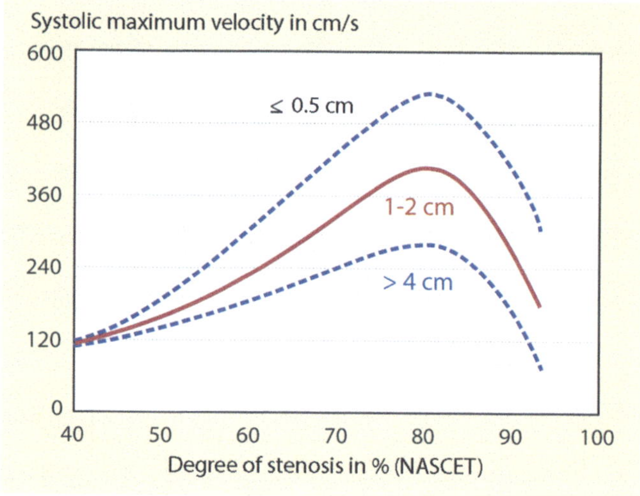

Fig. 13.7 Relationship between the degree of stenosis and the expected maximum systolic flow velocity as a function of the length of the stenosis. High-grade, short-distance stenoses lead to significantly higher flow velocities than long-distance stenoses. In contrast, the difference is not significantly noticeable in the case of less severe stenoses

Tandem Stenoses

Combined extra- and intracranial stenoses of the internal carotid artery can lead to extracranially lower flow velocities than would normally be expected. An additional, more severe stenosis of the intracranial carotid artery should always be considered if the other criteria for assessing the stenosis are more "pathological" than the local findings in the area of the extracranial carotid stenosis (color coded visible narrowing, systolic flow velocity) (**"stenosis mismatch"**). ◀

Narrow Vessels

Slim people, but also smokers, often have narrow vessels with relatively high flow velocities. However, these can be seen throughout the entire course of the vessel and generally do not exceed the tolerance range specified in Chap. 28. In case of doubt, it is helpful to determine the flow volume, which shows normal values. ◀

Color Coded Imaging of the Poststenotic Vessel

In addition to the assessment of the stenosis maximum, the assessment of the poststenotic vessel diameter also plays an important role in the evaluation of carotid stenoses. In comparison to standard values (see Chap. 28), a narrow-caliber poststenotic internal carotid artery with a diameter of 3.5 mm or less (Fig. 13.8) makes one think of two situations.

Carotid Dissection

Not infrequently, extracranial carotid stenoses represent only the visible part of an elongated dissection of the internal carotid artery. Since the therapeutic consequences of this are significantly different from those of the described internal carotid stenosis, such findings should be further clarified by MR angiography in the case of narrow-lumen internal carotid stenosis. ◀

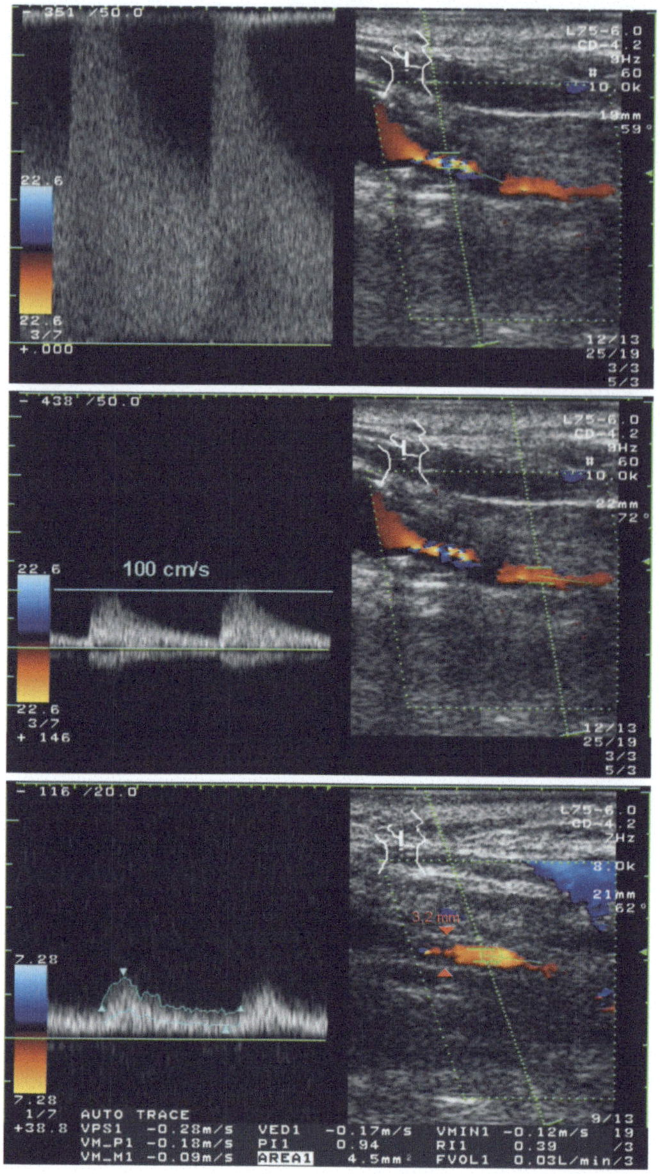

Fig. 13.8 Very severe stenosis at the origin of the internal carotid artery with poststenotic pronouncedly swollen, "collapsed" vessel lumen (3.2 mm) and a reduced flow volume of only 30 ml/min. Note the poststenotic seemingly "inconspicuous" maximum velocity

Collapsed Vessel

If the stenosis is isolated and there is no evidence of dissection (possibly MRA!), a poststenotic lumen indicates that the affected internal carotid artery contributes only insignificantly to the blood supply of the ipsilateral hemisphere (flow volume measurement!) and a significant part of the perfusion is carried out via collaterals. ◀

Note

When assessing carotid stenoses, the diameter of the poststenotic internal carotid artery should always be taken into account in order to exclude a long dissection or an already "collapsed" vessel.

Poststenotic Flow Velocity

The detailed assessment of very high grade stenoses is the domain of poststenotic flow velocity. The determination of the flow velocity at the stenosis maximum fails here and both high and low values can occur (Fig. 13.6). The influence of the poststenotic flow velocity can be calculated in two ways.

Expected Poststenotic Velocities

The maximum poststenotic systolic velocity is typically above 60 cm/s for stenosis grades up to 50%, but drops below this value from a stenosis grade of 70% (Fig. 13.6). To avoid falsification of the measured values due to flow disturbances, the determination should be made as far cranially as possible (at least 3–4 cm distal to the stenosis). ◀

Comparison with Intrastotic Flow Velocity

The nomogram described by Ranke et al. (1995) (Fig. 13.9) was originally developed for the graduation of peripheral arteries, but it can also be usefully applied to the brain-supplying arteries. However, its use requires that the originally unstenosed vessel diameter in the stenosis is identical to the pre–/post-stenotic vessel diameter. Graphic interpolation between the intra- and prestenotic systolic flow velocity results in a concrete degree of stenosis, which can be regarded as quite reliable within the limitations already mentioned. Due to the continuity law described in Sect. 2.3, pre- and poststenotic flow velocities are to be equated. This is particularly important in the case of stenoses at the origin of the internal carotid artery, since the flow velocity in the common carotid artery cannot be used as a reference here due to the different diameter. ◀

13.1.3 Additional Criteria for Stenosis Grading

The main significance of the "additional criteria" mentioned in the following is, on the one hand, to increase examination safety by ensuring that the additional criteria "fit" the main findings and, on the other hand, to achieve reliable results even under inadequate examination conditions (uncooperative patients, unfavorable anatomical conditions).

Periorbital Arteries

Pathological findings in the periorbital arteries (supratrochlear artery) are not to be expected until the

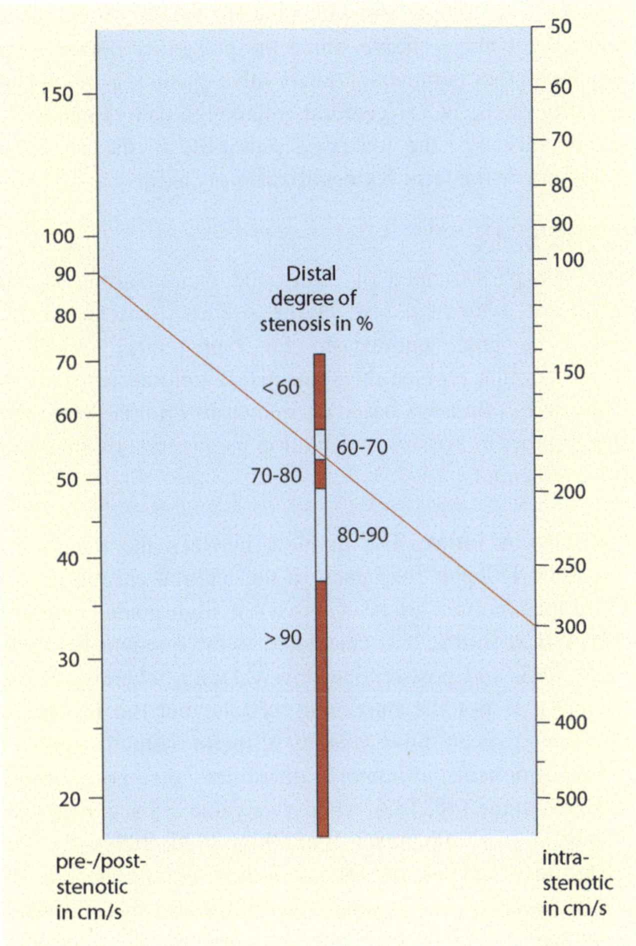

Fig. 13.9 Nomogram for the graduation of stenoses based on the graphic interpolation of the pre- or poststenotic as well as the intrastotic systolic maximum velocity. (According to Ranke et al. 1995). In the example determination of a 70% stenosis at flow velocities of 300 cm/s within and 90 cm/s behind the stenosis

physiological pressure gradient between inside and outside is reduced or even reversed at higher stenosis levels. Experience shows that this is the case from a stenosis level of approx. 70%. With diameter restrictions above this level, a pathological flow signal can almost always be expected.

Inconspicuously derivable periorbital arteries are a rarity in cases of occlusion of the internal carotid artery (and open external carotid artery). Conversely, however, in the context of an anatomical variant, these vessels may show an apparently pathological signal in completely inconspicuous extracranial conditions. Correspondingly, a sensitivity of almost 100% can be assumed here with a somewhat lower specificity.

Common Carotid Artery

From a stenosis level of about 70% onward, the prestenotic common carotid artery shows an increasingly increased pulsatility, which is particularly noticeable when comparing the sides. The comparison with standard values, on the other hand, is not very reliable, since the pulsatility depends on numerous other parameters (heart valve closure, elasticity of the aortic arch, pCO_2 cerebral microangiopathy) can vary considerably. For the increased pulsatility in the common carotid artery the term **Externalization** is used.

Stenosis Indices

Since the performance of ultrasound examinations is not considered a medical task in the Anglo-American world, there is a great enthusiasm for (apparently) objective parameters that replace the subjectively colored assessment of the overall findings based on numerous criteria. From the large number of possible calculation parameters, two indices appear essential:

- **ICA/CCA index.** The quotient between the maximum systolic Doppler frequency in the internal carotid artery and the common artery is above 4 in high-grade stenoses.
- **ICA/ICA index.** It is calculated as the quotient between the intra- and poststenotic flow velocity, whereby, however, it is not the maximum systolic but the intensity-weighted mean flow velocity (**"mean value"**) applies. This quotient ultimately quantifies the correlations shown in the Fig. 13.6, whereby a value >5 is considered to be proof of the presence of a high-grade stenosis.
- The uncritical use of stenosis indices entails the risk of false results if, for example, one of the two measurement parameters cannot be reliably measured due to an "acoustic shadow" or a high bifurcation or if complex vascular conditions, for example, with long-distance dissections, are present.

> Note
>
> **The use of stenosis indices is an aid to stenosis grading, but does not replace the individual evaluation of all existing diagnostic criteria.**

The stenosis indices mentioned are important in four cases.

Progress Observations

Since the absolute Doppler frequencies measured when examining the same patient with different devices can vary by 10–20% for technical reasons, quotient formation has the advantage of providing (approximately) the same value for each device. Especially if different devices are used, it is therefore possible to observe the course of stenoses more reliably. ◀

Primary Narrow Vessels

In adolescents and very slim persons, but not infrequently also in long-term smokers, an increased flow velocity is found in all examined vessels due to generally narrow vessels. The stenosis indices are not affected by this, as they are relative measures independent of the absolute flow velocity.

Tandem Stenoses

In consecutive extracranial and intracranial stenoses, the systolic maximum frequency in the area of the extracranial internal carotid artery may indicate lower values than would be expected based on the actual degree of stenosis. An important component for the detection of a **stenosis mismatch** are pathological stenosis indices in this case with only a moderately increased intrastotic flow velocity. For further details see Table 13.4. ◀

Hyperperfusion

As expected, hyperperfusion, for example, due to a collateral supply in the case of contralateral carotid occlusion, an AV fistula (Sect. 20.4) or after subarachnoid hemorrhages (Sect. 22.2), increases the flow not only in the internal carotid artery but also in the common carotid artery, so that the quotient of the flow velocity is not increased. ◀

Flow Disturbances

As already discussed several times, the – predominantly subjective – recording of flow disturbances is of essential importance in two cases, despite the undoubted preference for quantifiable measured values, also in the area of the carotid bifurcation.

Maximum of a Stenosis Not Detected

At the carotid bifurcation, this situation is particularly prevalent when the assessment is complicated by calcification in the vessel wall facing the transducer (Fig. 13.10). In this case, the assessment must be based on the sonographic findings in front of and behind the acoustic shadow, with the latter being of primary importance. Thus, starting at a degree of stenosis of about 50%, immediately behind stenoses there are regular detachment phenomena which are acoustically impressive in the loudspeaker of the device as "steps in the gravel" and can also be recognized in the Doppler spectrum in a characteristic way. Conversely, a higher degree of stenosis can be ruled out if no relevant flow disturbance is found immediately following an acoustic shadow. ◀

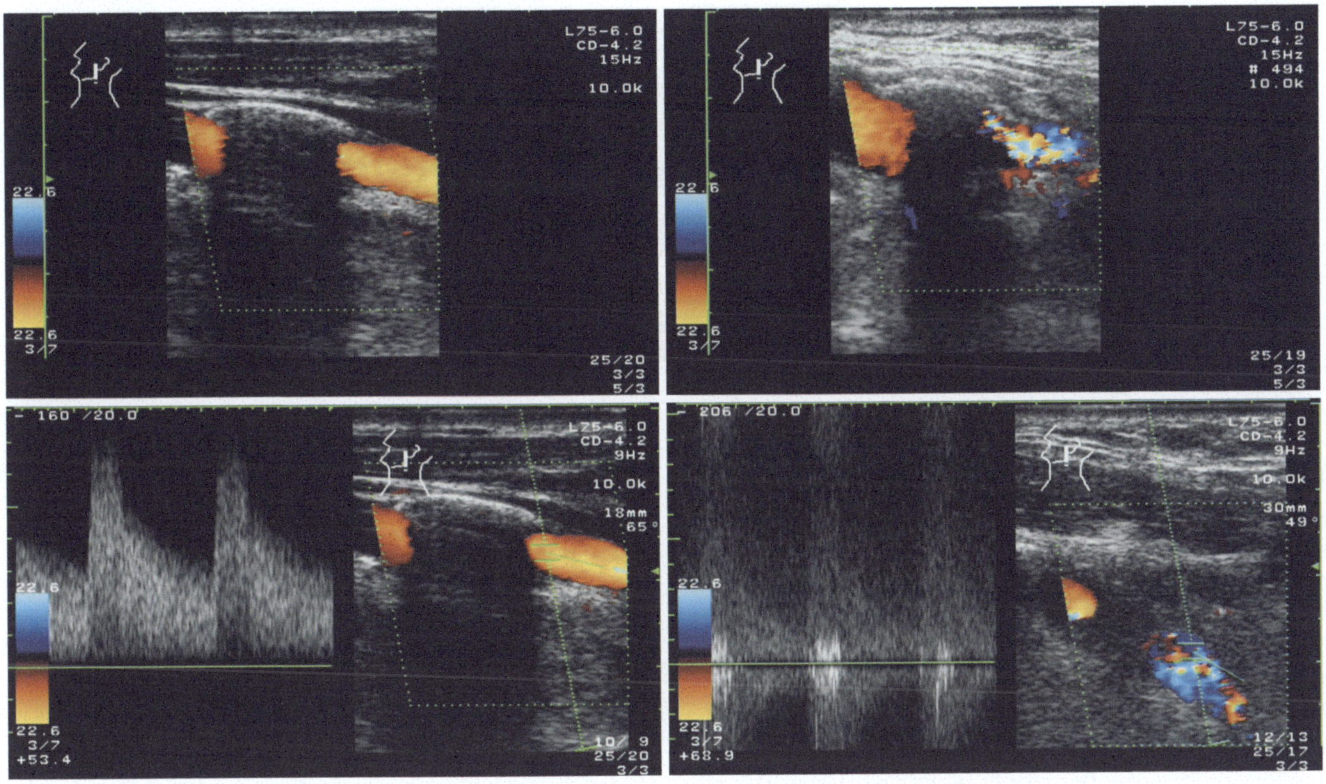

Fig. 13.10 Investigation problems with the internal carotid artery exit covered by sound cancellation ("acoustic shadow"). Exclusion of a high-grade stenosis (left): The absence of a detectable flow disturbance both in the color coded image and in the Doppler spectrum immediately distal to the "acoustic shadow" rules out a high-grade stenosis of 50% or more. Evidence of a high-grade stenosis (right): Alias phenomena in the color coded image and flow disturbances in the Doppler spectrum distal to the "acoustic shadow" indicate with a high degree of certainty a high-grade stenosis in the non-visible vessel area

Heavily Curved Vessel Course

In this case (e.g., with kink or loop formations or with eccentric stenoses) the adjustment of the angle correction cannot be carried out reliably (Fig. 13.11). Correspondingly, additional criteria such as the presence of flow disturbances are necessary to obtain a reliable statement. ◀

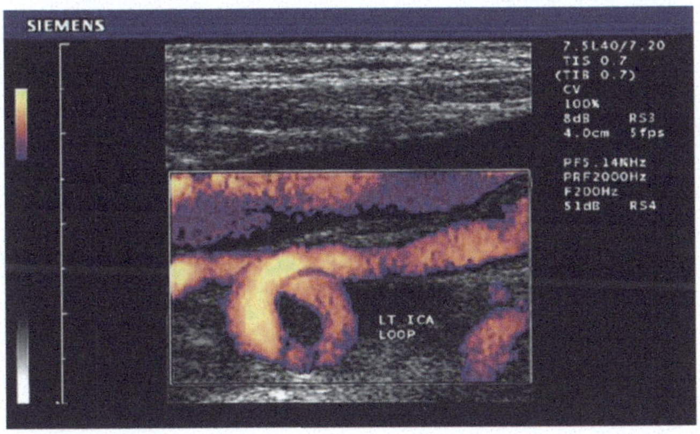

Fig. 13.11 Pronounced loop formation in the course of the internal carotid artery

Confetti Effect

Closely related to high-energy flow disturbances in high-grade carotid stenoses is the occurrence of the so-called **Confetti effect.** These are vibrations of the vessel walls, which are represented as a colorful spectrum of colored dots ("confetti") in the perivascular soft tissue (Fig. 13.12). The color dots typically begin immediately distal to the maximum of the stenosis and spread out distally in a fan shape (**Delta Formation**). According to investigations by Arning et al. (2010), the proof of a "confetti effect" has a very high predictive value for the presence of a high-grade stenosis (or hyperperfusion due to an AV fistula). However, only about 70% of all high-grade stenoses show such an effect.

Intracranial Findings

Due to the usually good collateral supply, a reduction of the flow velocity in the anterior basal arteries of the brain with reduced pulsatility is to be expected at best in very severe stenoses. The evidence of collateralization via the anterior and/or posterior common artery underlines the finding of a very severe stenosis. The determination of the cerebrovascular reserve capacity (Chap. 12) can be helpful in assessing the hemodynamic significance of a stenosis.

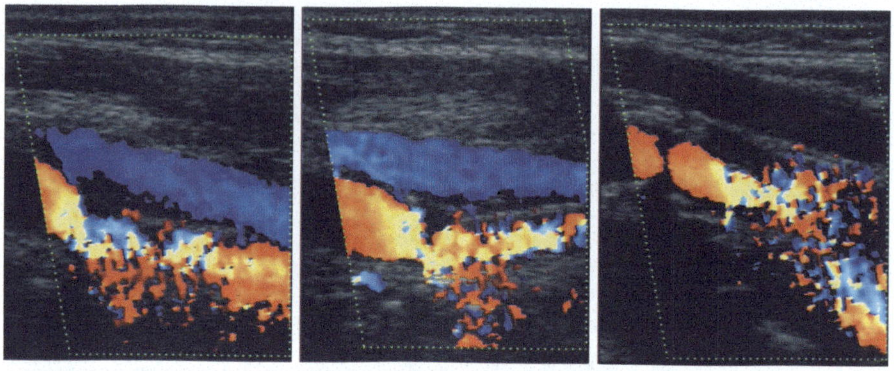

Fig. 13.12 Perivascular tissue vibrations ("confetti effect") in the area of high-grade carotid stenoses

13.1.4 Comparison with Other Methods

For the detection and quantification of extracranial carotid stenoses, various methods are available, each with their own advantages and disadvantages. The sensitivity and specificity of the different methods are summarized in Table 13.2 (Wardlaw et al. 2006).

Ultrasound
Even with simple Doppler methods, the quantification of the degree of stenosis and the localization of the extracranial vascular process can be reliably performed. Using B-mode imaging and color coded duplex techniques, the morphology and extent of the pathology causing the stenosis can also be assessed. In addition, transcranial Doppler/duplex sonography allows the assessment of hemodynamic compensation.

CT Angiography (CTA)
The CTA measures the morphological diameter of the carotid stenosis and is therefore not based on a flow phenomenon, in contrast to ultrasound and MRA. It requires the application of relatively high doses of contrast medium and is therefore subject to restrictions. Due to the high contrast between the vessel lumen, vessel wall and surrounding soft tissue, occlusions can be better identified with CTA than with ultrasound or MRA, but stenoses are overestimated, especially in the case of high calcium content.

MR Angiography (MRA)
MRA is also a non-invasive and therefore harmless method. The susceptibility to artifacts caused by bone and air is less than with CTA and less dependent on the examiner than ultrasound. However, the spatial resolution is limited and both the extent and length of the stenosis can be overestimated. The introduction of contrast-enhanced techniques has increased the informative value (Table 13.2).

Digital Subtraction Angiography (DSA)
In principle, the DSA continues to be the reference standard. However, as an invasive, also contrast-agent-dependent technique, the risk even of purely diagnostic angiography should not be neglected.

13.1.5 Follow-up Monitoring

There are no uniform criteria in the literature for observing the course of internal carotid stenosis. There is only agreement that the most sensitive and most reproducible parameter, the maximum systolic flow velocity, should be used to assess the possible progression of stenoses. This is least influenced by the device used. In contrast, color coded vascular lumen imaging is considered much less reproducible for higher-grade stenoses, although systematic studies on this are hardly ever available.

Table 13.2 Sensitivity and specificity of non-invasive diagnostic procedures for the quantification of carotid stenosis in comparison to digital subtraction angiography (AI confidence interval; according to Wardlaw et al. 2006)

Degree of stenosis	Ultrasound	CTA	MRA	MRA with contrast medium
70–99%				
Sensitivity (95% KI)	0.89 (0.85–0.92)	0.77 (0.68–0.84)	0.88 (0.82–0.92)	0.94 (0.88–0.97)
Specificity (95% KI)	0.84 (0.77–0.89)	0.95 (0.91–0.97)	0.84 (0.76–0.97)	0.93 (0.89–0.96)
50–69%				
Sensitivity (95% KI)	0.36 (0.25–0.49)	0.67 (0.3–0.9)	0.37 (0.26–0.49)	0.77 (0.59–0.89)
Specificity (95% KI)	0.91 (0.87–0.94)	0.79 (0.63–0.89)	0.91 (0.78–0.97)	0.97 (0.93–0.99)

Table 13.3 Misinterpretation in the Doppler and duplex sonographic assessment of stenoses at the origin of the internal carotid artery

Assessment	Error source
Stenosis degree too high estimated	Hyperperfusion (e.g., for contralateral carotid occlusion)
	Total narrow vessels
	Very short stenosis
Degree of stenosis underestimated	Oblong stenosis
	Additional intracranial stenosis (“tandem stenosis”)
	Reduced cardiac output per minute

13.1.6 Possible Errors

In order to correctly classify ultrasound findings, it is important to know possible sources of error during stenosis grading. These can be caused by the patient and his specific vascular situation as well as by the examiner. Ultimately, the only ones to be avoided are those resulting from incorrect handling of the examination equipment. In all other cases it is important for the examiner to know the possible errors in order to be able to clarify them reliably by using other examination criteria and/or methods.

Patient-Related Sources of Error

In addition to a corpulent neck, an immobile cervical spine and lack of compliance, these include above all anatomical norm variants and various complex vascular situations that can lead to an over- or underestimation of stenoses (Table 13.3).

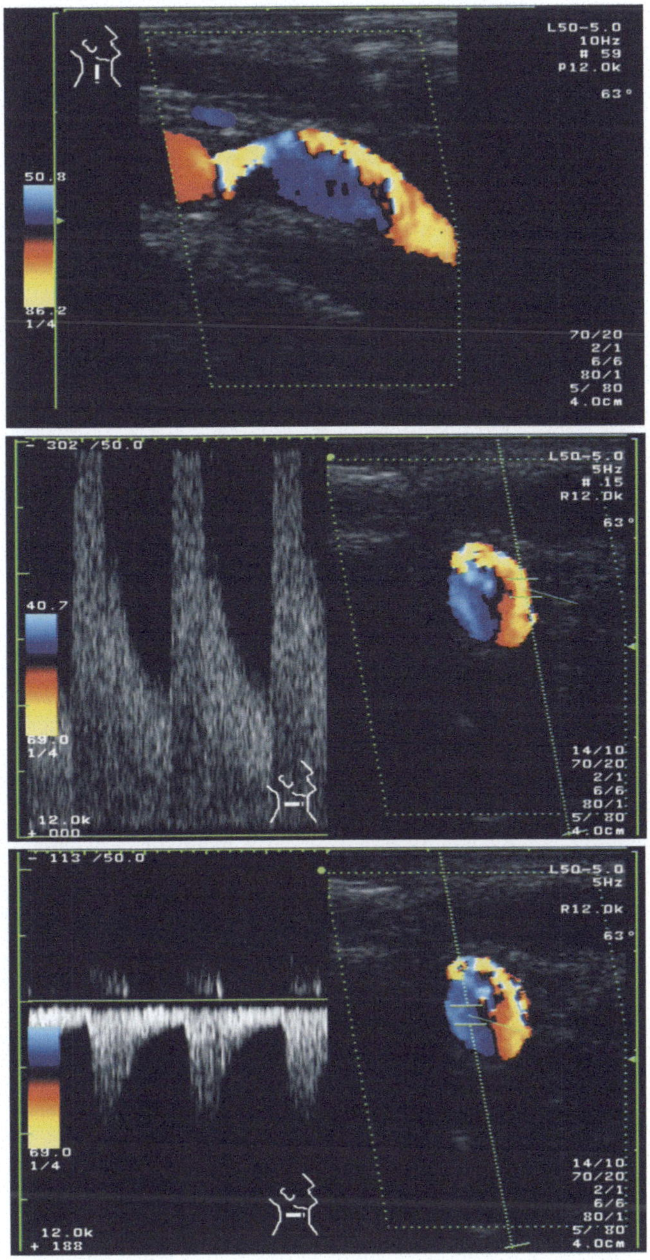

Fig. 13.13 Pronounced twisted flow behind a very short carotid stenosis in longitudinal and cross-sectional view. Note the “jet” with high flow velocity still detectable 2–3 cm distal to the stenosis and the lower frequency “twisted” component

Short-Distance Stenosis

High-grade, very short-distance stenoses with a total length < 1 cm are often overestimated because they can lead to significantly higher flow velocities compared to long-distance stenoses with the same degree of constriction (Fig. 13.7). In addition, very short-stretched stenoses are regularly characterized by a pronounced, narrowly limited **jet flow** reaching far into the poststenotic lumen with a slow, twisted flow in the remaining vessel lumen (Fig. 13.13). Especially in cross section, this situation can be confused with local vascular dissection. ◀

Acoustic Shadow

As already described several times, sound cancellation phenomena can prevent the view of the stenosis maximum. In this case, a classification of the degree of stenosis into “higher grade” and “not higher grade” is only possible on the basis of the evaluation of poststenotic flow disturbances (Fig. 13.10). ◀

Tandem Stenosis

Additional stenoses upstream or downstream of the carotid artery may lead to an underestimation of the local narrowing at the extracranial internal carotid artery. In this

Table 13.4 Indications of a high-grade intracranial tandem stenosis, which, in the case of a not yet high-grade exit stenosis of the internal carotid artery, indicate a high-grade distal flow obstruction ("stenosis mismatch")

Local findings	Not yet high-grade appearing stenosis with an intrastotic systolic flow velocity <250 cm/s
Mismatch criteria	Pathological periorbital arteries
	Increased pulsatility in the common carotid artery compared to the sides
	ICA/CCA index ≥4
	Poststenotic flow velocity <60 cm/s
	Reduced flow volume in the poststenotic internal carotid artery

case, the two stenoses are to be regarded as a series of two flow resistances. The more pronounced the additional stenosis is, the more there is a drop in flow velocity in the constriction to be assessed. Indications for the most important case of a higher degree of intracranial tandem stenosis are given by the already mentioned "**stenosis mismatch**" with non-matching sonographic findings (Table 13.4). ◄

Collateralisation

As expected, the flow velocity in carotid stenosis increases when the affected vessel contributes to the collateral supply of the contralateral hemisphere. In this case, the degree of stenosis is overestimated if the maximum flow velocity is considered uncritically. ◄

Primary Slim Vessel

If the vessel is already primarily slender or narrow, the graduation of stenoses based on the flow velocity leads to an overestimation (Fig. 13.14). The stenosis indices, which are independent of absolute values of the flow velocity, are helpful in this situation. ◄

Eccentric Stenosis

In the case of eccentric, short-distance stenoses, considerable problems can arise with the correct setting of the angle correction. In this case, all conceivable variants of the angle correction should be "played through" in order to obtain an impression of the error width when determining the flow velocity (Fig. 13.15). ◄

Investigator-Related Sources of Error

The three most important avoidable errors are:

Incorrect Insonation Angle

Forgetting (!) an angle correction, the use of a insonation angle of 70° and more as well as an incorrect setting of the angle correction are probably the most common mistakes in practice. The latter are most likely to occur if either the vessel is not shown in longitudinal section as a band over a sufficiently long distance (Fig. 13.15), or if the angle correction is placed without critical examination of various angle settings in the case of curved vessel courses and eccentric stenoses (Fig. 13.16). ◄

Inconclusive Findings

A further important quality criterion of ultrasound examination of the arteries supplying the brain is the combination of numerous direct and indirect diagnostic parameters. Taking only one parameter into account without considering the actually self-evident requirement that findings must be conclusive in themselves can lead to considerable misinterpretations, which then wrongly discredit the method. This point, too, can be regularly checked on the basis of the image and findings documentation and represents a building block of formal quality control.

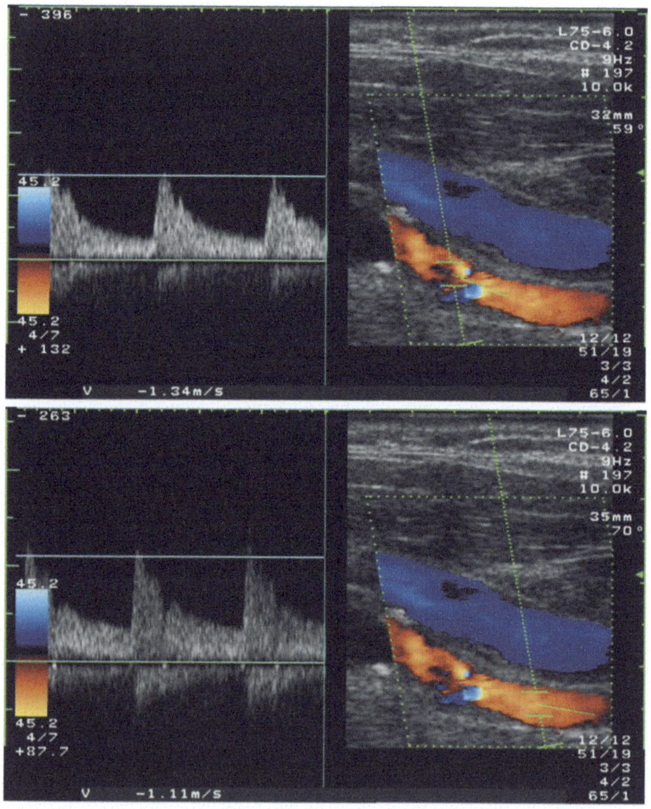

Fig. 13.14 "Pseudostenosis" of the internal carotid. A slight aliasing effect – probably caused by a steeper insonation angle in the color window – suggests the presence of a stenosis. Determination of the maximum systolic flow velocity results in about 135 cm/s, which could correspond to a moderate stenosis according to the Table 13.1. However, a comparison with the flow velocity further distal shows that relatively high flow velocities are present overall, so that the findings of a relevant stenosis cannot be confirmed with certainty (ICA/CCA-Index <2)

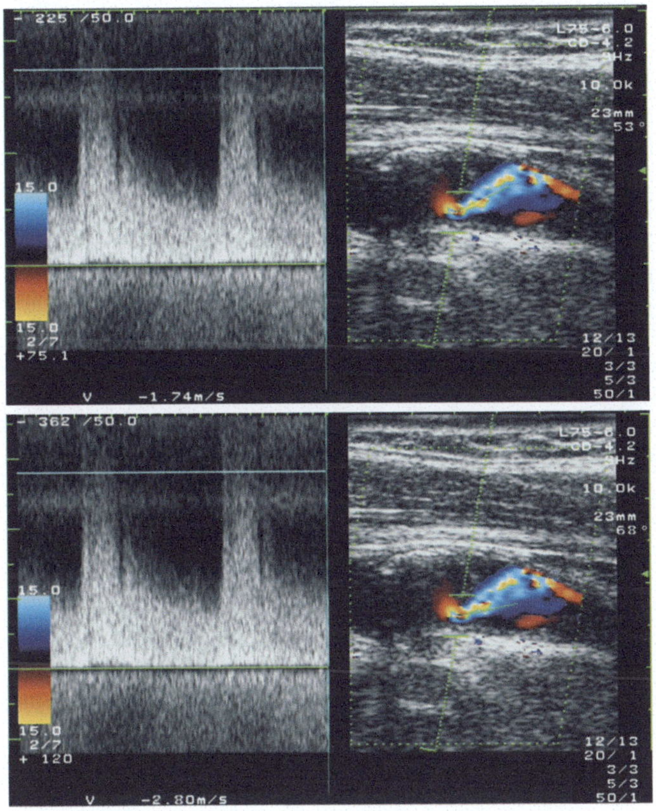

Fig. 13.15 Short, eccentric stenosis at the outflow of the internal carotid artery. Even with a caudally tilted color window and a "favorable" angle of incidence, flow velocities of between 170 and 280 cm/s are obtained, depending on the assessment of the course of the stenosis. With this unavoidable problem, it is essential for the examiner to know the possible "margin" of the flow values and to interpret them together with other criteria

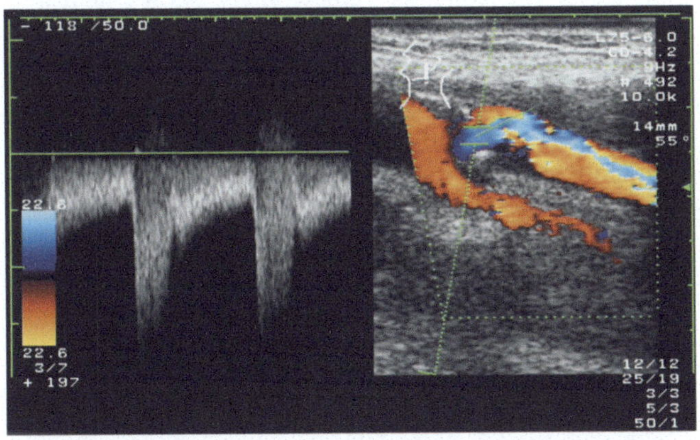

Fig. 13.16 Determination of the flow velocity at the maximum of a short-stretched stenosis with a lateral outlet of the internal carotid artery. With the "usual" cranially tilted sound window, an insonation angle of approximately 90° would be expected, which is why in this case a caudal tilting of the Doppler sound beam seems to be reasonable

Overestimating Color Coding

Although color coded vessel imaging is the method of choice for the visualization of low and moderate stenoses, the Doppler spectrum is the much more valid parameter for higher grade stenoses and should be evaluated accordingly. ◄

Note

All errors caused by the examiner can be easily recognized by means of the image documentation and thus represent the most important criterion in the quality control of sonographic findings.

Summary

Today, ultrasound diagnostics is the method of choice for the detection of stenoses in the area of carotid bifurcation; in terms of accuracy, it corresponds approximately to CTA or MRA. According to the revised DEGUM recommendations, the degree of stenosis should be indicated according to the NASCET criteria. The combination of different Doppler and duplex sonographic parameters is decisive for a reliable assessment. The main criteria are the constriction of the vessel lumen visible in the color coded duplex sonogram, the flow velocity at the maximum of the stenosis and the remaining poststenotic flow velocity. Various additional criteria, such as the findings at the periorbital arteries, the flow curve in the common carotid artery, the presence of flow disturbances or special stenosis indices, serve above all to check the plausibility of the findings and help in difficult examination conditions.

13.2 Stenoses of the Internal Carotid Artery Close to the Skull Base

For clinical and sonographic reasons, stenoses with a cranial location of the first 2–3 cm distal to the origin of the internal carotid artery (Fig. 13.17) should be considered separately from processes close to the bifurcation.

Other Etiology

In contrast to internal carotid stenoses, which are predominantly caused by arteriosclerosis (Chap. 16), more cranially located stenoses occur mainly in the case of kinking of the vessel (Sect. 20.1), fibromuscular dysplasia (Sect. 19.1) and vascular dissections (Chap. 18). Often there is an overlap,

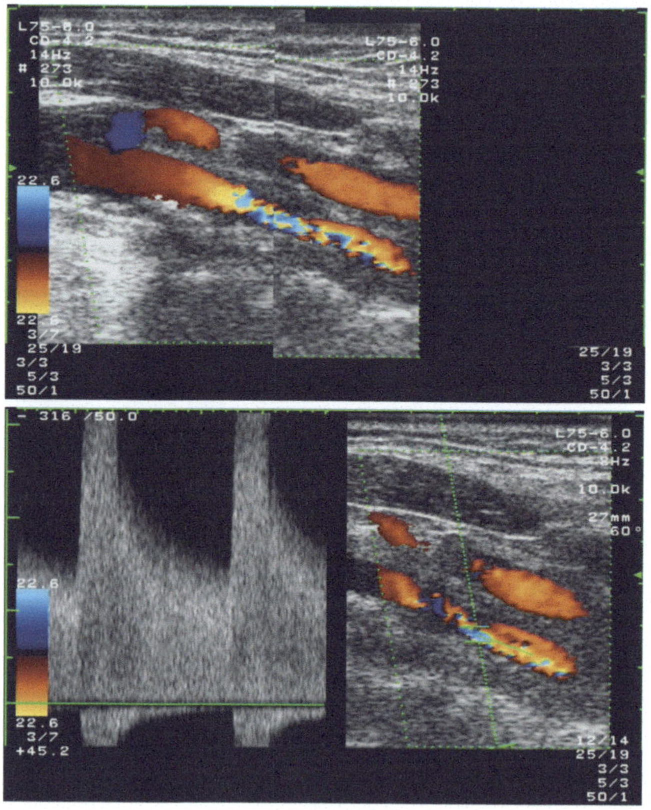

Fig. 13.17 Long-distance high-grade stenosis of the internal carotid artery, located about 2 cm cranially of the carotid bifurcation in a 58-year-old patient with ipsilateral recurrent amaurosis fugax. The etiology is unclear in an otherwise completely inconspicuous vascular system and lack of significant vascular risk factors (differential diagnosis dissection, fibromuscular dysplasia, arteriosclerotic)

since kink formations and fibromuscular dysplasias represent a risk for the occurrence of dissections.

Special Examination Problems

Since the entire course of the internal carotid artery up to the base of the skull can only rarely – in very slender persons – be adequately assessed with the usual linear sound probes, the direct assessment of stenoses ("main criteria," Sect. 13.1.2) is often difficult, and the "additional criteria" are of decisive importance.

> **Practical Tips**
> If available, the "curved array" probes designed primarily for the abdominal area can also be used for stenoses close to the base of the skull. Due to the low transmission frequency of 3–3.5 MHz, the penetration depth is considerably higher, but limitations in resolution must be accepted.

13.2.1 Diagnostic Criteria

In diagnostics, a distinction must be made as to whether the maximum stenosis can be sufficiently assessed by duplex sonography or not.

Maximum Stenosis Assessable by Color Coded Imaging

In this situation, in principle, all the criteria already mentioned in Sect. 13.1 apply. However, there are two special features to be considered.

Prestenotic Flow Velocity

Since the poststenotic flow velocity can often no longer be reliably measured in skull base stenoses, the prestenotic flow velocity should be determined as an alternative. ◀

Search for Multiple Stenoses

Since cranial stenoses of the internal carotid artery are often caused by vascular dysplasia, the entire visible course of the vessel should always be assessed in detail for the presence of (further) constrictions. The technique of "optimized flow imaging" (Sect. 6.3.2) is particularly suitable for this purpose. ◀

Maximum Stenosis Not Assessable by Color Coded Imaging

As already described above, indirect findings are of major importance in this case. As such are to be mentioned:

- **Periorbital arteries.** Pathological findings in the periorbital arteries are regularly found in high-grade stenoses.
- **Common carotid artery.** In severe stenoses, the flow signal of the common carotid artery shows increased pulsatility ("externalization") compared to the sides.
- **Prestostic flow velocity.** In high-grade stenoses, the flow velocity (and the flow volume) in the upstream vessel course is significantly reduced in lateral comparison. In addition, the flow signal shows an increased pulsatility.
- **Intracranial vessels.** A further component for the indirect detection of high-grade stenoses close to the skull base is the proof of collateralization via the anterior and/or posterior communicating artery.

> **Practical Tips**
> Side comparisons of the flow velocity are only useful if the vessel diameter is identical. As vessels are often narrow not only from behind but also in front of high-grade stenoses, the flow volume (Sect. 5.3.3) should preferably be determined.

13.2.2 Possible Errors

If the stenosis area cannot be directly visualized, only high-grade stenoses can be detected using the indirect hemodynamic criteria ("additional criteria"). The sonographic examiner should always be aware of this limitation and, if there is a corresponding clinical suspicion, should additionally use other imaging examination procedures.

> Note
> **If stenoses cannot be directly deduced, only high-grade constrictions can be recorded using indirect criteria.**

Other important sources of error are:

Kinking
In the area of a kinking, the assessment of the flow velocity is more difficult because the angle correction often cannot be reliably adjusted. In this case, the findings must be based primarily on the (non-)presence of flow disturbances (Sect. 13.1.3).

Narrow Vessels
As mentioned above, a reduction of the original vessel diameter regularly occurs not only after but also before very severe stenoses. The cause of this is unknown. It is possible that physiological adaptation phenomena are involved when the blood flow through a vessel decreases. In this case, incorrect assessments of the blood flow can only be avoided if the flow volume is determined by side comparison.

Long-Distance Stenoses
According to hemodynamic laws, long-distance stenoses lead to lower intrastotic flow velocities than would be expected based on the degree of stenosis (Fig. 13.7). This applies in particular to long-distance dissections, in which apparently "normal" flow velocities are often found (Fig. 13.8). The determination of the flow volume is also helpful here.

External Collaterals
If the appearance in the color coded duplex sonogram is approximately the same, a collateral vessel (e.g., ascending pharyngeal artery, occipital artery) originating from the proximal internal carotid artery can be confused with a long-distance dissection when the vessel is closed (see Case Study 18.5). This error can only be avoided if additional MRI and MRA images are taken when there is sonographic evidence of a vessel dissection.

Summary
Internal carotid stenoses located cranially of the carotid bifurcation are usually caused by vascular dysplasia and/or dissections. Provided that their maximum lies in the sonographically representable neck area, the same diagnostic criteria and accuracy apply as for stenoses close to the bifurcation. In contrast, stenoses located directly below the base of the skull can only be detected – on the basis of indirect criteria – if they are already high grade.

13.3 Occlusions of the Internal Carotid Artery

Occlusions in the bifurcation area of the internal carotid artery are the most important extracranial vascular findings besides stenoses. Due to the different therapeutic consequences, the differentiation between occlusions and (filiform) stenoses is of practical importance.

13.3.1 Main Diagnostic Criteria

The method of choice for differentiating between occlusion and high-grade, filiform stenosis (synonymous with pseudo-occlusion, subtotal stenosis) is color coded duplex sonography. The diagnosis is based on the following three examination conditions or criteria.

Low-Flow Setting
The basic prerequisite for the differentiation between existing and non-existing blood flow is that even slow flow can still be adequately detected by adjusting the device parameters (Fig. 13.18).

Demarcable Vessel Walls
The second, equally important prerequisite for the diagnosis of occlusion is that the vascular walls of the open or occluded internal carotid artery can be clearly (!) delineated on the first 2–3 cm in the B-mode image.

Distal Color Filling
Since the residual lumen may be so small or obscured by a "acoustic shadow" that it is not displayed in color coded form, the diagnosis is ultimately based on the exclusion or detection of blood flow in the further course of the vessel. An open vessel can be assumed if the distal carotid artery is completely (!) filled with color information over a distance of at least 1.5–2 cm between the two visible vessel walls. However, the appearance of individual color dots in the internal carotid artery cannot be regarded as evidence of an open vessel, since after carotid occlusions vessels regularly shoot into the occluded lumen and projection phenomena are

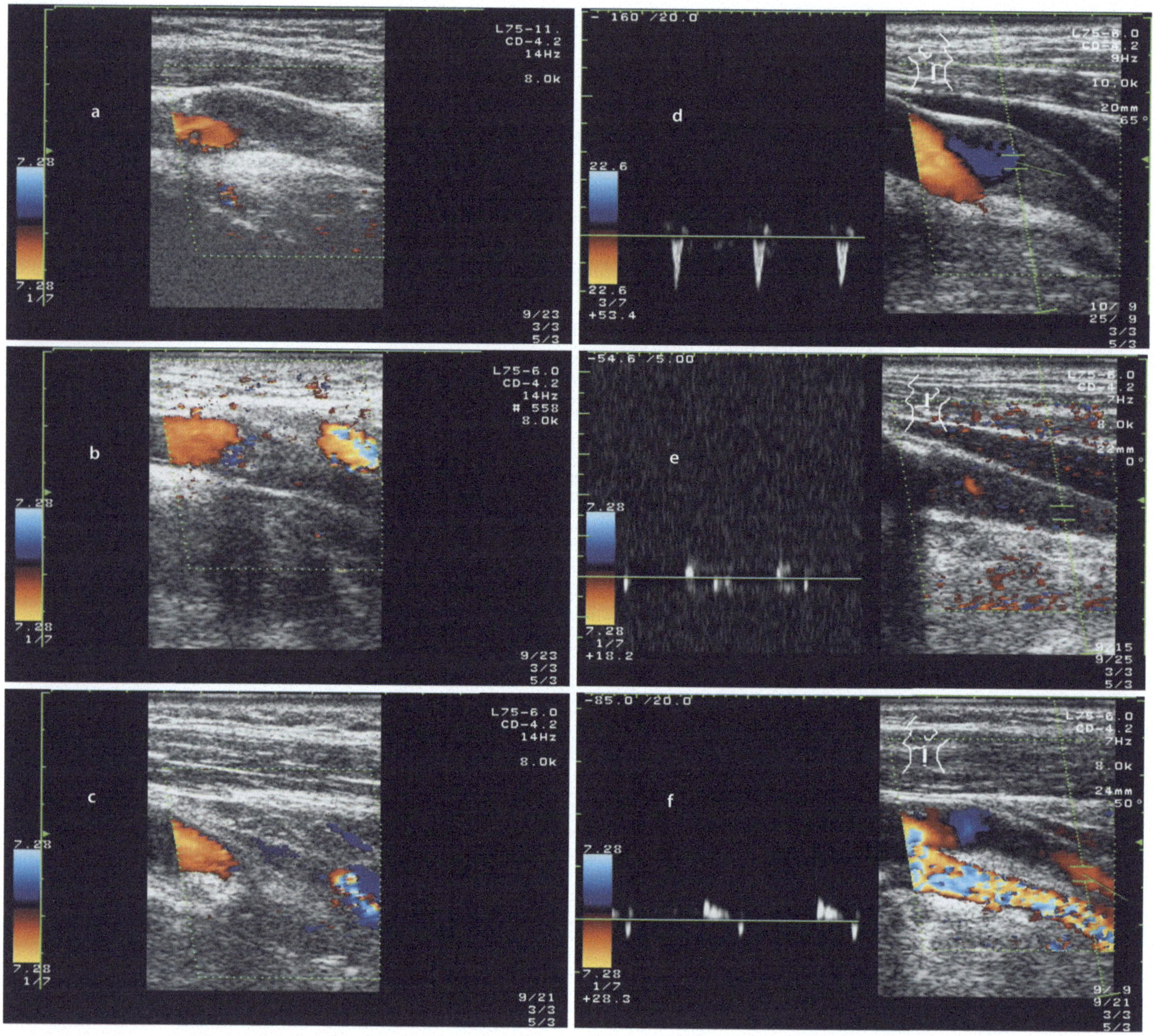

Fig. 13.18 (**a**–**f**) Color duplex sonographic diagnosis of occlusions of the internal carotid artery. (**a, b, d, e**) Vessels that can be clearly assessed as closed; (**c**) in the absence of vessel walls, the situation cannot be clearly clarified; (**d**) "Blunt signal" in a short carotid stump; (**e**) signals oscillating around the zero line, caused by longitudinal pulsations of the vessel; (**f**) Low flow signal with more distal vessel occlusion

possible due to the limited resolution of the sound probe (see overview).

Causes of color coded flow artifacts in an occluded internal carotid artery

- Projection of flow signals of a vessel running next to the internal carotid artery into the occluded lumen
- Lateral sprouting of small supply vessels into the occluded lumen
- Supply of the occluded lumen through an open "branch canal" (especially for dissections) (Fig. 13.19)

Practical Tips

A special case are dissections in which the visible outer wall of the vessel is constricted over a long distance by

(continued)

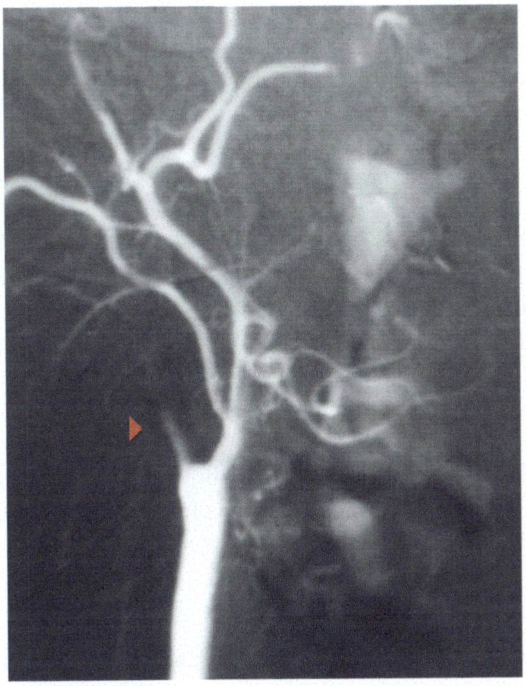

Fig. 13.19 Angiographic evidence of a short "canaliculus" in occlusion of the internal carotid artery following dissection

a dissection not visible in the sectional image. Thus the above mentioned criterion of "distal color filling" is by definition not fulfilled. However, false results are not to be expected, since in dissections, in contrast to filiform stenoses, the color coded residual lumen can be regularly followed over the entire extracranial course of the internal carotid artery.

Background Information

With CW-Doppler sonography, occlusions can be suspected but cannot be distinguished with certainty from high-grade stenoses, since in this case both the intra- and poststenotic Doppler signal may be very variable or not detectable at all. In particular, flow signals that appear relatively "normal" should be viewed with some skepticism (Fig. 13.20), while a low flow signal with greatly reduced pulsatility ("**pseudo vein**") or a slowed systolic acceleration ("**Delta signal**") rather indicate a still open vessel distal to a filiform stenosis (Fig. 13.21).

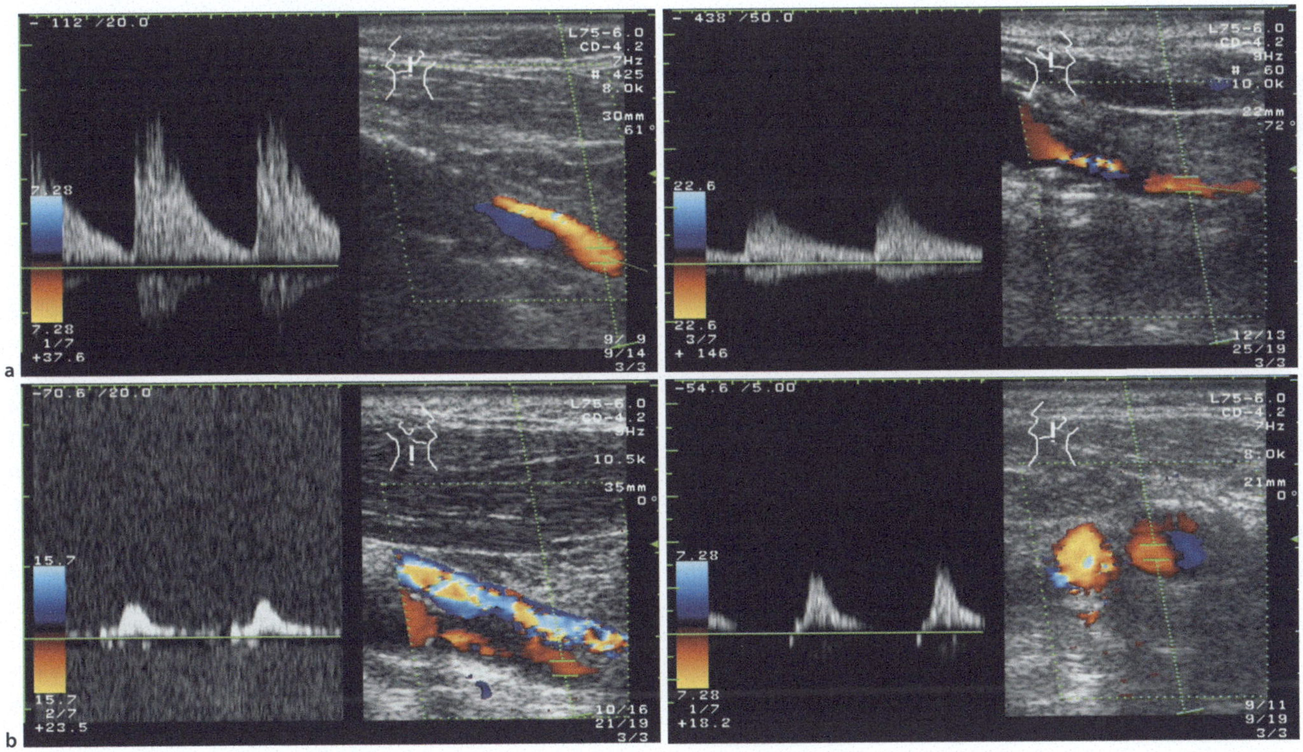

Fig. 13.20 (**a**–**d**) Variable flow signals behind filiform stenoses of the internal carotid artery. (**a**) "helix flow" behind a stenosis obscured by acoustic shadow with a low end diastolic flow component; (**b**) "delta signal" behind a high-grade stenosis without any discernible jet flow at the stenosis maximum; (**c**) apparently normal flow signal in "collapsed" poststenotic vascular lumen; (**d**) "delta signal" in cross section after a filiform stenosis, note the strongly depicted external carotid artery (left in the picture)

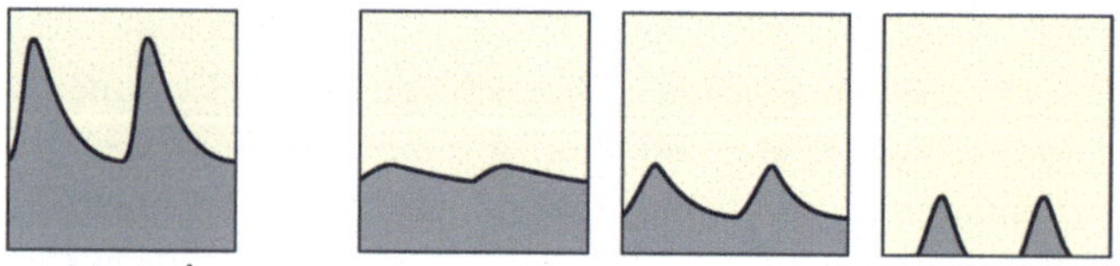

Fig. 13.21 Synopsis of possible flow signals distal to a high-grade stenosis (pseudo-occlusion). (**a**) low flow signal with greatly reduced pulsatility ("pseudo vein"), (**b**) slowed systolic acceleration with a relatively "normal" configured pulsatile course, (**c**) slowed systolic rise without diastolic flow ("Delta signal")

13.3.2 Additional Criteria for Occlusion Diagnosis

In addition to the goal of increasing redundancy already mentioned several times (see overview below), the "additional criteria" in the clarification of carotid occlusions have the primary task of ruling out a higher degree of flow obstruction in the event of unfavorable examination conditions and unclear local findings.

Diagnostic criteria for occlusion of the extracranial internal carotid artery
(for maximum redundancy, all criteria should be met)

- Main criteria
  - Absence of flow in the internal carotid artery over a longer distance with a vessel clearly visible in the sectional image and "low-flow setting" in the color coded duplex sonogram
- Secondary criteria
  - Pathological findings in the periorbital arteries
  - Reduced flow velocity and increased pulsatility in the lateral comparison in the common carotid artery
  - Reduced pulsatility in the ipsilateral middle cerebral artery
  - Evidence of collateralization via the circle of Willis

On the other hand, they do not contribute to the differential diagnosis between occlusion and pseudo-occlusion, since these are exclusively hemodynamic criteria, which in both cases are associated with a pathological finding. The most important "secondary criteria" are:

- **Periorbital arteries.** Periorbital arteries almost always show a pathological finding with zero or retrograde flow.
- **Common carotid artery.** Typically, when the internal carotid artery is occluded in there is an "externalization" with increased pulsatility and a reduction of the flow volume compared in the ipsilateral common carotid artery as compared to the contralateral one.
- **Intracranial findings.** Due to the usually good collateral supply via the circle of Willis, carotid occlusions in the affected brain base arteries are only relatively seldom accompanied by a pronounced reduction in flow. Typically, however, there is a reduced pulsatility in the ipsilateral middle cerebral artery compared to the sides, which can contribute to the differentiation between an occlusion and an open vessel that can only be inadequately drained in the case of unclear extracranial findings as an indirect criterion (see following overview). The same applies to the findings of hyperperfusion of the anterior communicating artery and/or retrograde flow in the A1 section of the anterior cerebral artery with color coded duplex sonography, which demonstrate a collateral supply via the anterior section of the circle of Willis.

Indirect evidence of a non-occluded internal carotid artery in unfavorable sonographic examination conditions in the area of carotid bifurcation

- Antegrade, equal-sided periorbital arteries
- Equal-sided common carotid artery
- Equal-sided middle cerebral artery
- Antegrade flow through the anterior cerebral artery
- No evidence of collaterals across the anterior and/or posterior communicating artery

13.3.3 Differential Diagnostic Aspects

In addition to the possibility of diagnostic clarification, the sonographic appearance of carotid occlusions provides some additional information.

Etiology
A homogeneous occlusion reaching directly to the outflow of the internal carotid artery indicates an embolus from the heart or aortic arch obstructing the vessel (Fig. 13.22). Although inhomogeneous structures in the cross-sectional image of the carotid bifurcation – possibly together with an acoustic shadow – are certainly no evidence of thrombotic occlusion of an arteriosclerotic stenosis of the internal carotid artery, they do make such an occlusion likely. A visible carotid stump, on the other hand, rather points to a cranial to caudal thrombotic occlusion. The causes are more widespread in this case. If the stump is broad and roundish, it is most likely a cardiac embolic or primary arteriosclerotic occlusion of the

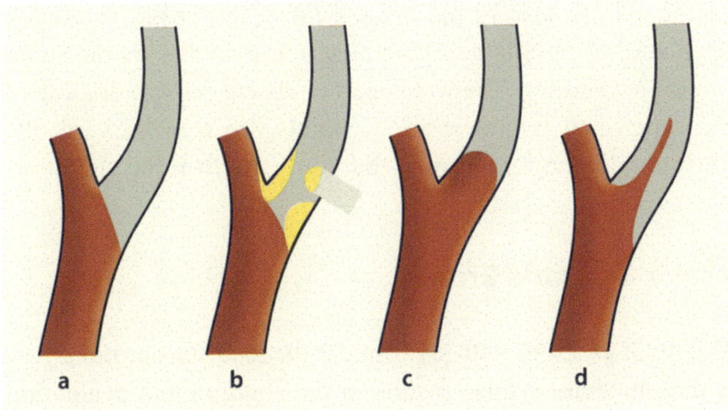

Fig. 13.22 (**a–d**) Indications of the cause of carotid occlusion based on the appearance of the carotid bifurcation in the ultrasound slice. (**a**) homogeneous closure in cardiac embolism, (**b**) inhomogeneous wall changes in arteriosclerotic occlusion, (**c**) broad "carotid stump" in the case of a cranial to caudal thrombosis, (**d**) tapered stump for carotid dissection

proximal carotid siphon, while a vessel with a pointed tip suggests dissection.

Time of Occlusion

To a limited extent, the cross-sectional sonogram provides information on when the vessel occlusion occurred. In older occlusions, for example, the vessel wall is typically remodeled into connective tissue and can only be recognized schematically (Fig. 13.18c). In contrast, no conclusions about the "age" of the occlusion can be drawn from the (non-) presence of internal reflections, since these change several times in the course of vascular occlusions.

13.3.4 Possible Errors

When differentiating between high-grade carotid stenoses and occlusions, all ultrasound methods with the exception of color coded duplex sonography are ultimately overtaxed. Errors will only occur when using this technique if the criteria mentioned in the overview on p. 165 are not reliably fulfilled. In this case, it is the task of the responsible examiner to recognize the limitations of the method and to use other diagnostic procedures (e.g., CTA/MRA).

Summary

Color coded duplex sonography is suitable for reliable detection of occlusions of the extracranial internal carotid artery and for differentiation of filiform stenoses. The prerequisites for this are that the occluded vessel must be clearly defined in the sectional image and that slow blood flows can be reliably detected by selecting suitable "low-flow parameters" If the conditions are unclear, indirect extra- and intracranial parameters and – in individual cases – compression maneuvers of the common carotid artery can help.

13.4 Stenoses and Occlusions of the External Carotid Artery

Stenoses and occlusions of the external carotid artery generally represent secondary findings without clinical significance. They are only relevant in 3 cases:

- As **confusing findings** in the sonographic evaluation of the internal carotid artery.
- Within the framework of **ophthalmic collaterals** in case of an occlusion or a very severe stenosis of the ipsilateral internal carotid artery. In the case of ocular or cerebral circulatory disorders, the possibility of spreading emboli from a stenosed external carotid artery must be considered in this case.
- In the preoperative examination before the application of an **extracranial bypass** in the case of a hemodynamically insufficiently compensated occlusion process in the area of the internal carotid artery or the carotid T.

13.4.1 Diagnostic Criteria in Stenoses

Color Coded Imaging

The same rules apply here as for the detection of stenosis of the internal carotid artery. It is not uncommon for high-grade stenoses of the external carotid artery to produce a "confetti effect," which then makes it difficult to examine the internal carotid artery.

Doppler Findings

Due to the high peripheral resistance, only very pronounced stenoses show hemodynamic effects, so that a stenosis of the external carotid artery that can be grasped in the Doppler spectrum is usually already quite severe. Because the blood flow in the external carotid artery is already highly variable in non-pathological cases, a maximum systolic flow rate of 150–200 cm/s (or a maximum systolic frequency of approx. 6 kHz at 4 MHz transmission frequency) can be assumed as a safe limit between normal and pathological (Fig. 13.23; Table 13.5). The finding of a stenosis is supported if there are pronounced flow disturbances.

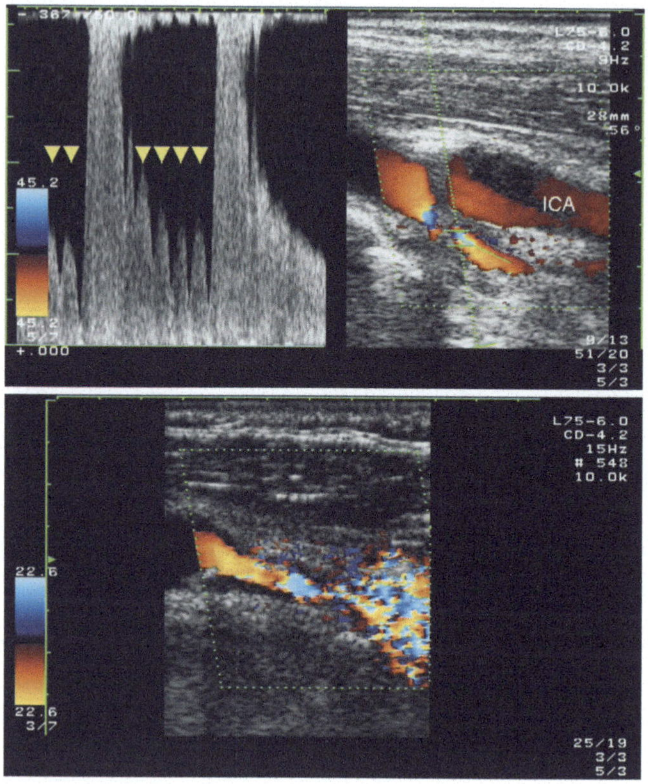

Fig. 13.23 Examples of high-grade stenosis of the external carotid artery. Note the response to intermittent compression of the ipsilateral superficial temporal artery (6) as a decisive criterion for differentiating it from internal carotid stenosis (top). Pronounced "confetti effect" in the lower picture for an external stenosis

Practical Tips

Due to the low clinical significance of stenoses of the external carotid artery, graduation in concrete percentages makes no sense and a descriptive classification into low, medium and high should be used.

13.4.2 Diagnostic Criteria in Occlusions

Occlusions of the external carotid artery generally have no clinical significance, since the external branches have an extensive collateral network. Only the occlusions can be diagnosed sonographically, since vascular occlusions located further cranially are regularly overlooked due to the possible anatomical variations.

Exit closures of the external carotid artery are characterized by the fact that it is almost always only a segmental closure. In the distal course, the vessel is usually open and retrogradely collateralized, especially via the superior thyroid artery. The weakened or absent pulse palpation of the superficial temporal artery points the way forward; the ultrasound examination will then only confirm the situation.

13.4.3 Possible Errors

The main problem with stenoses of the external carotid artery is that they cause false results in the sonographic evaluation of the internal carotid artery. Two situations can be observed.

External-Internal Confusion

Mutual confusions of stenoses of the external and internal carotid arteries are not uncommon. With careful identification of the carotid branches using compression maneuvers of the external branches, however, such errors can be largely ruled out.

Influence on the Periorbital Arteries

Due to their influence on the pressure equilibrium in the periorbital vessels (Sect. 7.3.4), combined internal and external anastomoses in particular – as well as occlusions of the common carotid artery – can lead to Doppler findings that are difficult to predict. The weakened or missing pulse palpation of the superficial temporal artery may help in individual cases.

Summary

Stenoses and occlusions of the external carotid artery are only of minor clinical importance. The same rules apply for their detection as for occlusion processes of the extracranial internal carotid artery, but only high-grade stenoses are hemodynamically conspicuous. In the case of occlusions, the pulse palpation findings of the superficial temporal artery contribute significantly to the diagnosis.

13.5 Stenoses and Occlusions of the Common Carotid Artery

13.5.1 Diagnostic Criteria in Stenoses

While low-grade plaques in the course of the common carotid artery are a frequent concomitant finding of occlusion processes of the internal carotid artery, isolated, higher-grade

Table 13.5 Maximum systolic flow velocities in stenoses of the external carotid artery. (after Päivänsalo et al. 1996)

Normal range	80 ± 40 cm/s
Moderate stenosis	140 ± 49 cm/s
High grade stenosis	230 ± 95 cm/s

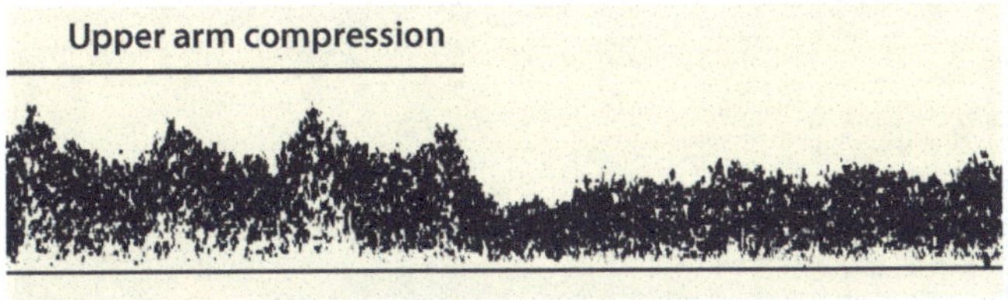

Fig. 13.24 "Pseudo vein" in Doppler sonography of the right common carotid artery with and without compression of the upper arm. This is caused by a high-grade stenosis in the area of the brachiocephalic trunk

stenoses of the vessel are rather rare. There are three localizations with different findings.

Stenoses at the Origin

Minor and moderate stenoses at the origin of the common carotid artery are regularly overlooked sonographically, since the vessel origin is generally not accessible to direct sonographic examination and there are (still) no indirect hemodynamic effects of the stenosis. An examination of the common artery origing is normally only considered in 2 situations:

- in the case of local bruit by **auscultation** in the area of the supraclavicular pit and/or
- in the case of a **reduced pulse rate ("pseudo vein")** in the Doppler spectrum of the distal common carotid artery (Fig. 13.24).

Stenoses in the Course

Stenoses in the course of the common carotid artery can be easily recognized and located in the B-mode image due to the usually very good image quality in this area (Fig. 13.25). Only very low-echo plaques can be overlooked in individual cases. As expected, color coded imaging helps here.

High-grade stenoses in the course of the common carotid artery are rare and usually indicate an expired traumatic lesion of the vessel wall (e.g., blow to the neck, strangulation), vasculitis or a consequence of radiation (radiation angiopathy). Typically, even very severe stenoses show only relatively small changes in the Doppler spectrum. The method of choice here is color coded duplex sonography, which reliably displays the stenoses regularly in both longitudinal and cross-sectional views.

Stenoses in the Bifurcation Area

Stenoses of the distal carotid artery are usually easy to localize in B-mode color coded ultrasound images (Fig. 13.26). Only extremely rarely is it a stenosis affecting only the common carotid artery. In most cases there is a "bifurcation stenosis" which also affects the internal and external carotid arteries. The findings in the Doppler spectrum correspond to those obtained with isolated stenoses of the two carotid branches.

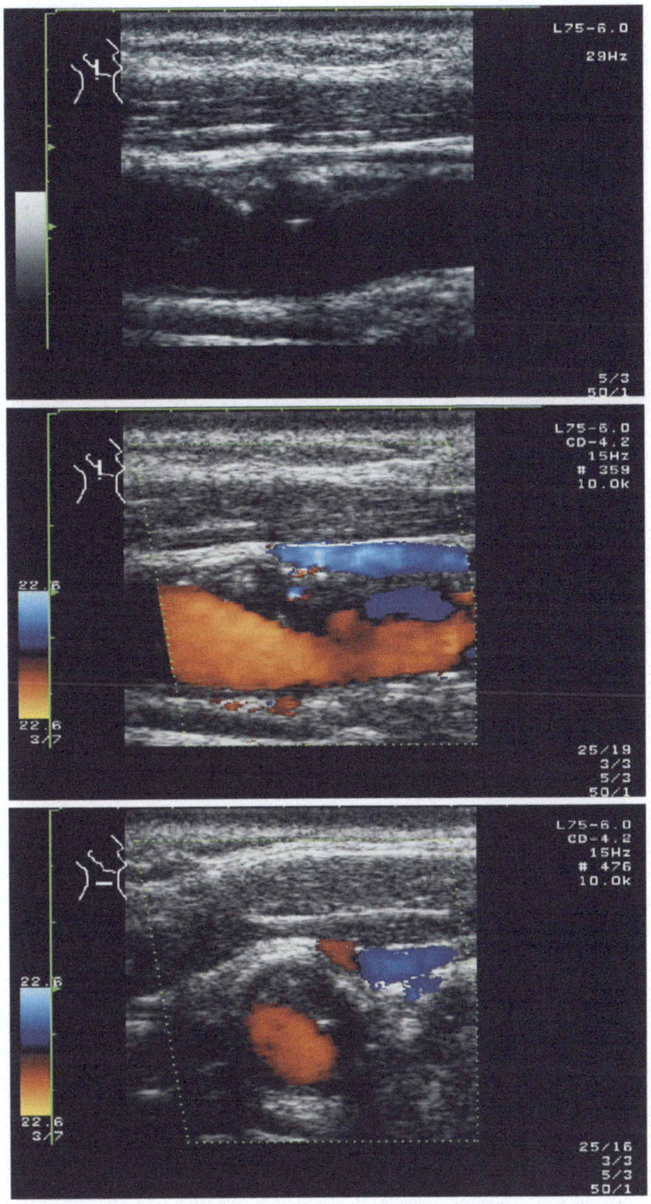

Fig. 13.25 Moderate, 40–50% stenosis of the right common carotid artery immediately below the carotid bifurcation in a 70-year-old patient with ipsilateral recurrent transient ischemic attacks. Due to the low-echogenic, inhomogeneous appearance of the plaque, it is a possible cause of cranially spreading embolisms

13.5.2 Diagnostic Criteria in Occlusions

Occlusions of the common carotid artery are usually caused by retrograde thrombosis of an occlusion of the internal carotid artery or by the fixation of a cardiac thrombus in the

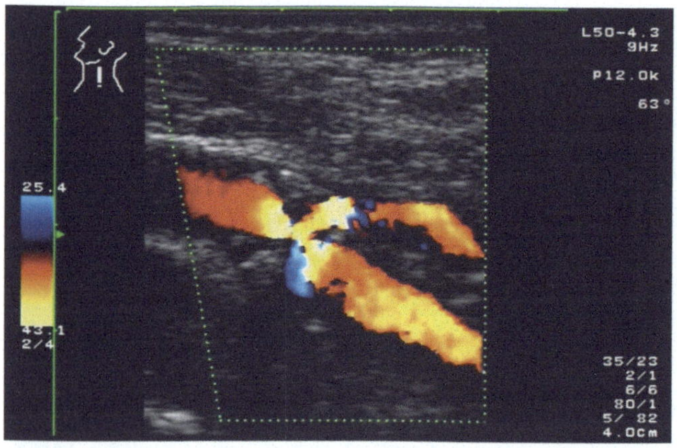

Fig. 13.26 Bifurcation stenosis of the distal carotid artery

area of the carotid bifurcation. In some of the latter cases the internal carotid artery remains open. It is then supplied retrogradely via the external carotid artery, which also receives its blood retrogradely from its branches (Fig. 13.27).

Duplex sonography is the method of choice for detecting occlusions of the common carotid artery. The diagnosis is considered confirmed when the three typical findings can be identified:

- **Missing "color fill"** of the vessel with "low-flow setting" in the color coded display
- **Missing flow signal** in the Doppler spectrum of the vessel with the wall filter set as low as possible
- **Narrow vessel** in the case of imaging in side comparison with clear internal reflections in the vascular lumen.

Summary

Stenoses at the origin of the common carotid artery are generally only detected sonographically if they are of a higher grade and lead to typical poststenotic flow changes. For stenoses in the rest of the vessel, the rules known from the internal carotid artery apply. Doppler sonography of occlusions of the common carotid artery leads to confusing findings, while color coded duplex sonography usually allows a clear diagnosis at first glance. It is not uncommon for the external and internal carotid arteries to remain open when the common carotid artery is occluded and to be treated retrogradely via the superior thyroid artery.

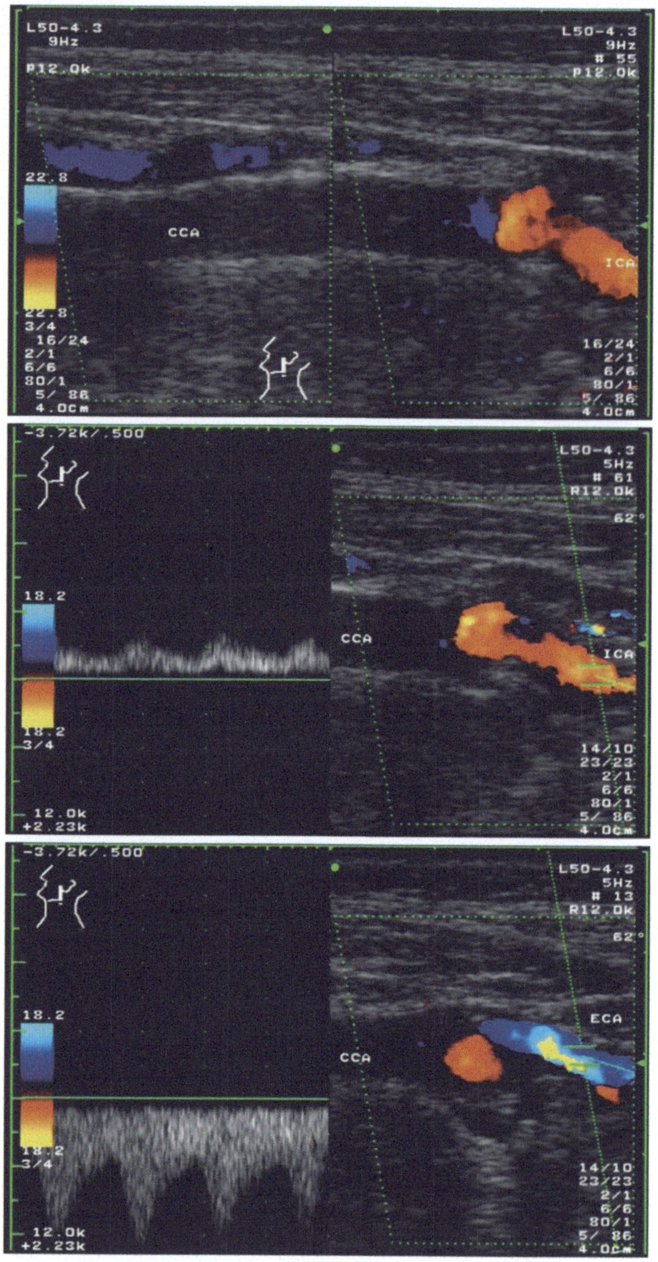

Fig. 13.27 Closure of the common carotid artery with the internal carotid artery supplied retrogradely via the external carotid artery

References

Arning C, Widder B, von Reutern GM, Stiegler H, Görtler M (2010) Ultraschallkriterien zur Graduierung von Stenosen der A. carotis interna – Revision der DEGUM-Kriterien und Transfer in NASCET-Stenosierungsgrade. Ultraschall in Med 31:251–257

Busutill SJ, Franklin DP, Youkey JR, Elmore JR (1996) Carotid duplex overestimation of stenosis due to serve contralateral disease. Am J Surg 172:144–147

de Weerd M, Greving JP, de Jong AW, Buskens E, Bots ML (2009) Prevalence of asymptomatic carotid artery stenosis according to age and sex: systematic review and metaregression analysis. Stroke 40: 1105–1113 de Weerd M, Greving JP, Hedblad B et al (2010) Prevalence of asymptomatic carotid artery stenosis in the general population: an individual participant data meta-analysis. Stroke 41:1294–1297

Eliasziw M, Rankin RN, Fox AJ, Hynes RB, Barnett HJ (1995) Accuracy and prognostic consequences of ultrasonography in identifying severe carotid artery stenosis. North American symptomatic carotid endarterectomy trial (NASCET) group. Stroke 26:1747–1752

European Carotid Surgery Trialists' Collaborative Group (1991) MRC European carotid surgery trial: interim results for symptomatic patients with severe (70–99%) or with mild (0–29%) carotid stenosis. Lancet 337:1235–1243

Henderson RD, Steinman DA, Eliasziw M, Barnett HJ (2000) Effect of contralateral carotid artery stenosis on carotid ultrasound velocity measurements. Stroke 31:2636–2640

Hill AB (1998) Should patients be screened for asymptomatic carotid artery stenosis? Can J Surg 41:208–213

Päivänsalo M, Leinonen S, Turunen J et al (1996) Quantification of carotid artery stenosis with various Doppler velocity parameters. Röfo 164:108–113

Ranke C, Rieder M, Creutzig A, Alexander K (1995) Ein Nomogramm zur duplexsonographischen Quantifizierung peripherer Arterienstenosen. Med Klinik 90:72–77

Ringleb P, Görtler M, Nabavi DG, Arning C, Sander D, Eckstein H-H et al (2012) S3-Leitlinie Extracranielle Carotisstenose. Gefässchirurgie 17:502–519

Wardlaw JM, Chappell FM, Best JJK, Wartolowska K, Berry E, NHS Research and Development Health Technology Assessment Carotid Stenosis Imaging Group (2006) Non-invasive imaging compared with intra-arterial angiography in the diagnosis of symptomatic carotid stenosis: a metanalysis. Lancet 367:1503–1512

Stenoses and Occlusions of the Main Cerebral Arteries

14

Bernhard Widder and Gerhard F. Hamann

14.1 Special Features of Intracranial Vascular Diagnostics

Similar to the extracranial brain-supplying arteries, the recognition of intracranial stenoses and occlusions is also not based on a single parameter, but on the combination of different extracranial and intracranial findings. In comparison to the diagnosis of the extracranial internal carotid artery, however, there are two major differences which will be discussed in more detail below.

14.1.1 Numerous Causes of Intracranial Occlusions

While extracranial occlusive processes are mainly caused by arteriosclerosis, a wide range of causes can be found intracranially (Table 14.1). In addition to arteriosclerotic vascular processes, which often occur isolated intracranially in diabetes mellitus, and the frequent dissections near the skull base (Chap. 18), these include vascular dysplasias (Chap. 19), vasculitis, vascular processes associated with infections, partially recanalized embolic occlusions, vasospasms and moyamoya syndromes (Chaps. 20 and 21). For details please refer to the corresponding chapters.

14.1.2 Limitation to Flow Parameters

As already mentioned in Sect. 6.1.4, the resolution of transcranial duplex sonography is not sufficient to display the intracranial vessel walls and to determine the vessel diameter. Vessel imaging is the domain of neuroradiological methods, especially MRA and CTA (Brinjikji et al. 2016). Color coded vessel imaging is therefore mainly used to demonstrate the course of the vessel, whereas stenoses can only be detected and assessed on the basis of increased flow velocities and/or flow disturbances. However, the exclusive application of flow parameters involves two basic problems.

Detection of Only Higher Grade Stenoses
Flow parameters only lead to pathological findings in higher grade stenoses. Comparable to "simple" extracranial Doppler sonography without additional imaging, intracranial stenoses are therefore only detectable if the degree of stenosis reaches 50–60% – in the case of the distal carotid artery even from about 70% (Sect. 14.2.1).

Differentiation Between Stenosis and Hyperperfusion
Increased flow velocities (and the associated flow disturbances) are a non-specific phenomenon and can be caused not only by vasoconstrictions but also by primarily narrow vessels, for example, in cases of long-term nicotine abuse, but above all by hyperperfusion:

- In the case of an occluded large cerebral artery, the **collateral vessels** show an increased flow velocity.
- According to **recanalization** of vascular occlusions, a temporary hyperperfusion occurs in the reopened vessels due to disturbed autoregulation (Sect. 21.2.2).
- Comparable flow accelerations can be found in other causes of **disturbed autoregulation.** This is the case, for example, after craniocerebral trauma (Kramer et al. 2013; Ogami et al. 2017) or in the context of pregnancy-induced hypertension (Zunker et al. 2000).
- **Arteriovenous malformations and fistulas** lead to increased flow volumes in the so-called "feeder vessels" with correspondingly increased flow velocity.

B. Widder (✉)
Expert Opinion Institute, District Hospital, Guenzburg, Germany
e-mail: bernhard.widder@bkh-guenzburg.de

G. F. Hamann
Clinic of Neurology and Neurological Rehabilitation, District Hospital, Guenzburg, Germany

B. Widder, G. F. Hamann (eds.), *Duplex sonography of the brain-supplying arteries*, https://doi.org/10.1007/978-3-662-65566-5_14

Table 14.1 Differential diagnosis of intracranial occlusive processes

Cause	Differential diagnostic findings
Dissection (overview at Debette et al. 2015)	String sign in the extracranial internal carotid artery
	(Minor) trauma in the medical history
	Acute occurred, half-sided headache
	Anisocoria (Miosis, less frequently also mydriasis)
	Sickle-shaped vascular wall hematoma at MRI
	Connective tissue disease
Vasculitis (overview at Dutra et al. 2017)	Inflammatory lab results
	Headache, mental changes, seizures
	Inflammatory swelling of extracranial arteries (carotid artery, vertebral artery, superficial temporal artery)
	Several vascular segments affected, therefore also multifocal cortical/subcortical Lesions at MRI
	Focal inflammation at MRT (e.g., sinusitis) in focal vasculitis
Arteriosclerotic process (overview at Reith et al. 2015)	Additional extracranial vascular changes
	Isolated intracranial stenoses mainly in diabetes mellitus
(Partially recanalized) cardiogenic thrombus	Short-stretched stenosis, only concerning one vascular segment
	Localization mainly at vascular bifurcations
	Cardiac changes (e.g., thrombus, aortic plaques)
	No vascular wall lesion at high-resolution MRI
Congenital vascular dysplasia	Concerning the carotid T area
	Frequently accompanied by dissections
	Further extracranial developmental disorders
Vasospasm (overview at Macdonald 2016, Findlay et al. 2016)	In the case of spontaneous vasospasms fluctuating findings with recurrences
	Migraine history
	Typical disease (Subarachnoidal hemorhage, purulent meningitis)
Idiopathic moyamoya syndrome (overview at Kim 2016, Bang et al. 2016)	Localisation on both sides, slowly progressive occlusive processes in the carotid T area with an abnormal vascular network (rete mirabile)
	Beginning in the childhood or youth
	Other causes excluded
Reversible cerebral vasoconstriction syndrome (overview at Wolff and Ducros 2016)	Mostly accompanied by thunderclap headache with reversible vascular constrictions mainly in the middle cerebral artery, frequently triggered by stress, sympathicomimetics etc.

– In the case of an **anemia** increased flow velocities are observed in all brain-supplying arteries as a function of hematocrit value (Brass et al. 1988). The most likely cause of this is the reduced oxygen binding capacity of the blood with correspondingly increased blood demand.

14.2 Stenoses of the Intracranial Carotid Artery

14.2.1 Diagnostic Criteria

The detection of stenoses in the intracranial course of the internal carotid artery is based to a considerable extent on the evaluation of indirect criteria (extracranial internal carotid artery, periorbital arteries, anterior cerebral artery), which only provide noticeable findings in high-grade stenoses (Table 14.2). For anatomical reasons, the transtemporal Doppler examination of the vessel above the carotid siphon is performed at an extremely unfavorable insonation angle of approximately 90° (Fig. 14.3), and the insonation angle is completely unknown in transorbital Doppler sonography. Accordingly, the determination of flow velocity, which is useful in other vascular regions, does not yield reliable results. Only flow disturbances are usable, which, however, only occur in high grade stenoses. Accordingly, in the region of the distal carotid artery only stenoses with a stenotic degree of approx. 70% and more can be detected sonographically.

> **Note**
> **Stenoses in the intracranial course of the internal carotid artery can only be reliably detected by sonography from a stenosis level of approx. 70%.**

Extracranial Internal Carotid Artery

As far as the extracranial course of the internal carotid artery is not directly affected (in dissections), there is indirect evidence of a more distal stenosis only in the case of high-grade stenoses,. Typical characteristics are:

Table 14.2 Synopsis of Doppler sonographic findings in high-grade stenoses in the intracranial course of the internal carotid artery

	Between skull base and ophthalmic artery	Between ophthalmic artery and posterior communicating artery	Between posterior communicating artery and carotid T
Extracranial internal carotid artery	Reduced flow volume, reduced flow velocity, increased pulsatility		
Periorbital arteries	Mostly retrograde	Inconspicuous	Inconspicuous
Transorbital	Distinct flow disturbance	Possible flow disturbance	Inconspicuous
Distal internal carotid artery	Variable findings (inconspicuous to not derivable)	Possible poststenotic flow disturbance	Distinct flow disturbance
Middle cerebral artery (M1)	Reduced pulsatility in the case of an inadequate collateral supply		Flow disturbance
Anterior cerebral artery (A1)	In very high grade stenoses possibly retrograde, but also not detectable vessel		Antegrade flow with flow disturbance or retrograde

- **Reduction of flow volume.** The side-by-side comparison of flow volume in the extracranial internal carotid arteries is particularly suitable for assessing unclear flow conditions in the distal internal carotid artery. However, physiological asymmetries of flow volume must be taken into account, which generally do not exceed or fall below 20–30%.
- **Increased pulsatility.** High-grade distal stenoses show an increased pulsatility in the internal (and common) carotid artery in comparison to the contralateral side. In extreme cases, in the case of a high-grade stenosis, there is no longer any significant blood flow during diastole or there is even an **oscillating flow** (Fig. 14.2) with early diastolic retrograde component. Minor and moderate stenoses, on the other hand, do not lead to extracranial abnormalities.

Practical Tips
In the case of intracranial carotid stenosis, a side-by-side comparison of flow velocity in the extracranial internal carotid artery is only of limited value.

Frequently, there are long-distance dissections whose lumen constriction extend extracranially that show an "inconspicuous" flow velocity there. However, even isolated intracranial carotid stenoses, if they are very severe, may lead to a "collapse" of the extracranial vessel lumen (Fig. 14.1).

Periorbital Arteries
The examination of the periorbital arteries is essential for the localization of high-grade stenoses in the intracranial carotid artery:

- **Stenoses proximal to the ophthalmic artery** behave like comparable processes in the extracranial section of the internal carotid artery for blood supply in the ophthalmic and periorbital arteries. The findings already mentioned there apply analogously (Sect. 7.3).
- **Stenoses distal to the ophthalmic artery** on the other hand, do not lead to any changes in the flow signal of the periorbital arteries.

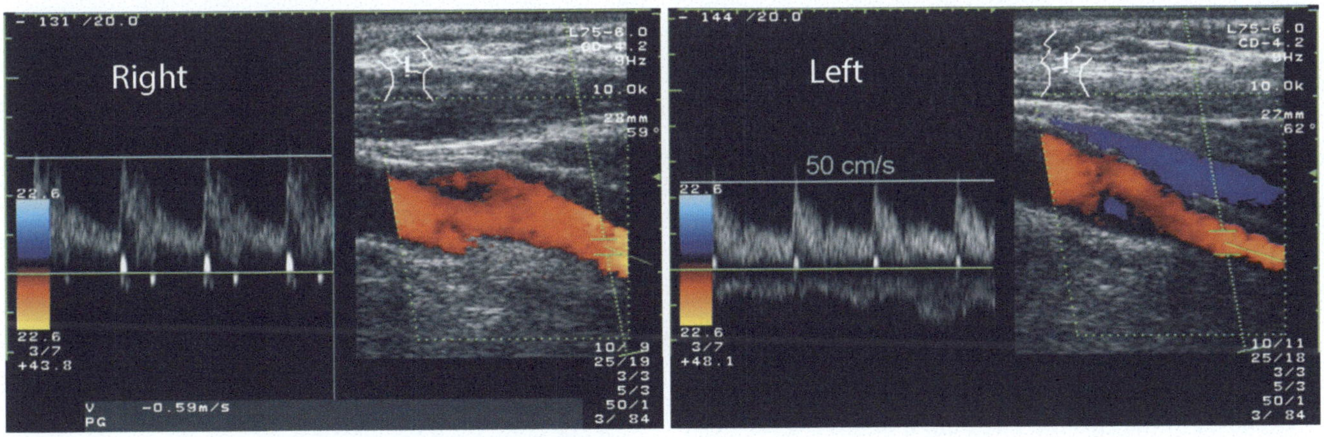

Fig. 14.1 Flow findings in the extracranial internal carotid artery in a high-grade stenosis of the left carotid siphon. Note the approximately identical flow velocity on both sides. On the left side, however, the diameter of the carotid artery appears significantly reduced (right 5.0 mm, left 3.5 mm). Accordingly, on the left side there is only a flow volume of 100 ml/min

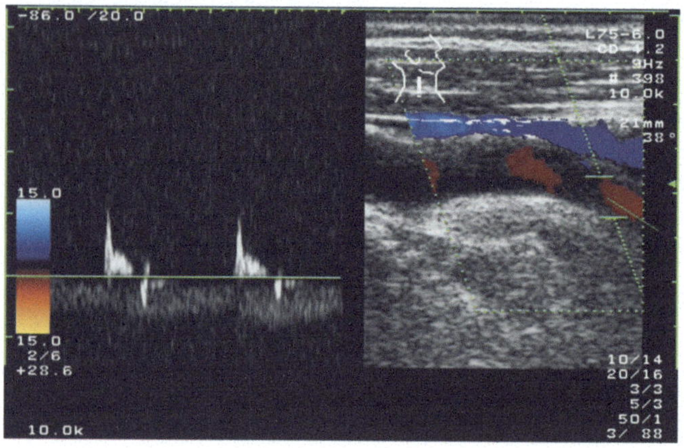

Fig. 14.2 Oscillating flow in the extracranial internal carotid artery in the case of a severe stenosis in the ipsilateral carotid siphon

Transorbital Doppler Findings

High-grade carotid artery stenoses located directly at the origin of the ophthalmic artery can be easily recognized by a local flow disturbance. Due to the undefined insonation angle, the absolute flow velocity cannot be detected accurately, which is why minor and moderate stenoses are overlooked. If the maximum stenosis is located more caudal in the area of the skull base, even higher grade stenoses usually do not show poststenotic phenomena reaching into the carotid siphon. The reason for this is that in this case the main blood flow in the distal carotid artery usually runs via the retrograde ophthalmic artery.

Findings in the Internal Carotid Artery

A reliable detection of the distal internal carotid artery is only possible by color coded duplex sonography (Fig. 14.4). Depending on the localization of the stenosis, three findings can be distinguished:

- **Stenoses proximal to the ophthalmic artery** usually do not lead to flow abnormalities in the distal vessel unless they are of the highest degree, since the poststenotic flow disturbances have returned to normal by then. In the case of extremely severe stenoses, the findings are variable and range from an apparently normal flow (with collateralization via the ophthalmic and/or posterior common artery) to a vessel that cannot be detected by color duplex sonography.
- **Stenoses in the upper carotid siphon** often are only recognizable by its poststenotic flow disturbances. In this case, however, it is not uncommon that the vessel cranially of the origin of the posterior communicating artery is no longer derivable at all.
- **Stenoses in the carotid T region,** if they are severe, can be easily recognized by the pronounced flow disturbances that typically continue into the middle as well as anterior cerebral artery (Fig. 14.3).

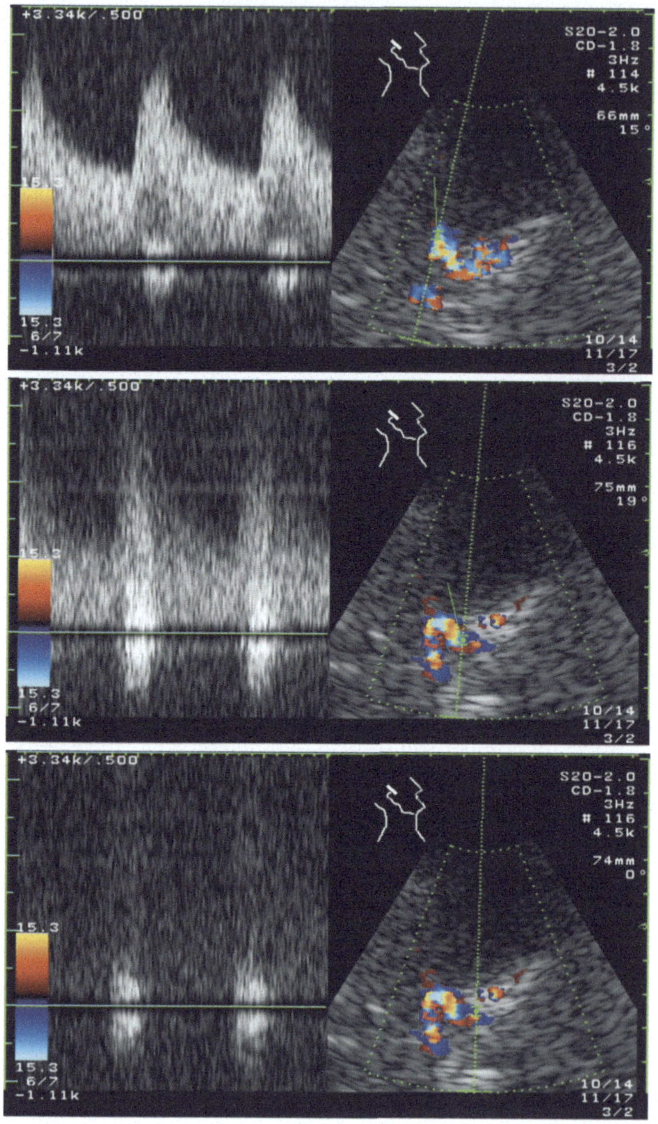

Fig. 14.3 Color coded coronary view in a high-grade stenosis of the distal internal carotid artery a few cm caudally of the carotid T. Maximum stenosis with flow disturbance without recognizable systolic maximum frequency (bottom); immediately poststenotic (middle); origin of the middle cerebral artery (top)

Practical Tips

The differentiation from physiological flow disturbances in the carotid T area can be difficult in individual cases. However, as a general rule, flow disturbances that can be detected in the middle cerebral artery and anterior more than 5–6 mm after their origin can be considered pathological.

Main Stem of the Middle Cerebral Artery (M1)

Depending on the location of the flow obstruction in the internal carotid artery, the poststenotic flow disturbances extend into the middle cerebral artery. In the case of very severe stenoses and insufficient collateralisation via the anterior common artery, the middle cerebral artery shows reduced pulsatility and reduced flow velocity compared to normal values.

Initial Section of the Anterior Cerebral Artery (A1)

The Doppler sonographic findings in the A1 section of the anterior cerebral artery are extremely variable and depend first of all on the degree of stenosis of the affected internal carotid artery. If the degree of stenosis is not yet high, flow in the anterior cerebral artery is usually antegrade. In the case of high-grade stenoses in the carotid siphon the anatomical situation in the anterior communicating artery is important. If the vessel is normplastic, there is a retrograde flow through the anterior cerebral artery. In the other case, the anterior cerebral artery is usually not visible or can only be derived with highly reduced flow.

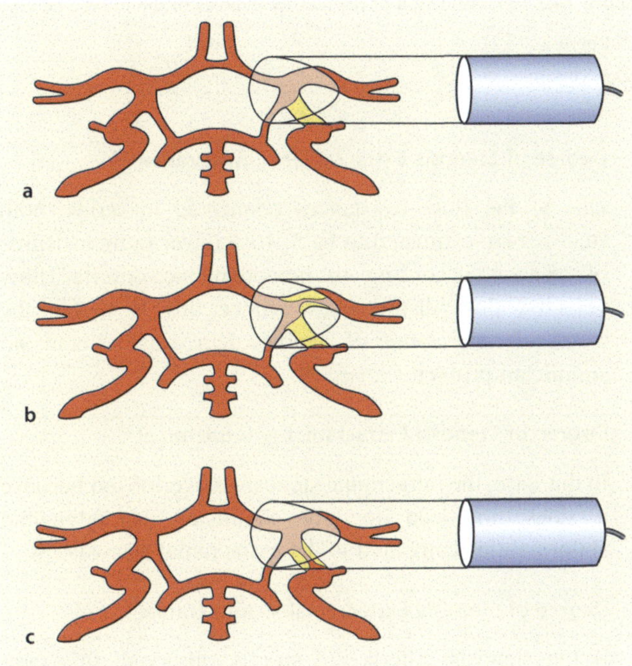

Fig. 14.4 (a–c) Problems in differentiating flow disturbances by "simple" transcranial Doppler sonography in an examination depth of 60–70 mm. Occlusion of the internal carotid artery with turbulent hyperperfusion in the collaterals in the case of a hypoplastic anterior cerebral artery and/or posterior communicating artery (**a**); occlusion of the internal carotid artery with well-developed circle of Willis, but additional high-grade stenosis in the middle cerebral artery (**b**); high-grade stenosis of the distal internal carotid artery resulting in local turbulence (**c**)

14.2.2 Accuracy and Possibilities of Error

A very high-grade, isolated stenosis of the intracranial internal carotid artery can hardly be overlooked if all (!) diagnostic criteria are observed. However, problems can occur in subsequent constellations.

Insufficient Temporal Window

"Standard problem" of every intracranial vascular examination is a missing or insufficient temporal sound window, since the diagnosis must then be limited to the available indirect criteria.

Other Causes of Flow Disturbance

Due to the unspecific character of flow disturbances, their exact localization is of essential importance. Thus, in the presence of a flow disturbance in the area of the distal carotid artery (examination depth 60–70 mm), a high-grade stenosis of the vessel appears possible using "simple" transcranial Doppler sonography, but two other findings cannot be excluded (Fig. 14.4):

- **Occlusion of the distal internal carotid artery** with turbulent collateral supply via the anterior and/or posterior communicating artery. The flow direction and the examination depth alone cannot be used as a criterion, since the collateral supply runs equally toward the Doppler probe and it is not possible to differentiate exactly between the signals of the internal carotid and middle cerebral artery as well as to possible collateral vessels (anterior cerebral artery, posterior communicating artery muscle) due to the restricted selectivity of the measurement volume.
- **Stenosis at the origin of the middle cerebral artery** whose maximum stenosis can often also be derived at 60–70 mm.

Note

A reliable differential diagnosis in the depth range of 60–70 mm always requires the use of color coded duplex sonography, which can be used to reliably differentiate the vessels in the carotid T-section – provided that there is a sufficient temporal sound window.

Tandem Stenoses

Combined extra – and intracranial stenoses as well as long-distance stenoses, which are not uncommon in the course of the internal carotid artery, can lead to misinterpretation of the degree of stenosis. Four cases with different extra – and intracranial degrees of stenosis can be distinguished.

Table 14.3 Classification of degrees of stenosis of the middle cerebral artery and other intracranial vessels

Numeric	≤40%	45–65%	≥70%
Description	Low grade	Medium grade	High grade

Degree of Stenosis Extracranial = Intracranial

Due to the flow resistances connected in series, both stenoses are estimated to be 5–10% lower in their degree of stenosis according to hemodynamic criteria (flow velocity, flow disturbances). Since this is within the usual tolerance range of stenosis degree assessment, no significant problems arise. ◀

Degree of Stenosis Extracranial > Intracranial

In this case, the intracranial stenosis is overlooked because it does not lead to any significant hemodynamic abnormalities compared to the extracranial stenosis. ◀

Degree of Stenosis Extracranial < Intracranial

If the stenosis criteria are strictly observed, this case should already be noticed during extracranial duplex sonography by **"stenosis mismatch"** (Table 13.4). ◀

Long-Distance Extra-/Intracranial Stenosis (Dissection)

As already described in Sect. 13.2.2, in this case "normal" flow velocities can be found by color coded imaging despite visible constriction of the vessel lumen. If indirect criteria are carefully considered, false results can be avoided by side-by-side comparison of the vessel lumen and especially by determining blood flow volume. ◀

Minor and Moderate Stenoses

Due to the lack of indirect evidence, moderate stenoses up to a degree of approx. 70% are difficult to diagnose and are generally overlooked. This is particularly true if the stenosis maximum is located directly at the skull base and flow disturbances have already returned to normal at the level of the ophthalmic artery origin.

Practical Tips

Increased flow velocities and flow disturbances can also occur in narrow intracranial vessels (e.g., in smokers, young women) and in the presence of anemia. In this case, side-by-side comparison and comparison with the other extra – and intracranial vessels are decisive.

However, even severe stenoses may be diagnostically problematic, but can be reliably confirmed or excluded by combination of extra – and intracranial ultrasound criteria. A mandatory prerequisite is the use of transcranial color coded duplex sonography with the possibility of visualizing the distal internal carotid artery in the coronary view. The flow direction in the periorbital arteries also indicates the location of stenoses before or after the origin of the ophthalmic artery.

Summary

Minor and moderate stenoses in the intracranial course of the internal carotid artery are regularly overlooked.

14.3 Stenoses of the Middle Cerebral Artery

14.3.1 Definition of the Degree of Stenosis

In contrast to vascular diagnostics of the extracranial internal carotid artery (Sect. 13.1), similar complex scales have not become established for the middle cerebral artery and other intracranial arteries. There are two main reasons for this.

Problem of the Standard of Comparison

Since the middle cerebral artery is significantly smaller in caliber than the carotid artery, it is difficult to give exact percentage values for stenotic degrees even when using high-resolution intra-arterial DSA. This applies increasingly to procedures such as CTA and MRA. Last but not least, no intraoperative findings are available as a "gold standard".

Lack of Predictive Significance

Statements on the clinical significance of extracranial carotid stenosis are mainly based on percentages of the degree of stenosis. No comparable studies are available for intracranial vessels.

In view of this situation, it has become common practice for sonographic vascular examinations of the intracerebral arteries to only roughly classify stenoses (Table 14.3), although flow velocity of the cerebral arteries provides a very sophisticated parameter, especially for follow-up examinations.

14.3.2 Diagnostic Criteria

Stenoses in the main stem of the middle cerebral artery (M1) can be easily assessed by Doppler and duplex sonography due to the favorable examination conditions with a small insonation angle. However, here too there is the fundamental limitation that increased flow velocities in a vessel can be caused by both stenosis and hyperperfusion.

Intrastenotic Flow Velocity

Duplex sonographically measured flow velocity at the maximum stenosis has proven to be the most reliable parameter for detection of stenoses in the main stem of the middle cerebral artery. With minor limitations, this also applies to the determination of the systolic maximum frequency using "simple" transcranial Doppler sonography (Sect. 9.4), since in about 80% of all cases the middle cerebral artery runs at an insonation angle of less than 30° and measurement errors are therefore minimal (Table 9.6).

Beginning at a degree of stenosis of approx. 50%, stenoses of the middle cerebral artery lead to a significant increase in flow velocity (Table 14.4). However, due to intra-individually increased flow velocities in slender or narrow vessels (e.g., in young, slim women or long-term smokers), stenosis can only be assumed with sufficient certainty from a maximum systolic velocity of 160 cm/s and more (Fig. 14.5). In the borderline area, more reliable values can be obtained by side-by-side comparison, which normally does not exceed 30 cm/s. A prerequisite in this case is a reliable angle-corrected measurement of flow velocity by color coded duplex sonography.

> **Practical Tips**
> The main significance of color coded duplex sonography is the exact localization of stenoses in the middle cerebral artery. The occurrence of a local alias phenomenon in the course of the vessel with circumscribed flow velocity acceleration verifies the presence of a stenosis (Fig. 14.6).

Pre/Poststenotic Flow Velocity

Comparable to the ultrasound examination of extracranial vessels, the poststenotic flow velocity provides additional information for assessing the severity of stenosis (Sect. 13.1.2). Also comparable to the extracranial examination, however, it should be possible to measure at least 1–2 cm distal to the stenosis in order to obtain results not impaired by local flow disturbances. In the case of stenoses located somewhat further distal, the prestenotic flow velocity can also be used as a reference according to the continuity law (Fig. 2.4), since the influence of the lenticulostriatal branches on the flow volume is negligible. A reduction of the pre- or postenotic flow velocity by more than half compared to the unaffected side indicates a very high degree of flow obstruction (Sect. 10.5.5; asymmetry index).

Flow Disturbances

High-grade stenoses from approx. 70% lead to flow disturbances within the maximum stenosis, sometimes also with a "confetti effect" (Fig. 13.12). Here, too, the rule applies that the longer the distance over which poststenotic flow disturbances can be detected, the higher the degree of stenosis. However, there are no detailed studies available in the literature.

Further Findings

Stenoses of the middle cerebral artery usually do not show abnormal extracranial ultrasound findings, since their hemodynamic effect on the total blood supply of the hemisphere is relatively small. Only in individual cases – in hypoplastic A1 segment of the anterior cerebral artery – very severe stenoses result in a reduced flow velocity with increased pulsatility in the ipsilateral internal carotid artery.

14.3.3 Differentiating Increased Flow Velocities

As already described above, increases in flow velocity and flow disturbances are an unspecific phenomenon that can be

Table 14.4 Criteria for the detection of stenoses in the middle cerebral artery. Frequency values related to a transmission frequency of 2 MHz

degree of stenosis	Normal	Borderline	Medium grade	High grade
Maximum stenosis				
Systolic maximum velocity	<120 cm/s	≥120 cm/s	≥160 cm/s	≥220 cm/s
Systolic maximum frequency	<3 kHz	>3 kHz	>3.5 kHz	>6 kHz
Side-by-side difference		<30 cm/s	>30 cm/s	
Flow disturbances	–	–	?	++
Poststenotic (for proximal stenoses)				
Systolic maximum velocity			Normal	Diminished
Flow disturbances			–	++
Confetti effect			–	+
Prestenotic (for distal stenoses)				
Systolic maximum velocity			Normal	Diminished
Stenotic indices				
MCA/ICA index		<2	≥2	≥3

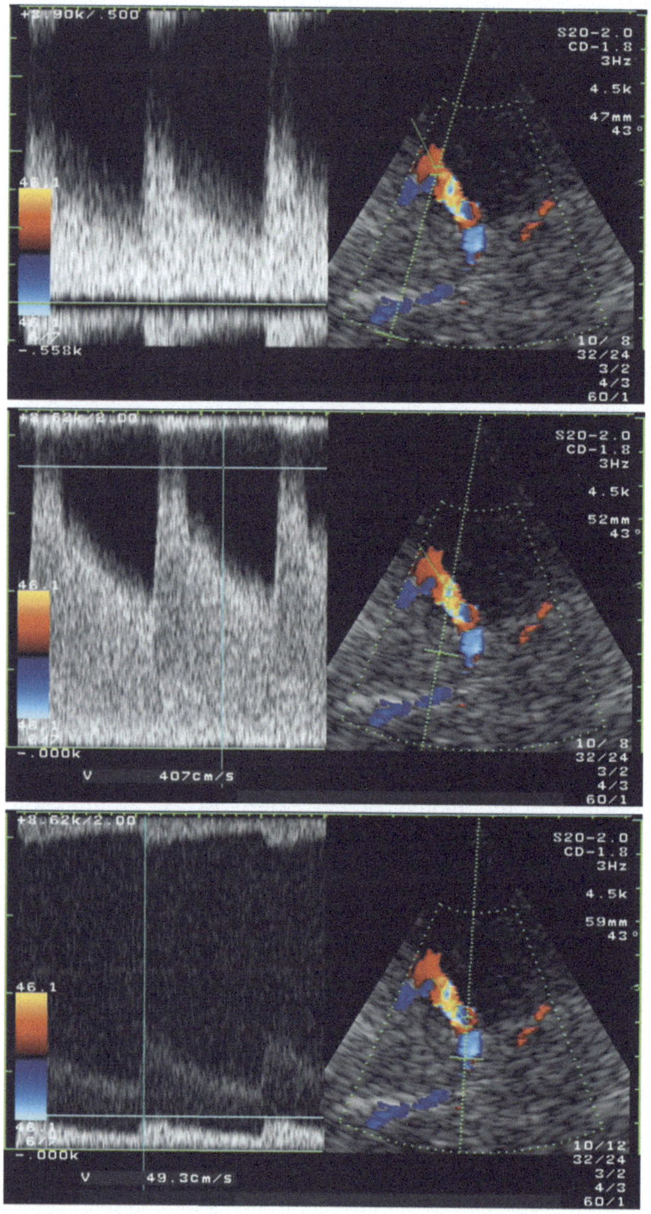

Fig. 14.5 Duplex findings in a high-grade stenosis in the M1 segment of the middle cerebral artery. Maximum systolic flow velocity around 400 cm/s (middle); associated pre- (bottom) and post-stenotic (top) findings

caused by stenoses as well as by hyperperfusion – for example, "luxury perfusion" in acute cerebral ischemia. A reliable differentiation is only possible if the vessel diameter is known at the same time, which cannot be determined by transcranial duplex sonography for methodological reasons (Sect. 6.1.4). Two approaches offer a useful way out of this dilemma.

MCA/ICA Index

The ratio between the flow velocities in the middle cerebral and the extracranial internal carotid artery can differentiate

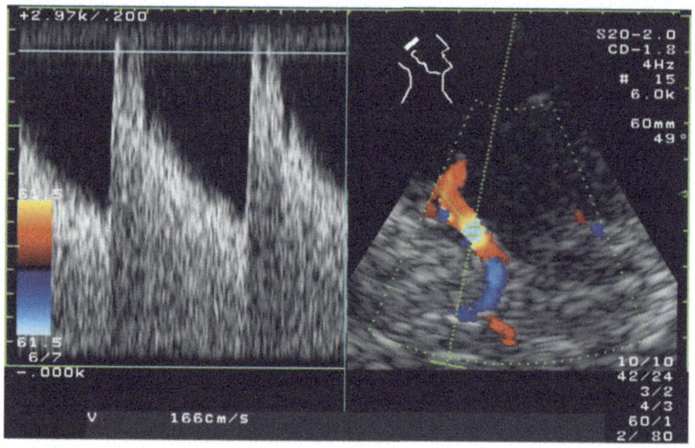

Fig. 14.6 Local aliasing phenomenon in the course of the middle cerebral artery with "optimized flow imaging" as an indication of a moderate stenosis

increased flow velocities in the middle cerebral artery as hyperperfusion (MCA/ICA $\leq$2) or as stenosis (MCA/ICA $\geq$3). However, if the internal carotid artery is equally affected by a stenosis (e.g., dissection with lumen constriction of the extracranial internal carotid artery), a misinterpretation may occur.

Limited Flow Velocity

In the case of hyperperfusion, an increase in cerebral blood flow by usually 100% is not exceeded. Due to the linear relationship between blood flow volume and blood flow velocity, there is therefore also a maximum doubling of the normally expected flow velocities. Systolic flow velocities in the middle cerebral artery exceeding 160–180 cm/s, however, can only be explained by a stenosis (quadratic relationship to the degree of stenosis) (Fig. 14.7).

$$\textbf{Hyperfusion}: V = \nu \frac{\text{CBF Hyperperfusion}}{\text{CBF normal}}$$

CBF cerebral blood flow
V pathological flow rate
ν normal flow rate

$$\textbf{Stenoses/Vasospasm}: \quad V = \nu \left(\frac{d}{D}\right)^2$$

d unstenosed diameter
D stenosed diameter

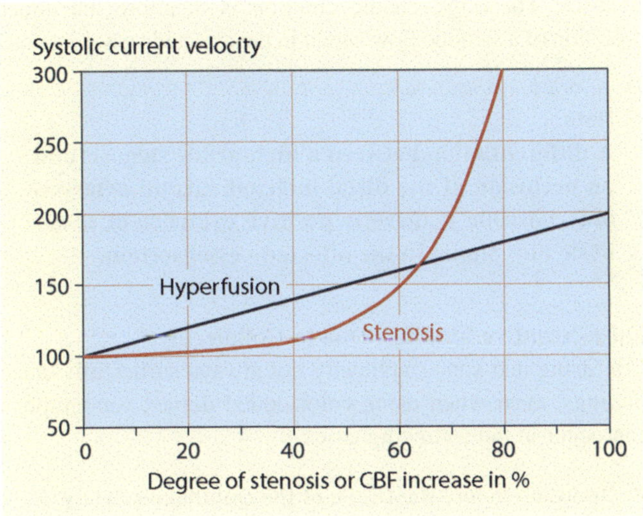

Fig. 14.7 Differentiation between hyperperfusion and stenosis/vasospasm in the middle cerebral artery based on measuring the maximum systolic flow velocity. Due to the quadratic relationship with the degree of stenosis, much higher flow velocities are to be expected in high-grade stenoses than in hyperperfusion

14.3.4 Accuracy and Possibilities of Error

The main stem of the middle cerebral artery can be assessed very reliably by Doppler and duplex sonography. The accuracy of the examination is largely equivalent to extracranial duplex examination with regard to the detection of medium and high-grade stenoses. Beyond the M1 segment, however, the accuracy decreases rapidly. Stenoses in the M2 segment can – if at all – only be detected by color coded duplex sonography. Although the positive predictive value is high (a positive ultrasound result confirms a stenosis), conversely, a negative ultrasound result cannot exclude a stenosis in this segment. In addition, two basic problems of ultrasound diagnostics of the intracranial vessels must be considered.

Confusion with Hyperperfusion

In the first 4–6 weeks after a major stroke, caution is required, as the hyperperfusion in the affected vessels following spontaneous lysis of an intracranial artery occlusion can simulate the findings of a (moderate) stenosis. The same applies to subarachnoid hemorrhages and inflammatory brain diseases, which can be accompanied by considerable cerebral hyperperfusion.

Problems of the Temporal Sound Window

If one relies exclusively on the systolic maximum velocity for the detection of a middle cerebral artery stenosis – which extracranially makes sense – false-negative findings may occur. This is due to the fact that the often insufficient temporal sound window prevents the acquisition of low energy frequency components, as they regularly occur in high-grade stenoses (Fig. 5.9). In contrast to extracranial Doppler and duplex recordings, it is therefore of decisive importance in intracranial examinations to consider also the presence of flow disturbances.

Summary

If the temporal sound window is sufficient, medium and high-grade stenoses in the proximal section of the middle cerebral artery can be reliably detected using both Doppler and color coded duplex sonography. A systolic maximum velocity of approx. 160 cm/s and higher confirms the presence of a stenosis. Very severe stenoses can sometimes only be recognized by the massive flow disturbance, while the expected high flow velocities are not (no longer) visualized due to the damping by the cranial bone.

14.4 Occlusions of the Intracranial Internal Carotid Artery

14.4.1 Diagnostic Criteria

The detection of an intracranial occlusion of the internal carotid artery is first and foremost the domain of extracranial ultrasound examination, while intracranial examination usually contributes little to further clarification (Table 14.5). On the basis of the findings, two localizations can be distinguished.

Table 14.5 Synopsis of sonographic findings in the case of an occlusion in the intracranial course of the internal carotid artery

	Before the origin of the ophthalmic artery	After the origin of the ophthalmic artery
Main criteria		
Extracranial internal carotid artery	Mostly also extracranial occlusion	Distinctive flow reduction and increased pulsatility
Periorbital arteries	Retrograde	Antegrade
Secondary criteria		
Transorbital	No trend-setting findings	
Distal internal carotid artery	Variable (not derivative or diminished)	
Middle cerebral artery (M1)	In the case of inadequate collateral supply possibly reduced pulsatility	

Occlusions Before the Origin of the Ophthalmic Artery
A complete occlusion of the internal carotid artery before the origin of the ophthalmic artery almost always leads to the thrombus "growing down" to the carotid bifurcation within a short time. In principle, such an occlusion can no longer be distinguished from a primarily extracranial occlusion. However, the presence of a **carotid stump** and the absence of significant arteriosclerotic changes in B-mode imaging of the carotid bifurcation indicate a primary intracranial occlusion (Fig. 13.23). The intracranial findings correspond to the findings of an extracranial carotid occlusion with collateral supply, especially via the anterior communicating artery.

Occlusions After the Origin of the Ophthalmic Artery
The diagnosis here is based on the combination of two findings:

- Extracranial evidence of a very high degree of flow obstruction in the distal internal carotid artery
- Antegrade, usually strong flow in the ophthalmic and periorbital arteries.

A reliable differentiation between an occlusion and a very severe stenosis is not possible if the stenosis is not directly detectable by sonography. For example, a non-derivable distal internal carotid artery can also be caused by a too low flow velocity and/or an unfavorable insonation angle.

Additional Information
A clinically significant special case is the so-called carotid T occlusion in which both the cranial segment of the internal carotid artery and the origins of the middle and anterior cerebral arteriy are occluded – usually by a thrombus coming from the cardiac system. Due to the important differential diagnosis to an isolated occlusion of the middle cerebral artery, the diagnostic criteria are discussed in the Sect. 14.5.1.

14.4.2 Accuracy and Possibilities of Error

When detecting distal carotid occlusions, there are essentially two basic problems that should be known to the examiner.

Differentiation Occlusion/Stenosis
As already mentioned above, occlusions and high-grade stenoses of the distal internal carotid artery cannot be reliably differentiated. An increased pulsatility in the extracranial internal carotid artery occurs in both cases. The absence of a detectable flow or, conversely, a reduced flow is found in the distal internal carotid artery in both occlusions and stenoses. The only reliable criterion is therefore the direct detection of a stenotic flow signal in the affected vessel section.

Note
A differentiation between a high-grade stenosis and an occlusion of the distal internal carotid artery is only possible if there is positive evidence of a stenotic flow signal in the affected vessel section.

False-Negative Findings Due to Collaterals
Confusing and sonographically not always sufficiently clear findings, even when using color coded duplex sonography, can occur in the following cases.

Occlusion Before the Origin of the Ophthalmic Artery

Branches of the external carotid artery that come out of the internal carotid artery and persistent embryonic vessels can keep the proximal section of the internal carotid artery open and in individual cases even cause a remarkably "normal" flow signal. ◀

Occlusion Before the Origin of the Posterior Communicating Artery

The distal internal carotid artery can be supplied from behind by large-scale posterior communicating artery and appears "normal" sonographically. ◀

Occlusion After the Origin of the Posterior Communicating Artery

In the case of an embryonic variant with supply of the posterior circulation via the internal carotid artery, extracranially "normal" flow conditions may also be present in cases with carotid T occlusion. ◀

Summary
Occlusions of the internal carotid artery proximal to the origin of the ophthalmic artery show identical findings as extracranial carotid occlusions. Occlusions distal to the ophthalmic origin are usually not distinguishable from high-grade stenoses in this area. In addition, collateral vessels of the internal carotid artery can lead to confusing findings.

14.5 Occlusions of the Middle Cerebral Artery

Occlusions of the middle cerebral artery are almost always associated with severe neurological deficits. Accordingly, if an ultrasound examination is indicated, there is already a corresponding clinical suspicion which must be substantiated

Table 14.6 Synopsis of the findings in occlusions of the middle cerebral artery at different localizations

	Carotid T-occlusion	Proximal M1-occlusion	Distal M1-occlusion	Main branch (M2-) occlusion	Pripheric branch occlusion
Main criteria					
Middle cerebral artery (M1 proximally)	Not derivable	Not derivable	Mean < 20 cm/s, increased pulsatility	Mean < 40 cm/s, possibly increased pulsatility	Normal (mean > 40 cm/s)
Middle cerebral artery (M1 distal)	Possibly low residual flow	Possibly low residual flow	Not derivable	Diminished	Normal
Asymmetry index (AI_{mod})	100%	100%	>50–100%	>20%	<20% (normal)
Side-by-side comparison	–	–	≥30% ipsilateral reduction in mean flow velocity	≥30% ipsilateral reduction in mean flow velocity	Normal
Secondary criteria					
Internal carotid artery (extra-cranial)	Diminished	Possibly moderately diminished	Possibly moderately diminished	Normal	Normal
Anterior cerebral artery	Not derivable	Mostly increased flow	Mostly increased flow	Mostly Normal	Normal
Posterior cerebral artery	Increased flow	Possibly increased flow	Possibly increased flow	Normal	Normal

or rejected. For the special features of sonographic diagnostics in acute stroke, please refer to the Chap. 21 on "Ultrasound diagnostics in acute stroke."

14.5.1 Diagnostic Criteria

Main Criteria

Due to their clinical significance, five localizations can be distinguished, which will be considered in the following (Table 14.6).

Carotid T-occlusion

The occlusion of the distal internal carotid artery in the area of its division into the middle und anterior cerebral artery (**carotid T**) represents clinically the most unfavorable case, since all arteries of the anterior circulation are affected and collateralization can only occur via the usually insufficient leptomeningeal anastomoses. Duplex sonographic criterion is an unrecognizable middle and anterior cerebral artery in otherwise well-visualized arteries of the posterior circulation and the opposite side. In individual cases, multiple vessels are found in the clivus region, which may correspond to **Heubner collateral** vessels. ◀

Proximal Main Stem Obstruction of the Middle Cerebral Artery

Typically, a strongly perfused anterior cerebral artery is found here in the absence of evidence of the middle cerebral artery (Fig. 21.3). ◀

Practical Tips

The diagnosis of a complete occlusion of the middle cerebral artery by color coded imaging is based almost exclusively on the lack of a visualization of the vessel. However, since intracranial vessels, in contrast to extracranial examination, cannot be reliably depicted on the basis of B-mode imaging, a clear statement can only be made if a sufficient temporal sound window can be demonstrated on the basis of the ability to examine other cerebral arteries. It is not sufficient to rely on the visualization of the ipsilateral posterior cerebral artery. It is not uncommon for the bone window to be so limited under poor examination conditions that only the posterior circulation can be visualized. Therefore, the detection of either the ipsilateral anterior cerebral arteries or – in the case of carotid T-occlusion – the contralateral cerebral arteries must always be requested.

Distal Main Stem Obstruction of the Middle Cerebral Artery

The characteristic finding is a strongly reduced flow velocity in the main stem of the middle cerebral artery (**mean value** in flow velocity <20 cm/s, **asymmetry index** > 50% with markedly increased pulsatility (lack of diastole or oscillating flow). The detectable flow in the initial section of the middle cerebral artery is due to the fact that the occlusion is distal to the origin of the lenticulostriate arteries. If there is reduced pulsatility, on the other hand, a proximally located obstruction of flow with possibly insufficient collateral supply must be considered. Color coded imaging shows a short media stump which breaks off after 1–2 cm length. ◀

Main Branch Occlusion of the Middle Cerebral Artery

Depending on the size of the affected vessel, a more or less pronounced reduction of flow velocity in the middle cerebral artery is shown compared to the contralateral side (**mean value** <40 cm/s, **asymmetry index** >20%) (Sect. 10.5.5). Color coded imaging alone does not point the way forward. ◀

Practical Tips
For practical concerns in the treatment of acute strokes, a simple side-by-side comparison is generally sufficient. If flow velocity in the affected middle cerebral artery is reduced by 30% or more, there is a high probability that the distal artery or one of its main branches is occluded.

Occlusion of a Smaller Branch of the Middle Cerebral Artery

Such occlusions cannot be detected reliably by ultrasound. ◀

Secondary Criteria
Since the middle cerebral artery is the largest intracranial vessel, hemodynamic effects on the ipsilateral internal carotid artery are regularly found in its total occlusion – at least in acute cases – in the form of a reduced flow velocity and an increased pulsatility compared to the contralateral side. In contrast, branch occlusions of the middle cerebral artery show no extracranial abnormalities, which can be used for differential diagnosis in acute stroke.

14.5.2 Accuracy and Possibilities of Error

The absence of the middle cerebral artery under good examination conditions and a clearly definable internal carotid artery or anterior cerebral artery ensures the finding of a main stem occlusion of the middle cerebral artery. With comparable accuracy, carotid T-occlusions can be recognized by the absence of the middle an anterior cerebral artery while at the same time the ipsilateral posterior cerebral artery and the contralateral cerebral arteries can be visualized by color coded imaging.

A major source of error is the failure to observe the requirement that not only the ipsilateral posterior cerebral artery but also the contralateral cerebral vessels must always be shown. Since only the combination of detectable and undetectable vessels can be used as a diagnostic criterion, "simple" transcranial Doppler sonography is methodically overtaxed here.

Summary
Provided that sufficient examination conditions are available, occlusions in the main stem of the middle cerebral artery, including so-called carotid T-occlusions, can be reliably detected using color coded duplex sonography. Smaller branch occlusions are regularly overlooked. Although transcranial Doppler sonography can suggest such occlusive processes, it is not able to secure them.

14.6 Stenoses and Occlusions of the Other Cerebral Base Arteries

14.6.1 Stenoses and Occlusions of the Anterior Cerebral Artery

Diagnostic Criteria
Stenoses in the sonographically assessable A1 segment of the anterior cerebral artery are rare compared to the above mentioned localizations. The diagnosis is based on two criteria.

Examination of the Anterior Cerebral Artery

Stenoses together with an intact anterior communicating artery are generally overlooked, since with higher stenotic levels the collateral supply "springs up" from the contralateral side. The ipsilateral stenosis then does not lead to noticeable local flow phenomena due to the lack of hemodynamic needs. Similarly, color coded duplex examination is also overtaxed with regard to the detection of occlusions in the initial section of the anterior cerebral artery. Since hypoplasia is quite common in this region (Sect. 1.7.2), it is not possible to reliably differentiate between an occlusion and an anatomical variant in a non-visualized vessel. ◀

Examination of the Anterior Communicating Artery

The sonographic detection of occlusive processes of the anterior cerebral artery or its exclusion is therefore based almost exclusively on the assessment of the anterior communicating artery. If an isolated hyperperfusion is found in this vessel without higher grade stenoses or occlusions of the internal carotid artery explaining a possible collateral supply, this can be interpreted as an indication of an occlusion of the vessel – if the anterior cerebral artery cannot be visualized. Conversely, a non-derivable A1 section of the anterior cerebral artery without local flow acceleration and turbulence in the region of the anterior communicating artery is more likely to indicate a congenital anomaly than a vascular occlusion. ◀

> **Note**
> **The flow findings in the area of the anterior communicating artery can contribute to the differential diagnosis between occlusion and hypo-/aplasia in the case of a non-visualized anterior cerebral artery.**

Accuracy and Error Possibilities
The detection of isolated hyperperfusion in the anterior communicating artery has a high positive predictive value for the presence of a flow obstruction of the anterior cerebral artery. Conversely, however, no useful statement can be made in the absence of such a finding.

Caution is required if a severe stenosis or occlusion of an internal carotid artery is present at the same time. In this case there is the problem that increased flow velocities and flow disturbances may occur not only in stenoses but also in the context of collateral supply via the anterior communicating artery. However, the flow disturbances that can be drained at a depth of 70–80 mm are then always associated with an ipsilateral retrograde perfusion of the anterior cerebral artery (A1 section).

14.6.2 Stenoses and Occlusions of the Posterior Cerebral Artery

Diagnostic Criteria
Stenoses of the posterior cerebral artery are relatively frequent. Often this is a residual finding in a partially recanalized "migration thrombus" of the vertebrobasilar vascular system. Depending on the rather variable formation of the posterior communicating artery, two different Doppler and duplex sonographic findings can be distinguished.

Normal Posterior Communicating Artery

In this case, the same situation applies to the initial section of the posterior cerebral artery (P1 segment) as described above for the anterior cerebral artery with intact anterior common anterior artery: Stenoses do not lead locally to pathological flow phenomena and are therefore overlooked. Even occlusions in the P1 segment can only be indirectly recognized by this, if a measurable hyperperfusion occurs in the posterior communicating artery. For the P2 segment, the criteria mentioned below apply. ◄

Hypoplastic Posterior Communicating Artery

In the absence of an influence of the anterior cerebral circulation, stenoses in both the P1 and P2 segments are detected with high reliability according to the sufficiently known criteria on the basis of an increased flow velocity with or without additional flow disturbance (Fig. 14.8). The expected flow velocities are approx. 30–40% lower than the values occurring in comparable findings in the middle cerebral artery (Table 14.4). Due to the variable course of the vessel, color coded duplex sonography should always be preferred. ◄

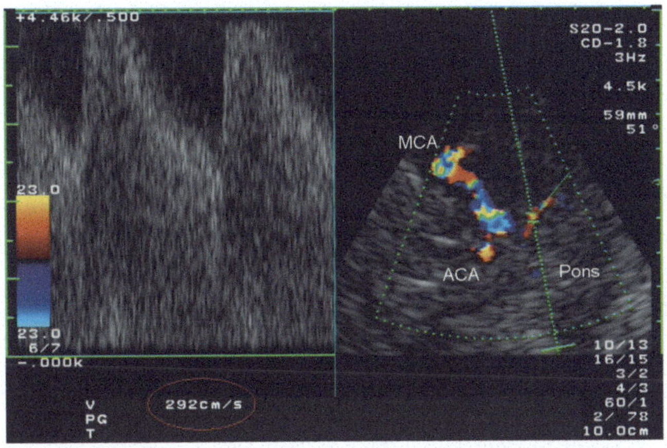

Fig. 14.8 High-grade stenosis of the posterior cerebral artery at the transition between the P1 and P2 segments with a sonographically unrecognizable posterior communicating artery

Accuracy and Error Possibilities
Under sufficient examination conditions, higher grade stenoses of the posterior cerebral artery can be diagnosed quite reliably by color coded duplex imaging; the same applies to the exclusion of a stenosis. Due to the numerous anatomical variations and the close proximity of different vessels, transcranial Doppler sonography can only be regarded as a rough screening method to exclude abnormal vascular findings. The diagnosis of an occlusion of the posterior cerebral artery is unreliable both in terms of Doppler and duplex sonography.

> **Summary**
> Due to the numerous anatomical variations, occlusions of the anterior and posterior cerebral arteries can only be diagnosed with uncertainty using sonography. The same applies to stenoses of the anterior cerebral artery. In contrast, isolated stenoses of the posterior cerebral artery are often recognizable by its typical flow abnormalities.

References

Bang OY, Fujimura M, Kim SK (2016) The pathophysiology of moyamoya disease: an update. J Stroke 18:12–20

Brass LM, Pavlakis SG, DeVivo D, Piomelli S, Mohr JP (1988) Transcranial Doppler measurements of the middle cerebral artery. Effect of hematocrit. Stroke 19:1466–1469

Brinjikji W, Mossa-Basha M, Huston J, Rabinstein AA, Lanzino G, Lehman VT (2016) Intracranial vessel wall imaging for evaluation of steno-occlusive diseases and intracranial aneurysms. J Neuroradiol. pii: S0150-9861(16)30173-0

Debette S, Compter A, Labeyrie MA, Uyttenboogaart M, Metso TM, Majersik JJ et al (2015) Epidemiology, pathophysiology, diagnosis, and management of intracranial artery dissection. Lancet Neurol 14: 640–654

Dutra LA, de Souza AW, Grinberg-Dias G, Barsottini OG, Appenzeller S (2017) Central nervous system vasculitis in adults: an update. Autoimmun Rev 16:123–131

Findlay JM, Nisar J, Darsaut T (2016) Cerebral vasospasm: a review. Can J Neurol Sci 43:15–32

Kim JS (2016) Moyamoya disease: epidemiology, clinical features, and diagnosis. J Stroke 18:2–11

Kramer DR, Winer JL, Pease BA, Amar AP, Mack WJ (2013) Cerebral vasospasm in traumatic brain injury. Neurol Res Int 2013:415813. https://doi.org/10.1155/2013/415813. Epub 2013 Jun 19

Macdonald R (2016) Origins of the concept of vasospasm. Stroke 47(1): e11–e15

Ogami K, Dofredo M, Moheet AM, Lahiri S (2017) Early and severe symptomatic cerebral vasospasm after mild traumatic brain injury. World Neurosurg 101:813.e11–813.e14. https://doi.org/10.1016/j.wneu.2017.03.039. Epub 2017 Mar 16

Reith W, Berkefeld J, Dietrich P, Fiehler J, Jansen O (2015) Diagnosis and treatment of intracranial stenoses. Clin Neuroradiol (Suppl 2): 307–316

Wolff V, Ducros A (2016) Reversible cerebral vasoconstriction syndrome without typical thunderclap headache. Headache 56:674–687

Zunker P, Georgiardis AL, Louwen F, Georgiardis D, Ringelstein EB, Holzgreve W (2000) Maternal cerebral hemodynamics in pregnancy-related hypertension. A prospective transcranial Doppler study. Ultrasound Obstet Gynecol 16:179–187

Stenoses and Occlusions in the Vertebrobasilar System

15

Bernhard Widder and Gerhard F. Hamann

The vertebrobasilar vascular system consists of a complex branching of numerous vessels. For didactic reasons the individual arterial sections are discussed separately in the following. Without considering the possible clinical significance, this is done in the order from caudal to cranial.

15.1 Stenoses and Occlusions of the Subclavian Artery

15.1.1 Auscultation and Palpation

The method of choice for the detection of relevant subclavian artery stenoses and occlusions is not ultrasound, but the clinical combination of auscultation of the cervical vessels and palpation of the radial pulse or the side-by-side comparison of blood pressure of the arms. The finding of a local stenosic bruit in the supraclavicular area in combination with an ipsilateral blood pressure reduction largely secures the diagnosis of a higher grade stenosis of the subclavian artery. Conversely, if no bruit can be auscultated and no reproducible blood pressure difference of more than 20% (usually at least 30 mmHg) is present, an occlusion of the vessel can be considered largely certain.

Practical Tips

The problem of a negative auscultation in very high-grade stenoses, which is known from the carotid arteries, does not occur in the area of the subclavian artery. Due to the usually good collateral supply via the vertebral artery and the cervical vessels, the blood flow "turns over" to the collaterals when the degree of stenosis continues to increase, analogous to the situation in the parallel vertebral arteries, so that high-grade stenoses here turn directly into an occlusion without the intermediate stage of a "pseudo-occlusion".

Possible Errors

A false-positive auscultation result may be obtained in the case of a bruit transmitted from the aorta. In this case, however, a positive auscultation result is found in both supraclavicular areas. In principle, false-positive findings can also occur in the case of a high-grade stenosis at the origin of the common carotid artery. However, the sonographic examination will clarify the situation here.

The false-positive finding of a subclavian occlusion can be made if not the subclavian artery, but the axillary artery or the brachial artery is stenosed or occluded. However, careful auscultation and palpation of the vessel course will help in this case. In addition, the subclavian artery can usually be investigated by Doppler and duplex sonography.

Practical Tips

Comparative blood pressure measurement in the arms can lead to apparently pathological side differences, especially in patients with highly fluctuating blood pressure values. Although not quantifiable, comparative pulse palpation is often more reliable in this case, since with some exercise, blood pressure differences can be "felt" with astonishing accuracy by increasing pressure with the finger on the radial artery. Last but not least, in many cases even the delayed arrival of the pulse wave at the affected arm can be feeled.

(continued)

B. Widder (✉)
Expert Opinion Institute, District Hospital, Guenzburg, Germany
e-mail: bernhard.widder@bkh-guenzburg.de

G. F. Hamann
Clinic of Neurology and Neurological Rehabilitation, District Hospital, Guenzburg, Germany

B. Widder, G. F. Hamann (eds.), *Duplex sonography of the brain-supplying arteries*, https://doi.org/10.1007/978-3-662-65566-5_15

Alternatively, in cases of doubt, simultaneous blood pressure measurement on both arms using two devices is recommended.

15.1.2 Sonographic Findings in the Subclavian Artery

Only with its proximal section the subclavian artery belongs to the brain-supplying arteries. Accordingly, the following informations are limited to this part of the vessel.

Diagnostic Criteria

In comparison to the arteries of the neck, the sonographic evaluation of the subclavian artery is limited to few criteria.

Doppler Spectrum

Due to the high peripheral resistance at rest in arteries supplying skin and muscles, stenoses of the subclavian artery only have a hemodynamic effect when they are already quite severe. Accordingly, subclavian stenoses with stenotic degrees below 60–70% – at least at rest – do not lead to flow changes that can be detected by Doppler and duplex sonography. But even higher stenotic degrees often cause diagnostic problems if the maximum of the stenosis cannot be localized. In this case, the assessment must be limited to the detection of poststenotic changes. Last but not least, the exit of the subclavian artery can often only be evaluated for parts of the cardiac cycle due to movement artifacts of the aota and breathing-dependent excursions, and superimposed venous signals cause further confusion, so that occlusions are ultimately difficult to secure. ◀

Note

The sonographic diagnosis of a subclavian occlusion should only be made with caution, since its origin cannot be evaluated accurately.

Color Coded Imaging

Although color coded duplex sonography allows the subclavian artery to be displayed regularly in its course, the above mentioned limitations apply with regard to the detection of stenoses and occlusions. For example, the large number of cervical collaterals in the case of a subclavian artery occlusion often leads to confusing vascular findings. In addition, the exit of the subclavian artery can usually only be visualized in slim patients using the linear array probes usually used on extracranial vessels. Superimposed vein signals additionally complicate the examination. ◀

Accuracy and Error Possibilities

Unless characteristic flow signals of a stenosis in the form of a pronounced flow disturbance are positively detectable, the Doppler and duplex sonographic clarification of stenoses of the subclavian artery generally fails. Even the finding of a moderate flow disturbance is not usable, since the loss of the **systolic window** cannot be detected accurately due to overlay effects. Previously used criteria such as the loss of the **diastolic return flow** as a criterion have not proved to be valid either.

An increased angle-corrected measured flow velocity can be used if it is possible to reliably follow the vessel over a sufficiently long distance both at the stenosic maximum and pre- or poststenotically. However, this seems only rarely feasible. In this case the nomogram shown in Chap. 13 (Fig. 13.9) may be used as criterion. Due to the extremely variable blood requirement in the arm, absolute velocity values are not useful for grading stenoses and must always be set in relation to the unstenosed vessel. It goes without saying that, in view of the unclear angular relationships, determining the maximum systolic Doppler frequency with the simple Doppler pen probe without simultaneous angular correction does not lead to any meaningful results.

Equally unsatisfactory is the sonographic evidence or exclusion of occlusions of the subclavian artery. An attempt can be made to display the vessel stump by color coded imaging and also to generate a corresponding flow signal (**blunt signal**). However, in view of the fact that a subclavian occlusion is not difficult to prove clinically in the absence of an auscultating bruit and an blood pressure difference >30 mmHg, further diagnostic measures are unnecessary.

15.1.3 Sonographic Findings in the Vertebral Artery

The main domain of ultrasound diagnostics for occlusive processes of the subclavian artery is to answer the question whether and to what extent the vertebrobasilar blood flow is impaired by such an event.

Subforms of the Subclavian Steal Effect

In the pathological case, three constellations of findings with smooth transitions are detectable (Fig. 15.1).

Beginning Subclavian Steal Effect

If the lumen of the subclavian artery is no longer sufficient for an adequate supply of both the vertebral artery and the arm as the result of a stenosis, the flow signal of the

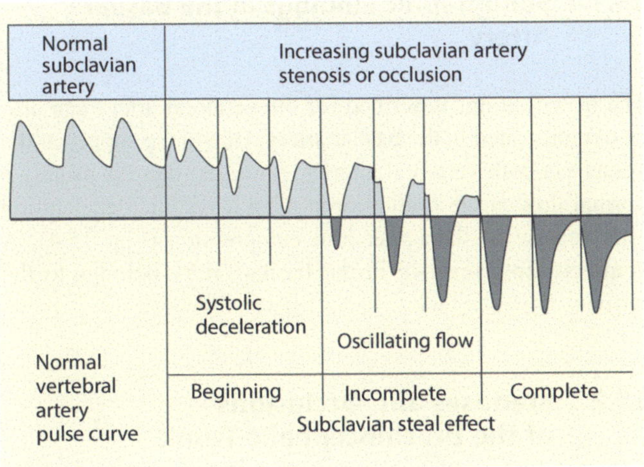

Fig. 15.1 Pulse curves of the vertebral artery with increasing hemodynamic effect of a stenosis or occlusion at the origin of the subclavian artery. If only a Doppler probe is available for diagnosis, the vascular pathology can be assessed with the aid of the **Upper Arm Compression Test** already described in Sect. 7.5.1. After the end of a 20–30 s lasting upper arm compression, a "worsening" of the pulse curve typically occurs by 1–2 categories to the right due to reactive hyperemia in the arm (Fig. 15.2). Further explanations in the text

vertebral artery initially shows a brief collapse of the systolic flow component with maintained diastolic flow. This effect is described as **systolic deceleration**. ◀

Practical Tips

A clear distinction must be made between a subclavian steal effect and a subclavian steal syndrome. Both have the common basis of a flow obstruction in the proximal subclavian artery affecting the blood supply in the vertebral artery. The subclavian steal effect describes only the hemodynamic abnormality, whereas the subclavian steal syndrome means the occurrence of clinical symptoms in the form of dizziness and other neurological abnormalities during physical exertion of the affected arm.

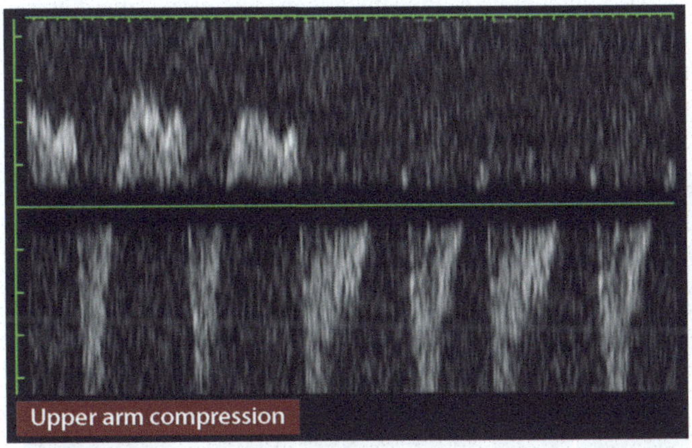

Fig. 15.2 At rest (during upper arm compression) incomplete subclavian steal effect, at exertion after end of compression complete subclavian steal effect

Incomplete Subclavian Steal Effect

If the degree of stenosis continues to increase, the systolic flow drop reaches zero or even changes to the other flow direction. This finding, in which the blood flows from cranial to caudal during systole in the vertebral artery, while it flows again from caudal to cranial during diastole, is referred to as **oscillating flow**. Such flow phenomena can cause confusion in other imaging procedures (CTA, MRA) if the systolic blood flow is approximately identical to the diastolic and the affected vertebral artery is not or only very little contrasted. ◀

Complete Subclavian Steal Effect

This is the case when, in very severe subclavian artery stenosis or occlusion, the direction of flow in the ipsilateral vertebral artery is retrograde, that is, directed toward the arm, both during systole and diastole. ◀

Accuracy and Error Possibilities

Due to the possibility of assessing hemodynamic phenomena, Doppler and duplex sonography is the easiest and most reliable method compared to (other) imaging procedures (CTA, MRA) to clarify the influence of occlusive processes of the subclavian artery (and the brachiocephalic trunk, see below) on cerebral perfusion. Vertebral arteries not shown in MR angiography when a subclavian steal effect is detected in ultrasound must be interpreted as false findings of MRA if no sequential image sequence was performed during contrast medium administration.

Note

Compared to (other) imaging techniques, Doppler sonographic imaging of the vertebral artery is the method of choice for the evaluation of a subclavian steal effect and its subforms in occlusive processes of the subclavian artery.

When using the simple Doppler probe, false results can occur if the occlusion or hypoplasia of the vertebral artery does not result in a subclavian steal effect with vertebro-vertebral overflow, but rather in a co-supply of the arm via the occipital artery. Due to the close proximity of vertebral artery and occipital artery in the mastoid region, confusion is possible if only CW Doppler sonography is available and the

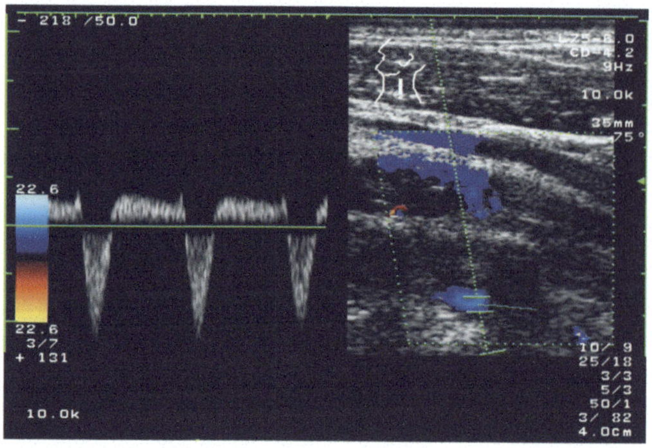

Fig. 15.3 Duplex sonographic detection of an incomplete subclavian steal effect with oscillating flow in the intertransversal course of the left vertebral artery in the case of a high-grade stenosis of the ipsilateral proximal subclavian artery (without upper arm compression)

occipital artery shows the same increase in flow in upper arm compression test as would be expected from the vertebral artery in a complete subclavian steal effect. In the case of color coded imaging of the vertebral artery in the intertransversal course, such misinterpretations do not occur (Fig. 15.3).

Summary

The contribution of Doppler and duplex sonography to the detection of stenoses and occlusions of the subclavian artery is relatively small, since the accuracy of the examination is limited due to the often unfavorable examination conditions. In addition, such occlusive processes are usually much easier to diagnose by auscultation and side-by-side blood pressure measurement (or pulse palpation). The main purpose of sonography is to determine the influence on the vertebral artery and thus on the blood flow in the posterior cerebral circulation. Based on the flow findings in the vertebral artery, subclavian steal effects and their pre-forms can be assessed in a differentiated manner.

15.1.4 Sonographic Findings in the Basilar Artery

The flow findings described for the vertebral artery can also be demonstrated in the basilar artery. Due to the supply of the vessel via both vertebral arteries, however, there is usually a normal flow curve finding or at most a systolic deceleration after release of the upper arm compression (Fig. 15.4). A complete flow reversal in the basilar artery belongs to the rarities.

15.2 Stenoses and Occlusions of the Brachiocephalic Trunk

Higher grade stenoses and occlusions of the brachiocephalic trunk are relatively rare, so that they can be mentioned only briefly. It is important to think of them in case of a blood pressure difference to the disadvantage of the right arm and/or an auscultation bruit in the right supraclavicular area. The same applies if the flow signal of the right carotid artey appears to be noticeably altered. If stenoses or occlusions of the brachiocephalic trunk are suspected, the presence of Takayasu arteritis should always be considered (Seyahi 2017).

Diagnostic Criteria

Typical flow findings in the carotid arteries in the case of a high-grade stenosis or occlusion of the brachiocephalic trunk are

- **Reduced pulsatility** in the sense of a poststenotic flow curve and/or
- **Carotid steal effect** analogous to the subclavian steal effect with its various forms (especially systolic deceleration and incomplete steal effect). A complete carotid steal effect, however, is only observed in rare cases.

Also analogous to the subclavian steal effect, the diagnosis is based on the flow reaction in the carotids using the **upper arm compression tests** (Sect. 7.5.1). It is remarkable that often each carotid artery branch shows a different steal

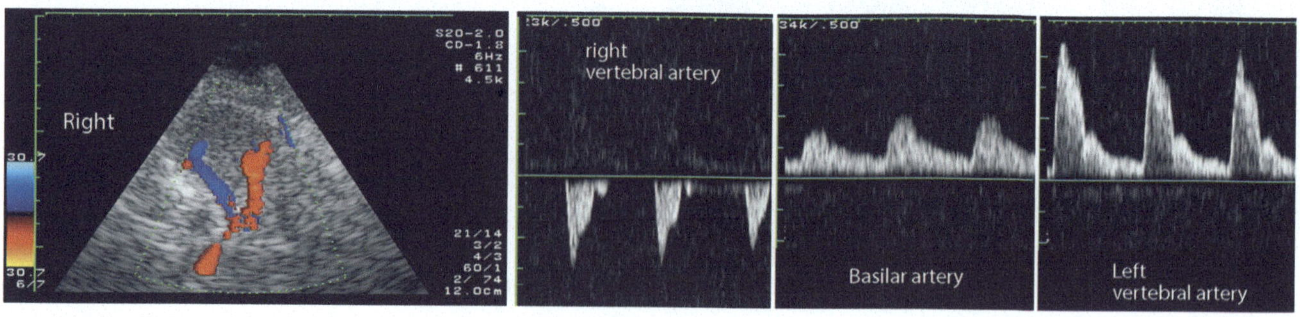

Fig. 15.4 Findings in a subclavian steal effect on the right side. Transnuchal sonography with normal basilar artery

subform. The vertebral artery usually also shows one of the forms of a subclavian steal effect.

Additional Information

Occlusions of the brachiocephalic trunk are often accompanied by quite extraordinary supply routes of the cerebral blood flow. Thus, a vertebro-vertebral overflow with retrograde supply of the right vertebral artery can lead to a further antegrade filling of the right internal carotid artery. In individual cases, however, also the reverse way with filling of the vertebral artery via the carotid artery or via the thyrocervical and external carotid artery can be found. An interventional therapy of these stenoses is possible, which is why a distinct clarification of the vascular situation should be intended. (Bradaric et al. 2015).

Accuracy and Error Possibilities

A poststenotic flow signal in the common carotid artery similar to a vein (**"pseudovein"**) can lead to confusion when using the simple Doppler probe without imaging. Therefore, duplex sonography is the method of choice for assessing the hemodynamic effects of stenoses and occlusions of the brachiocephalic trunk, comparable to the sonographic clarification of the subclavian steal effect.

> Note
>
> **In the case of a high-grade stenosis or occlusion of the brachiocephalic trunk, poststenotic changes with reduced pulsatility or curve forms known from the subclavian steal effect can be found in both the right carotid and vertebral artery** (Fig. 15.5).

15.3 Stenoses of the Vertebral and Basilar Artery

15.3.1 Special Features of Vascular Diagnostics in the Vertebral Artery

Paired Attachment of the Vertebral Arteries

Due to the paired course of the vertebral arteries with intracranial connection to the unpaired basilar artery, there are significant hemodynamic differences to the other brain-supplying arteries. In terms of flow physiology, this is a parallel connection of vascular resistances, for which the **Kirchhoff Laws** apply. The second Kirchhoff law states that when resistors are connected in parallel, the currents in the individual branches behave in reverse to the individual branching resistors:

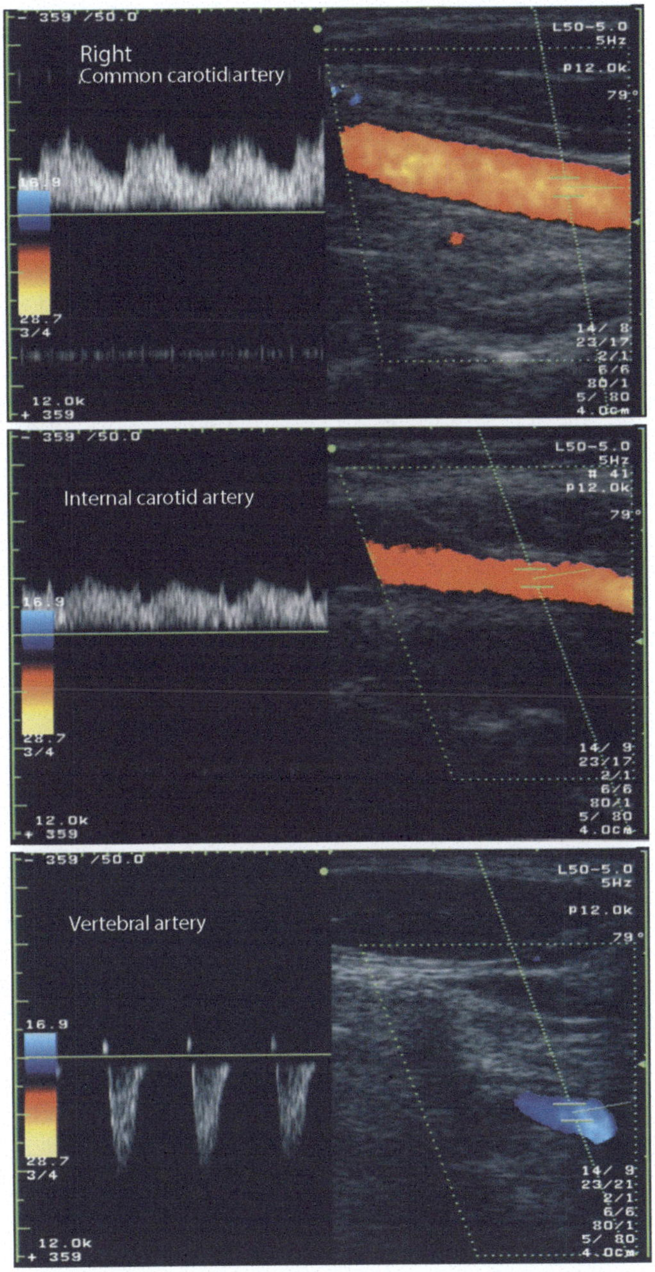

Fig. 15.5 Ipsilateral flow signals in the branches of the carotid artery (pseudovein) and vertebral artery (subclavian steal effect) in a high-grade stenosis of the brachiocephalic trunk

$$I_1/I_2 = R_2/R_1$$

I Current

R Vascular resistance

If, instead of the vessel resistances, their diameter is taken into account according to the **Hagen-Poiseuille law** (Sect. 2.3), there results the relationship

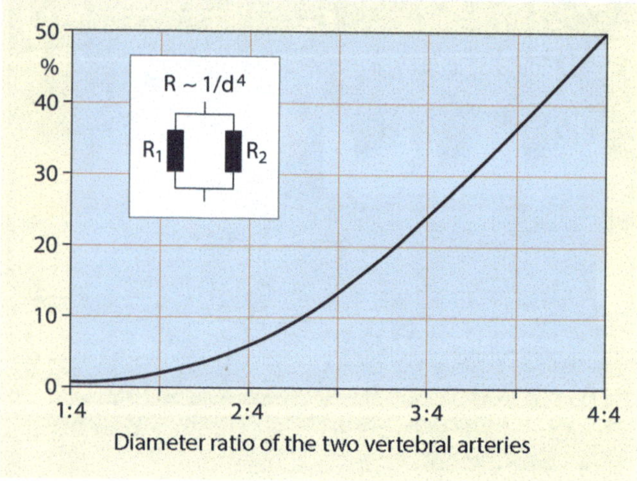

Fig. 15.6 Calculated proportion of the hypoplastic or stenosed vertebral artery on total blood flow of the basilar artery depending on the diameter ratio of the two vessels. The disproportionately strong decrease is due to the fact that the vertebral arteries are – from a flow physiological point of view – a parallel connection of two flow resistances. According to the law of Hagen-Poiseuille, the flow resistance R is inversely proportional to the diameter of the vessels to the fourth power

$$I_1/I_2 = (d_1/d_2)^4$$

d Vessel diameter

Since the vessel diameter enters the equation in the fourth power, this results in the fact that even relatively small hypoplasias or stenoses of one vertebral artery lead to a considerable decrease in blood flow in the affected vessel (Fig. 15.6).

In the case of largely symmetrical diameters of the vertebral arteries, a critical reduction in blood flow in the poststenotic vessel of only 1–2% of the original blood flow is achieved even with a one-sided stenosis of 70%, that is, the contralateral vertebral artery has taken over the nearly complete blood supply of the posterior cerebral circulation. Due to the remaining minimal flow in the pre- or poststenotic vessel, spontaneous thrombosis in the affected segment can be expected – at least in the case of further progression of the stenosis. High-grade stenoses of vertebral artery are therefore remarkably rare and generally only to be expected if the contralateral vertebral artery is hypoplastic, occluded or also stenosed to a higher degree.

Lack of Benefit of CW Doppler Sonography

As already mentioned in Sect. 7.1, CW Doppler sonography of the vertebral artery is no longer of any practical significance today. The systolic maximum frequency is not very useful due to the very variable and unknown insonation angle at the two Doppler sonographic recording points at the origin of the vertebral artery and at the atlas loop. Other flow parameters such as pulsatility depend to a large extent on the vessel diameter which cannot be recorded by Doppler sonography due to the hemodynamic peculiarities mentioned above.

> Note
> **The Doppler sonographic examination of the vertebral arteries is considered obsolete today – with the exception of the clarification of a clinically suspected subclavian steal effect.**

15.3.2 Stenoses at the Origin of the Vertebral artery (V0)

The duplex sonographic diagnosis of such stenoses is problematic for two reasons.

Limited Representability

When using the "usual" linear array probe, the origin of the vertebral artery, especially on the left side and in obese patients with short neck, cannot always be reliably visualized.

Kinkings and Coilings

As already described in Sect. 1.3.1, kink and loop formations at the origin of the vertebral artery are the rule rather than the exception, which makes it difficult to differentiate between stenosis and an anatomical variant in individual cases. In particular, it should be taken into account that moderate flow disturbances at the origin of the vertebral artery are physiological due to the fact that the vessel outlet is usually rectangular.

Diagnostic Criteria

Color coded imaging is often not very trend-setting in the outlet area of the vertebral artery, since no optimal "color filling" of the vessel is achieved due to the already physiologically existing flow disturbance. Accordingly, lumen constrictions can only be directly assessed if the vessel is normo- or even hyperplastic and the vessel walls can be clearly delineated.

As far as possible in view of the often strong systolic-diastolic excursions of the supraaortic vessel outlets, an angle-corrected measurement of **flow velocity** should be sought (Fig. 15.7). Since no standard values are available due to the variable hemodynamic conditions, stenosis can be graded using the nomogram presented in Chap. 13 (Fig. 13.9). As a reference for the unstenosed vessel, the poststenotic flow velocity in the V1 section of the vessel is determined.

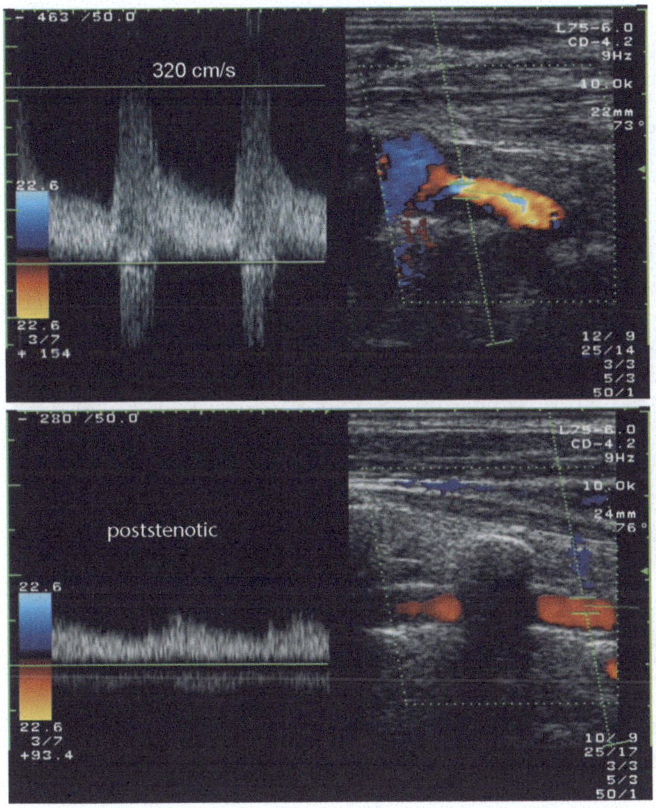

Fig. 15.7 Stenosis at the origin of the vertebral artery (top). Notice the reduced pulsatility ("pseudovein") in the poststenotic V2 section of the artery (bottom)

As already mentioned above, moderate **flow disturbances** at the origin of the vertebral artery must be considered physiological. Pathologically, therefore, only pronounced flow disturbances can be utilized which then indicate an already higher degree of stenosis of the vertebral artery.

Accuracy and Error Possibilities

As in various other areas of the vertebrobasilar system, ultrasound diagnostics has a very high positive predictive value, that is, if a stenosis is detected positively, it is actually present. In differential diagnosis, vasculitis must be considered in addition to arteriosclerotic lesions and dissections (Chap. 17). Conversely, however, the negative predictive value is relatively low. This is particularly true for low and moderate stenoses, which are almost regularly overlooked.

15.3.3 Stenoses in the Prevertebral Course of the Vertebral Artery (V1)

Stenoses in the prevertebral course between the vessel origin and the entry into the transverse foramina represent only a hypothetical localization of stenoses. The authors are not aware of any case of such a stenosis. Since the vessel is regularly stretched in this section, also no stenotic kinkings are to be expected.

15.3.4 Stenoses in the Intertransversal Course of the Vertebral Artery (V2)

Diagnostic Criteria

Higher grade stenoses in the intertransverse course of the vertebral arteries are also rare and usually only found in connection with kinking and dissections of the vessel (Sect. 20.1). A reliable diagnosis is easily possible by color coded duplex sonography, which detects the elongation of the vessel or the narrowing of the lumen with locally increased flow velocity and the presence of flow disturbances.

Accuracy and Error Possibilities

A frequent problem is the differentiation between a long dissection and a primary hypoplasia. Three diagnostic criteria help here in individual cases.

Unstenosed Lumen Visible

In principle, simple clarification can be achieved when, under good examination conditions, the (original) lumen of the vertebral artery is visible in the B-mode image, and the color filled lumen is clearly narrower (Fig. 15.8). However, it should be noted that false results can result if color coding is not optimized according to a low-flow setting (Sect. 6.3.1). ◄

Comparison with the V0/V1 Section

Even long-distance dissections of the vertebral artery almost always do not involve the V0/V1 area. Accordingly, the prevertebral findings should be compared with the intertransversally recognizable lumen. ◄

Vertebrobasilar Transition

The course of the vertebral arteries into the basilar artery usually follows regularities, which allow conclusions to be drawn about hypoplasia. Thus, symmetrically positioned vertebral arteries regularly run largely symmetrically into the basilar artery, whereas in asymmetrical positioning, the larger caliber vessel usually describes an arc toward the contralateral side immediately before it enters the basilar artery. It goes without saying that this situation is best visualized by MR angiography. Under favorable examination conditions, however, color coded duplex sonography can also adequately depict the vertebrobasilar transition region. ◄

15.3.5 Stenoses in the Area of the Atlas loop (V3)

Stenoses in the area of the atlas loop are usually not caused by arteriosclerosis, but mainly by dissections, more rarely also by kinkings. In addition, the rule already mentioned above

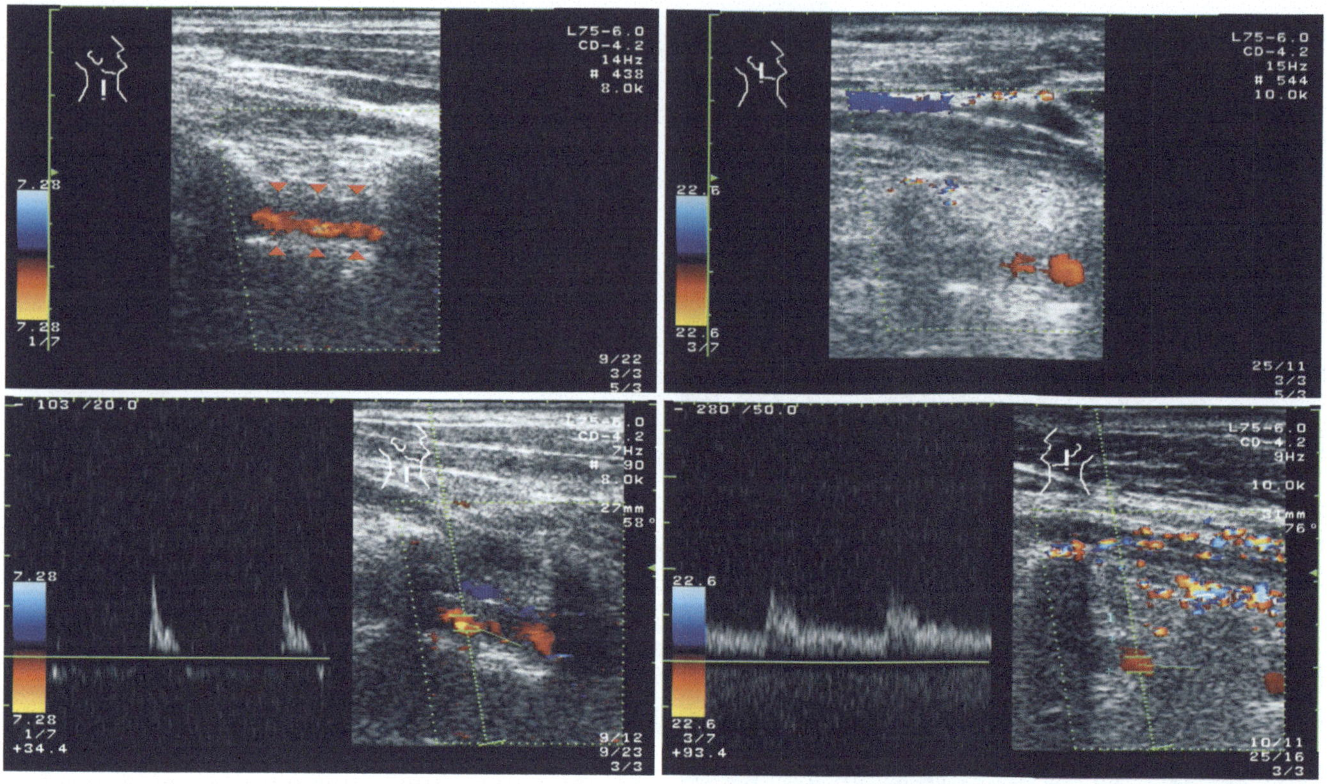

Fig. 15.8 Clearly definable original lumen of the vertebral artery in the V2 section of a long dissection (left). In comparison, only insufficient "color filling" of the vertebral artery under reduced examination conditions (right). In this case, the typical flow signal (below) is decisive for differentiation

applies, according to which higher grade stenoses only occur if a hypoplastic or likewise stenosed vessel is present contralaterally. Otherwise, complete occlusion in the affected segment regularly occurs.

Diagnostic Criteria

In the best case, color coded duplex sonography can be used to directly visualize the cause of the stenosis (kinking or dissection) due to the typical course of the vessel or the change in diameter of the vertebral artery. Using B-mode imaging, however, the original vessel wall is only recognizable in isolated cases due to the often reduced image quality in this area. Otherwise, the usual criteria for determining the angle-corrected flow velocity and assessing flow disturbances apply.

Accuracy and Error Possibilities

The main problem is the identification of hypoplastic vessels, especially in obese patients, with correspondingly reduced imaging possibilities. It is not uncommon in this case to find several small arteries which, however, cannot be reliably assigned to the vertebral artery. In contrast, the detection of stenoses in normal sized and hyperplastic vessels is usually not difficult.

15.3.6 Stenoses of the Intracranial Vertebral artery (V4) and Basilar Artery

Diagnostic Criteria

The sonographic diagnosis of stenoses of the vertebrobasilar junction is based on the direct and indirect assessment of the vessel.

Direct Assessment

Intracranial stenoses can be recognized by a local flow acceleration with the occurrence of flow disturbances during transnuchal insonation. It goes without saying that this is only true for higher grade stenoses. Since the flow velocities in the posterior cerebral circulation are lower than in the anterior cerebral circulation, the limit between normal and pathological systolic maximum velocities of 100–120 cm/s (or 2.5–3 kHz) should be considered (Table 15.1). ◄

Indirect Assessment

Indirect criteria in the extracranial vertebral artery for a stenosis in the vertebrobasilar transition area are only found if there is a very high flow obstruction. In this case an ipsilateral increased pulsatility with a proximally

Table 15.1 Criteria for the detection of stenosis of intracranial vertebral and basilar arteries Frequency values related to a transmission frequency of 2 MHz

Degree of stenosis	Normal findings	Borderline	Stenosis
Direct assessment			
Systolic maximum velocity	<100 cm/s	≥100 cm/s	≥120 cm/s
Systolic maximum frequency	<2.5 kHz	>2.5 kHz	>3 kHz
Flow disturbances		–	Distinctive
Indirect assessment			
Pulsatility		Normal	Increased

inconspicuous vessel lumen is indicative. A prerequisite for this is a largely symmetrical vessel diameter, otherwise pulsatility as a criterion fails (Fig. 20.8). ◀

Practical Tips
In individual cases, the transtemporal duplex sonographic examination also helps to detect stenoses of the basilar artery. Under good examination conditions, the vessel can often be traced caudally from the basilar head over 1–2 cm in the coronary view, so that higher-grade stenoses in the distal part of the basilar artery can be both detected and reliably excluded.

Accuracy and Error Possibilities
Stenoses of the posterior inferior cerebellar artery (PICA) can simulate the local findings of a stenosis of the intracranial vertebral artery. In most cases, this vessel runs retrograde in the direction of the sound probe during transnuchal insonation, but anatomical variants are not uncommon. Since PICA stenoses, on the other hand, lead to similar therapeutic consequences, such false findings cannot be classified as serious.

While a stenosis can be predicted with a high degree of certainty if a systolic maximum velocity of 120 cm/s (or a maximum frequency of 3 kHz) is exceeded, the reverse conclusion is not possible. Due to the numerous anatomical variations and the hardly predictable collaterals in the vertebrobasilar area, "normal" Doppler frequencies cannot reliably exclude a flow obstruction. The only exception is when under good examination conditions the vertebrobasilar vascular system can be clearly (!) visualized in its entire course by color coded duplex sonography.

Summary
Slight and moderate constrictions of the vertebral and basilar arteries are not detectable by sonography. The combination of high flow velocity and flow disturbance reliably detects a high-grade stenosis (high positive predictive value) in transnuchal sonography (Doppler or duplex sonography). However, due to the numerous anatomical variants, a reliable exclusion of stenosis is only possible if the entire course of the vessel can be continuously displayed by color coded imaging without circumscribed alias phenomena.

15.4 Occlusions of the Vertebral and Basilar Arteries

Due to the numerous spinal collaterals, thrombosis in the course of the vertebrobasilar vascular system leads only relatively rarely to an occlusion of the entire vertebral or basilar artery. Rather, depending on the flow physiology and the width of the respective collaterals, individual vessel sections usually remain open. Due to the different findings 4 occlusion localizations can be distinguished.

15.4.1 Occlusions of the Proximal Vertebral Artery (V0–V1)

Occlusions of the vertebral artery before entry into the transverse foramina are not uncommon and are usually a random finding, since they are regularly collateralized by spinal vessels. Due to the segmental limitation and the collateral supply they usually do not cause brainstem infarctions. On the question of their involvement in **vertebrobasilar insufficiency** see Sect. 20.3.2.

Diagnostic Criteria
The leading finding is an "atypical" flow signal in a normal sized vertebral artery. Due to the complex flow conditions with variable collaterals, this signal can ultimately show any form of flow reduction with normal, increased or decreased pulsatility. Characteristically, the signal shape changes over the course of the vertebral artery at the neck. In individual cases there is also a systolic deceleration or an oscillating flow.

Accuracy and Error Possibilities

If the above mentioned flow signals are found in the intertransversal course of the vertebral artery and the proximal vessel section cannot be visualized, there is no doubt about the diagnosis of an occlusion at the origin of the vessel. A diagnostic problem that cannot be solved, however, are primarily hypoplastic vertebral arteries. In this case, it is not uncommon for the proximal section of the vessel to be unreliably displayed, and variable flow signals may also be detectable in the course of the vessel. For a vessel diameter < 2.5 mm, the diagnosis of a proximal occlusion should therefore not be made.

15.4.2 Occlusions in the Middle Section of the Vertebral Artery (V2–V3)

Diagnostic Criteria

Segmental occlusions of the vertebral artery in the course between two transverse processes probably belong to the rarities and are not familiar to the authors from their own practice. In contrast, long-distance vascular occlusions occur mainly in the course of dissections. In such a case, the main finding is a normal caliber vertebral artery that can be clearly defined by B-mode imaging without corresponding blood flow when a low-flow setting is used (Sect. 6.3.1).

Accuracy and Error Possibilities

The main source of error is the description of an occlusion that could not be visualized by B-mode imaging. In principle, confusion with the vertebral vein, which runs directly next to the vertebral artery, is also possible. If the flow signal is derived from this vessel, however, differentiation is not difficult to achieve.

> **Practical Tips**
> Since Doppler signals from smaller veins often have a pulsatile character, it can be difficult in individual cases to distinguish pathologically altered arteries from veins. This can be remedied by performing a short-term Valsalva maneuver, which characteristically leads to a temporary cessation of venous blood flow.

15.4.3 Occlusions of the Distal Vertebral Artery (V4)

Diagnostic Criteria

The diagnosis of an intracranial occlusion of the vertebral artery is essentially based on 3 findings:

- Evidence of markedly increased pulsatility in a vertebral artery during extracranial insonation (often also an oscillating flow)
- Exclusion of hypoplasia as the cause of increased pulsatility on the basis of the vessel imaging
- Lack of evidence for a higher degree of stenosis of the vertebral artery in transnuchal insonation.

> **Note**
> **An oscillating flow is also to be regarded as pathological in a hypoplastic vertebral artery, since such a flow behavior cannot be explained physiologically.**

Accuracy and Error Possibilities

In case of corresponding clinical failures (e.g., **Wallenberg syndrome**) and observance of the above criteria, the diagnosis is considered certain (high positive predictive value). However, the reverse conclusion is not possible. Due to the numerous anatomical variants and the possibly high outflow into a dilated posterior inferior cerebral artery (PICA), a normal Doppler signal in the vertebral artery cannot exclude an occlusion distal to the PICA.

A repeatedly discussed cause of intermittent vertebral circulation disorders is the so-called **Bow Hunter's syndrome** in which the ipsilateral vertebral artery is compressed by massive rotation of the head under exertion (Duan et al. 2016). In most cases there are additional bony or degenerative changes as an additional pathology near the vertebral artery (osteophytes, spondylosis, abnormal tendon attachments or tumors). Ultrasound examination can provide first indications of an abnormal reduction of the ipsilateral vertebralis flow. The diagnosis is confirmed by dynamic CTA and/or DSA.

> **Practical Tips**
> Caution is required when describing increased pulsatility in the vertebral artery. If there is an angle of approximately 90° between the sound beam and the vessel, which is often unavoidable due to the vertebral arteries usually lying quite deep in the tissue, only relatively low Doppler frequencies are shown on the screen. In such a case, the diastolic flow component can be cut off by the wall filter, which leads to the misdiagnosis of high pulsatility (Fig. 5.14).

15.4.4 Occlusions of the Basilar Artery

Diagnostic Criteria

The criteria mentioned for intracranial occlusion of the vertebral artery apply equally to occlusions of the basilar artery,

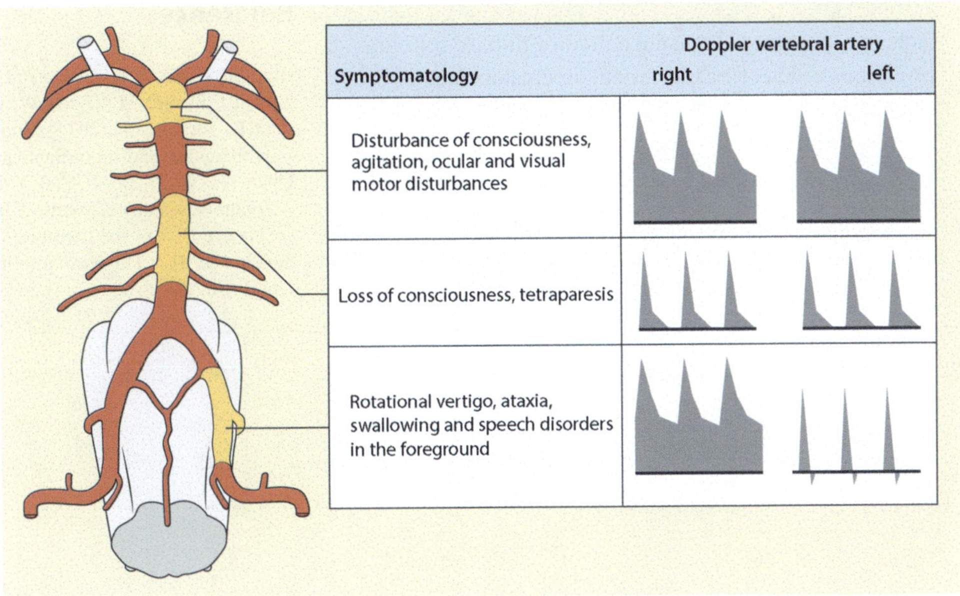

Fig. 15.9 Synopsis of clinical findings and typical flow signals in the extracranial vertebral artery when the distal vertebral artery and the basilar artery are occluded

whereby in this case both vertebral arteries typically show conspicuous Doppler signals (Fig. 15.9).

Accuracy and Error Possibilities

Again, though the positive predictive value is high, a basilar occlusion cannot be excluded if the extracranial flow signals of the vertebral arteries show normal findings (low negative predictive value). This applies in particular to slowly developing and older basilar artery thromboses as well as to "top of basilar occlusions" which are clinically difficult to detect, since psychological abnormalities are the main concern.

> **Note**
>
> **The accuracy of the sonographic detection of basilar occlusions decreases,**
> - **the more distal the occlusion is,**
> - **the slower the occlusion has developed,**
> - **the longer the occlusion occurred.**

Transnuchal sonography with color coded duplex sonography provides additional certainty only with regard to the exclusion of basilar thrombosis. If the vertebrobasilar transition in Y-form can be shown continuously (!) and without alias phenomena, such a basilar thrombosis can be excluded.

The transtemporal insonation in the coronary view helps here additionally. A non-visualized basilar artery can be caused both by an occlusion and by unfavorable examination conditions. However, an inconspicuously displayed posterior circulation without evidence of a posterior communicating artery perfused from the anterior circulation is a strong indication against basilar occlusion (see overview).

> **Duplex sonographic criteria in occlusions of the basilar artery (basilar thrombosis)**
> - Basilar thrombosis likely
>   - Markedly increased pulsatility compared to the anterior cerebral vessels or oscillating flow in **both** vertebral arteries and/or the basilar artery by transnuchal insonation
> - Basilar thrombosis unlikely
>   - Vertebrobasilar transition can be **continuously** tracked with an inconspicuous flow signal to a depth of at least 100 mm by transnuchal insonation
>   - Posterior cerebral artery on both sides during transtemporal insonation with inconspicuous flow signal and without evidence of a posterior communicating artery perfused from the anterior circulation.

Summary

After exclusion of hypoplasia, occlusions of the distal vertebral or basilar arteries typically show a markedly increased pulsatility or oscillating flow even extracranially. The accuracy of the diagnosis decreases the further cranially the occlusion is located, the slower it has developed and the longer ago the cerebral

(continued)

ischemia occurred. Transnuchal color duplex sonography cannot detect basilar artery occlusion, but if the typical Y-shape of the vertebrobasilar transition is shown, thrombosis in this area can be largely ruled out.

References

Bradaric C, Kuhs K, Groha P, Dommasch M, Langwieser N, Haller B, Ott I, Fusaro M, Theiss W, von Beckerath N, Kastrati A, Laugwitz KL, Ibrahim T (2015) Endovascular therapy for steno-occlusive subclavian and innominate artery disease. Circ J 79:537–543

Duan G, Xu J, Shi J, Cao Y (2016) Advances in the pathogenesis, diagnosis and treatment of Bow Hunter's syndrome: a comprehensive review of the literature. Interv Neurol 5:29–38

Seyahi E (2017) Takayasu arteritis: an update. Curr Opin Rheumatol 29:51–56

Part IV

Findings in Special Questions

Arteriosclerotic Vascular Diseases

16

Dirk Sander

16.1 Diffuse Arteriopathies

16.1.1 Diffuse Thickening of Vessel Walls

Sonographic Assessment

The sonographic appearance of the normal vessel wall is composed of several layers: From the inside to the outside, the low-echo vascular lumen is followed by a narrow, echo-rich lamella, then a usually somewhat wider, low-echo layer and finally a seam, which is often blurred on the outside and rich in echo (Fig. 16.1). These layers are not, as one might initially assume, the three parts of the vessel wall, intima, media and adventitia, but are physically caused reflection phenomena at border zones of different sound impedance ("border zone reflex"). On the basis of experimental investigations, according to which the reflection near the lumen represents the lumen-intima boundary layer and the second echogenic band the media-adventitia boundary layer, the term "lumen-intima reflection" has been developed for this purpose. The term **Intima-Media Thickness (IMT)** has become generally accepted for this. For the technique of IMT assessment in the area of the common carotid artery as the best assessable vessel of the brain-supplying arteries, please refer to Sect. 8.3.3.

Importance of IMT as an Arteriosclerosis Marker

The IMT was established over many years as a marker of subclinical arteriosclerosis and was used in numerous intervention studies (e.g., for statins) as a surrogat parameter for the success of therapeutic intervention. In healthy people it is in the range of 0.5 mm until the age of 30–40 years and shows an increase of about 0.1 mm per decade of life. Correspondingly, values of around 0.8 mm can be expected in healthy older people. An intima-media thickness of 1 mm and above is generally considered pathological; from a value of approx. 1.5 mm, a pronounced change in the vessel wall can be assumed (Fig. 16.2).

However, large meta-analyses showed that IMT **progression** is not a predictor of an increased cardiovascular risk – also in diabetics – and therefore does not appear suitable as a surrogate marker for vascular events (Lorenz et al. 2012). In contrast, however, it was found that the **unique** determination of the IMT is certainly suitable for estimating vascular risk: Compared to the first quintile, the risk of a vascular events was significantly increased in people with IMT in the top quintile (Lorenz et al. 2012). Recently, the importance of an IMT determination for risk classification in primary prevention in addition to classical risk factors has been controversially discussed and is no longer recommended in the guidelines (Bots et al. 2014, Goff et al. 2014). Even with different risk populations, no clinically significant improvement in risk stratification could be achieved for IMT in the context of primary prevention (Table 16.1).

Adherence and IMT Measurement

Using IMT measurement, early stages of arteriosclerosis can already be visualized, which is often impressive for patients. It has been shown that the inclusion of IMT in an educational interview for risk optimization in patients after TIA or stroke can positively influence adherence to medication as well as risk factors (Näslund et al. 2019). Thus, after four years, drug adherence was significantly better in patients who included the annual IMT measurement in the treatment and prevention discussion (Sander et al. 2020) (Fig. 16.3). The higher drug adherence was associated with a significantly better adjustment of HbA1c, blood pressure and LDL.

Other Markers of Diffuse Arteriopathy

In addition to the IMT, other surrogate markers were examined with regard to their suitability as risk parameters. The Nixdorf recall study showed that both the Ankle-Brachial-Index (ABI) as a subclinical marker of PAD and the

D. Sander (✉)
Benedictus Hospital, Department of for Neurology, Tutzing, Germany
e-mail: psander@imm.uzh.ch

B. Widder, G. F. Hamann (eds.), *Duplex sonography of the brain-supplying arteries*, https://doi.org/10.1007/978-3-662-65566-5_16

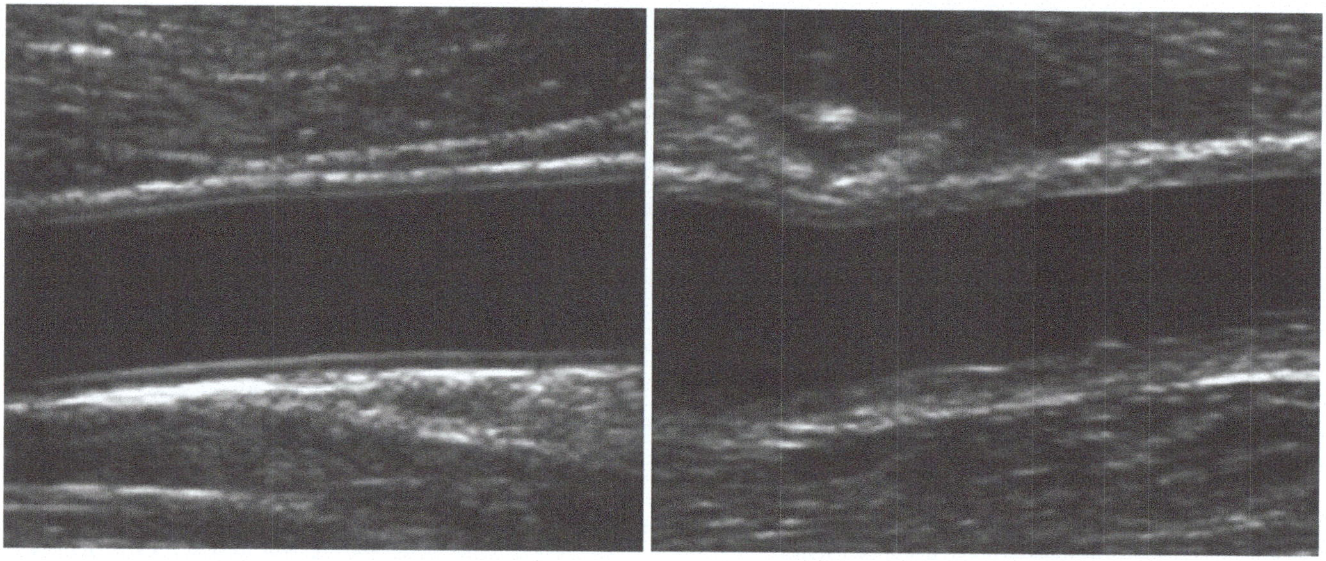

Fig. 16.1 Illustration of a normal (0.6 mm) and pathologically thickened IMT (1.5 mm) of the common carotid artery

measurement of coronary calcium are more reliable risk predictors than IMT (Gronewold et al. 2014). For the ABI measurement it could be shown that, independent of the clinical risk, a more precise risk stratification was possible in previously healthy people in addition to the Framingham risk score (Kröger et al. 2013).

Risk factors for IMT Thickening

In recent years, numerous risk factors for the occurrence of increased IMT have been described (overview p. 202). As expected, the presence of several vascular risk factors also increases IMT (Baldassarre et al. 2000). Furthermore, it has been shown that inflammation markers (e.g., hsCRP) are associated with increased IMT and a stronger progression of IMT (Willeit et al. 2014). The combination of inflammation and subclinical diabetes showed the clearest IMT progression and was associated with an increased risk of new cardiovascular events (Sander et al. 2006).

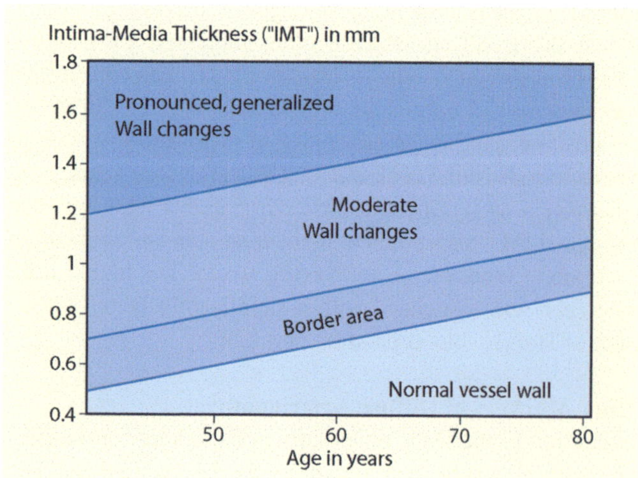

Fig. 16.2 Evaluation of intima-media thickness ("IMT") in the common carotid artery as a function of age

If a diffuse wall thickening is only slightly echogenic and has a homogeneous structure, an inflammatory process must be considered in addition to an arteriosclerotic change (Chap. 17). However, a reliable differentiation based on the sonographic appearance is not possible. Based on the latest findings on the inflammatory (co-)causation of arteriosclerotic vascular lesions, a considerable overlap can be expected here anyway.

Irregular thickening of the vascular wall in the form of a focal arteriosclerosis (additional) and usually defined as plaques (Fig. 16.4). The border between increased intima-media thickness and plaques is fluid. A proposal for the delimitation was published at several consensus conferences in 2012 (Touboul et al. 2012): **Plaques** are defined as focal thickenings of the vessel wall by at least 0.5 mm or more than 50% of the surrounding IMT or as thickening >1.5 mm measured from the media-aventitia boundary to the intima lumen boundary.

Risk Factors Described in the Literature for the Occurrence of Increased IMT in the Common Carotid Artery

- Higher age
- Diabetes mellitus
- Overweight (increased body mass index, BMI)
- Increased total cholesterol/reduced HDL cholesterol

(continued)

Table 16.1 Importance of IMT measurement for risk stratification in different populations in primary prevention

Study	Participants	N	End point	Meaning IMT measurement
Elias-Smale et al. (2012)	Men vs. women (middle age 65 years)	3580	CHD, stroke	None for men, low for women regarding 10-year risk
Yoshida et al. (2012)	Hypertensives (middle age 61 years)	17,254	Heart attack, stroke	None for 10-year risk forecast
Bots et al. (2014)	Type 2 diabetics	783	Heart attack, cardiovascular death, cerebral infarction, TIA	Low for 5-year risk forecast
Gardin et al. (2014)	Older people (middle age 72 years)	4384	CHD, heart failure, stroke	If necessary low for 10-year risk forecast

- Elevated triglycerides
- (systolic) Hypertension
- Longstanding nicotine abuse
- Past infection with chlamydia pneumoniae
- Past infection with cytomegalovirus (CMV)
- ACE polymorphism
- eNOS Polymorphism
- Elevated hs-CRP
- Periodontosis
- Elevated homocysteine
- Increased inflammation values (BSG, CRP)
- Vasculitis
- Sleep apnea syndrome
- Family history of stroke and heart attack.

With a corresponding IMT or comparable plaques in the common carotid artery, it can be assumed with a high degree of certainty that relevant and potentially embolisable vascular wall changes are also found in the aortic arch. However, the reverse conclusion is not possible: an inconspicuous IMT does not exclude aortic plaques. In contrast, circumscribed stenoses at the exit of the internal carotid artery are not suitable as a predictor of aortic plaques. They correlate much more closely with the presence of stenoses in the area of the coronary arteries (Hulthe et al. 1997) and with calcifications of the mitral ring (Adler et al. 1998).

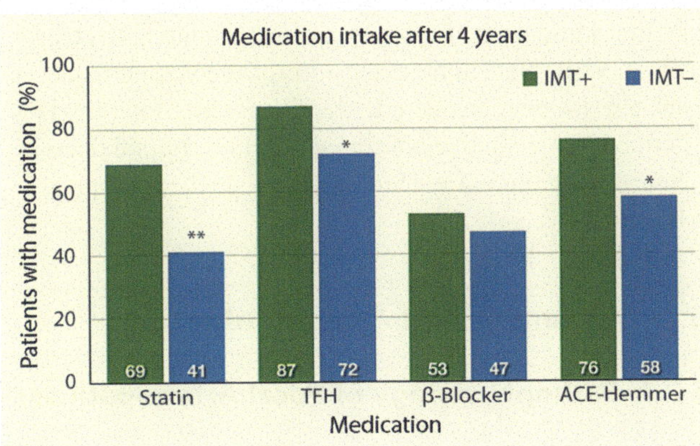

Fig. 16.3 Adherence of statin, TFH, ß-blocker and ACE inhibitor intake after 4 years depending on the inclusion of the annual IMT measurement in the treatment interview (IMT +) or non-inclusion (IMT-) in 254 patients after TIA or stroke

Note

An IMT (or plaque thickness) in the common carotid artery of 1.5 mm and more indicates relevant aortic plaques, but a "normal" common carotid artery does not exclude aortic plaques.

16.1.2 Dilated Arteriopathies

Sonographic Assessment

Sonographically, statements on dilated arteriopathies can be made with equal preference in the common carotid artery, since here the vessel diameter can be assessed most reliably and in adults normally shows only a low age dependency (Sass et al. 1998). As expected, however, there are considerable gender differences (Table 16.2).

In the literature, both the outer diameter between the two media-adventitia boundary layers (interadventitial diameter) and the inner vessel lumen are considered as measurement parameters (Fig. 16.5). Since the latter can be affected by plaques or inflammatory vascular changes, the assessment of dilated arteriopathies should preferably be based on the outer diameter. For exact measurements, the M-mode image at the time of final diastole can also be used.

Table 16.2 Standard values (mean values and standard deviation) of the outer and inner diameter of the common carotid artery in the ultrasound image

	Men	Women
Outer diameter	8.2 ± 0.9	7.3 ± 0.8
Interior diameter	6.5 ± 0.9	5.8 ± 0.7

According to Crouse et al. (1996)

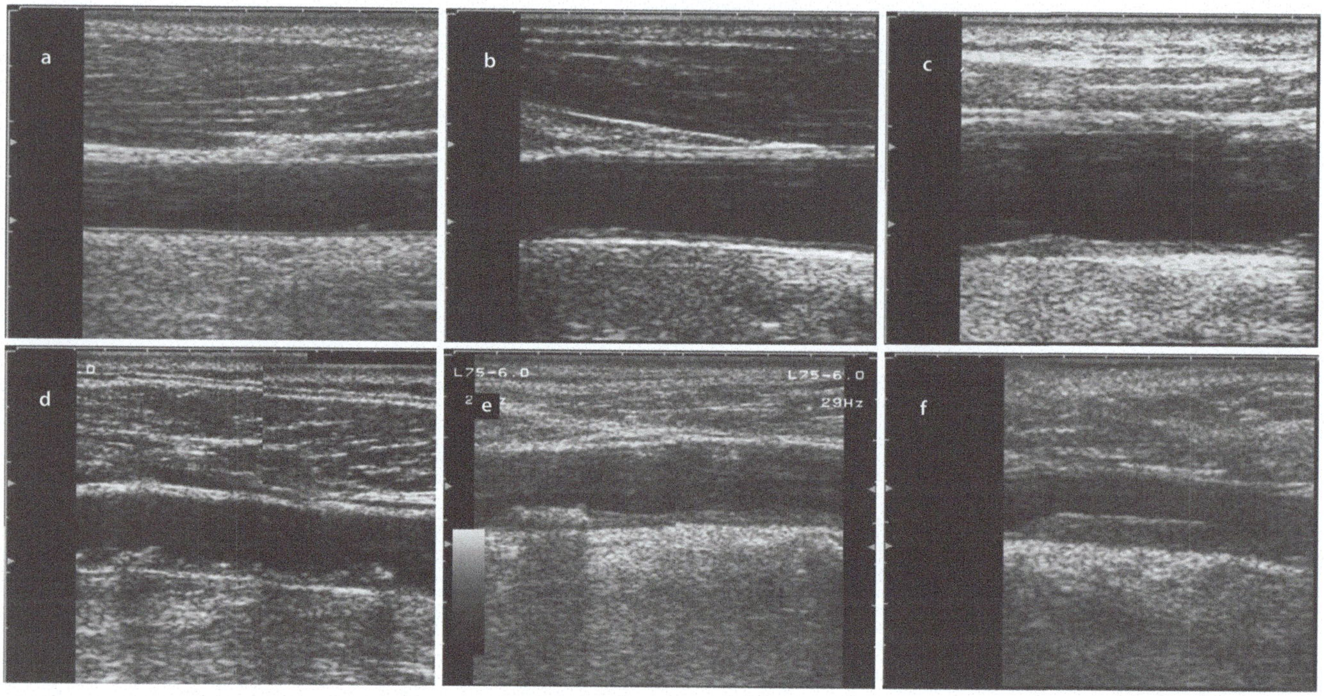

Fig. 16.4 (**a**–**f**) Examples for the formation of the vascular wall in the common carotid artery. Inconspicuous vessel in younger (**a**) and higher (**b**) age, generalized wall thickening (**c**), additionally circumscribed plaques (**d, e**), isolated, long-stretched plaque (**f**)

Clinical Significance

A dilated arteriopathy in the narrow sense is defined as a dilated arteriopathy if the vessel diameter exceeds the average value by more than two times the standard deviation.

Note

A dilated arteriopathy can be assumed if the external diameter of the common carotid artery is greater than 10 mm.

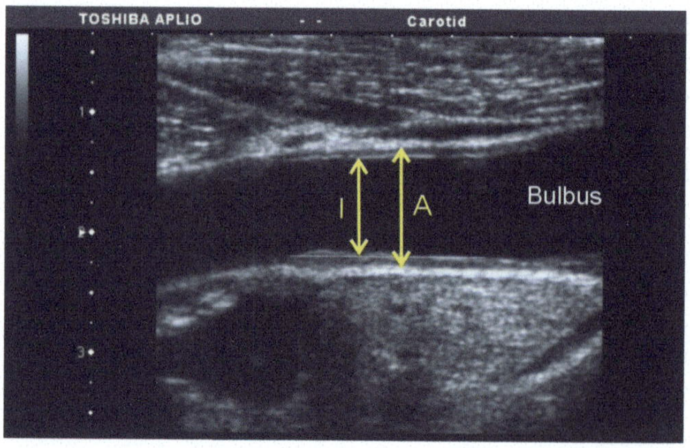

Fig. 16.5 Determination of the outer (A) and inner (I) vessel diameter in a black and white longitudinal sectional image of the common carotid artery

Summary

The intima-media thickness is a sonographic parameter for the evaluation of diffuse arteriosclerotic – in individual cases also inflammatory – vascular wall changes. It is best assessed in the common carotid artery. Depending on age, values above 0.8–1 mm are considered pathological. Values over 1.5 mm correlate additionally with the presence of (generalized) plaques in the aortic arch. Probably as a secondary effect of vessel wall thickening, extensions of the vessel diameter are to be considered. A dilated arteriopathy is defined as a dilatative arteriopathy if the external diameter of the common carotid artery exceeds approx. 10 mm.

16.2 Circumscribed Arteriopathies

16.2.1 Pathophysiology of Focal Arteriopathies

For hemodynamic reasons, the predilection sites of circumscribed vascular changes are located at vascular branches and junctions, since turbulence with increased shear forces in the blood flow occurs here, which promotes the formation of deposits as well as vascular migration erosions.

The data on absolute frequencies fluctuate considerably in the literature, which is probably mainly related to the different composition of the patient groups investigated. It can only be stated that in 100 patients with circumscribed occlusion processes of the brain-supplying arteries, isolated stenoses and occlusions of the carotid bifurcation are found in about 1/3 of the cases; about 1/3 are intracranial, the remaining third are distributed over the aortic arch branches (overview).

Frequency Distribution of Focally Circumscribed, Arteriosclerotic Vascular stenoses and Occlusions

- 1/3 branches of the aortic arch
- 1/3 carotid bifurcation
- 1/3 intracranial vessel branching

Development of Arteriosclerosis

Starting from a normal vessel wall (Fig. 16.6a), arteriosclerotic vessel wall changes initially occur due to a pathophysiologically altered endothelial function caused by irritative stimuli such as dyslipidemia, hypertension or pro-inflammatory substances (Libby et al. 2011). The expression of adhesion molecules and altered endothelial permeability play an important role in this early phase of arteriogenesis (Fig. 16.6b). Furthermore, the formation of an early atheroma with migration of smooth muscle cells from the media into the intima and the production of collagen, elastin and proteoglycans (Fig. 16.6c). In the course of the disease an activated plaque with a large lipid core and thin or ruptured fibrous cap with thrombus formation results (Fig. 16.6d; Fig. 16.7).

Practical Tips

The term plaque is used in many places only for low-grade arteriosclerotic vascular deposits, while higher-grade changes are known as stenoses can be designated. In this book plaque describes always the morphological substrate of a vascular constriction, while stenosis characterizes the hemodynamic findings of a vasoconstriction.

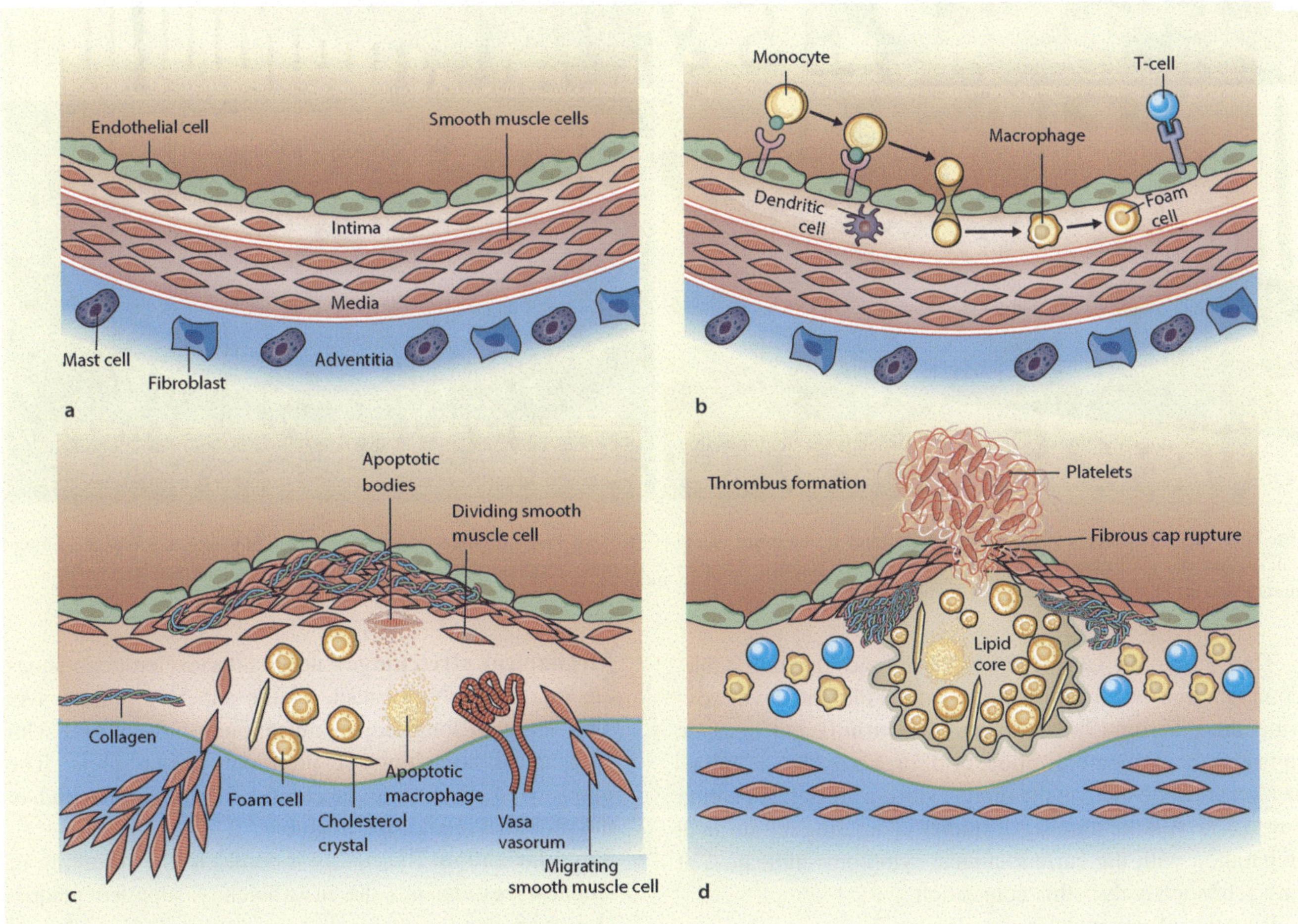

Fig. 16.6 (**a**–**d**) Stages of arteriosclerosis (according to Libby et al. 2011). (**a**) normal vessel wall; (**b**) endothelial activation; (**c**) stable atheroma; (**d**) activated plaque

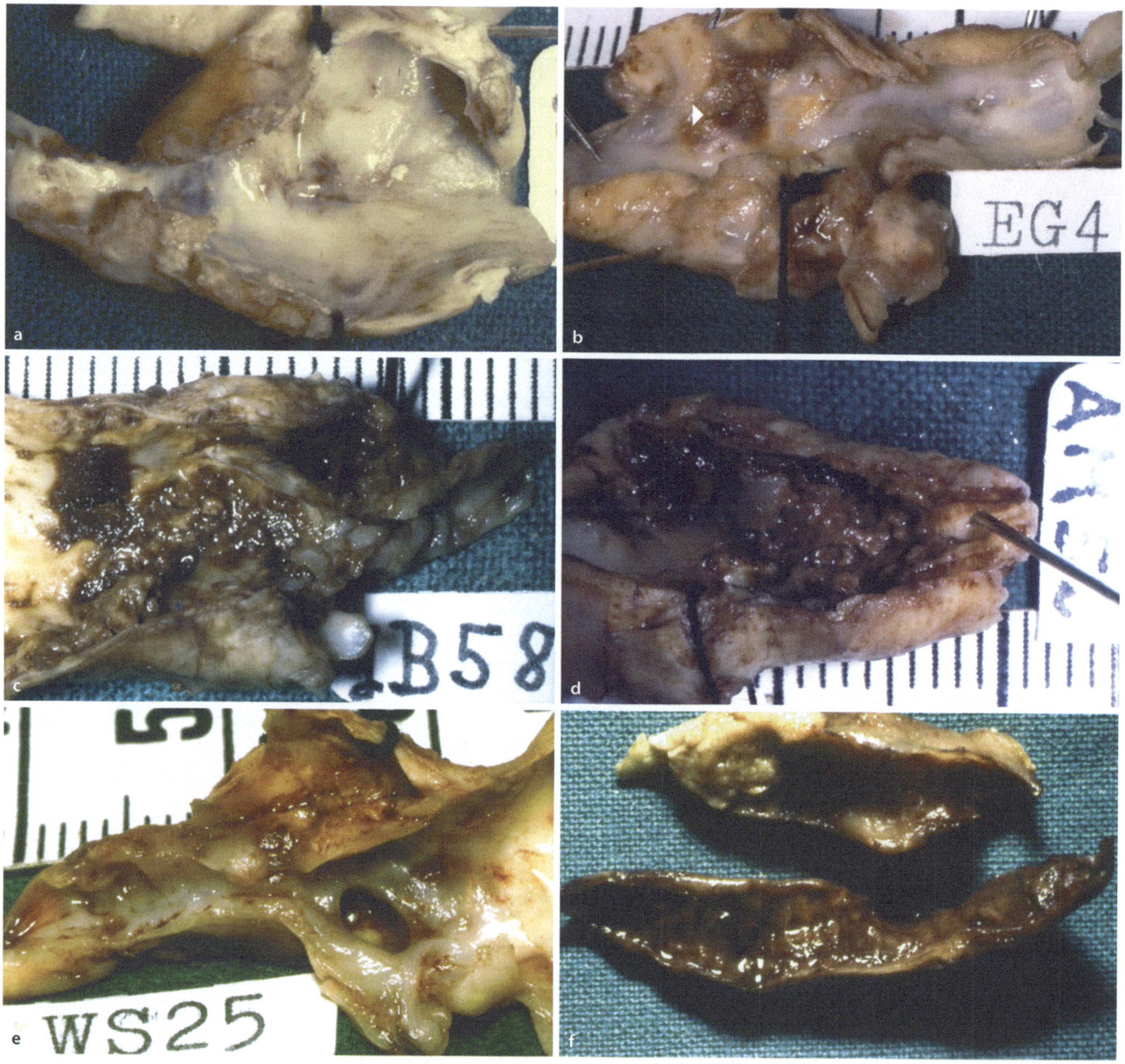

Fig. 16.7 (a–f) Examples of characteristic findings of the inner vessel wall of operated carotid stenoses. Smooth surface (**a**); scarring (7) after rupture (**b**); thrombotic deposits (**c**); broken, distinctly ulcerated surface (**d**); washed out ulcer niche (**e**); extraction preparation of a long-distance, organized thrombus from the internal carotid artery (**f**)

This atheroma can organize itself and remain stable. Complications occur, however, when the intimate layer covering the atheroma breaks open (**ulceration**) and necrotic parts after cranial embolization, or thrombi capable of embolization are deposited on the rupture site during defect healing (Fig. 16.7). A large number of studies comparing the surgical preparation with the current clinical symptoms indicate – at least retrospectively – this connection.

Rupture of atherosclerotic plaques is favored by two factors:

- **Mechanical stretching.** Larger arteriosclerotic plaques are a considerable obstacle to the adhering pulse wave. This leads to longitudinal pulsations of the vessel with mechanical stretching of proximal plaque parts. The majority of ulcerations in carotid stenoses are found in the proximal area of the plaque.
- **Vascularization.** Reactively it comes to the sprouting of smallest vessels into the insufficiently supplied plaque. However, these vessels are considerably vulnerable and tend to rupture, especially under increased mechanical

stress. The result can be the so-called **intramural bleeding** into the plaque, which relatively suddenly increases the volume of the plaque and also further increases the risk of intima rupture due to necrosis near the surface.

> Note
> **Arteriosclerotic plaques are subject to dynamic development and often change their structure over time.**

16.2.2 Sonographic Assessment of the Degree of Stenosis

The sonographic techniques for assessing the degree of stenosis in the carotid artery have already been described in detail in Chap. 13 and need not be discussed further here.

16.2.3 Sonographic Assessment of Plaque Morphology

Statements on the sonomorphological appearance of plaques can be made either descriptively or by means of a graded classification.

Descriptive Parameters
In order to avoid confusion and misinterpretation, the sonographic description of the plaque structure should always be limited to what is actually visible in the ultrasound image. Pathoanatomical terms such as "fibrous," "friable" and "ulcerated" are not included. In detail, sonographic statements can be made on 3 parameters (Table 16.3).

> Note
> **When describing plaques, pathoanatomical terms such as "fibrous," "friable" or "ulcerated," which simulate a confirmed sonographic-morphological context, should not be used.**

Table 16.3 Parameters for the sonomorphological description of plaques

Parameters	Sonomorphological description
Surface	Good/moderate/bad delimitable – Not visible
	Sectional view criterion: Continuously – Interrupted
	Color duplex criterion: Regularly – Irregularly
Internal echoes	Rich Echo – Poor Echo – Not visible
	Homogeneous – Inhomogeneous
Acoustic shadow	Distinctive – Low – Not available

Information on Plaque Surface

The boundary layer of a stenosis directed toward the open vascular lumen is called the plaque surface. If such a layer is visible at all, or at least presumably so, it is possible to describe the delimitability, shape and interruptions of the contour (Fig. 16.8). ◀

Information on Plaque Structure

The "inside" of a plaque can also be described using several criteria. Since the base often has a significantly different echo structure than the rest of the plaque, this is neglected and only the part of the plaque that is directed toward the lumen and is more significant for possible embolization is assessed. The echo density can be described in different gradations as echo rich to echo poor. Reference structures are the blood flow (minimum echo) and the unstenosed vessel wall away from the transducer (maximum echo). Furthermore, the distribution of the bright pixels in a plaque can be used to classify between homogeneous and inhomogeneous. Of particular importance is the detection of circumscribed low-echo areas in the middle of a echo rich plaque as an indication of a hemorrhage or an atheroma nucleus (Fig. 16.9). ◀

Information on Acoustic Shadowing

So-called acoustic shadows are of particular importance. If such a shadow is recognizable, it is the only situation in which the sonographic image allows direct conclusions to be drawn about the pathoanatomical structure, since acoustic shadows are almost always caused by an increased calcium content in the plaque (**"Calcification"**). ◀

16.2.4 Clinical Significance of Sonographic Plaque Parameters

In the case of extracranial carotid stenoses, which are accessible to interventional procedures both in the form of carotid surgery and stent placement, reliable criteria are needed to provide an indication for such procedures. Besides the occurrence of fresh ipsilateral neurological symptoms and the general condition, the degree of stenosis has proven to be the most important parameter. In individual cases, however, other criteria contribute to the assessment of the indication.

Significance of the Degree of Stenosis
Numerous studies over the past 30 years have demonstrated a correlation between the degree of carotid stenosis and the risk of suffering an ipsilateral stroke (Fig. 16.10). The risk is

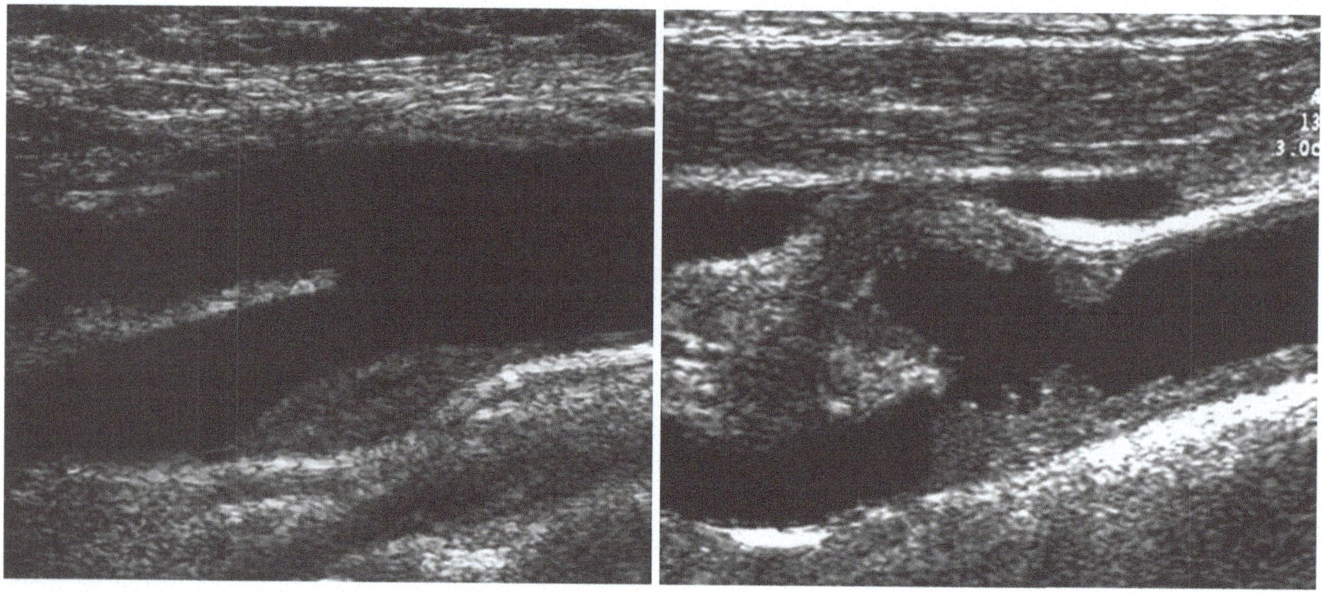

Fig. 16.8 Sonographic imaging of plaques. **Left:** Homogeneous, well delimited, regular, smoothly bounded and moderately echogenic plaque. **Right:** Slightly inhomogeneous, well defined, irregular plaque with contour interruption

additionally increased when stenoses show a progression. Furthermore, studies indicate that sonographically high local flow velocities of more than 400 cm/s are associated with a higher probability of plaque ulceration and thus with an additionally increased risk of stroke (Beach et al. 1993).

Significance of Sonomorphology
The morphological description of plaques in the ultrasound image is desirable for the detection of unstable stenoses. The studies available for this purpose considered two comparison parameters.

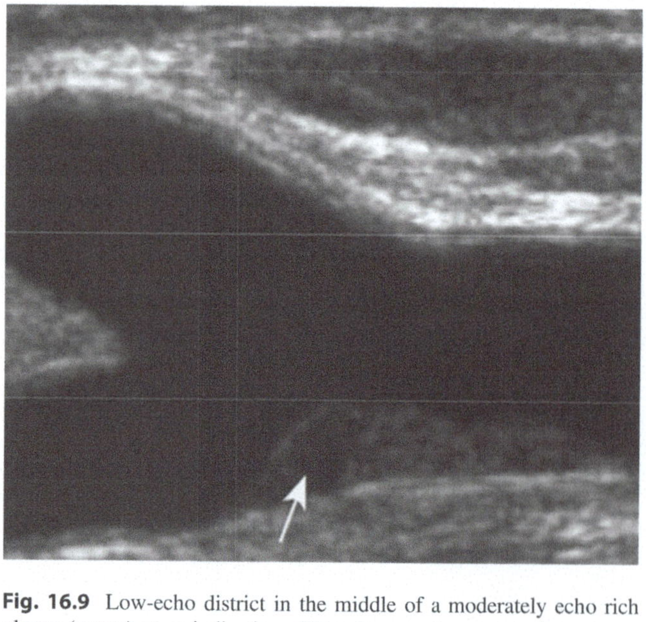

Fig. 16.9 Low-echo district in the middle of a moderately echo rich plaque (arrow) as an indication of bleeding or atheroma nucleus

Sonomorphology Versus Surgical Specimen

Numerous studies, especially from the 1990s, have unanimously established an at least indirect connection between sonographic criteria and morphological findings. For example, low-echo, heterogeneous plaques were found to be significantly more frequent intraoperatively than ulcerations and/or "crumbly" mixed atheromas, while echo rich, homogeneous plaques with regular contours showed a smooth surface more frequently (Fig. 16.11). However, this statement is qualified by the fact that heterogeneous plaques are more frequent in higher-grade stenoses, for which an increased risk of stroke is already known. A recent study emphasizes the additional importance of the sonomorphological appearance (Topakian et al. 2011). ◀

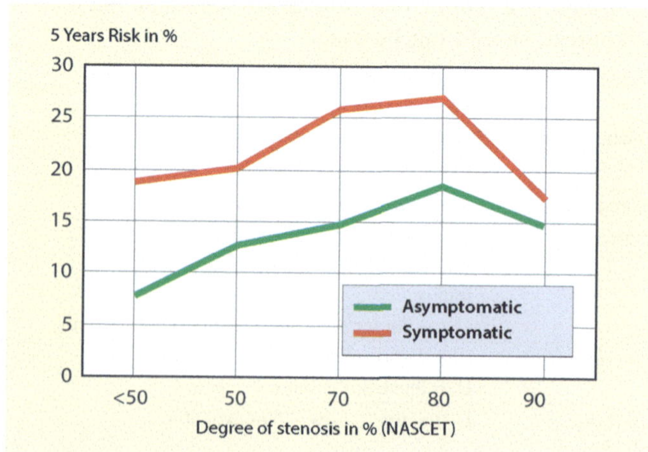

Fig. 16.10 Degree of stenosis of the internal carotid artery and risk of ipsilateral cerebral infarction

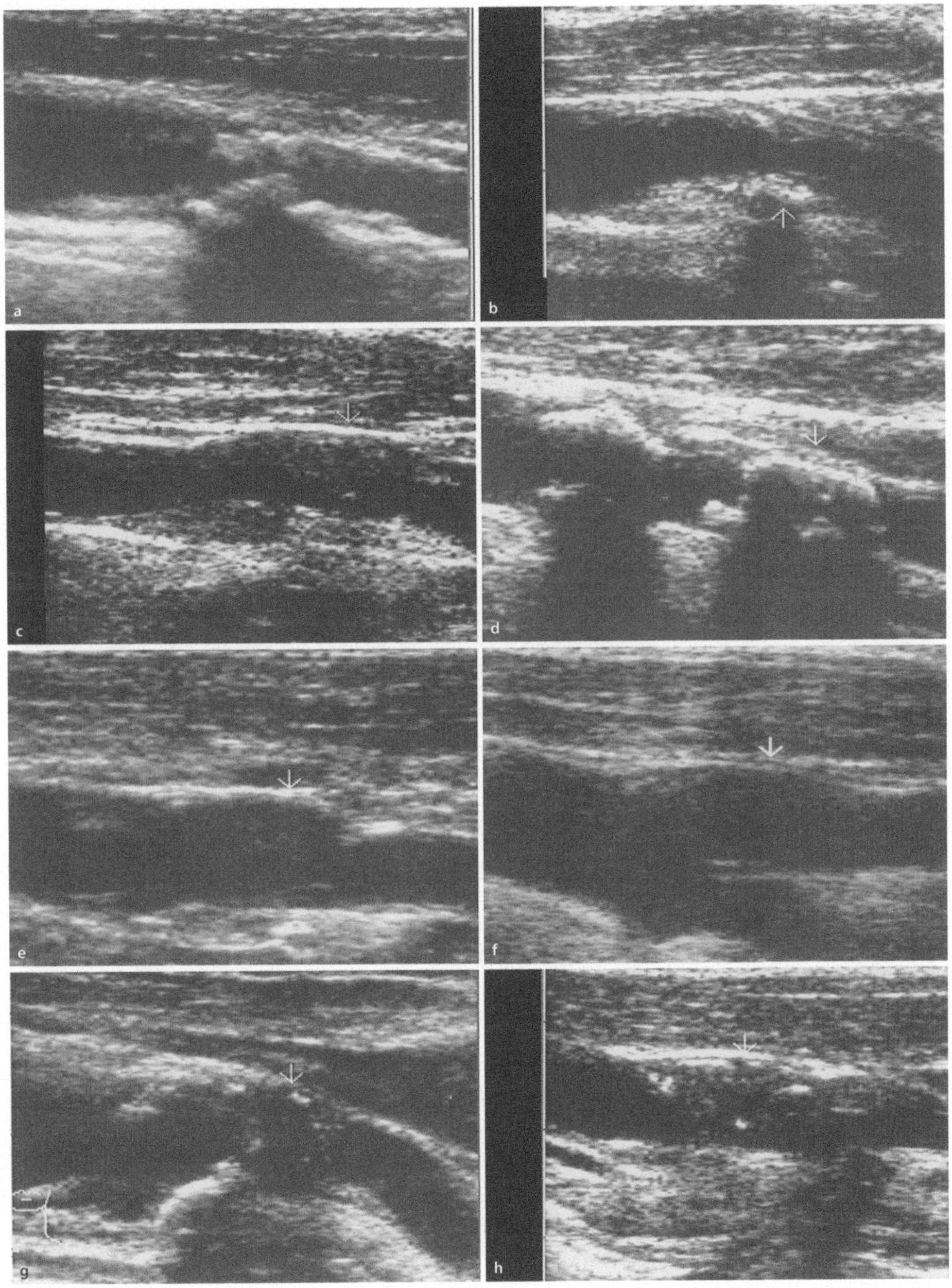

Fig. 16.11 Examples of intraoperatively correlated ultrasound images of carotid stenoses. Surgical findings: (**a**) smooth, fibrous plaque, (**b**) fibrous plaque with a rough but not ulcerated surface, (**c**) mixed atheroma, partly fibrous, partly ulcerated with disintegrating, atheromatous debris, (**d**) pronounced ulcerated plaque with calcifications, (**e**) smooth, fibrous plaque, (**f**) massive ulcerated mixed atheroma, (**g**) "crumbly," partially calcified atheroma with moderate ulceration, (**h**) fresh intramural hemorrhage with extensive ulceration

Sonomorphology Versus Spontaneous Course

It has been shown that patients with low-echo, heterogeneous plaques are more likely to suffer ipsilateral ischemic events. However, a sufficiently reliable differentiation between "stable" and "complex" plaques (Table 16.4) appears possible only in a small proportion of the stenoses sonographically. In contrast, calcifications appear more significant. According to Hunt et al. (2002), the risk decreases with increasing calcification of the plaque.

The analysis of the plaque morphology is more successful with MRI (Albuquerque et al. 2007). Especially

Table 16.4 Morphological classification of carotid plaques with a degree of stenosis of 50% and more based on the sonographic image

"Stable plaque"	Clear delimitable plaque surface, echoing, homogeneous structure
"Complexe plaque"	Irregular plaque surface, echo-poor, heterogeneous structure with individual echoing points (*echogenic spots*)
None statement	Ultrasound slice image not delimitable, homogeneous echo-poor plaque

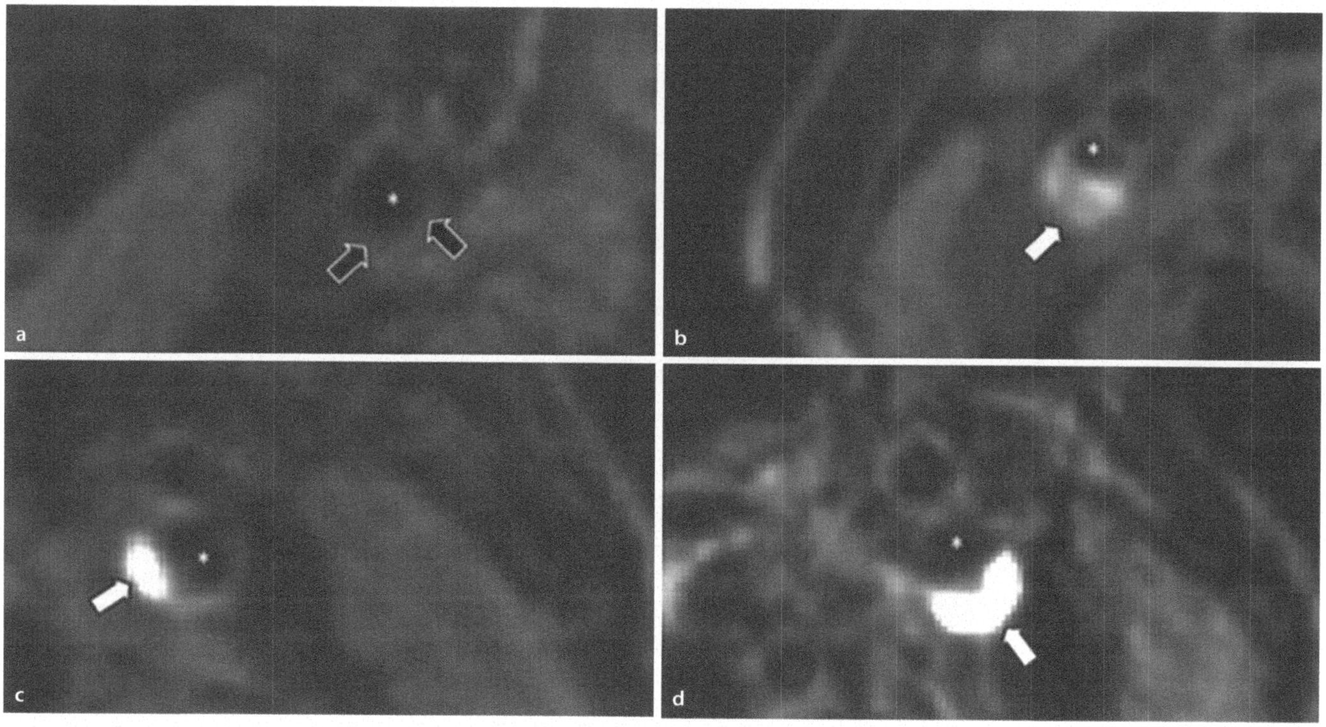

Fig. 16.12 Axial high-resolution MRI imaging of a plaque shown with different sequences: Hyperintense signals (white arrows) indicate bleeding

Table 16.5 Morphological parameters for assessing the risk of stroke

Method	Increased risk	Diminished risk
CT	–	Strong calcified stenosis
MRI	Detection of intramural hemorrhage	–
PET	Inflammation (enrichment ^{18}FDG) Microcalcification (enrichment ^{18}F-sodium fluoride)	–
Ultrasound	Inhomogeneous, echo-poor stenosis	Homogeneous, echo-rich stenosis, strong calcified stenosis

high-resolution carotid coils allow a detailed representation of the plaque. Hosseini et al. (2017) were able to show that this method can be used to detect intraplaque hemorrhages, which identify an unstable plaque with a significantly increased risk (Fig. 16.12; Table 16.5). Also by means of PET-CT and corresponding ligands (inflammation: e.g., ^{18}F-fluorodeoxyglucose; microcalcification: ^{18}F-sodium fluoride), plaques can be specified more precisely (Evans et al. 2016). ◀

Summary
Focal arteriopathies are mainly characterized by their circumscribed localization mostly at vascular branches or junctions, by the extent of the associated lumen constriction (degree of stenosis) and the morphological structure. The ultrasound image is able to provide information on the morphology to a limited extent. Homogeneously echo rich plaques, especially in the presence of more pronounced calcification (acoustic shadow), are rather stable, whereas heterogeneously echo poor plaques are often associated with ulcerations and/or intramural bleeding (complex plaques). However, the prognostic significance of plaque characterization by MRI is significantly better.

16.2.5 Ultrasound Parameters for the Indication of Carotid Surgery

The optimal treatment of the high-grade asymptomatic stenosis of the internal carotid artery is still controversially discussed. Although the optimal drug therapy is increasingly favored, surgery and stenting are available as interventional procedures, but no convincing data are available to compare these two methods (Spence and Naylor 2016). The discussion whether stenting (CAS) or surgery (CEA) of symptomatic carotid stenosis should be performed will certainly continue

Table 16.6 Assessment of the need for intervention and the method to be used, if necessary, in two steps

For intervention Higher-grade stenosis Ipsilateral symptomatology in the last days to weeks Progression of stenosis within the last months Contralateral carotid occlusion (?) Morphological signs of unstable plaque (biological) younger age	**Is there any need for an intervention?**	**Against intervention** Peri-interventional risk ≥2% for asymptomatic and ≥ 4% for symptomatic stenoses Filiform stenosis with "collapsed" poststenotic vessel Female gender More difficult comorbidities Generalized arteriosclerosis Somoking continued
For CAS Younger age (<65) Far cranial located carotid bifurcation Slim vessel	**Which method should be used?**	**For CEA** Calcified stenosis Kinking Generalized plaques Age > 65

According to Widder (2014)

in the coming years. Various studies have shown that age affects the complication rate, with older patients having a higher risk after stenting (Howard et al. 2016). Currently, an individual clarification in two steps is recommended in the daily routine (Table 16.6). In the first step, it should be clarified whether an intervention is indicated in a specific case at all. The second step is to find the most suitable method for the individual. Several anatomical factors must be taken into account:

- Since the beginnings of CEA, it has been known that the risk of surgery increases the further cranially the carotid bifurcation lies below the lower jaw. This concerns both the occurrence of recurrent stenosis at the distal end of the suture and postoperative cranial nerve loss. For obvious technical reasons, the risk of recurrent stenosis is also increased in very small vascular lumina. The expectation of **difficult surgical conditions** therefore rather speaks in favor of the use of CAS, the relevant clarification can usually be carried out without difficulty on the basis of an ultrasound examination of the neck vessels.
- Conversely, the existence of a relevant **kinking** in the immediate vicinity of the carotid stenosis to be removed favours CEA, since there is a risk of developing kink-stenosis due to the rather stiff stent.
- A technical problem for CAS also poses a pronounced **calcified stenoses** which cannot be expanded or can only be expanded incompletely. The assessment in this regard can be easily carried out within the framework of a CT angiography or ultrasound examination; MR angiography fails here for methodological reasons.
- In the end, also **generalized arteriosclerotic changes** – if any intervention is considered at all – favour the use of the CEA. Rosenkranz et al. (2010) were able to show that, in addition to old age, the presence of a sonographically measured intima media thickness (IMT) of 1.5 mm and more is associated with a significantly increased rate of peri-interventional DWI lesions after CAS. This corresponds to the experience that an IMT exceeding 1.5 mm indicates generalized arteriosclerotic changes already in the aortic arch. In CAS, the arch have to be passed with the catheter, which possibly detaches emboli.
- A histological analysis of CEA preparations showed (Wendorff et al. 2016) that men with asymptomatic carotid stenosis are significantly more likely than women to have unstable plaques and thus have a higher risk and may explain why men with asymptomatic high-grade carotid stenosis benefit more from an intervention than women. It would be interesting to compare these histological findings with ultrasound or plaque MRI.

References

Adler Y, Shohat-Zabarski R, Vaturi M, Shapira Y, Ehrlich S, Jortner R et al (1998) Association between mitral annular calcium and aortic atheroma as detected by transesophageal echocardiographic study. Am J Cardiol 81:784–786

Albuquerque LC, Narvaes LB, Maciel AA, Staub H, Friedrich M, Filho JR, Marques MB, Rohde LE (2007) Intraplaque hemorrhage assessed by high-resolution magnetic resonance imaging and C-reactive protein in carotid atherosclerosis. J Vasc Surg 46:1130–1137

Baldassarre D, Amato M, Bondioli A, Sirtori CR, Tremoli E (2000) Carotid artery intima-media thickness measured by ultrasonography in normal clinical practice correlates well with atherosclerosis risk factors. Stroke 31:2426–2430

Beach KW, Hatsukami T, Detmer PR, Primozich JF, Ferguson MS, Gordon D et al (1993) Carotid artery intraplaque hemorrhage and stenotic velocity. Stroke 24:314–319

Bots ML, Groenewegen KA, Anderson TJ, Britton AR, Dekker JM, Engström G et al (2014) Common carotid intima-media thickness measurements do not improve cardiovascular risk prediction in individuals with elevated blood pressure: the USE-IMT collaboration. Hypertension 63:1173–1181

Crouse JR, Goldbourt U, Evans G, Pinsky J, Sharrett AR, Sorlie P et al (1996) Risk factors and segment-specific carotid arterial enlargement in the atherosclerosis risk in communities (ARIC) cohort. Stroke 27: 69–75

Elias-Smale SE, Kavousi M, Verwoert GC, Koller MT, Steyerberg EW, Mattace-Raso FU et al (2012) Common carotid intima-media thickness in cardiovascular risk stratification of older people: the Rotterdam study. Eur J Prev Cardiol 19:698–705

Evans NR, Tarkin JM, Chowdhury MM, Warburton EA, Rudd JHF (2016) PET imaging of atherosclerotic disease: advancing plaque assessment from anatomy to pathophysiology. Curr Atheroscler Rep 18:1–13

Gardin JM, Bartz TM, Polak JF, O'Leary DH, Wong ND (2014) What do carotid intima-media thickness and plaque add to the prediction of stroke and cardiovascular disease risk in older adults? The cardiovascular health study. J Am Soc Echocardiogr 27:998–1005.e2

Goff DC, Lloyd-Jones DM, Bennett G, Coady S, D'Agostino RB, Gibbons R et al (2014) 2013 ACC/AHA guideline on the assessment of cardiovascular risk: a report of the American College of Cardiology/American Heart Association task force on practice guidelines. J Am Coll Cardiol 63:2935–2959

Gronewold J, Bauer M, Lehmann N, Mahabadi AA, Kälsch H, Weimar C et al (2014) Coronary artery calcification, intima-media thickness, and ankle-brachial index are complementary stroke predictors. Stroke 45:2702–2709

Hosseini AA, Simpson RJ, Altaf N, Bath PM, MacSweeney ST, Auer DP (2017) Magnetic resonance imaging plaque hemorrhage for risk stratification in carotid artery disease with moderate risk under current medical therapy. Stroke 48:678–685

Howard G, Roubin GS, Jansen O, Hendrikse J, Halliday A, Fraedrich G et al (2016) Carotid stenting Trialists' collaboration. Association between age and risk of stroke or death from carotid endarterectomy and carotid stenting: a meta-analysis of pooled patient data from four randomised trials. Lancet 387:1305–1311

Hulthe J, Wikstrand J, Emanuelsson H, Wiklund O, de Feyter PJ, Wendelhag I (1997) Atherosclerotic changes in the carotid artery bulb as measured by B-mode ultrasound are associated with the extent of coronary atherosclerosis. Stroke 28:1189–1194

Hunt KJ, Pankow JS, Offenbacher S, Kritchevsky SB, Duncan BB, Shahar E et al (2002) B-mode ultrasound-detected carotid artery lesions with and without acoustic shadowing and their association with markers of inflammation and endothelial activation: the atherosclerosis risk in communities study. Atherosclerosis 162:145–155

Kröger K, Lehmann N, Moebus S, Schmermund A, Stang A, Kälsch H et al (2013) Impact of atherosclerotic risk factors on different ankle-brachial-index criteria – results of the Heinz Nixdorf RECALL study. Vasa 42:120–126

Libby P, Ridker PM, Hansson GK (2011) Progress and challenges in translating the biology of atherosclerosis. Nature 473:317–325

Lorenz MW, Polak JF, Kavousi M, Mathiesen EB, Völzke H, Tuomainen T-P et al (2012) Carotid intima-media thickness progression to predict cardiovascular events in the general population (the PROG-IMT collaborative project): a meta-analysis of individual participant data. Lancet 379:2053–2062

Näslund U, Ng N, Lundgren A, Fhärm E, Grönlund C, Johansson H, Lindahl B et al (2019) Visualization of asymptomatic atherosclerotic disease for optimum cardiovascular prevention (VIPVIZA): a pragmatic, open-label, randomised controlled trial. Lancet 393:133–142

Rosenkranz M, Thomalla G, Havemeister S, Wittkugel O, Cheng B, Krutzelmann A, Fiehler J, Gerloff C (2010) Older age and greater carotid intima-media thickness predict ischemic events associated with carotid-artery stenting. Cerebrovasc Dis 30:567–572

Sander D, Schulze-Horn C, Bickel H, Gnahn H, Bartels E, Conrad B (2006) Combined effects of hemoglobin A1c and C-reactive protein on the progression of subclinical carotid atherosclerosis: the INVADE study. Stroke 37:351–357

Sander D, Gnahn H, Poppert P, Bickel H (2020) IMT measurement as a tool for improved risk factor control and medication adherence after ischemic stroke. Circulation, under revision

Sass C, Herbeth B, Chapet O, Siest G, Visvikis S, Zannad F (1998) Intima-media thickness and diameter of carotid and femoral arteries in children, adolescents and adults from the Stanislas cohort: effect of age, sex, anthropometry and blood pressure. J Hypertens 16: 1593–1602

Spence JD, Naylor AR (2016) Endarterectomy, stenting, or neither for asymptomatic carotid-artery stenosis. N Engl J Med 374: 160218110019005–160218110011088

Topakian R, King A, Kwon SU, Schaafsma A, Shipley M, Markus HS et al (2011) Ultrasonic plaque echolucency and emboli signals predict stroke in asymptomatic carotid stenosis 77:751–758

Touboul P-J, Hennerici MG, Meairs S, Adams H, Amarenco P, Bornstein N et al (2012) Mannheim carotid intima-media thickness and plaque consensus (2004-2006-2011). An update on behalf of the advisory board of the 3rd, 4th and 5th watching the risk symposia, at the 13th, 15th and 20th European stroke conferences, Mannheim, Germany, 2004, Brussels, Belgium, 2006, and Hamburg, Germany, 2011. Cerebrovasc Dis 34:290–296

Wendorff C, Wendorff H, Kuehnl A, Tsantilas P, Kallmayer M, Eckstein H-H, Pelisek J (2016) Impact of sex and age on carotid plaque instability in asymptomatic patients-results from the Munich vascular biobank. Vasa 45:411–416

Widder B (2014) Therapie von Karotisstenosen: Endarterektomie oder Stent? NeuroTransmitter 25:56–59

Willeit P, Willeit P, Thompson SG, Thompson SG, Agewall S, Agewall S et al (2014) Inflammatory markers and extent and progression of early atherosclerosis: meta-analysis of individual-participant-data from 20 prospective studies of the PROG-IMT collaboration. Eur J Prev Cardiol 23:194–205

Yoshida M, Mita T, Yamamoto R, Shimizu T, Ikeda F, Ohmura C et al (2012) Combination of the Framingham risk score and carotid intima-media thickness improves the prediction of cardiovascular events in patients with type 2 diabetes. Diabetes Care 35:178–180

Inflammatory Vascular Diseases

17

Bernhard Widder and Gerhard F. Hamann

Inflammatory vascular diseases represent an inhomogeneous collective, which is usually divided into primary and secondary vasculitides. The common feature is an inflammatory infiltration of the vessel wall with intimal thickening, but in individual cases also aneurysmatic vasodilatation. Both arteries and veins are affected, the latter generally occurring before the arteries.

Primary vasculitides are chronic inflammatory vascular diseases that occur without a recognisable cause. In addition to histological characteristics and pathogenetic findings, they are differentiated according to the size of the affected arteries (Table 17.1; Jennette et al. 2013). In clinical practice, however, there are overlaps in terms of size, since occlusive processes of the larger and thus sonographically detectable arteries have also been described in vasculitides, which primarily affect smaller vessels (Schmidt et al. 2001).

The numerically much more frequent **secondary vasculitides** occur in autoimmune diseases, infections and malignant syndromes, but also when taking drugs (see following overview). Although secondary vasculitides preferentially affect the small vessels, there are at least casuistics in the literature indicating (co-)affection of large arteries in almost all of these diseases The extracranial carotid artery and vertebral artery may also be involved.

Histologically there are intimate changes with swelling and inflammatory exudate formation, which are reversible in the initial stage. They are often sickle-shaped or crescent-shaped and can therefore be confused with dissections if T2-weighted MRI imaging is used exclusively (Chap. 18). If all layers of the vessel wall are affected, infectious vasculitides can lead to the formation of "mycotic" aneurysms. Frequently, focal necroses also occur, which can be confused sonographically with arteriosclerotic lesions. In addition, secondary thromboses can bei found in inflammatory intimal diseases.

Causes of Secondary Systemic Vasculitis

- Collagenoses (e.g., lupus erythematosus, Sjögren's syndrome)
- Rheumatic systemic diseases (e.g., rheumatoid arthritis)
- Infections (e.g., bacterial meningitis, borreliosis, zoster, hepatitis, HIV)
- Malignant diseases (e.g., carcinomas, lymphoproliferative diseases)
- Drug abuse (e.g., heroin, cocaine)
- Medication (e.g., hydralazine, penicillamine)
- Other causes (e.g., monoclonal gammopathy).

17.1 Takayasu Arteritis

This vascular disease mainly affects younger women up to about 40 years of age. The name goes back to the ophthalmologist Mikito Takayasu, who first described the clinical picture in detail in 1905 (Seyahi 2017). It denotes a chronically progressing vasculitis, especially of the aortic arch and the vascular trunks originating from the aortic arch (**"aortic arch syndrome"**), also called "pulseless disease".

After unspecific initial symptoms with fever, dizziness and a general feeling of illness, which often precede the palpable onset of the disease by months, an inflammatory swelling of the inner wall of the vessels originating form the aortic arch occurs with long-distance stenoses up to occlusions. From the brain-supplying arteries the subclavian and common carotid arteries are particularly affected; only rarely the disease does exceed the carotid bifurcation. In

B. Widder (✉)
Expert Opinion Institute, District Hospital, Guenzburg, Germany
e-mail: bernhard.widder@bkh-guenzburg.de

G. F. Hamann
Clinic of Neurology and Neurological Rehabilitation, District Hospital, Guenzburg, Germany

B. Widder, G. F. Hamann (eds.), *Duplex sonography of the brain-supplying arteries*, https://doi.org/10.1007/978-3-662-65566-5_17

Table 17.1 Classification of vasculitides according to the size of the affected vessels

Large arteries	Medium sized arteries	Medium-sized – small vessels	Small vessels
Takayasu arteritis	Panarteritis nodosa	Wegener's granulomatosis	Henoch-Schönlein-purpura
Cranial arteritis	Kawasaki syndrome	Churg-Strauss syndrome	Leucocytoclastic purpura
	Isolated CNS angiitis	Microscopic polyangitis	Cryoglobulin-associated vasculitis

According to Jennette et al. (2013)

individual cases there is also a general dilatation of the aortic arch branches or a circumscribed aneurysmatic dilatation, which can lead to tracheal compression with swallowing difficulties. Only rarely the findings are symmetrical, usually one side of the neck is affected dominantly.

Sonographic Assessment

In B-mode imaging of the common carotid artery, the diagnosis can easily be performed by the typical concentric thickening of the inner wall of the vessel (intima-media thickness) (Taniguchi et al. 1997; Case Study 17.1). The inflammatory process of the wessel wall appears homogeneous, relatively low-echogenic and has a predominantly smooth surface running parallel to the outer wall of the vessel (so-called "**macaroni sign**"). The same applies to subclavian artery, which is often more severely affected.

A reliable differentiation to arteriosclerotic changes is not possible. However, diffuse atherosclerotic wall thickenings in lipid metabolism disorders and diabetes mellitus usually appear more echogenic, have a more irregular surface and are focally differently pronounced.

The findings in the initial section of the vertebral artery are not very indicative caused by the usually insufficient visualization of the vessel by B-mode imaging. On the basis of the flow behavior, however, statements can be made about a possible complete or incomplete subclavian steal effect or an occlusion of the vessel.

Clinical Significance

Ultrasound diagnostics is of essential importance in the diagnosis and follow-up of Takayasu syndrome.

Early Diagnosis

According to the substantial investigations of Schmidt et al. (2002), sonography is excellently suited for the early diagnosis of Takayasu arteritis in patients with fatigue, arthralgias and inflammatory laboratory signs. ◀

Monitoring of Progress

Several long-term studies confirmed the usefulness of sonography for follow-up examinations (Fukudome et al. 1998; Park et al. 2001; Sun et al. 1996). To what extent the sonographic findings can be used as a marker for the success of an immunosuppressive therapy, however, seems contradictory. ◀

Cerebral Hemodynamics

The determination of cerebrovascular reserve capacity provides quantitative information about a possible impairment of cerebral hemodynamics. ◀

Summary

Takayasu arteritis is found mainly in younger women and affects the branches of the aortic arch. Sonographically, a concentric, low-echo vascular wall thickening (macaroni sign) is typical. The ultrasound examination is suitable for control examinations during the course of the disease.

17.2 Cranial Arteritis

Cranial arteritis (synonymous **Horton arteritis**, **giant cell arteritis**, **temporal arteritis**) is the most common immune vasculitis of old age. The term temporal arteritis is misleading, because although the disease mainly affects the branches of the external carotid artery including the ophthalmic artery, it can also affect other extra- and intracranial vessels such as the vertebral artery, subclavian artery and axillary artery (Reinhard et al. 2003). Correspondingly there is a broad range of possible symptoms, ranging from visual disturbances to cerebral ischemias and ischemias in the arm region. Frequently, the disease is found together with polymyalgia rheumatica associated with generalized muscle pain. Laboratory tests regularly show a strongly increased erythrocyte sedimentation rate (ESR) and an increased C-reactive protein (CRP).

A recent review by Buttgereit et al. (2016) summarizes the diagnostic, pathophysiological and therapeutic aspects of this disease, which is particularly important in terms of differential diagnosis. The relationship to the polymyalgia rheumatica is described. Essential diagnostic points of the American College of Rheumatology (Hunder et al. 1990) are

- Emerging headache (in more than 2/3 of patients)
- Age over 50 years
- ESR >50 mm in the first hour
- Clinical abnormalities of the temporal artery (painfulness under pressure, thickening)
- Positive biopsy.

Table 17.2 Normal flow velocities in the proximal and distal superficial temporal arteries and pathological changes in patients with cranial arteritis (mean velocity and standard deviation)

	Proximal	Distal
Normal findings	57 ± 2 cm/s	43 ± 2 cm/s
Temporal arteritis	31 ± 6 cm/s	6 ± 4 cm/s

According to Lauwerys et al. (1997)

17.2.1 Findings in the Superficial Temporal Artery

Sonographic Assessment

The examination should be carried out with an ultrasound probe of a transmission frequency as high as possible (ideally a linear transducer with a transmission frequency of up to 18 MHz), the focus should be adjusted to approx. 5 mm. The superficial temporal artery is first identified in the area of its main stem in front of the tragus by color coded imaging in a longitudinal and/or cross-sectional view and then traced cranially into its branches. The pressure of the probe on the skin surface should be kept as low as possible. In the vast majority of cases there is a bifurcation with division into a frontal and lateral branch (Fig. 1.5), only relatively rarely is there no division or a trifurcation. When occipital headache is reported, an attempt should also be made to investigate the occipital artery above the mastoid. An infestation of the vertebral artery has also been described (Reinhard et al. 2004), so that here too, attention should be paid to the presence of inflammatory abnormalities.

In the case of a focal infestation of the superficial temporal artery, various sonographic findings are described in the literature as characteristic:

Halo Sign

Concentric, often multisegmental constriction of the superficial temporal artery in color coded imaging with a low-echogenic vascular wall thickening of 0.3–1.2 mm in the B-mode image (Schmidt et al. 1997; Fig. 17.3) – comparable to the findings in the carotid artery in Takayasu's arteritis. ◀

Absence of Vascular Pulsations

According to investigations of Reinhard et al. (2004), the (extensive) absence of visible vascular pulsations of the superficial temporal artery in the M-mode image (Fig. 5.25) – respectively their reduction in side to side comparison – has a high predictive value for the presence of an inflammatory vascular swelling. ◀

Presence of a Vessel Occlusion

As known from X-ray angiographies, the evidence of an occlusion of the superficial temporal artery is a strong indicator of arteritis. It is problematic, however, that such findings can only be made if the occluded vessel can be clearly (!) delineated as a low-echogenic band in the B-mode image. In the experience of the authors, this is only relatively rarely the case. ◀

Reduced Flow Velocity

So far only one study has reported a pronounced, distally emphasized reduction of mean flow velocity in the superficial temporal artery in patients with cranial arteritis compared to normals (Lauwerys et al. 1997; Table 17.2). ◀

Visible Vessel Wall during Compression

Normally, when the vessel is mechanically compressed by the transducer, the vessel wall can no longer be separated from the surrounding tissue. If it remains visible, this indicates the presence of vasculitis (Buttgereit et al. 2016). ◀

Clinical Significance

In a meta-analysis of 10 studies involving a total of 696 patients, Buttgereit et al. (2016) described a sensitivity of duplex sonography of the superficial temporal artery with halo signs between 55 and 100% and a specificity between 78% and 100%. Stenoses or occlusions of the superficial temporal artery could be detected with a similar specificity (73–100%) but a significantly lower sensitivity (8–80%) in five studies with 316 patients. The visible wall sign after mechanical compression of the vessel showed a sensitivity of 73–78% and a specificity of 100%. The authors saw ultrasound as an ideal method for follow-up examinations. Thus, in 95% of the treated patients a previously detected halo sign disappeared after a median of eight weeks.

Case Study 17.1: Takayasu Arteritis

Upon admission, the 18-year-old commercial employee complained diffuse dizziness and insecure gait that had increased in the weeks before. The ESR was borderline increased, pathological findings were also found for C-reactive protein. The other inflammatory parameters were negative.

(continued)

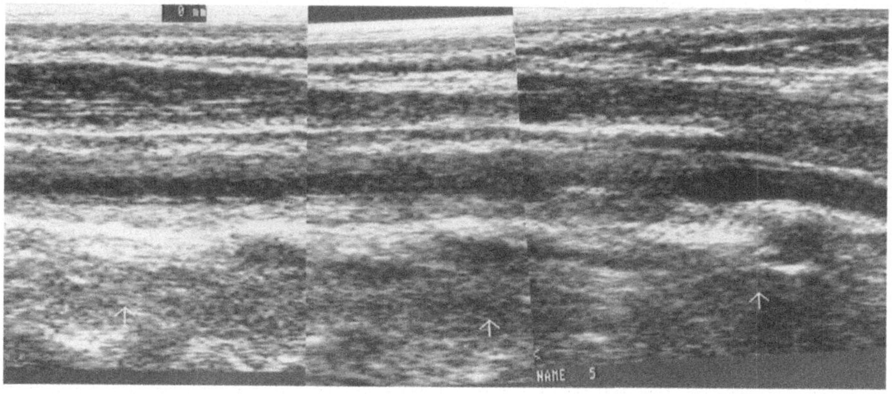

Fig. 17.1 Longitudinal section through the left common carotid artery (left) and internal carotid artery (right). Note the inconspicuous presentation of the internal carotid artery

Case Study 17.1 (continued)

B-mode imaging of the left common carotid artery showed a pronounced, concentric thickening of the inner wall of the vessel, whereas the internal carotid artery was normal (Fig. 17.1). The maximum systolic flow velocity in the area of the constriction was 200 cm/s. The right carotid artery as well as the vertebral arteries showed normal findings.

Long-term corticosteroid therapy resulted in a certain reduction of dizziness, no further complaints occurred. Sonographic examination two years later revealed an unchanged long-distance narrowing of the right common carotid artery. In addition, an approx. 50% constriction of the vessel lumen was also visible in the area of the left carotid artery (Fig. 17.2).

17.2.2 Findings on the Other Vessels

As already mentioned at the beginning, vasculitic changes can also be found in individual cases in other extracranial arteries, especially in the vertebral artery (Case Study 17.2).

Summary

Cranial arteritis (giant cell arteritis, temporal arteritis) is a common immunovasculitis of older age and can affect all extra- and intracranial vessels. Comparable to the findings in Takayasu's arteritis, at least in some patients a concentric thickening of the inner wall of the superficial temporal artery (halo sign) is shown sonographically. Further diagnostic criteria are the absence of vascular pulsation, reduced blood flow, detectable occlusion of the vessel and a still visible vessel wall when the vessel is compressed.

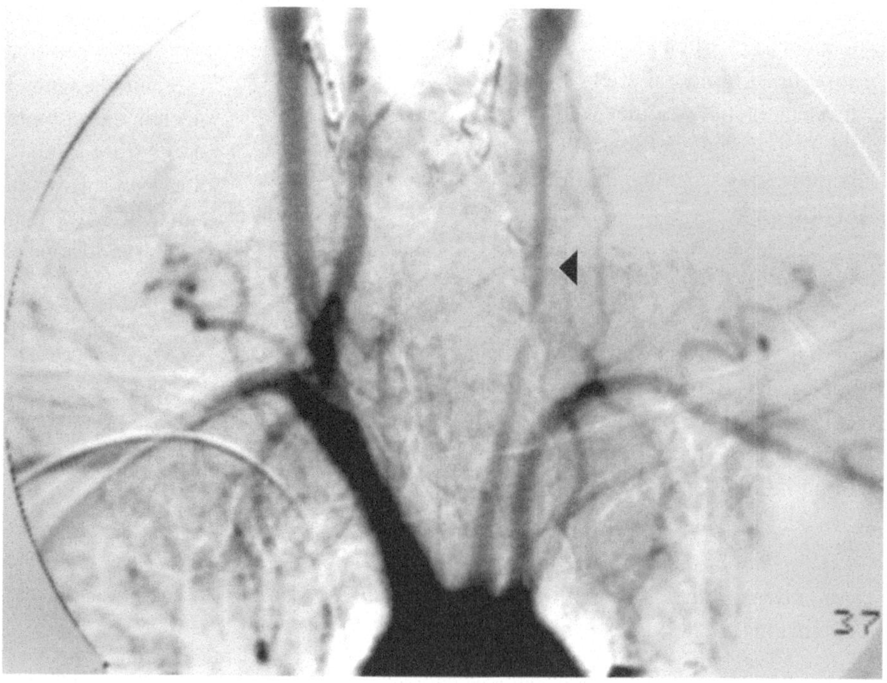

Fig. 17.2 Aortic arch DSA with evidence of a pronounced constriction of the left carotid artery

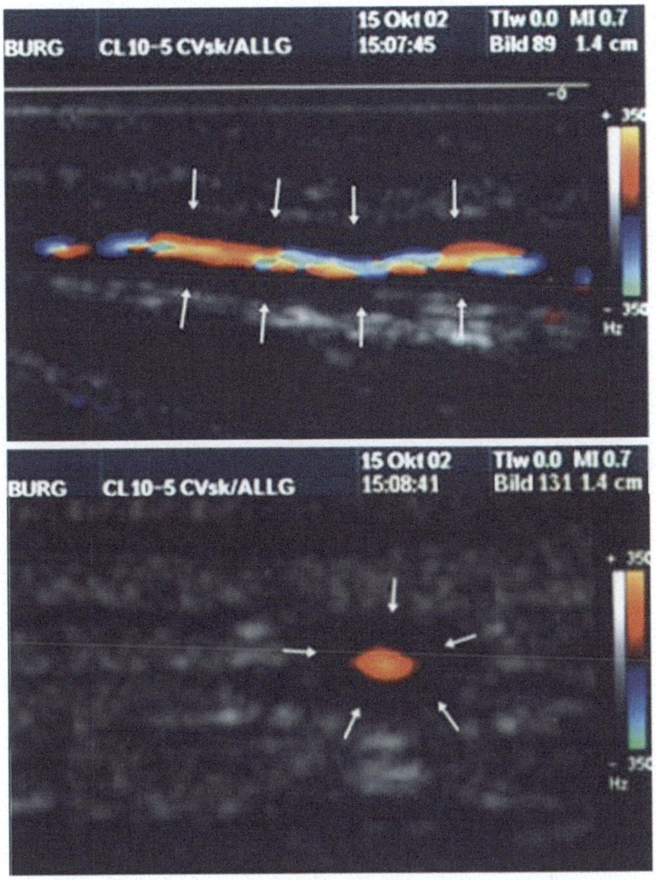

Fig. 17.3 Concentric constriction of the superficial temporal artery in cranial artitis in longitudinal (top) and cross-sectional (bottom) view (Prof. Dr. A. Hetzel, Bad Krozingen)

17.3 Primary Cerebral Vasculitis

The contribution of ultrasound diagnostics in primary cerebral vasculitis is generally small. However, if the large cerebral arteries are (co-)affected, the stenoses present there can be detected in individual cases and, in particular, observed in the course of the disease (Case Study 17.3).

17.4 Secondary Cerebral Vasculitis

Infectious and parainfectious vasculitides represent an inhomogeneous group of secondary vascular complications. However, the findings in the large arteries are generally remarkably uniform. Only purulent meningitides represent a particular case, which will be considered separately in the following.

17.4.1 Vasculitis in Purulent Meningitis

Unlike other vasculitides, vascular complications in purulent meningitis are characterized by three pathomechanisms:

- **Vasculitis.** As with other vasculitides, there is a subintimal infiltration of inflammatory cells into the arterial wall. This results in an intimal thickening or edema, which can lead to the occlusion of the vessel.
- **Purulent walled enclosure.** The purulent exudate in the subarachnoid space can cause a mechanically induced constriction of the large cerebral arteries.
- **Vasospasm.** Probably due to the release of vasoconstrictive mediators, a functional constriction of the vessels running in the subarachnoid space can develop, as it is well known from subarachnoid hemorrhage (Sect. 22.2).

However, despite different pathogenesis, the functional effects of all three mechanisms are identical by causing stenoses in the major cerebral arteries.

In addition, there are complications from the "vascular end section":

- **ICP elevation.** The regularly developing edema can lead to an increase in intracranial pressure with an increase in peripheral vascular resistance.
- **Hyperperfusion.** Re-opening of stenosed and/or occluded vascular areas can lead to segmental or generalized hyperperfusion caused by paralyzed cerebral autoregulation (Sect. 14.1.2).

Sonographic Assessment

The above mentioned vascular complications in combination with the problems of the vascular end section lead to four sonographic constellations (Table 17.3). A reliable differentiation only appears possible if, in addition to flow velocity in the cerebral arteries (especially middle cerebral artery), the MCA/ICA index (Sect. 14.3.3), the flow volume in the internal carotid artery and, if necessary, the pulsatility of the flow curves in the brain supplying arteries are also taken into account. Pulsatility is the least standardized and will only lead to a clear pathological finding if there is a marked increase in intracranial pressure (Sect. 23.1). In the case of positive evidence of increased flow velocities, the criteria for the assessment of the degree of stenosis apply (Sect. 14.2).

17.4.2 Other (Para)Infectious Vasculitis

Vasculitides not caused by purulent meningitides but by other infections are divided into two groups:

Table 17.3 Doppler/duplex sonographic findings in bacterial meningitis in comparison to standard values

	Stenosis without cerebral pressure	Stenosis with cerebral pressure	Stenosis with hyperperfusion	Hyperperfusion without stenosis
Local flow velocity	↑	±/↓	↑	↑
MCA/ICA index	↑	↑	↑	±
Flow volume of the internal carotid artery	±/↓	↓	±	↑
Pulsatility of the internal carotid artery	±/↓	↑	±	±/↓

- **Vasculitides with frequently multifocal stenoses** caused by systemic bacterial, viral or fungal infections (Case Study 17.4)
- **Accompanying focal vasculitides** caused by circumscribed inflammatory processes in the head and neck area, which only affect the immediately adjacent vessels.

Sonographic Assessment

For vasculitides not caused by purulent menigitides, the above mentioned sonographic criteria apply equally in principle. However, since there is usually no relevant increase in intracranial pressure, no vasospasm and no exudative walling of the vessels, the situation is much simpler and is reduced to the differentiation between stenosis and hyperperfusion. The criteria mentioned in Sect. 14.3.3 apply here.

Clinical Significance

The main significance of ultrasound diagnostics lies in the possibility of close monitoring the follow-up, while sonography can usually only make a minor contribution in the often difficult differential diagnosis.

Summary

Due to their systemic character, vasculitides in infectious diseases often occur multifocally, but can also remain isolated and are then difficult to assess. Vasculitides caused by purulent meningitis are a special form, since the sonographic flow findings in this case can be significantly influenced by an increase in intracranial pressure.

Case Study 17.2: Cranial Arteritis

81-year-old patient with longstanding unexplained pain symptoms. The pain was rather generalized and alternating, concerning the shoulders and the hip, but also the vertebral column. An ESR had not been determined so far. Various rheumatological and orthopedic examinations had remained without result. The patient was admitted to hospital with acute severe brainstem

(continued)

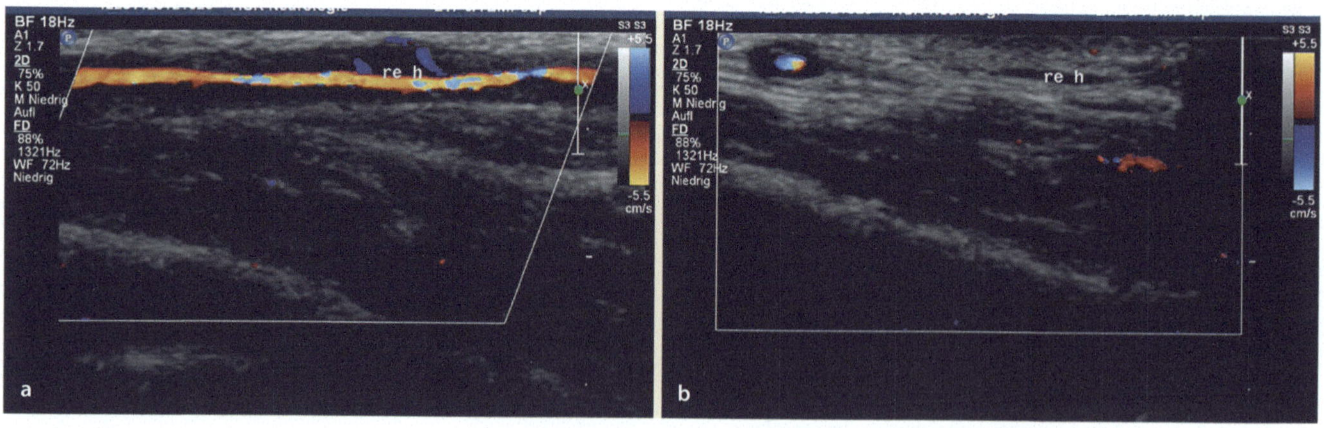

Fig. 17.4 Findings in cranial arteritis with involvzement of the vertebral artery

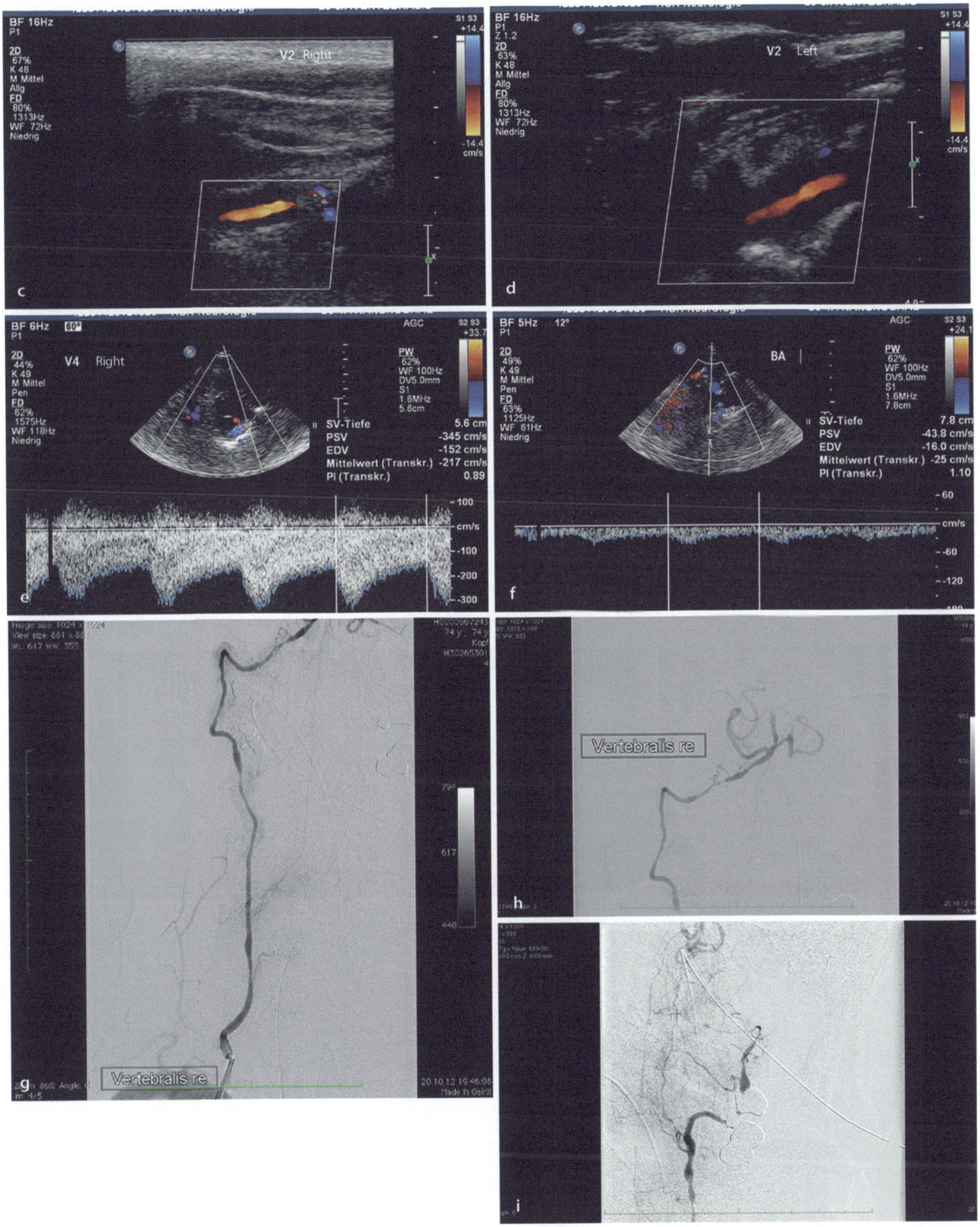

Fig. 17.4 (continued)

Case Study 17.2 (continued)
symptoms with double vision, skew-deviation and right hemiparesis.

On admission, a strongly accelerated ESR of 90 mm was observed in the first hour. The superficial temporal artery was strongly conspicuous using a high-resolution 18 MHz linear probe and showed a so-called macaroni sign (Fig. 17.4a); in cross-section, the so-called halo sign was visible (Fig. 17.4b). The vertebral arteries also showed a macaroni sign (Fig. 17.4c, d). Using in transcranial duplex sonography the flow velocity in the V4 segment of the right vertebral artery was significantly accelerated with values up to 300 cm/s indicating a high-grade vertebral stenosis (Fig. 17.4e). The basilar artery showed only a very low poststenotic flow (Fig. 17.4f).

MR angiography (TOF) showed no vertebrobasilar system except for a rudimentary right vertebral artery. A DSA revealed multiple stenoses in the vertebral artery and contrast medium uptake in the vessel wall, indicating a large vessel vasculitis (Fig. 17.4g, h), a high-grade stenosis of the left vertebral artery and an occlusion in the distal vertebrobasilar system (Fig. 17.4). In summary, this case shows the frequent involvement of the vertebrobasilar system in cranial arteritis and the high sensitivity of ultrasound in detecting vasculitic vessel wall changes.

Case Study 17.3: Primary Cerebral Vasculitis
The 45 years old patient was previously completely healthy. Acutely, an intracerebral hemorrhage occurred in the left hemisphere (Fig. 17.5a). Two days after the intracerebral hemorrhage, a disturbed sensibility on the right side was observed. In addition to intracerebral hemorrhage, MRI revealed multiple infarcts bihemispheric and in the left thalamus (Fig. 17.5b). The determination of vasculitis parameters in the blood showed negative findings for ANA, ANCA, CRP, and a normal ESR, the cerebrospinal fluid initially revealed pleocytosis with 60/3 cells. Cerebral angiography showed multiple vessel wall constrictions

(continued)

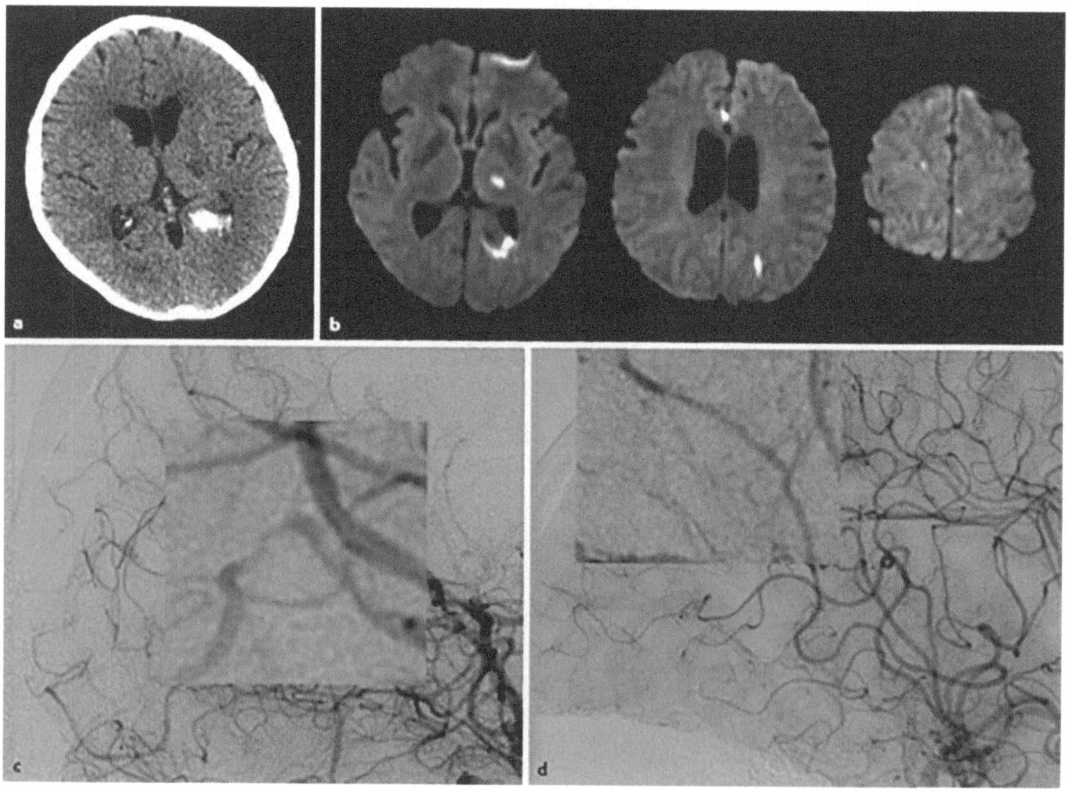

Fig. 17.5 Findings in primary cerebral vasculitis (explanations in text)

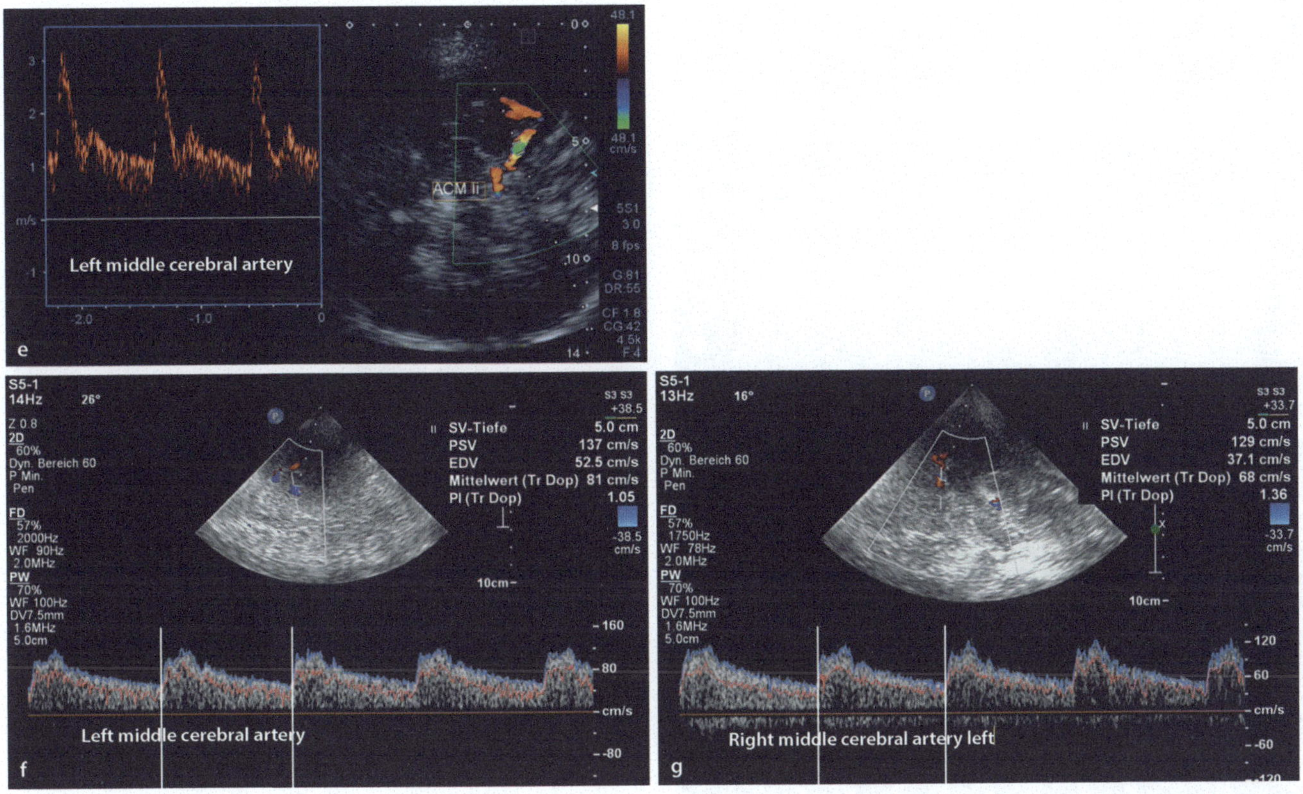

Fig. 17.5 (continued)

Case Study 17.3 (continued)

of the middle and smaller brain vessels indicating cerebral vasculitis (Fig. 17.5c, d).

In transcranial duplex examination, an increase in flow velocity in the main stem of both middle cerebral arteries up to 300 cm/s were observed (left side shown in Fig. 17.5e). Endoxan had not produced any significant change for six months, but with rituximab there was a significant decrease in intracranial stenosis. The last carried-out CSF control showed normal findings. Transcranial duplex sonography also revealed a decrease in stenosis of both middle cerebral arteries (Fig. 17.5f, g). In summary, a classic picture of primary cerebral vasculitis was obtained.

Case Study 17.4: Parainfectious Vasculitis

The 60-year-old patient experienced an increasing disturbance of consciousness 15 months ago after a holiday stay. CSF findings revealed a fungal meningoencephalitis (coccidioidomycosis), at that time stenoses of the middle cerebral artery were found on both sides. A fungicidal therapy led to a rapid improvement of the symptoms.

Later, the patient was admitted again because of a peracute onset of vertigo and severe occipital headaches. Transnuchal duplex examination revealed a high-grade stenosis of the basilar artery (8–9 cm depth of examination) with maximum systolic flow velocities of about 180 cm/s (Fig. 17.6), which could

(continued)

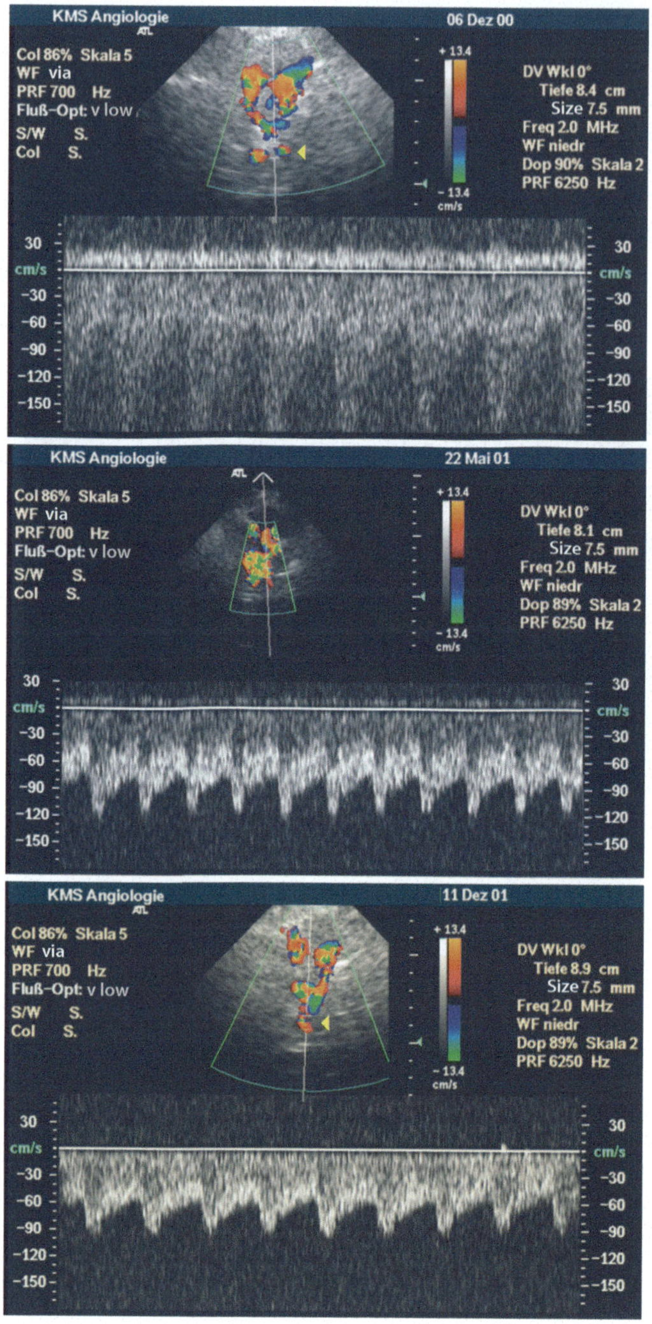

Fig. 17.6 Duplex sonographic recordings over the course of one year

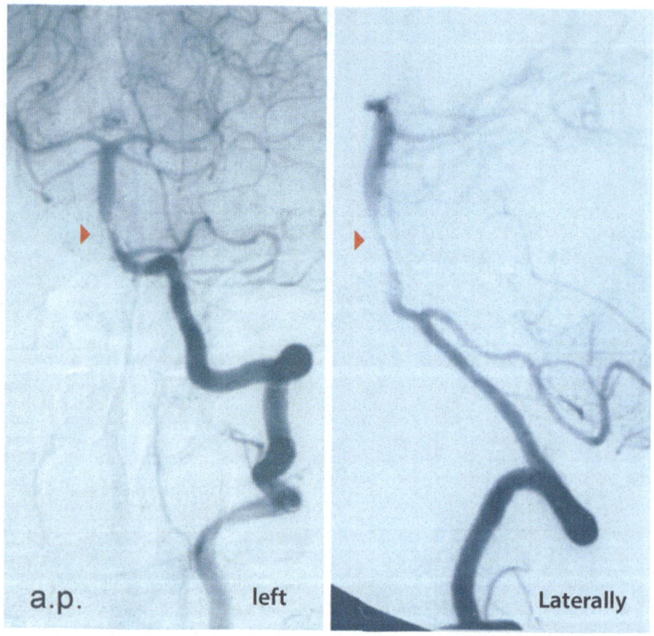

Fig. 17.7 Initial angiographic images

Case Study 17.4 (continued)

also be confirmed angiographically (Fig. 17.7). The stenoses in the middle cerebral arteries were no longer detectable. Under long-term fungicidal therapy and anticoagulation, the stenosis was largely reduced to values around 90 cm/s systolic in the course of several controls over the course of one year.

References

Buttgereit F, Dejaco C, Matteson EL, Dasgupta B (2016) Polymyalgia Rheumatica and Giant cell arteritis: a systematic review. JAMA 315: 2442–2458

Fukudome Y, Abe I, Onaka U, Fujii K, Ohya Y, Fukuhara M, Kaseda S, Esaki M, Fujishima M (1998) Regression of carotid wall thickening after corticosteroid therapy in Takayasu's arteritis evaluated by B-mode ultrasonography: report of 2 cases. J Rheumatol 25:2029–2032

Hunder GG, Bloch DA, Michel BA, Stevens MB, Arend WP, Calabrese LH et al (1990) The American College of Rheumatology 1990 criteria for the classification of giant cell arteritis. Arthritis Rheum 33:1122–1128

Jennette JC, Falk RJ, Bacon PA, Basu N, Cid MC, Ferrario F et al (2013) 2012 revised international Chapel Hill consensus conference nomenclature of Vasculitides. Arthritis Rheum 65:1–11

Lauwerys BR, Puttemans T, Houssiau FA, Devogelaer JP (1997) Color Doppler sonography of the temporal arteries in giant cell arteritis and polymyalgia rheumatica. J Rheumatol 24:1570–1574

Park SH, Chung JW, Lee JW, Han MH, Park JH (2001) Carotid artery involvement in Takayasu's arteritis: evaluation of the activity by ultrasonography. J Ultrasound Med 20:371–378

Reinhard M, Schmidt D, Hetzel A (2004) Color-coded sonography in suspected temporal arteritis – experiences after 83 cases 24:340–346

Reinhard M, Schmidt D, Schumacher A, Hetzel A (2003) Involvement of the vertebral arteries in giant cell arteritis mimicking vertebral dissection. J Neurol 250:1006–1009

Schmidt WA, Kraft HE, Vorpahl K, Völker L, Gromnica-Ihle EJ (1997) Color duplex ultrasonography in the diagnosis of temporal arteritis. N Engl J Med 337:1336–1342

Schmidt WA, Seipelt E, Molsen HP, Poehls C, Gromnica-Ihle EJ (2001) Vasculitis of the internal carotid artery in Wegener's granulomatosis: comparison of ultrasonography, angiography, and MRI. Scand J Rheumatol 30:48–50

Schmidt WA, Nerenheim A, Seipelt E, Poehls C, Gromnica-Ihle E (2002) Diagnosis of early Takayasu arteritis with sonography. Rheumatology 41:496–502

Seyahi E (2017) Takayasu arteritis: an update. Curr Opin Rheumatol 29: 51–56

Sun Y, Yip PK, Jeng JS, Hwang BS, Lin WH (1996) Ultrasonographic study and long-term follow-up of Takayasu's arteritis. Stroke 27: 2178–2182

Taniguchi N, Itoh K, Honda M, Obayashi T, Nakamura M, Kawai F, Irie T (1997) Comparative ultrasonographic and angiographic study of carotid aterial lesions in Takayasu' arteritis. Angiology 48:9–20

Arterial Dissections

18

Bernhard Widder and Gerhard F. Hamann

About 2% of all brain infarctions are caused by dissections (Ortiz and Ruland 2015). In adolescence and younger adulthood, however, arterial dissections are the most frequent cause of an occlusion of the brain supplying arteries and of cerebral infarctions (Ferro et al. 2010). Etiologically, a distinction is usually made between traumatic and spontaneous dissections. However, the transitions are fluid, as light traumas ("trivial traumas") or rapid head movements have often been described in connection with the occurrence of dissections (Debette et al. 2015, Engelter et al. 2013). Although dissections are usually unilateral, in about 20% of cases there are lesions on both sides, often in combination of the anterior and posterior circulation (Guillon et al. 2000).

Symptomatology

A regular leading symptom is an abrupt onset of unilateral neck or face pain or headache, which is often misinterpreted as a "cervical syndrome" or "migraine". However, also the other accompanying symptoms can lead to misinterpretation due to their ambiguity (Baumgartner and Bogousslavsky 2005). In addition to a ipsilateral Horner syndrome, which frequently occurs in carotid artery dissections due to direct damage of sympathetic fibers running in the carotid wall (38% of carotid dissections; Lyrer et al. 2014), ischemic cerebral infarctions, pulsatile tinnitus (16–27%) or direct compressive lesions in the peripheral course of cranial nerves (especially hypoglossal nerve, glossopharyngeal nerve, facial nerve and chorda tympani) can occur and may even be the only pathologic finding in individual cases (Fig. 18.1). Isolated lesions of the upper brachial plexus have also been described as a consequence of vertebral dissections (Eberhardt and Topka 2015).

> Note
> **Unilateral headaches associated with cranial nerve loss and/or Horner's syndrome should always make one think of a dissection of the brain-supplying arteries.**

The interval between the dissection and the appearance of clinical symptoms can range from minutes to several days, in some cases even weeks. The cause is usually an embolization of thrombi from the dissection. Only relatively rarely, especially in dissections extending to the intracranial carotid bifurcation (carotid T), hemodynamically caused cerebral infarcts occur. A typical clinical presentation of vertebral artery dissections is the Wallenberg Syndrome, caused by the secondary occlusion of the posterior inferior cerebellar artery (PICA). In individual cases, however, all failures attributable to the posterior circulation can occur (Bartels 2006).

Pathogenesis

According to current knowledge, dissections occur when two factors interact: On the one hand, genetic risk factors leading to wall weakness due to changes in the proteins of the extracellular matrix of the vessel wall, on the other hand "exogenous" factors such as inflammation of the vessel wall and the vasa vasorum and/or (minor) trauma (Ortiz and Ruland 2015; overview) (Table 18.1).

B. Widder (✉)
Expert Opinion Institute, District Hospital, Guenzburg, Germany
e-mail: bernhard.widder@bkh-guenzburg.de

G. F. Hamann
Clinic of Neurology and Neurological Rehabilitation, District Hospital, Guenzburg, Germany

B. Widder, G. F. Hamann (eds.), *Duplex sonography of the brain-supplying arteries*, https://doi.org/10.1007/978-3-662-65566-5_18

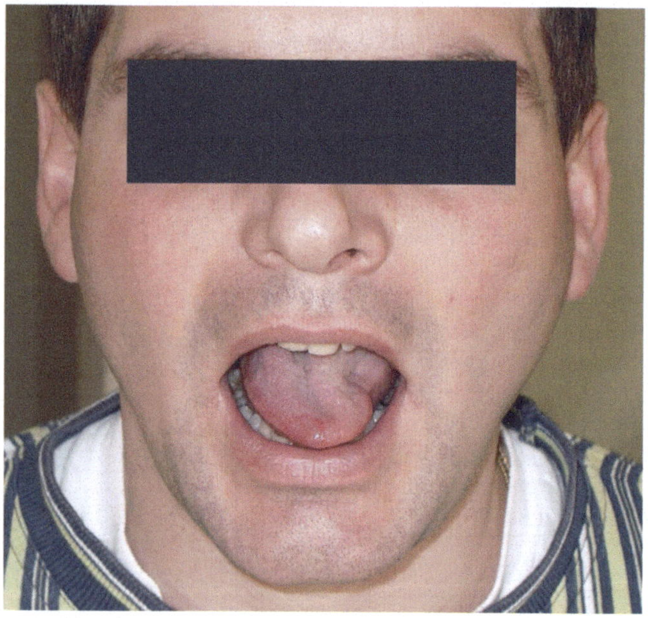

Fig. 18.1 Hypoglossal paresis on the left as the only symptom of a dissection of the left internal carotid artery with pronounced pseudoaneurysmatic dilatation of the vessel below the skull base

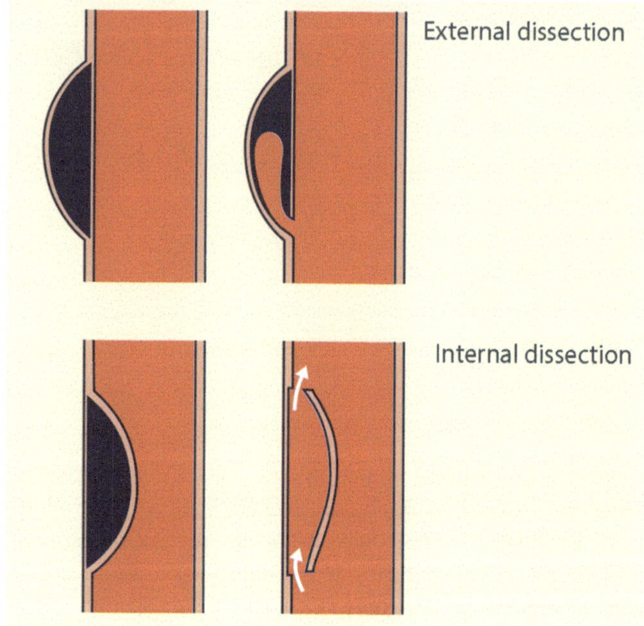

Fig. 18.2 Types of arterial dissections. External dissection (top) with possible formation of a "pseudoaneurysm" open to the vessel lumen. Internal dissection (bottom) with formation of a vascular stenosis. In individual cases a "false" lumen may be formed with blood flowing through it

Table 18.1 Risk Factors for the Occurrence of Vascular dissections (According to Ortiz and Ruland 2015)

Genetic factors	Acquired Factors
Fibromuscular dysplasia	Trauma (blunt or penetrating)
Marfan syndrome	Violent sneeze or cough
Ehlers-Danlos syndrome	Sports activities like weightlifting, tennis, golf
Turner syndrome	Chirotherapeutic manipulations
Willimas syndrome	Oropharyngeal infections
Pseudoxanthoma elasticum	Arterial hypertension
Hereditary hemochromatosis	Drug abuse
Menkes disease	Oral contraceptives
Osteogenesis imperfecta	Migraine
Alpha-1-antitrypsin deficiency	Aortic coarticulation
Cystic median necrosis	Vascular tortuosities
Down syndrome	Extended styloid processus (eagle syndrome)
Polycystic renal diseases	

Dissections occur preferentially at sites where the artery is fixed to a bone. Proximal and/or distal to it there is usually a considerable mobility of the vessel with increased mechanical stress. This situation affects the carotid artery when entering the skull base, but also when exiting the bony canal into the sinus cavernosus. In the region of the vertebral artery, the proximal V1 segment before entry into the transverse foramina and the cervicocranial transition (V3 segment) are particularly affected.

Morphologically, two types of lesions can be distinguished (Fig. 18.2), but they often occur in combination.

Internal Dissection

The bleeding into the vessel wall (intramural hemorrhage) causes a narrowing of the vessel lumen up to the complete occlusion of the vessel. This type of lesion occurs preferably near the skull base and often runs both cranially and caudally to the next larger vessel origin, where the dissection then generally comes to a halt. Thrombus embolization can occur during vessel occlusion, recanalization, and the formation of a false lumen with blood flow through proximal and distal intimal tears. The probability of a cerebral infarction increases with the degree of stenosis (Ortiz and Ruland 2015). ◀

External Dissection

Intramural hemorrhage can also lead to an outward dilatation of the vessel, which can be approximately symmetrical ("spindle-shaped") or asymmetrical ("bag-shaped"). This can lead to local compression of the cranial nerves located in close proximity. If the hemorhage cavity comes into contact with the vessel lumen, a so-called **pseudoaneurysm** can occur. Despite their impressive appearance in MR and/or CT angiography, external dissections rarely lead to cerebral ischemia (Baumgartner et al. 2001). ◀

Diagnostic Imaging

The method of choice for diagnosing dissections is MR imaging and angiography (MRI/MRA). Preferably after fat suppression, the axial T1-weighted sectional images show the usually crescent-shaped constriction or sacculation (**"crescent sign"**) of the vessel lumen. Diagnostic uncertainties of this technique, especially with regard to hemodynamic changes, can be overcome by combining it with ultrasound diagnostics.

> Note
> **MRI/MRA and ultrasound diagnostics are complementary methods for the diagnosis of dissections of the brain-supplying arteries.**

18.1 Primary Extracranial Carotid Dissections

Dissections in the area of the common carotid artery and the carotid bifurcation usually have two causes:

- **Traumatic dissections** after blunt neck injuries and iatrogenically by accidental puncture of the carotid artery when inserting a jugular catheter and by "impaling" the vessel wall with an arterial catheter, but also by hyperextension of the head, for example, in traffic accidents (Okada et al. 1999).
- **Spontaneous dissections** in dissections of the ascending aorta, which continue into the supraaortic vessels (Arning et al. 1995). (Case Study 18.1) Such dissections can be arteriosclerotic, but also inflammatory, especially in the context of syphilis. They often show a "false" lumen that is open over a long distance with ante- or retrograde blood perfusion.

Sonographic Assessment

Due to the localization favorable for ultrasound diagnostics, duplex sonography generally allows prima vista diagnostics. Four characteristic findings can be distinguished.

Intramural Bleeding

The finding of a circumscribed, non-arteriosclerotic thickening of the vessel wall in connection with a pressure-sensitive carotid artery indicates an intramural hemorhage. The differential diagnosis should include a "mycotic" aneurysm, in which, however, the aneurysmatic sacculation is typically in the foreground, and an arteriosclerotic plaque. The latter only affects the vascular intima, while the other vessel wall structures appear intact. ◀

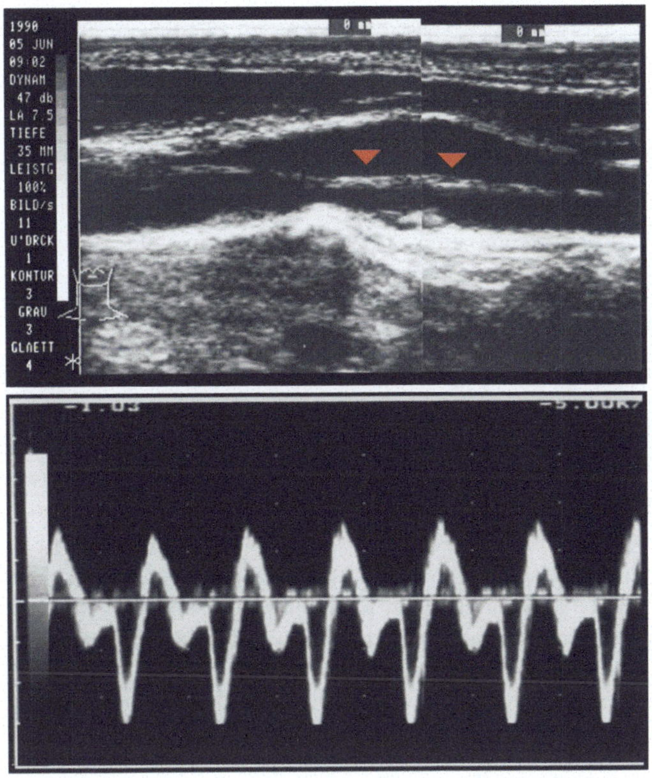

Fig. 18.3 Dissection in the area of the aortic arch caused by syphilis with detachment of the vessel wall extending into the common and internal carotid artery. In the B-mode image, an oscillating membrane is visible in the center of the vessel (top), which shows an oscillationg Doppler signal (bottom)

Detection of a "False Lumen"

In the presence of a perfused false lumen, B-mode imaging usually shows a transversely oscillating membrane that divides the vascular lumen into two compartments with different flow characteristics (Fig. 18.3). Depending on the individual hemodynamic constellation, the Doppler pulse curve shows an antegrade, alternating or even retrograde flow in the "wrong" lumen. In the "right" lumen, in addition to the "normal" flow signal, there are underlying, intensity-rich, alternating signals that are caused by the oscillation of the dissected membrane. ◀

Intimal Flap Detection

Short-distance, locally limited dissections often show intimal flaps that oscillate freely in the vessel lumen (Case Study 18.2). Experience shows that at least smaller dissections disappear with increasing temporal distance from the event or reattach themselves to the vessel wall, often "walled in" by a thrombus. The residual findings of older dissections often include circumscribed wall deposits in an otherwise completely inconspicuous vessel. ◀

Short-Distance, "Pointy" Stenoses (So-Called Bishop's Mitre)

As a result of vessel wall trauma (e.g., strangulation), but also after arterial catheterization with "impaling" of the vessel wall, short-stretched stenoses can develop, which can also be severe in individual cases (Case Study 18.3). The differentiation of congenital plicatures of the vessel wall, which look identical sonographically, can be difficult in individual cases. ◀

Clinical Significance

Dissections in the area of the proximal carotid artery are rare and are even less frequently accompanied by cerebral ischemia. Since the sonographic findings are usually very impressive, an isolated dissection that does not involve the aortic arch should not generate excessive actionism. Only in individual cases an interventional procedure with stent placement may be appropriate. Ultrasound diagnostics is the method of choice for monitoring the course of the disease.

18.2 Primary Intracranial Carotid Dissections

Internal carotid artery dissections from the base of the skull represent the vast majority of dissections of the brain-supplying arteries. In most cases, these are subintimal dissections with stenosis or occlusion of the vessel at the entry to the skull base. The dissection can extend over a long distance down to the carotid bifurcation. Dissections above the base of the skull occur mainly in children (Fullerton et al. 2001), but have not been studied much.

Sonographic Assessment

With regard to the sonographic findings, four constellations can be distinguished (Fig. 18.4).

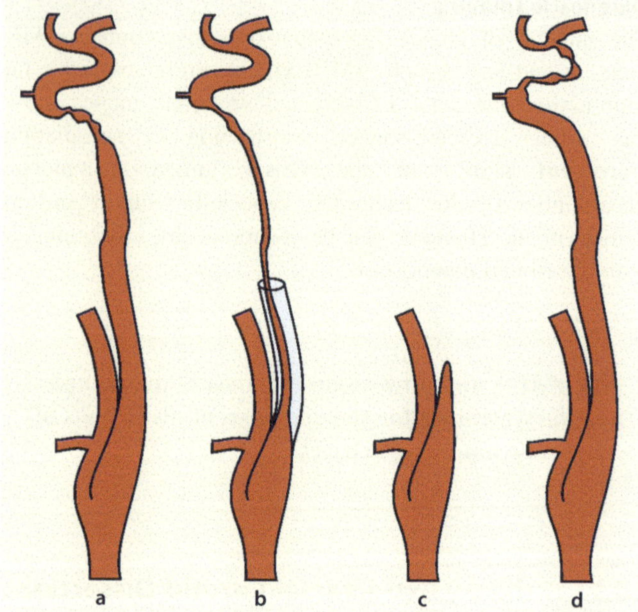

Fig. 18.4 (**a**–**d**) Typical vascular findings in dissections of the distal internal carotid artery. Short-distance dissection close to the skull (**a**); long-distance dissection extending down to the carotid bifurcation with "string sign" and the original vessel lumen visible in the extracranial ultrasound image (**b**); occlusion of the internal carotid artery with tapered vessel stump (**c**); dissection in the cranial section of the internal carotid artery ("carotid T") (**d**)

Case Study 18.1: Aortic Arch Dissection

54-year-old, extremely obese female patient with a BMI of 46 and acute chest pain. Clinical examination ruled out pulmonary embolism, heart attack and coronary heart disease. During the cardiological examination, it was noticed that the patient was tired, always fell asleep and moved the right side less.

At neurological investigation there was a somnolent patient who was only awake and oriented when spoken to. An initially detectable hemiparesis on the right side was no longer detectable, but after a short time a hemiparesis of the left side appeared. MRI was technically not possible due to the obesity of the patient, initial native CT imaging was inconspicuous. Duplex sonography showed a lang-distance membrane in the common carotid arteries on both sides indicating dissection (Figs. 18.5 and 18.6). The subsequent thoracic CT confirmed the diagnosis of an aortic dissection type A according to Stanford classification. The patient was transferred to cardiothoracic surgery for aortic replacement.

Short-Distance Dissection Close to the Skull Base

Since the dissection area is not accessible to direct sonographic examination, the findings do not differ from those in arteriosclerotic stenoses. The only differentiation criterion is the absence of other arteriosclerotic vascular wall changes in the extracranial vessels. For the constellations of findings see Sects. 14.2.1 and 14.4.1. It goes without saying that dissections near the base of the skull can only be diagnosed sonographically if they show a higher degree of stenosis. ◀

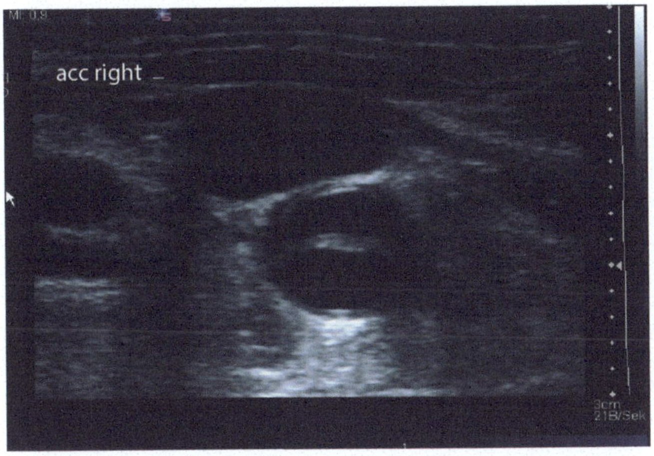

Fig. 18.5 Transversal section through the right common carotid artery

Case Study 18.2: Traumatic Dissection of the Common Carotid Artery

The 7-year-old girl suffered a slight accident a week ago when she crashed with her scooter and the handlebars pressed into her neck on the left. Immediately afterward she complained of nausea and vomited once. In the following days she reported left-sided temporal headaches in addition to a localized pressure pain on the left side of her neck. Neurological symptoms did not occur at any time.

Sonographically a short circular tear of the vascular intima in the left carotid artery was already visible by B-mode imaging. Cranially of it a "swinging" structure was visible. In the color coded image, signs of a high-grade stenosis were found, caused by a curling of the vascular intima. In the transversal image a sickle-

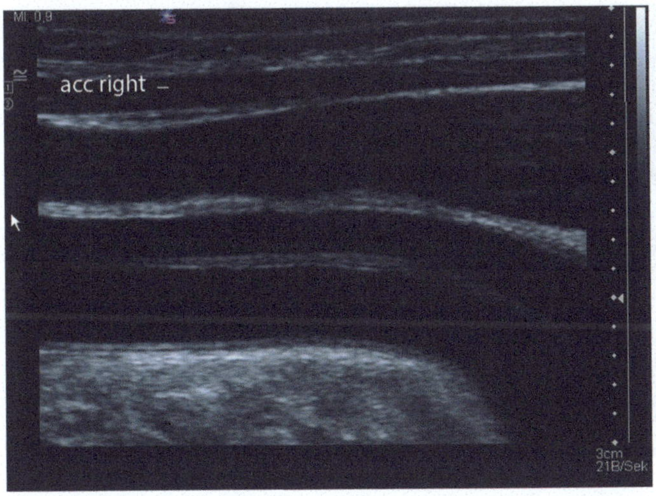

Fig. 18.6 Longitudinal section of the right common carotid artery

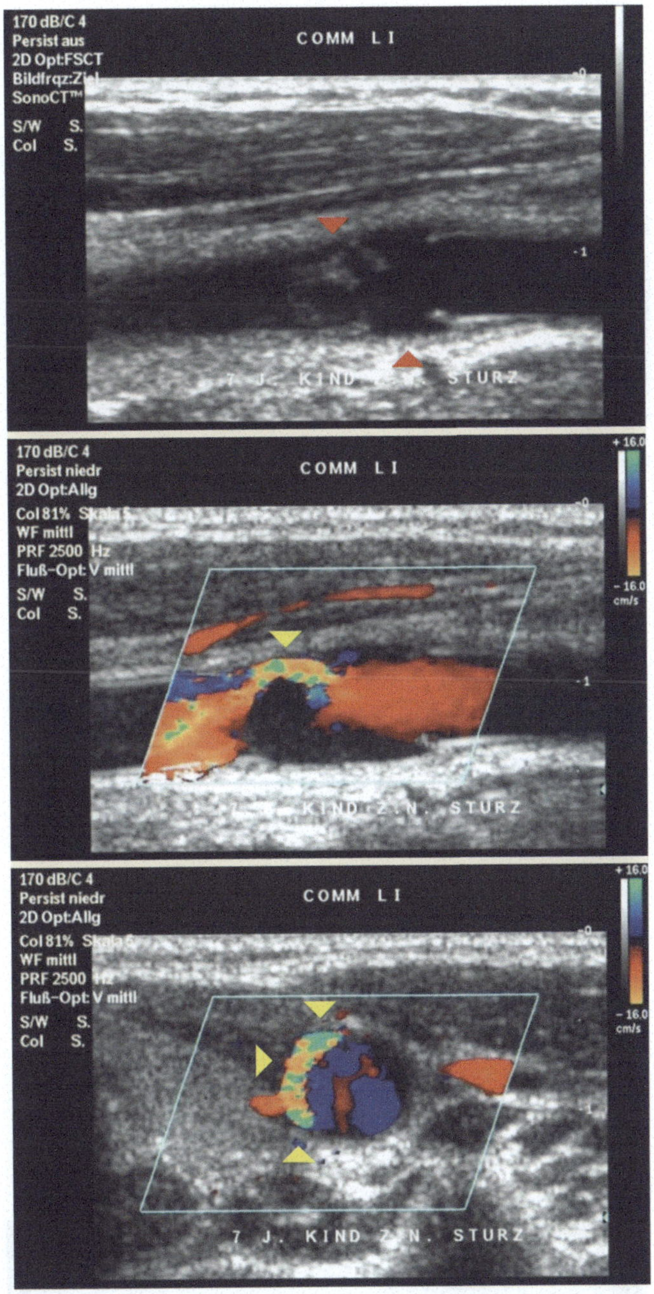

Fig. 18.7 Duplex sonographic findings of the left common carotid artery

Case Study 18.2 (continued)

shaped residual lumen was visible (Fig. 18.7). Due to the unstable vascular findings, a vascular surgical intervention with sewing of the dissection was performed (Fig. 18.8).

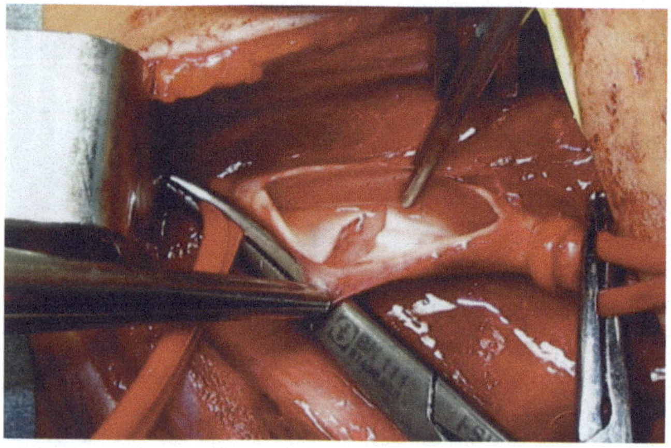

Fig. 18.8 Intraoperative site of the dissection

> **Note**
> **Dissections near the skull base with aneurysmatic sacculation and without significant stenosis of the vessel are usually not detectable sonographically.**

Long-Distance, Proximally Extending Dissection

In this case extracranial duplex sonography shows a tapering internal carotid artery immediately after the carotid bulb ("**string sign**") with a considerably reduced flow volume compared to the other side. However, since long-distance extracranial vascular narrowings can also occur when the vessel "collapses" in front of a high-grade flow obstruction affecting only the carotid siphon (Sect. 14.1), reliable (!) evidence of a dissection in this situation is only provided if the original, unstenosed vessel lumen can be identified as a low-echogenic structure around the stenosed lumen seen by color coding (Case Study 18.4). ◀

> **Case Study 18.3: Traumatic Dissection of the Extracranial Internal Carotid Artery**
> A 49-year-old doctor suffered a traffic accident as a car driver when another vehicle collided with the passenger side. In the first few days after the accident, there was a pulse-synchronous tinnitus in the left ear, which disappeared after about a week. Neurological deficits did not occur at any time. Sonographically and by DSA und MRA a dissection at the origin of the left internal carotid artery with a pseudoaneurysm could be detected (Figs. 18.9 and 18.10). In the controls six (Fig. 18.11) and twelve months later (Fig. 18.12), an increasing reduction of the aneurysm coud be seen, finally returning to a nearly normal vascular structure.

> **Case Study 18.4: Carotid and Vertebral Dissection After Marathon Run**
> The 48-year-old land surveyor took part in a marathon run; in the last third, calf cramps occurred due to a fluid imbalance. After the run, he noticed neck and throat pain on the right side, which was initially interpreted as cervical syndrome and muscular dysbalance. A few days later, a short episode with "white vision" of the right eye occurred inducing further investigations.
>
> Sonographically and in MRA a dissection of the right internal carotid artery with "string sign" as well as a dissection of the left vertebral artery in the upper V2 segment with congenital bilateral elongation of the vertebral artery and with kinking at about HWK 4 coud be found (Figs. 18.13 and 18.14). At the control two months later, the findings were largely unremarkable again (Fig. 18.15).

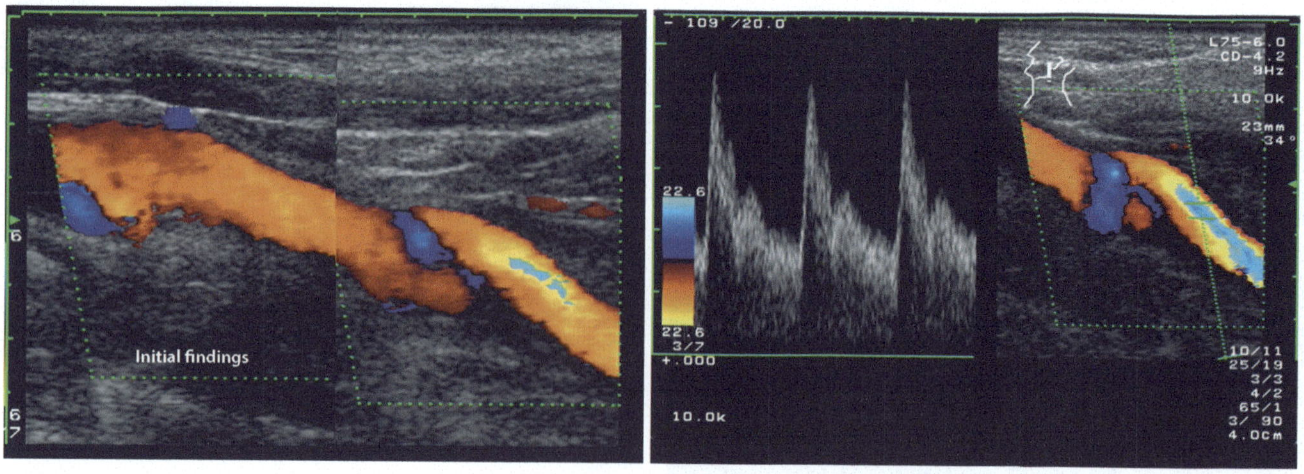

Fig. 18.9 Dissection approx. 3 cm distal to the origin of the left internal carotid artery

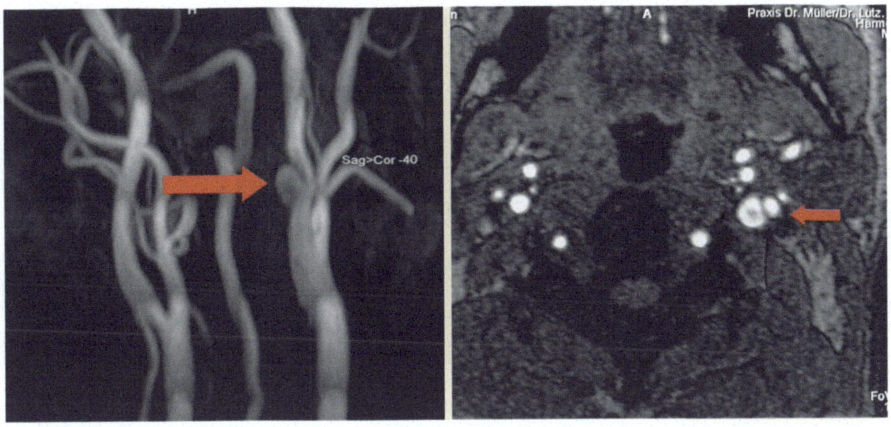

Fig. 18.10 DSA findings and MRI with fat-saturated transverse sectional image

> **Note**
> **Sonographically, a long-distance dissection of the carotid artery reaching from the skull base down to the carotid bifurcation can only be reliably diagnosed if the original, unstenosed vessel lumen can be visualized extracranially around the stenosed lumen.**

Vascular Occlusion Due to Dissection

Characteristically, in this case the extracranial color duplex image shows a non-perfused, tapering stump (Fig. 13.26). In the perfused initial section of the internal carotid artery there is usually a low pendulum flow ("**blunt signal**", Fig. 13.22d). ◀

Dissection in the Intracranial Carotid T-Area

Intracranial dissections are mainly found in childhood, the constellations of findings are described in Chap. 14. It is not uncommon that the initial section of the middle cerebral and/or anterior cerebral artery are affected as well. The differential diagnosis is primarily a moyamoya syndrome (Sect. 19.2) or vasculitis (Sect. 17). It is not possible to make a sonographic distinction; in any case, clarification requires a high-resolution MRI and MRA of the intracranial carotid artery. ◀

Diagnostic Pitfalls

Examining for dissections in the area of the skull base, it must always be taken into account that these can only be detected on the basis of indirect signs if they are accompanied by severe stenoses. Below a degree of stenosis of 70–75% they are overlooked. Therefore a dissection may be secured or at least made probable in the case of typical findings, but conversely, an inconspicuous finding does not exclude such a vascular lesion. This is why sonography should always be performed in combination with MRI in the case of such a clinical suspicion.

Even with an apparently typical **string sign** of the extracranial internal carotid artery, false findings cannot be ruled out. For example, if the internal carotid artery is occluded at the skull base, an ascending pharyngeal or occipital pharyngeal artery emerging from the internal carotid artery (Case Study 18.5) can feign an open vessel, the same applies to persistent primitive arteries (Fig. 1.10), rarely also strong vasa vasorum, which drain into the distal vessel and can be misinterpreted as a partial recanalization of a dissection (Kemeny et al. 1998).

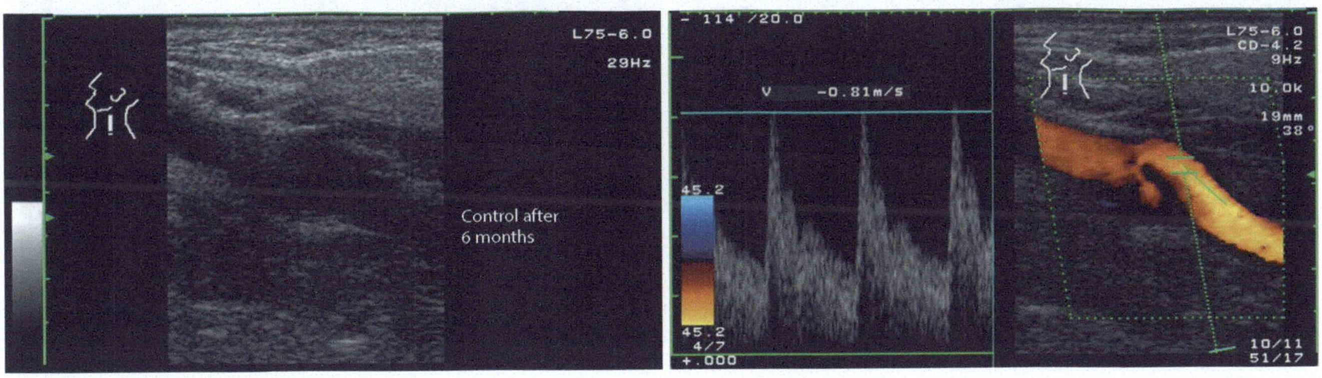

Fig. 18.11 Control after six months

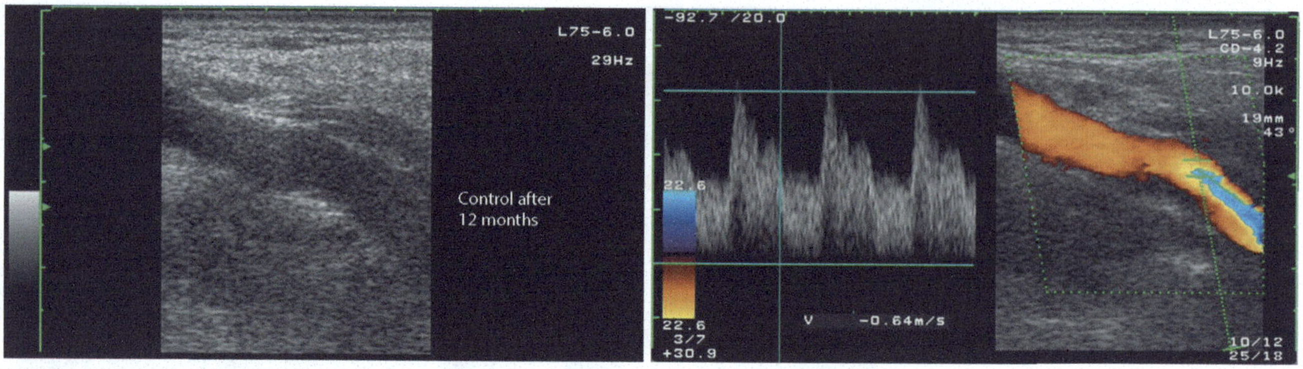

Fig. 18.12 Nearly normal vascular situation after twelve months

In contrast to arteriosclerotic vascular lesions, Doppler sonography of the periorbital arteries provides only limited information about the localization of the occlusive process in long-distance dissections. Although a retrograde flow through the supratrochlear artery suggests the maximum of the dissection proximal to the origin of the ophthalmic artery, it cannot be excluded that only the eye is retrogradely supplied by external carotid artery branches, since the ophthalmic artery may also be affected by the dissection.

An inconspicuous flow velocity in the extracranial internal carotid artery can lead to the oversight of a dissection in long-distance vessel narrowing if duplex sonography fails to detect the reduced vessel diameter in comparison to the contralateral side. In such case the flow volume should always be determined.

Clinical Significance

As already mentioned several times above, ultrasound examination should always be used in combination with MRI/MRA in the diagnosis of carotid dissections, as both procedures are complementary. In addition to the primary diagnosis, sonography is of major importance for follow-up examinations. Since the initially occluded or highly stenosed vessel often shows (partial) recanalization within days to weeks (Kremer et al. 2003), ultrasound is more suitable than any other method for following the course of the disease and thus provides important information for the therapeutic procedure. Due to the possible change in vessel diameter during the course of a dissection, the assessment should always be based on the determination of flow volume.

> Note
> **Due to the changing vessel diameter in dissections, follow-up examinations should always include flow volume measurements.**

> **Case Study 18.5: Incorrect Findings of a Carotid Dissection with Anatomical Variant**
> A 27-year-old soldier suffered from acute right brain infarction with mild hemiplegia on the left side. CT und MRI showed a small territorial infarction in the right insula area. Due to the apparently typical sonographic findings with a long-distance traceable, filiform vascular lumen (flow volume 20 ml/min) a dissection of the

(continued)

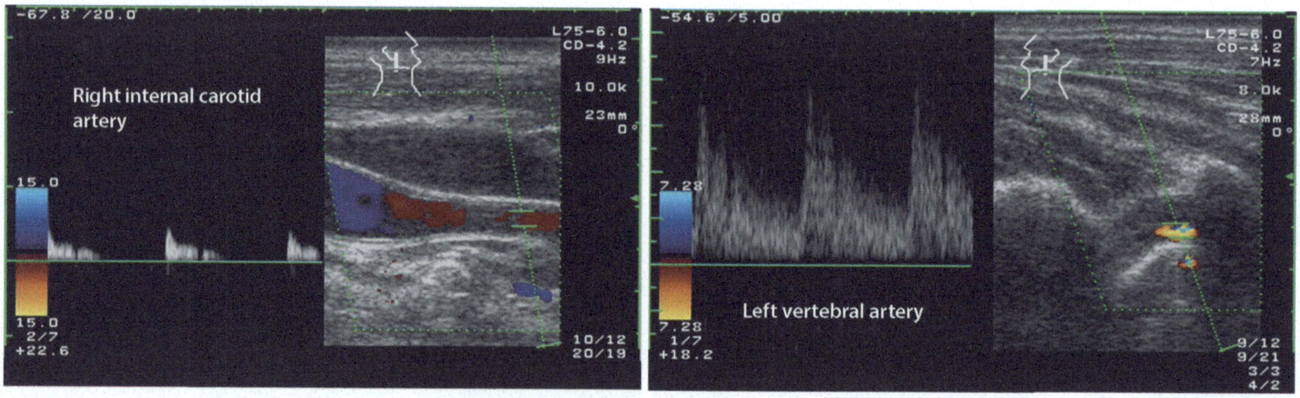

Fig. 18.13 String sign in the right internal carotid artery and short-distance macaroni sign in the left vertebral artery

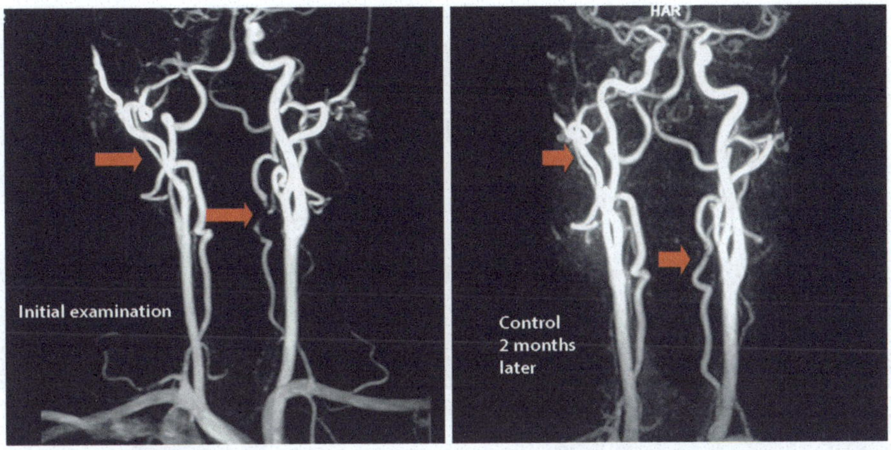

Fig. 18.14 MRA images in the course of the disease

> **Case Study 18.5** (continued)
> internal carotid artery was assumed to be the cause and anticoagulation was started.
>
> Due to recurrent, short-term tingling paresthesia of the left arm with spread to the left leg despite anticoagulation, an angiographic examination was performed several months later. Surprisingly, this revealed a complete occlusion of the right internal carotid artery distal to an anatomical variant with an occipital artery leaving the internal carotid artery about 3 cm above the bifurcation (Fig. 18.16). This vessel had been misinterpreted as a residual lumen of the internal carotid artery.
>
> The tingling paresthesias ceased under anticonvulsive therapy, so that focal seizures could be assumed as the cause. Transesophageal echocardiography (TEE) revealed an atrial septal defect with a large open foramen ovale indicating that the carotid occlusion was caused by a venous thrombus.

18.3 Dissections of the Vertebral Artery

Due to the course of the vessel with frequent changes between "free" course and fixation at the transverse processes and the skull, vertebral artery dissections can basically occur throughout the entire course of the vessel. Due to the particular hypermobility in these areas, however, there are two predilection sites:

- **V3 segment (Atlas loop)** until the vessel enters the skull through the foramen magnum. Dissections occur here in cases of sudden hyperextension of the head, but also in the context of chiropractic maneuvers (Case Study 18.6). Clinically problematic is the often uncharacteristic prodromal stage with uncharacteristic neck pain ("cervical syndrome") (Case Study 18.7).
- **V1-Segment** directly at the entrance of the vertebral artery into the transverse process of the (mostly) sixth cervical vertebra. Due to the good collateral supply via the spinal arteries, such dissections rarely lead to cerebral infarctions, but in individual cases they can be the cause of an acute ischemic cervical medullary lesion (Crum et al. 2000).

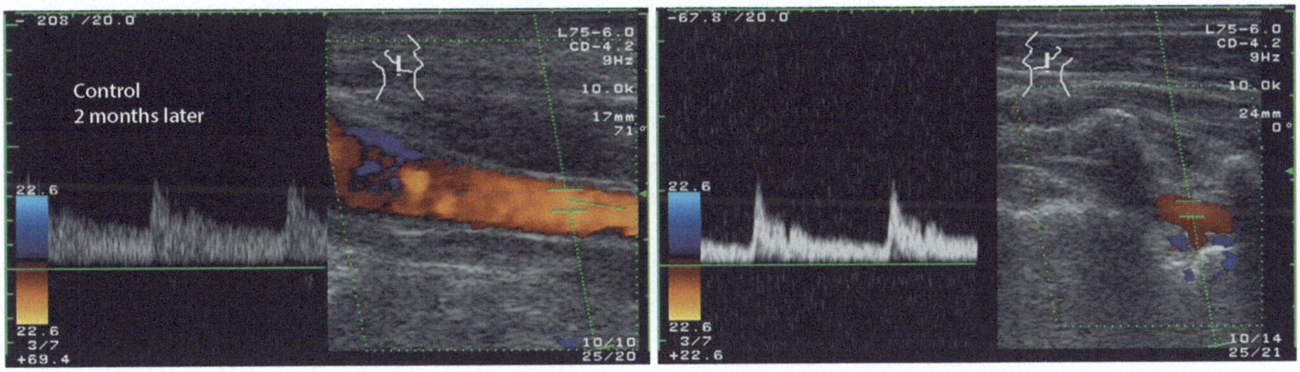

Fig. 18.15 Sonographic findings at control two months later

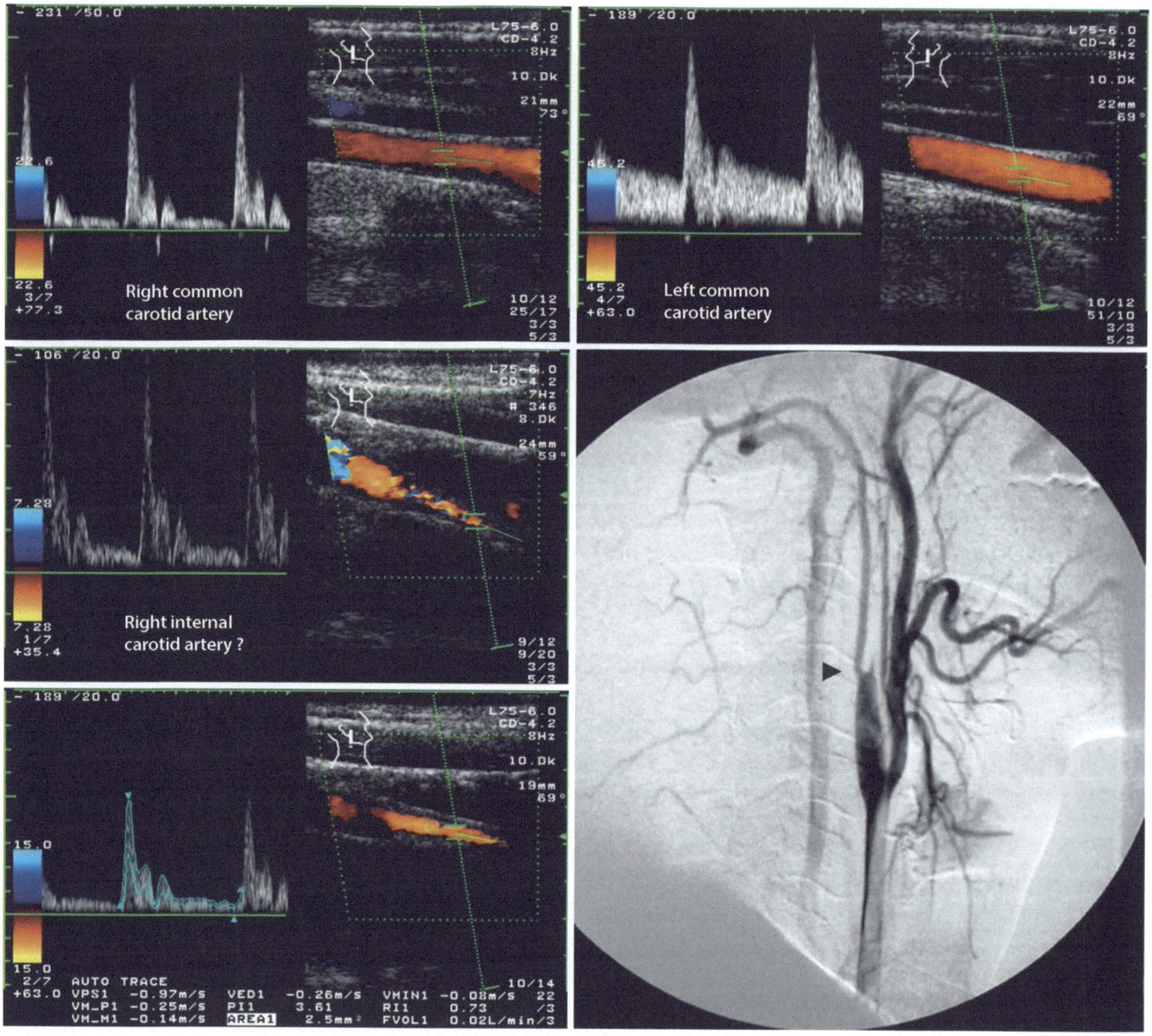

Fig. 18.16 Incorrect sonographic findings of an intracranial carotid dissection in the presence of carotid occlusion and an occipital artery originating from the internal carotid artery

Case Study 18.6: Vertebral Artery Dissection After Chiropractic Treatment

The 47-year-old patient with a history of migraine had frequent neck complaints and was chiropractically treated. After leaving the practice, she noticed a dizziness, which repeated several times in the following period. Under aspirin, a stabilization of the symptoms was finally achieved over 2 years. MRI, which was performed after a conspicuous Doppler and duplex sonography, showed an intravascular membrane in

Case Study 18.6 (continued)

the distal V2 segment as an expression of a vascular dissection (Fig. 18.17a). Duplex sonography revealed a normal flow signal in the right V2 segment (Fig. 18.17b), while a slightly increased pulsatility was observed in the left segment (Fig. 18.17c). On the left, a normal color coded image was obtained in the proximal section of the V2 segment (Fig. 18.17d), but a bilaminar vessel was detected in the distal V2 section (Fig. 18.17e).

(continued)

Case Study 18.6 (continued)

The intracranial flow signal of the right vertebral artery was inconspicuous (Fig. 18.17f); on the left side a flow-reduced vertebral artery was visible. The basilar artery was normal (not shown).

In summary, a distal V2 dissection with persistent presentation of a membrane in the V2 section of the vertebral artery was observed. To what extent the dissection was the cause of the neck pain or whether it was caused or worsened by the chirotherapeutic treatment remains to be discussed as well as the question whether a recurrent dizziness over 2 years can be an expression of the dissection.

Case Study 18.7: Spontaneous Vertebral Artery Dissection in the Distal V3 Segment

The 43-year-old warehouse worker was admitted to the hospital on New Year's Eve because of severe right-sided headaches and sore throats as well as a discreet feeling of dizziness. His medical history showed that he had hemiplegic headaches for 3 weeks, which the neurologist interpreted as atypical migraine. During the night after admission, acute rotational vertigo with nausea and vomiting occurred, which is why the patient was transferred to the next stroke unit. On admission there was also facial nerve palsy and a deviation of the

(continued)

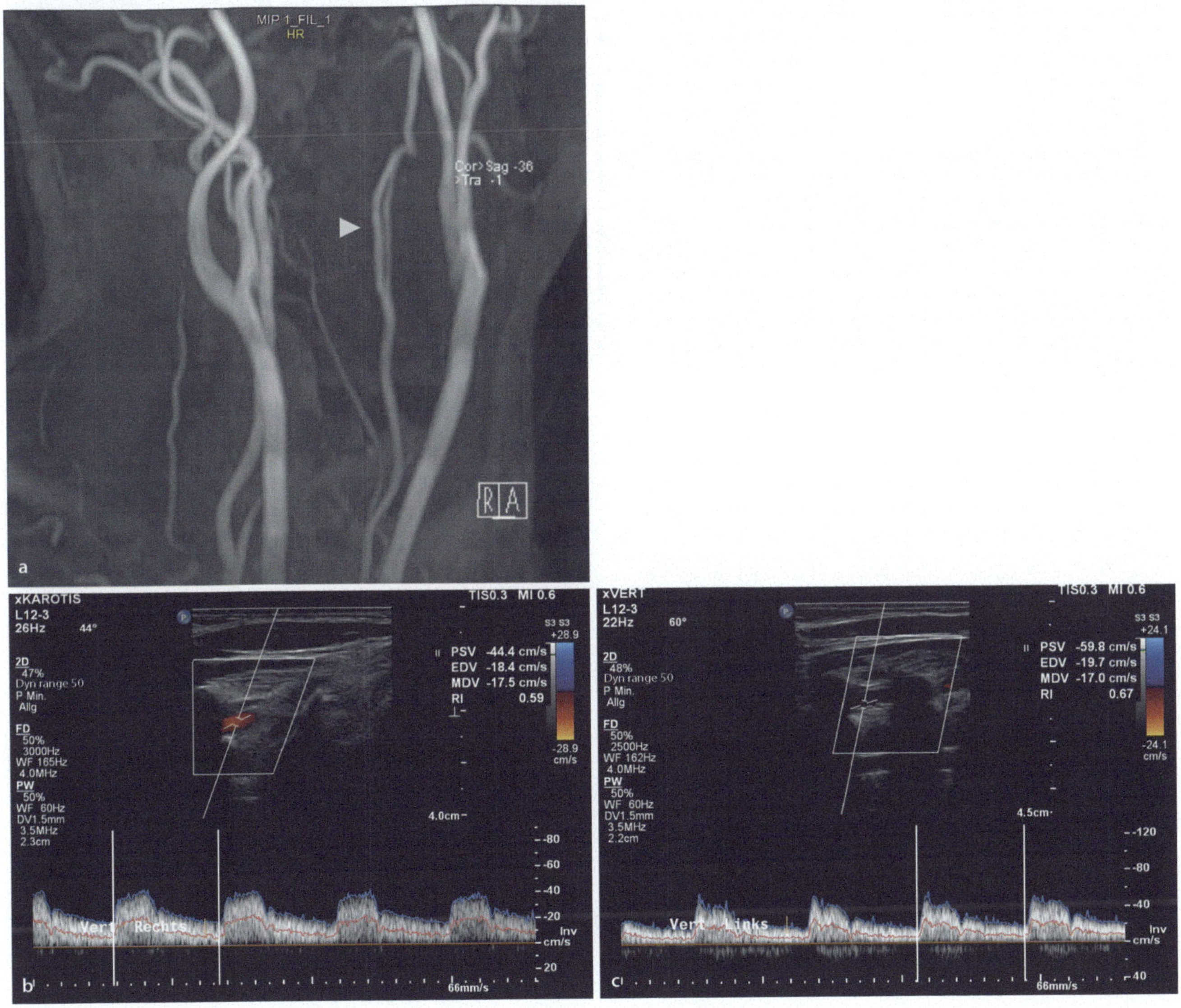

Fig. 18.17 Findings with left-sided vertebral artery dissection (explanations in the text)

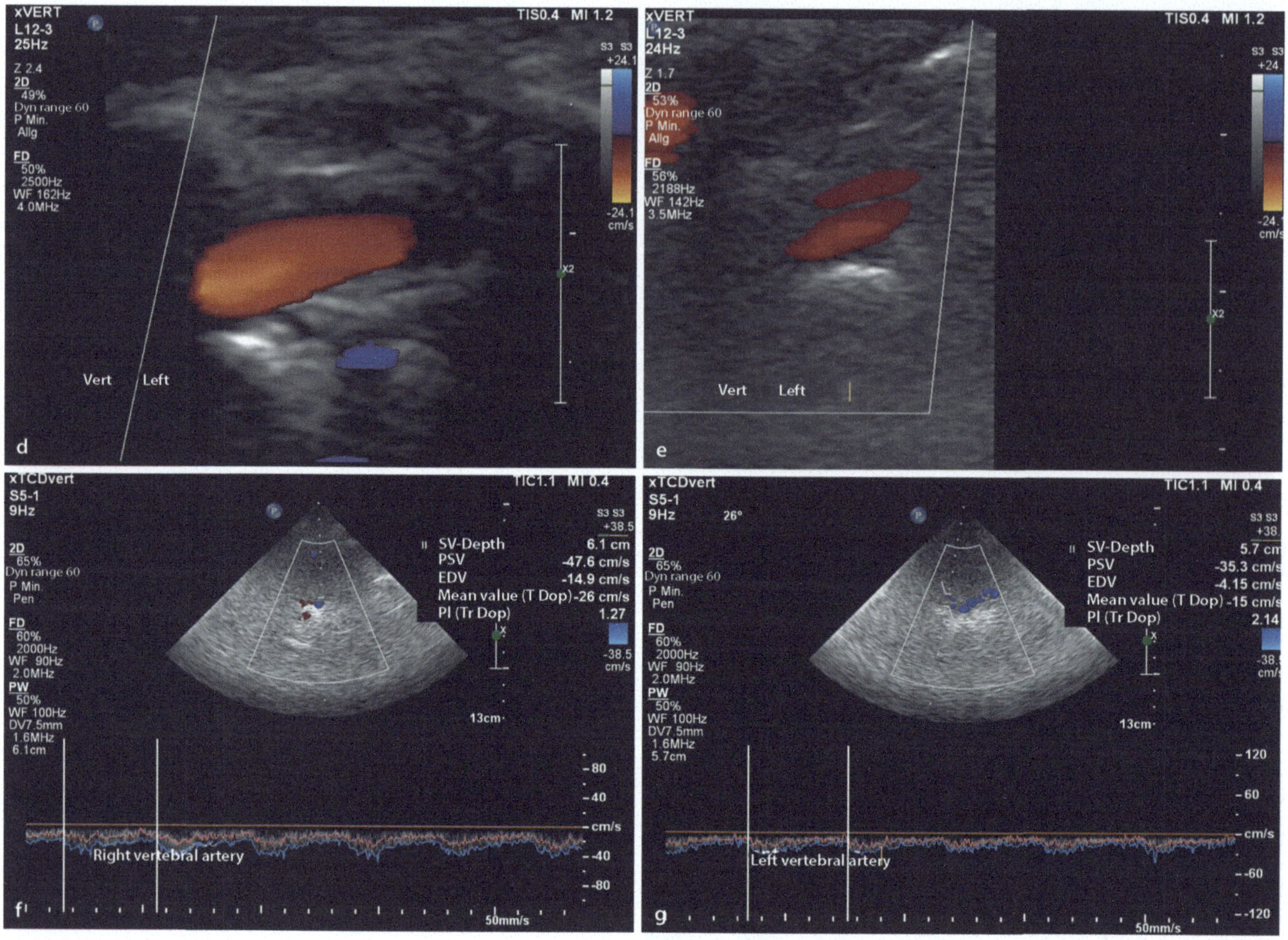

Fig. 18.17 (continued)

Case Study 18.7 (continued)
tongue to the right, a pronounced hemiataxia and slight hemiplegia on the right side and dysarthria.

The CT scan gave evidence of a cerebellar infarction on the right side. Sonographically, the vertebral arteries showed an approximately symmetrical diameter (Figs. 18.18 and 18.19), but an oscillating flow was found in the right V0 and V2 segment (Figs. 18.20 and 18.21). A few cm distal to the atlas loop, trans-nuchal duplex sonography showed an increased flow velocity, so that the diagnosis of a vertebral artery dissection was achieved (Fig. 18.22).

Under anticoagulation no new events occurred. Ten days later, the patient could be mobilized on the rollator for the first time. When the patient was transferred to the follow-up treatment at the end of January, there were only moderate neurological deficits. The last ultrasound examination showed no change in the findings.

Note
Traumatic dissections of the vertebral artery usually affect the area of the atlas loop (V3 segment). In contrast, other localizations are significantly less frequent.

Sonographic Assessment

In accordance with the two predilection sites, the vertebral artery should be followed cranially and caudally in the intertransversal course in case of clinical suspicion and/or conspicuous flow findings. In individual cases, however, dissections can also occur monosegmentally between two transverse processes (Hoffmann et al. 1993). For the diagnosis of such constrictions the sufficiently known sonographic criteria apply. In the context of aortic arch dissections, the vertebral arteries may also be affected and show a "false lumen," which leads to a multiphase signal already mentioned for the carotid artery.

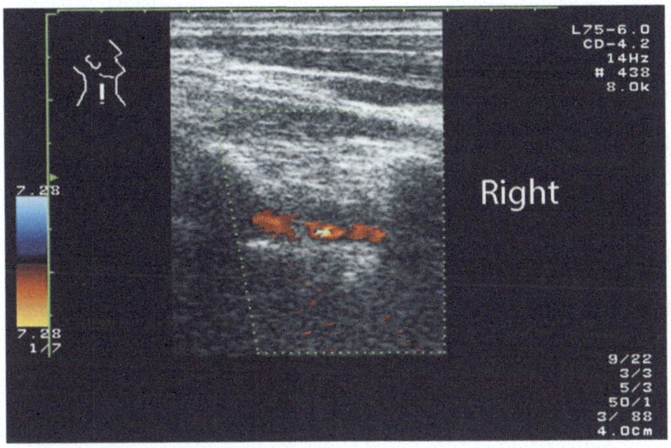

Fig. 18.18 Right vertebral artery

Diagnostic Pitfalls

Diagnostic problems arise when the vertebral artery cannot be imaged with certainty, especially in the area of the atlas loop. In this case, the first step is to use **low-flow parameters** (Sect. 6.3.1) to ensure that the lack of representability is not due to a technical problem. A problem that ultimately cannot be solved are pronounced degenerative spinal column changes that can prevent vessel imaging.

Only an apparent problem is the fact that in hypoplastic vessels the atlas loop is often not delimitable even in healthy vascular patients. In this situation, however, the flow signal in the V2 section is leading, which in dissections regularly shows an increase in pulsatility that exceeds the "normal" increase in pulsatility in hypoplasia, with a complete lack of diastolic flow. The reason for this is the observation that in the case of a primarily small vessel dissections rather immediately lead to a total occlusion.

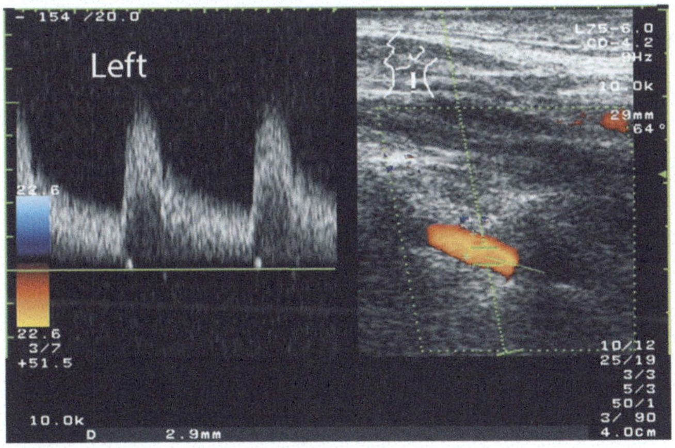

Fig. 18.19 Left vertebral artery

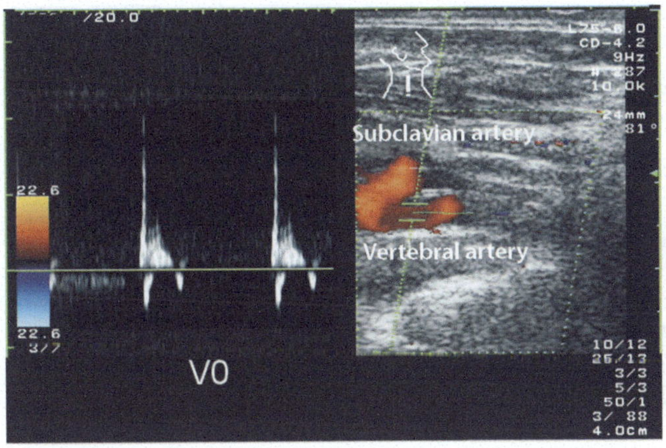

Fig. 18.20 Oscillating flow in V0 segment right

> **Practical Tips**
> Vertebral dissections can be confused with giant cell arteritis (Reinhard et al. 2003). Although arteriitides typically show a concentric lumen constriction ("halo sign"), while dissections are usually accompanied by an eccentrically located residual lumen, this differentiation is not always reliable. Especially in older patients with apparently clear "vertebral artery dissection", the presence of arteritis should be considered in the differential diagnosis and attention should be paid to signs of inflammation in the laboratory (increased ESR, C-reactive protein).

Clinical Significance

In the case of acute neck pain accompanied by dizziness or other – often diffuse – brain stem symptoms, color coded duplex sonography is the method of choice for quickly and accurately gaining an initial impression of the blood flow

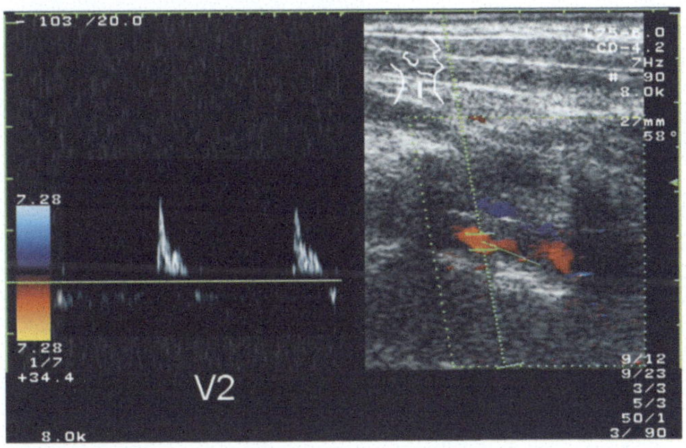

Fig. 18.21 Low oscillating flow in V2 segment right

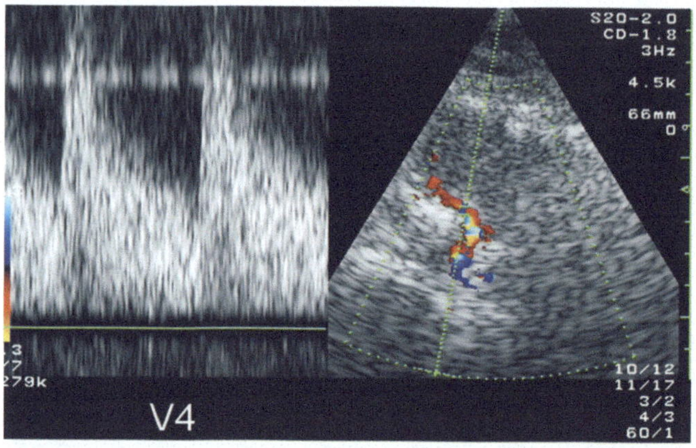

Fig. 18.22 V4 segment right

situation in the posterior cerebral circulation, from which the indication for further diagnostic measures can be derived.

Summary

Vascular dissections of the brain-supplying arteries are relatively common, but usually occur without serious complications. The main localization is the skull base. Clinically indicative are headaches as well as isolated cranial nerve deficits and/or a Horner's syndrome. Morphologically, hemorhage into the vascular wall with resulting vascular stenoses must be distinguished from "pseudoaneurysms" that extend outward. Often a combination of both lesion types is found. The sonographic findings vary depending on localization, severity and extent. The finding of a "string sign" in the area of the extracranial internal carotid artery is diagnostically indicative, but only conclusive if the original vascular lumen is still recognizable. Ultrasound diagnostics (including sonographic determination of the flow volume) is excellently suited for follow-up examinations of dissections.

References

Arning C, Oelze A, Lachenmayr L (1995) Eine seltene Schlaganfallursache: Die Aortendissektion. Akt Neurol 22:189–192

Bartels E (2006) Dissection of the extracranial vertebral artery: clinical findings and early noninvasive diagnosis in 24 patients. J Neuroimaging 16:24–33

Baumgartner RW, Bogousslavsky J (2005) Clinical manifestations of carotid dissection. Front Neurol Neurosci 20:70–76

Baumgartner RW, Arnold M, Baumgartner I, Mosso M, Gonner F, Studer A, Schroth G, Schuknecht B, Sturzenegger M (2001) Carotid dissection with and without ischemic events: local symptoms and cerebral artery findings. Neurology 57:827–832

Crum B, Mokri B, Fulgham J (2000) Spinal manifestations of vertebral artery dissection. Neurology 55:304–306

Debette S, Compter A, Labeyrie MA, Uyttenboogaart M, Metso TM, Majersik JJ et al (2015) Epidemiology, pathophysiology, diagnosis, and management of intracranial artery dissection. Lancet Neurol 14: 640–654

Eberhardt O, Topka H (2015) Compressive cervical radiculopathy due to vertebral artery dissection. J Stroke Cerebrovasc Dis 24:e115–e116

Engelter ST, Grond-Ginsbach C, Metso TM, Metso AJ, Kloss M, Debette S et al (2013) Cervical artery dissection: trauma and other potential mechanical trigger events. Neurology 80:1950–1957

Ferro JM, Massaro AR, Mas JL (2010) Aetiological diagnosis of ischaemic stroke in young adults. Lancet Neurol 9:1085–1096

Fullerton HJ, Johnston SC, Smith WS (2001) Arterial dissection and stroke in children. Neurology 57:1155–1160

Guillon B, Tzourio C, Biousse V, Adrai V, Bousser MG, Touboul PJ (2000) Arterial wall properties in carotid artery dissection: an ultrasound study. Neurology 55:663–666

Hoffmann M, Sacco RL, Chan S, Mohr JP (1993) Noninvasive detection of vertebral artery dissection. Stroke 24:815–819

Kemeny V, Droste DW, Nabavi DG, Schulte-Altedorneburg G, Schuierer G, Ringelstein EB (1998) Collateralization of an occluded internal carotid artery via a vas vasorum. Stroke 29:521–523

Kremer C, Mosso M, Georgiadis D, Stockli E, Benninger D, Arnold M, Baumgartner RW (2003) Carotid dissection with permanent and transient occlusion or severe stenosis: long-term outcome. Neurology 60:271–275

Lyrer PA, Brandt T, Metso TM, Metso AJ, Kloss M, Debette S et al (2014) Cervical artery dissection and ischemic stroke patients (CADISP) study group. Clinical import of Horner syndrome in internal carotid and vertebral artery dissection. Neurology 82: 1653–1659

Okada Y, Shima T, Nishida M, Yamane K, Kagawa R (1999) Traumatic dissection of the common carotid artery after blunt injury to the neck. Surg Neurol 51:513–519

Ortiz J, Ruland S (2015) Cervicocerebral artery dissection. Curr Opin Cardiol 30:603–610

Reinhard M, Schmidt D, Schumacher A, Hetzel A (2003) Involvement of the vertebral arteries in giant cell arteritis mimicking vertebral dissection. J Neurol 250:1006–1009

19 Other Vascular Diseases

Bernhard Widder and Gerhard F. Hamann

19.1 Fibromuscular Dysplasia (FMD)

Fibromuscular dysplasia (FMD) is a non-arteriosclerotic, non-inflammatory disease – probably quite common in abortive form – mainly of the renal arteries and the carotid and vertebral arteries (De Groote et al. 2017). Pathoanatomically, it is a mostly slowly progressive, often multifocal and bilateral fibrotic transformation of smooth muscle cells of the vascular media; more rarely, vascular intima is involved (Touzé et al. 2010). In the brain-supplying arteries, the changes in the area of the internal carotid artery are predominantly found below the base of the skull. Infestation of the intracranial internal carotid arteries and/or the large brain base arteries is rather rare. Those affected are mainly younger women, a hereditary component of the disease is likely. A specific therapy is not known.

Angiographically, Osborne and Anderson (1977) distinguish three types:

- **Type 1: Pearl cord** A series of short stretched vascular constrictions so called string beads, between the constrictions the lumen is normal or slightly aneurysmatically dilated.
- **Type 2: Tubular** Narrowing at a typical site with or without subsequent aneurysmatic dilatation.
- **Type 3:** Eccentric **crescent-shaped** constriction at a typical location.

B. Widder (✉)
Expert Opinion Institute, District Hospital, Guenzburg, Germany
e-mail: bernhard.widder@bkh-guenzburg.de

G. F. Hamann
Clinic of Neurology and Neurological Rehabilitation, District Hospital, Guenzburg, Germany

> **Additional information**
> From today's point of view, it is doubtful whether types 2 and 3 are actually fibromuscular dysplasia and not spontaneous or traumatic dissections. Individual, untypical constrictions can therefore only be interpreted as fibromuscular dysplasia if "pearl-cord" lesions can be detected in other vessel sections at the same time (Mettinger and Ericson 1982).

Sonographic Assessment
Fibromuscular dysplasia should always be considered by Doppler and duplex sonography if a circumscribed stenosis is not found at the exit area of the internal carotid artery but a few centimetres further cranially in the course of the vessel and no other significant arteriosclerotic vascular changes are detectable (**Case Study 19.1**). The finding of several constrictions confirms the diagnosis.

> **Note**
> **In the case of stenoses of the extracranial internal carotid artery distal to the carotid bifurcation and not accompanied by kinking or coiling, fibromuscular dysplasia should always be considered for differential diagnosis.**

The accuracy of the ultrasound examination for fibromuscular dysplasia is limited because such vascular processes are usually located far cranially below the base of the skull. Even when using low-frequency duplex probes, the image quality in this area is often already so poor that the findings can only be suspected.

B. Widder, G. F. Hamann (eds.), *Duplex sonography of the brain-supplying arteries*, https://doi.org/10.1007/978-3-662-65566-5_19

Clinical Significance

The most common clinical manifestation of fibromuscular dysplasia is renovascular hypertension. Only relatively rarely does such a vascular disease cause cerebral ischemia (Touzé et al. 2010). The most important complication of the brain-supplying arteries is probably the tendency to develop arterial dissections. It is not yet known whether there is also a risk due to thrombi adhering to the wall or additional arteriosclerotic changes. Also a part of Moya moya diseases (Sect. 19.2) might ultimately be fibromuscular dysplasia.

Practical Tips

In case of an (accidental) finding of a stenosis in the course of the internal carotid artery, which can be interpreted as fibromuscular dysplasia, it should be considered that such lesions are often accompanied by intracranial aneurysms, even in asymptomatic status. Accordingly, in this case cranial CT or MR angiography is recommended to detect a major such vascular malformation.

Case Study 19.1: Fibromuscular Dysplasia of the Internal Carotid Artery

The 51-year-old, until now completely healthy patient came to the examination because of an amaurosis fugax of the right eye, a neurological deficit could not be determined. In the color coded duplex sonogram of the right internal carotid artery, a twofold constriction (Fig. 19.1) with local alias phenomenon was found approx. 4 cm distal to the bifurcation. The maximum flow velocity in this area was 170 cm/s vs. 70 cm/s in the proximal carotid artery. In addition, a slight constriction with a maximum flow velocity of 140 cm/s was also observed on the left side below the jaw angle. Due to the multifocal findings, a suspicion of fibromuscular dysplasia was expressed, which could be confirmed angiographically (Fig. 19.2).

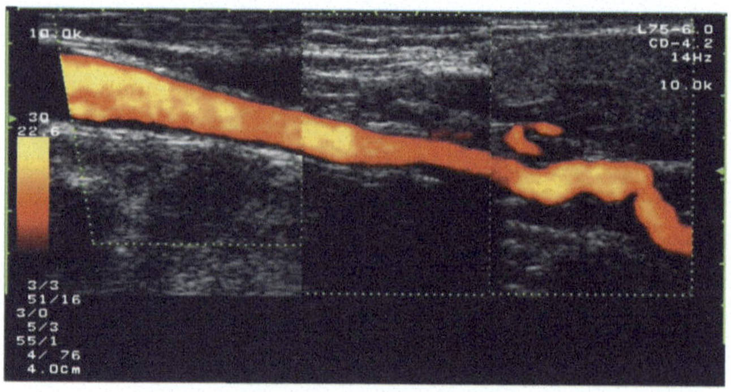

Fig. 19.1 Course of the right internal carotid artery

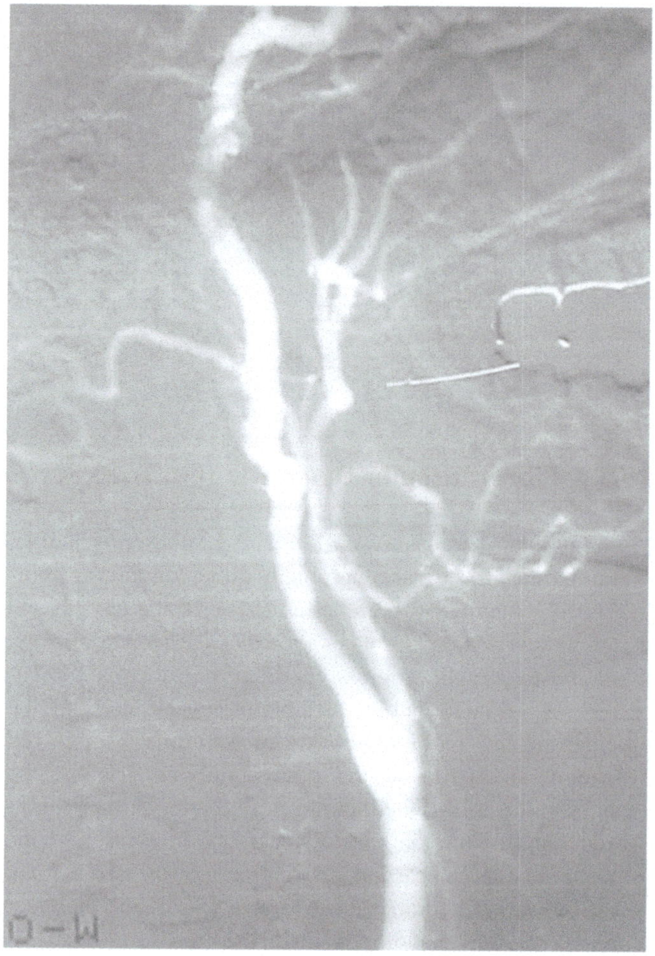

Fig. 19.2 Angiography of the right carotid artery

Under therapy with platelet aggregation inhibitors no further ischemic events occurred in the patient for several years.

Summary

Fibromuscular dysplasias are "pearl-cord," usually multiple retractions of the vessel wall, which are associated with an increased risk of dissection. In the extracranial color coded duplex sonogram they are impressive as short-stretched stenoses in the course of the internal carotid artery. Since dysplasias are often located directly below the base of the skull, they can only be detected under good examination conditions.

19.2 Moya Moya Disease

Moya moya disease, which is relatively common in East Asian countries and is also intensively studied there, is morphologically characterized by non-infectious and non-arteriosclerotic, progressive occlusion processes in the

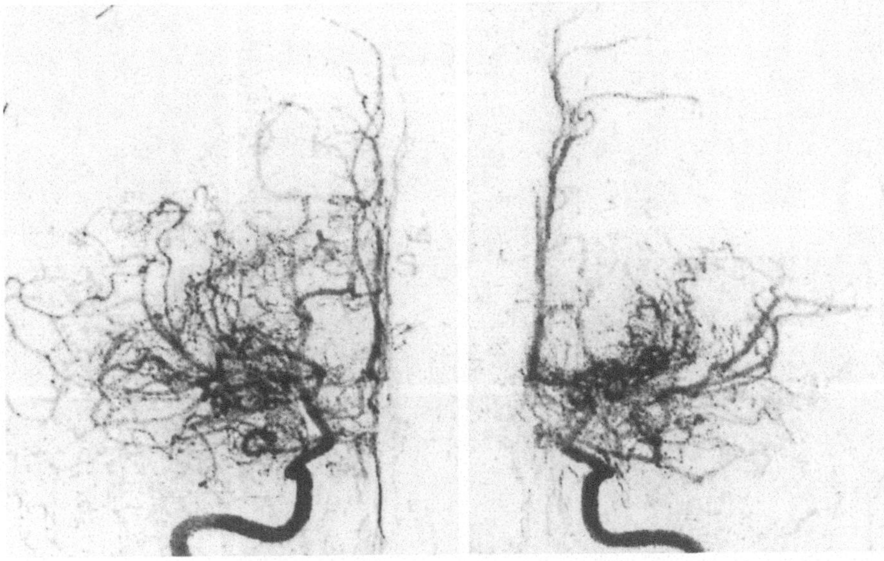

Fig. 19.3 "Moyamoya vessels" in the angiographic a.p. image of the carotid T-region on both sides

end section of the internal carotid artery on both sides immediately before it branches out (carotid T) (Fujimura et al. 2016). Frequently the initial sections of the middle cerebral artery and anterior as well as the posterior communicating artery are also affected. In the Asian literature, two frequency peaks are described, in childhood and in the fourth decade of life. In countries with a predominantly Caucasian population, in contrast, there seems to be an approximately equal distribution of the different age groups with a dominance of the female sex (Wenz et al. 2017). Moya moya disease was given its name because of the small collateral vessels in the area of the base of the skull (moya moya, Japanese smoke), which appear "smoky" in the angiographic image and which develop in the course of the disease (Fig. 19.3). It should be noted, however, that these are also only small collateral vessels ("pseudo-moyamoya") of a vascular occlusion slowly developing in the carotid T-region, for example, in the context of vasculitis or radiation angiopathy, so that the diagnosis of an idiopathic moyamoya disease is ultimately an exclusion diagnosis.

The clinical symptoms are characterized on the one hand by transitory and/or permanent cerebral ischemias, which are mostly of embolic nature, but may also be hemodynamically caused due to the unfavorable location of the occlusion localization. On the other hand, cerebral hemorrhages occur more frequently in these patients due to the pathological vascular network, which must be taken into account in the differential diagnosis of basal cerebral hemorrhages.

Sonographic Assessment

Sonographically, a moyamoya phenomenon can be spoken of if – in addition to the evidence of a higher degree of occlusion of the distal internal carotid artery – the color coded duplex sonogram shows indications of the presence of a pathological network in the outflow region of the middle cerebral artery (and anterior). The characteristic finding is a colorful image of various colored dots which cannot be assigned to a larger cerebral basal vessel and which show signals of different frequency and direction of flow in the Doppler recording (case examples 19.2–19.4). In contrast, the distal M1 segment of the Middle cerebral artery can usually be clearly delineated again – but often the flow velocity and pulsatility are significantly reduced.

Case Study 19.2: Moya Moya Syndrome on Both Sides

The onset of symptoms in the now 40-year-old geriatric nurse dates back 10 years. At that time recurrent weakness and furiness in the right arm as well as problems finding words. In the cranial CT a hypodense zone on the left frontal, parietooccipital and occipital was described, sonographically an occlusion of the left internal carotid artery was diagnosed. A cause of the symptoms could not be found. Medical history since the age of 15, taking of contraceptives, also 5–10 cigarettes/day.

In recent times now complaints of increasing fatigue, unsystematic dizziness and falling tendency. Sonographically low residual flow in the internal carotid artery on both sides (right 60 ml/min (a), left not measurable (b) (Fig. 19.4a, b)). With transtemporal sonication from the left, it is mainly the posterior circulation that shows a strong flow signal, whereas in the anterior circulation, flow signals can only be derived at points (Fig. 19.4c–f).

Pronounced borderline ischemia on the left side (Fig. 19.5) with left-sided "hemiatrophy" (Fig. 19.6).

(continued)

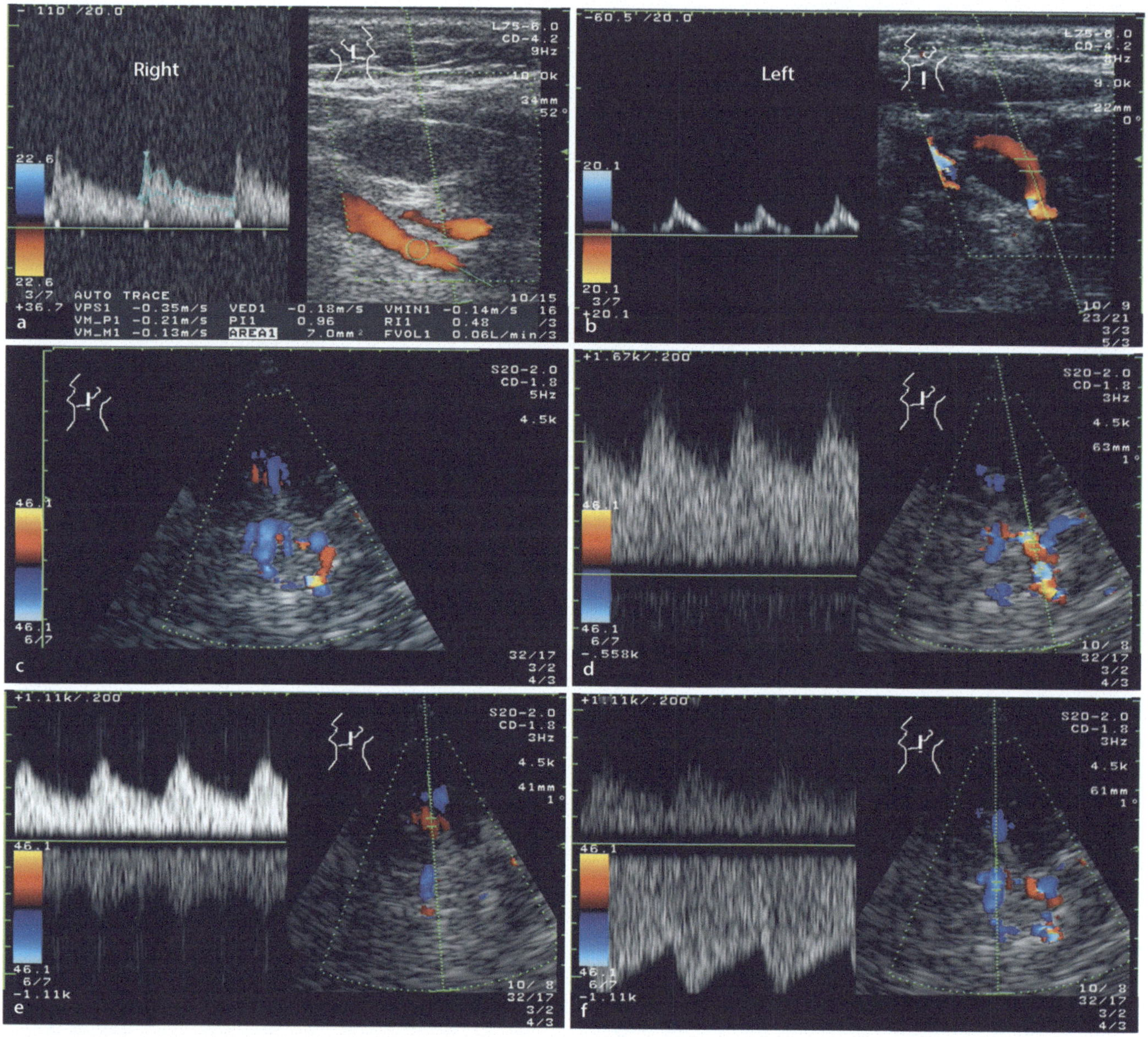

Fig. 19.4 Internal carotid artery right (**a**) and left (**b**), axial drains of the brain base arteries in case of transtemporal left sonication (**c–f**)

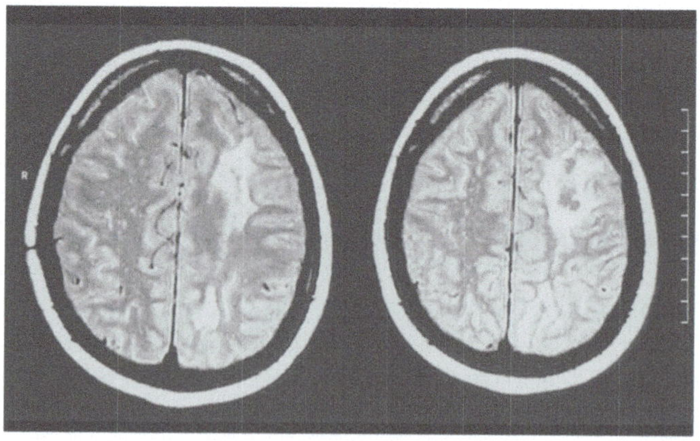

Fig. 19.5 Axial T2 sequence

> **Case Study 19.2** (continued)
> After gadolinium administration, a vascular network ("moyamoya network") appears at the basal right side, while such a network is not clearly visible at the left side (Fig. 19.6).

Clinical Significance

In addition to the primary diagnosis of the intracranial occlusion process – usually in combination with MRI and MRA – color coded duplex sonography enables follow-up examinations. These are essentially based on two findings:

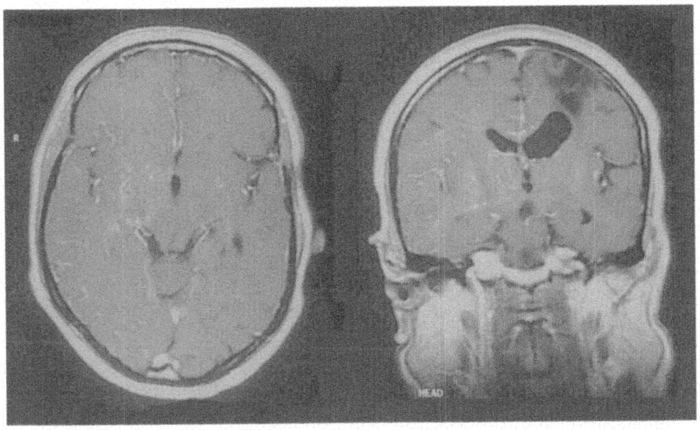

Fig. 19.6 MRI after gadolinium administration

- **Measurement of the flow volume** in all four of the extracranial arteries supplying the brain.
- **Determination of the cerebrovascular reserve capacity** in the affected middle cerebral artery in a side by side comparison. Doppler sonographic recording should be performed as far away as possible from the site of the occlusion (distal M1 or M2 segment) to ensure that the patient is not (no longer) in the area of the collateral vessels. The use of moyamoya vessels as a reference makes little sense, since changing findings are possible here.

Case Study 19.3: Moya Moya Syndrome with Bilateral Extra-intracranial Bypass

In the then 50-year-old patient recurrent transient ischemic attacks occurred, first in the supply area of the arteria cerebri media on the right, then intermittently also on the left. In addition, epileptic seizures with focal exudations in the area of the left hand occurred. In the course of an inpatient examination, a severe constriction of the distal internal carotid artery on both sides in the sense of a moyamoya disease was noticed. In hemodynamically induced changes on the right side (Fig. 19.7c), TIAs always occurred in the context of circulatory declines, an extra-intracranial bypass was performed on both sides at a distance of ½ year. Since then, no further recurrent transitory/ischemic attacks have occurred. However, with strong collateralization via the posterior communicating artery, the patient developed an aneurysm of the A. basilaris and a stenosis of the left posterior cerebral artery. The MR angiography (Fig. 19.7a) shows the bilateral bypass image and the collateralization of the mediastromal area via the posterior cerebral artery on both sides. The aneurysm of the basilar artery and the

Case Study 19.3 (continued)

stenosis of the left posterior cerebral artery are shown in the Fig. 19.7b.

The extra-intracranial bypass should ideally be investigated with the high-frequency linear probe, which is also used for imaging the arteria temporalis superficialis, here a linear probe 18–5 MHz. The right bypass is significantly more powerful than the left bypass (Fig. 19.8). In the extracranial internal carotid artery the patient showed only low flow velocities and a strongly tapering vessel. The right cerebral posterior artery showed a very high flow velocity in transcranial color duplex sonography, which is to be understood as a collateral flow. The flow in the cerebral media was weak and had a poststenotic effect; the arteria communicans posterior right appeared very strong.

The case shows an unusual bilateral moyamoya disease in a somewhat older patient without known genetic roots in East Asia. The extra-intracranial bypass was hemodynamically successful. Ultimately, however, the essential collateralization was achieved via the posterior communicating artery, which probably also led to the development of the basilar head aneurysm in the hemodynamically particularly stressed collateral flow area. Interestingly, this clinical course copies the experimental induction of basilar head aneurysms by bilateral carotid isobliteration (Tutino et al. 2014).

Case Study 19.4 Long-term Moya Moya Syndrome

The patient, who was 30 years old at the time of diagnosis, had recurrent TIAs and focal epilepsy with left-sided ejections. She was of German descent without genetically known roots in East Asia; strokes or neurological diseases were unknown in the family. Angiography revealed high-grade distal almost occlusion of the internal carotid artery on both sides with moyamoya-like miracle netting on both sides.

Under oral anticoagulation with a vitamin K antagonist and ASA, the patient was clinically stable for 19 years. She also received antiepileptic therapy with oxcarbazepine. The MR angiography shows the distal closure of the internal carotid artery on both sides with strong posterior communicating artery on both sides and P2 stenosis of the left posterior cerebral artery (Fig. 19.9a). There were smaller infarcts with medullary hypodensities at the beginning of the disease (Fig. 19.9b), no further TIAs or MRI changes occurred

(continued)

Case Study 19.4 (continued)
under the aggressive antithrombotic therapy. Since initially the diagnosis of a pseudo-moyamoya syndrome could not be excluded under the suspected diagnosis of cerebral vasculitis, a cortisone therapy followed by years of azathioprine therapy was performed. The anti-inflammatory therapies were discontinued after several years without clinical or vascular deterioration.

The internal carotid artery was extracranially dislocated on both sides and with low flow (Fig. 19.10). The left vertebral artery was very strong and contributed significantly to intracranial perfusion. The middle cerebral artery showed a poststenotic flow profile on both sides. The internal carotid artery showed highest intracranial flow acceleration with "musical murmurs" on both sides, flow velocities up to 450 cm/s were detected. The stenosis of the left posterior cerebral artery was also excellently visualized in color duplex sonography with flow velocities up to 210 cm/s systolic. The basilar artery was very strong due to the collateralization flow.

This is the more common picture in Germany of relatively young women with moyamoya alterations. Since the patient never had a carotid occlusion, but the highest grade stenoses remained unchanged, the indication for extra-intracranial bypass surgery was never given.

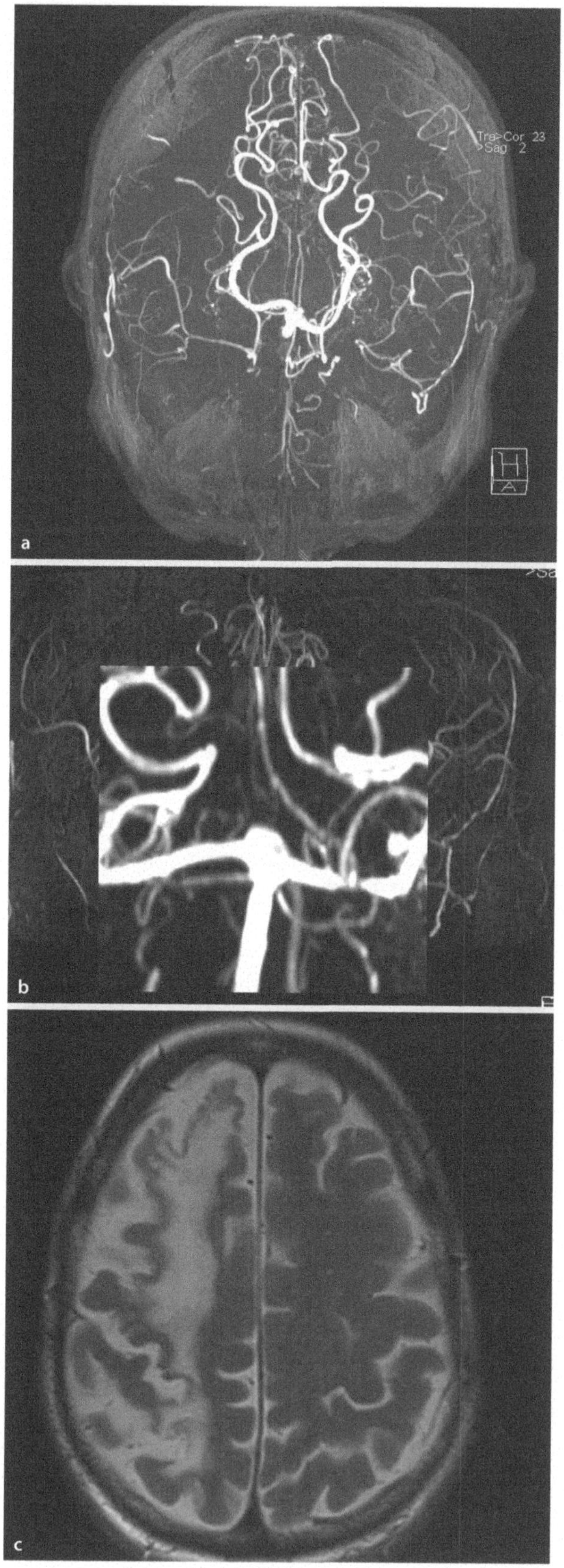

Fig. 19.7 (**a–c**) MRI images (explanations in the text)

Summary
Moyamoya alterations are characterized by multiple small collateral vessels in the area of the anterior basilar arteries of the brain, which develop in connection with a highly stenosed or occluded distal internal carotid artery. An independent moyamoya disease is only present if other causes (vasculitis, dissection, arteriosclerosis) are excluded. Duplex sonography shows – in addition to the actual vessel occlusion – a colorful picture of different colored dots with variable flow signals, which cannot be assigned to any larger brain basal vessel.

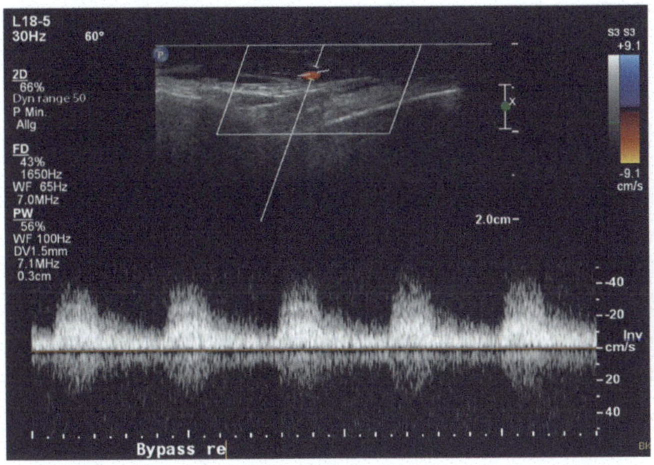

Fig. 19.8 Duplex sonographic recording of the right extra-intracranial bypass

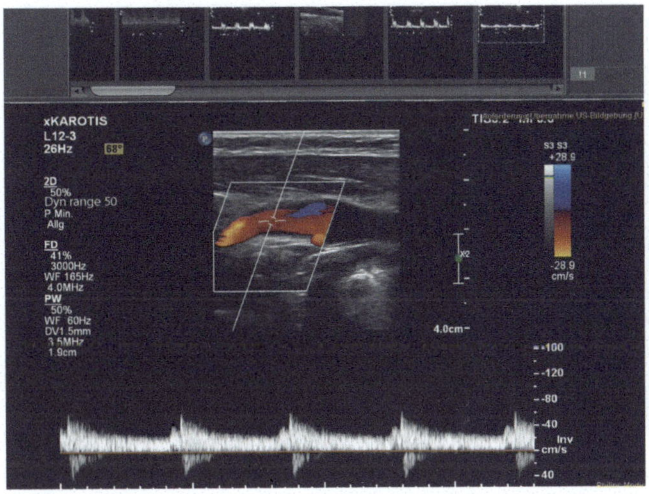

Fig. 19.10 Duplex sonogram of the right internal carotid artery

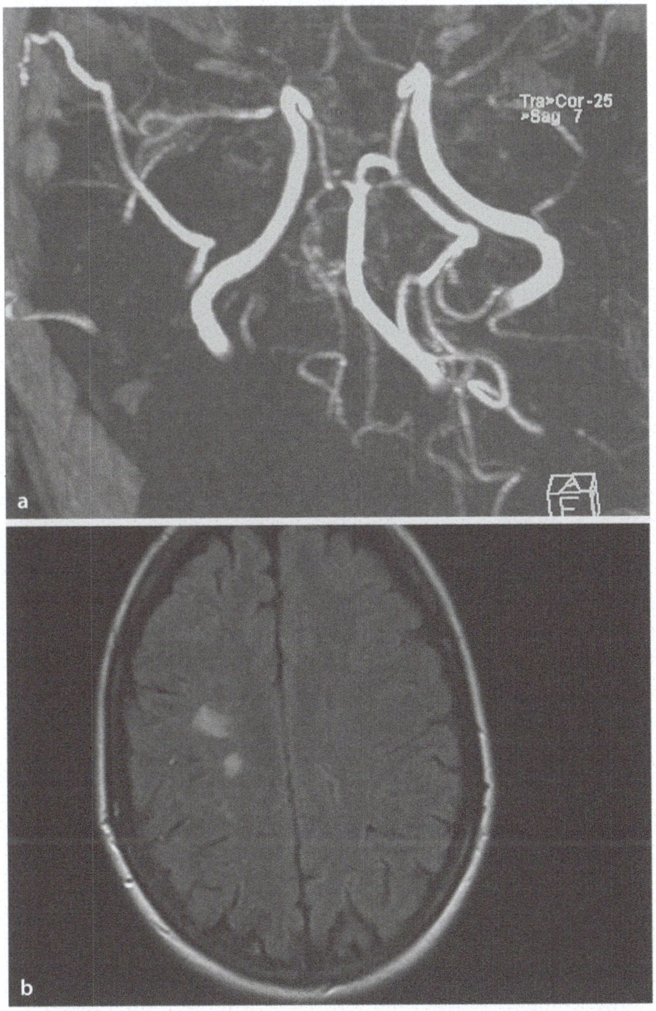

Fig. 19.9 (a, b) MRT images (explanations in the text)

19.3 Aneurysms

19.3.1 Extracranial Aneurysms

Aneurysms of the extracranial brain-supplying arteries are relatively rare. As verum **aneurysm** are called so, since all three vessel wall layers (intima, media, adventitia) are affected. Differential diagnoses are to be discussed:

- **Congenital aneurysm.** Relevant vascular sacculations at the extracranial arteries in the context of congenital connective tissue diseases are among the rarities. However, in the area of the carotid bulb, smooth transitions between a "normal" formation (Sect. 1.3.2) and a vascular dilatation that is considered a normal variant, but in individual cases also a pathological one, are not uncommon.
- **Inflammatory aneurysm.** Both bacterial and abacterial inflammatory reactions of the vessel wall can lead to local sacculation (Fig. 19.11). The most frequent causes of this are local inflammatory processes in the head and neck area including purulent dental diseases (Knouse et al. 2002; Nader et al. 2001), but in individual cases also hematogenic scattering, for example, in the context of endocarditis (Hubaut et al. 1997). The extent of the aneurysmatic dilatation is usually small, so that the findings can only be recognized by a thorough search in the black-and-white ultrasound image. Typically, inflammatory aneurysms are accompanied by a pressure painful carotid artery (Sect. 19.4).

In addition to the "aneurysma verum," three other constellations of findings are associated with the term "aneurysm."

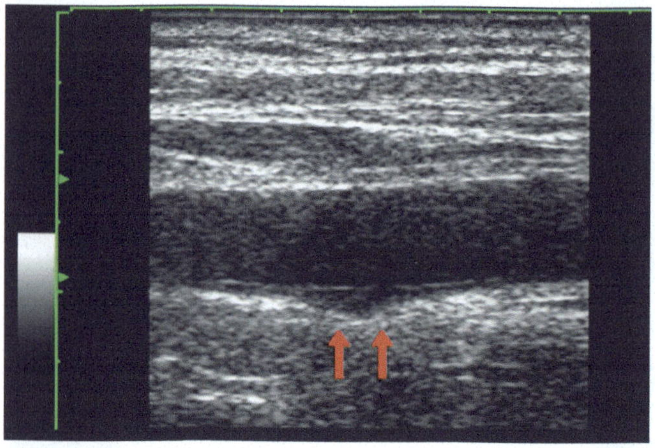

Fig. 19.11 Local vascular wall sacculation, accompanied by local pain, improvement on non-steroidal anti-inflammatory drugs

Secondary Aneurysm

Aneurysmatic dilatation after carotid surgery with patch insertion is relatively common. As this is an essential aspect of postoperative sonographic controls, they will be discussed in more detail in this Sect. 24.1.4. ◀

Pseudoaneurysm

Bleeding between the vessel walls in the course of an external dissection leads to local vascular dilatation without affecting the continuity of the inner vessel wall. Further details Sect. 19.1. ◀

"False" Aneurysm (Aneurysm Spurium)

This is a bleeding cavity in the tissue due to a leak in the vessel wall. This usually occurs traumatically after a vascular puncture or in the context of suture failure after carotid surgery (Sect. 24.1.4), but can also occur as a result of a spontaneous vascular rupture in the context of congenital vascular dysplasia. Typically, the color coded display and the Doppler signal show outflow and reflux phenomena in rapid alternation in the bleeding cavity (Anglo-American **to and fro sign**; Fig. 19.12). ◀

Sonographic Assessment
In the sonographic detection of aneurysms, two localizations can be distinguished:

Carotid Bulb

Based on the standard values for the carotid bulb shown in the table, the diagnosis of aneurysmatic dilatation appears justified from an outer diameter of 14–15 mm (mean value ± 2 times standard deviation). Alternatively – especially in dilated arteriopathies with altogether wide vessels – an individual orientation on the diameter of the common carotid artery is possible. If this is exceeded by 50% or more in the bifurcation area, an aneurysm is suspected. 1.5. ◀

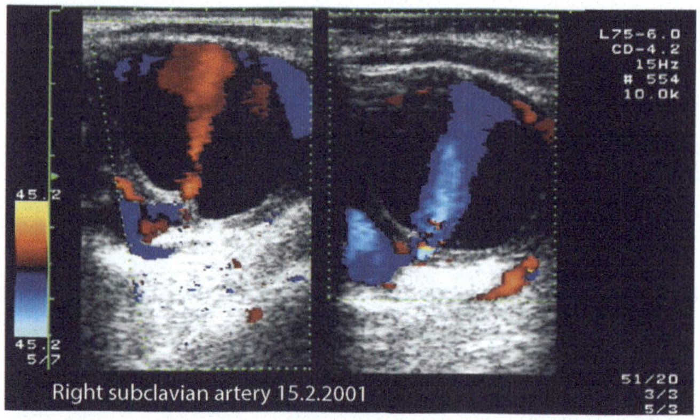

Fig. 19.12 "To and fro sign" for a false aneurysm due to spontaneous vascular rupture in the context of Ehlers-Danlos syndrome

Other Vessel Course

Aneurysms at other sites in the course of the extracranial carotid artery and vertebral artery are usually less pronounced and often only recognizable by subtle assessment of the vessel wall layers. It goes without saying that this is only possible where the intima-media complex can be assessed. Otherwise the assessment must be based on the in this case not very reliable color coded vessel representation, which only shows coarser abnormalities. ◀

Clinical Significance
Color coded duplex sonography is the method of choice for the clarification of pulsating tumors of the neck and for the exclusion of a spontaneous or "mycotic" aneurysm in carotid dydynia (Sect. 19.4). In most cases a "prima vista diagnosis" is possible.

19.3.2 Intracranial Aneurysms

In contrast to the situation with extracranial vessels, aneurysms are relatively common in intracranial vessels. They occur at congenital weak points of the vessel wall and can lead to subarachnoid hemorrhages in the event of rupture. The detection of aneurysms in color coded ultrasound images is based on the detection of a color-filled "appendage" on a vessel. The diagnostic accuracy is so low compared to CTA and MRA that sonographic procedures have no relevant clinical significance.

> **Summary**
> Aneurysms in the area of the extracranial arteries leading to the brain are relatively rare. Although dilatations

(continued)

of the carotid bulb are frequently found, they are usually standard variants and not aneurysms. With pressure painful carotid arteries, an inflammatory ("mycotic") aneurysm is to be considered. "False" aneurysms occur in ruptures of the vessel wall when the outflowing blood in the surrounding tissue causes a non- or only partially thrombosed bleeding cavity. Although intracranial aneurysms are occasionally visible sonographically, the diagnostic accuracy is marginal.

19.4 Carotidodynia

The painful carotid is a frequently reported problem, mostly the symptoms are transient and related to infections. Pain and sensitivity to pressure as well as a self-limiting course within a few days to weeks are the clinical characteristics. The ultrasound findings of carotidodynia are inhomogeneous. Arning (2004) provides a good overview of these findings. In 6 patients he showed a diffuse thickening of the wall of the common carotid artery, which had regressed well in control. In addition, there are reports of bleeding into the wall of the common carotid artery (Lim et al. 2012) or clear infectiological complications with vascular wall involvement in the sense of vasculitis (Cassone et al. 2013).

19.5 Reversible Cerebral Vasoconstriction Syndrome

Many different syndromes have been named in recent decades, which are now grouped together under the term reversible cerebral vasoconstriction syndrome (RCVS), among them postpartum angiopathy, eclampsia with vasoconstriction, drug-induced vasospasms, call or call-fleming syndrome, migraine angiitis, thunderclap headache with vasoconstriction, benign cerebral vasculitis and pseudo-CNS vasculitis. The diagnosis of RCVS requires after Ducros (2014):

1. Detection of multifocal vessel wall constrictions intracranially (CTA, DSA, MRA, TCCS)
2. Severe, unusual headaches without neurological deficits
3. Lack of evidence of subarchnoid hemorrhage
4. Normal CSF
5. Complete reversibility of multifocal vascular wall changes in the course of (within the next 12 weeks)
6. In the course of and by further examinations exclusion of other essential differential diagnoses, for example, vasculitis.

Since the first publication by Ducros et al. (2007), there are numerous publications describing the relationship of these "new" syndromes with known syndromes and also overlaps with RCVS, posterior reversible encephalopathy syndrome (PRES) and vasculitis (Sextro et al. 2012). Ultrasound is ideally suited to contribute to diagnosis and, above all, to monitoring during the course of the disease (Chen et al. 2008, Levin et al. 2013). The disease is not always benign, bleeding and secondary cerebral pressure increases, which can lead to death, are reported.

References

Arning C (2004) Die Karotidynie im Ultraschallbild: Mythos. Syndrom oder Krankheitsbild? 75:1200–1203

Cassone G, Colaci M, Giuggioli D, Manfredi A, Sebastiani M, Ferri C (2013) Carotidynia possibly due to localized vasculitis in a patient with latent mycobacterium tuberculosis infection. Case Rep Vasc Med 2013:585789

Chen SP, Fuh JL, Chang FC, Lirng JF, Shia BC, Wang SJ (2008) Transcranial color doppler study for reversible cerebral vasoconstriction syndromes. Ann Neurol 63:751–757

De Groote M, Van der Niepen P, Hemelsoet D, Callewaert B, Vermassen F, Billiouw JM, De Vriese A, Donck J, De Backer T (2017) Fibromuscular dysplasia – results of a multicentre study in Flanders. Vasa 3:1–8

Ducros A (2014) Reversible cerebral vasoconstriction syndrome. Handb Clin Neurol 121:1725–1741

Ducros A, Boukobza M, Porcher R, Sarov M, Valade D, Bousser MG (2007) The clinical and radiological spectrum of reversible cerebral vasoconstriction syndrome. A prospective series of 67 patients. Brain 130:3091–3101

Fujimura M, Bang OY, Kim JS (2016) Moyamoya Disease Front Neurol Neurosc 40:204–220

Hubaut JJ, Albat B, Frapier JM, Chaptal PA (1997) Mycotic aneurysm of the extracranial carotid artery: an uncommon complication of bacterial endocarditis. Ann Vasc Surg 11:634–636

Knouse MC, Madeira RG, Celani VJ (2002) Pseudomonas aeruginosa causing a right carotid artery mycotic aneurysm after a dental extraction procedure. Mayo Clin Proc 77:1125–1130

Levin JH, Benavides J, Caddick C, Laurie K, Wilterdink J, Yaghi S, Silver B, Khan M (2013) Transcranial Doppler ultrasonography as a non-invasive tool for diagnosis and monitoring of reversible cerebral vasoconstriction syndrome. R I Med J 99:38–41

Lim S, Khanafer A, Misselhorn D, Laing A (2012) Focal common carotid artery intramural haematoma. N Z Med J 126:82–85

Mettinger KL, Ericson K (1982) Fibromuscular dysplasia and the brain. I. Observations on angiographic, clinical and genetic characteristics. Stroke 13:46–52

Nader R, Mohr G, Sheiner NM, Tampieri D, Mendelson J, Albrecht S (2001) Mycotic aneurysm of the carotid bifurcation in the neck: case report and review of the literature. Neurosurgery 48:1152–1156

Osborne AG, Anderson RE (1977) Angiographic spectrum of cervical and intracranial fibromuscular dysplasia. Stroke 8:617–626

Sextro F, Klimpe S, Hamann GF (2012) Pregnancy-linked endotheliopathy. A disease with multiple variants? Nervenarzt 83: 510–513

Touzé E, Oppenheim C, Trystram D, Nokam G, Pasquini M, Alamowitch S, Hervé D, Garnier P, Mousseaux E, Plouin PF (2010) Fibromuscular dysplasia of cervical and intracranial arteries. Int J Stroke 5:296–305

Tutino VM, Mandelbaum M, Choi H, Pope LC, Siddiqui A, Kolega J, Meng H (2014) Aneurysmal remodeling in the circle of Willis after carotid occlusion in an experimental model. J Cereb Blood Flow Metab 34:415–424

Wenz H, Wenz R, Maros M, Ehrlich G, Al-Zghloul M, Groden C, Förster A (2017) Incidence, locations, and longitudinal course of cerebral microbleeds in European moyamoya. Stroke 48:307–313

Vascular Anomalies and Malformations

20

Bernhard Widder and Gerhard F. Hamann

20.1 Kinkings and Coilings

Curved vascular courses can basically occur in all extra- and intracranial arteries supplying the brain. Predilection sites for kinkings and coilings, however, are those areas of the vessels that require special flexibility to allow head rotations. These include the extracranial course of the internal carotid artery below the skull base and the origin and atlas loop of the vertebral artery. Less frequently affected are the course of the vertebral artery between the transverse processes and the origin of the common carotid artery. Major intracranial kinkings and coilings are equally rare.

The probability of kinkings and coilings increases with increasing age, concurrent changes concern the increase in the diameter of the bulb and the increase in the bifurcation angle of the carotid artery (Kamenskiy et al. 2015). The causes for this are the age-related loss of muscular tone of the vascular walls, cranial enlongation of the aortic arch probably due to hypertension, and the reduction in body size due to the collapse of the intervertebral discs. A considerably curved vascular course in the area of the internal carotid artery and at the origin of the vertebral artery is found in about half of the elderly. In most cases, however, these are only so-called **elongations or tortuosities**.

A kinking is defined as an angle between the two vessel legs is less than 90° (Fig. 20.1) and a defined kinking is visible in the ultrasound image. The transitions of what is called kinking or not are fluid and different kinking angles can occur depending on the head position. Women show such vascular changes much more frequently than men, the cause is unknown (Macchi et al. 1997).

B. Widder (✉)
Expert Opinion Institute, District Hospital, Guenzburg, Germany
e-mail: bernhard.widder@bkh-guenzburg.de

G. F. Hamann
Clinic of Neurology and Neurological Rehabilitation, District Hospital, Guenzburg, Germany

20.1.1 Sonographic Assessment

Localization in the Internal Carotid Artery
Color coded duplex sonography can be used to visualize curved courses of the internal carotid artery, provided these are present in the proximal section of the vessel (Fig. 20.2). By means of the angle-corrected measurement of the flow velocity over the course of the kinking formation, which is as continuous as possible, statements about the presence of a possible kinking stenosis can be made. The evaluation is based on the assessment of the degree of stenosis of the extracranial internal carotid artery (Chap. 13). The search for circumscribed wall thickenings, plicatures and dissections in black and white sections is also essential (Fig. 20.3), while functional examinations at different head rotations generally do not lead to usable results.

There are two basic difficulties to be considered in sonographic diagnostics.

Problem of Cranial Localization

The majority of kinkings and coilings are not found directly in the area of the carotid bifurcation, but further cranially below the base of the skull. However, in obese patients with a short neck this area is often not reliably assessable. ◄

Practical Tips
If the "usual" sound probe with a transmission frequency of 7.5 MHz is not sufficient to detect kink formations located cranially below the jaw angle, the use of a lower frequency 5 MHz or even 3.5 MHz probe often helps. The reduction in resolution to be expected from this is only minimal with regard to the color coded display.

B. Widder, G. F. Hamann (eds.), *Duplex sonography of the brain-supplying arteries*, https://doi.org/10.1007/978-3-662-65566-5_20

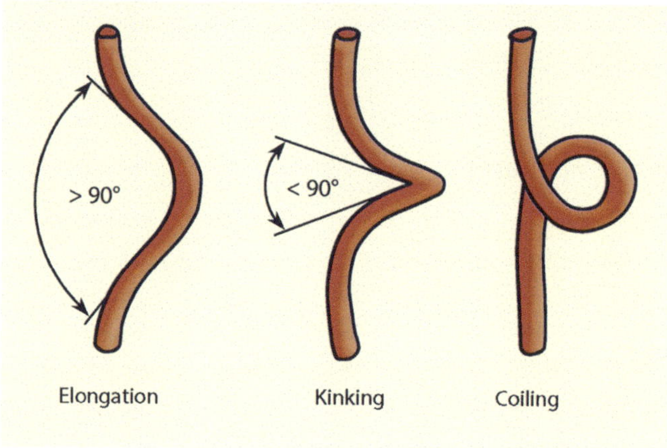

Fig. 20.1 Appearance of elongations, kinkings, and coilings

Problem of Angle Correction

The assessment of stenoses caused by kinking (**kinking stenoses**) cannot be reliably carried out by determining flow velocity, since no sufficiently accurate angle correction is possible directly in the area of kinking (Fig. 5.20). In this case, the occurrence of flow disturbances is of major diagnostic importance. Physiologically, such disturbances are also found in the area of kinking formations (Fig. 2.6), but they have disappeared again no more than 5–10 mm distal to the maximum kinking point. Flow disturbances that can be detected over a greater distance are to be regarded as proof of the existence of a higher degree of kinking stenosis. Conversely, however, this means that minor and moderate kinking stenosis are regularly overlooked. ◄

Other Localizations

Kinkings and coilings of the vertebral artery are relatively frequent (Fig. 20.4), but no experience is available on their clinical value. The rare case of a head rotation-dependent kinking in the vertebral artery is referred to in the following Sect. 20.3.2. Also relatively rare are kinking formations of the common carotid artery, possibly also of the brachiocephalic trunc or the subclavian artery (Fig. 20.5). They preferably occur in the context of pre-existing vascular anomalies, possibly intensified or induced by thyroid surgery or chronic bronchitis with prolonged coughing.

20.1.2 Clinical Significance

Kinkings as a Cause of Stroke

Kinkings and coilings of the internal carotid artery are often held responsible for the occurrence of cerebral ischemia. However, due to their frequent occurrence, their clinical significance is very controversial. There are also no prospective studies available.

While a hemodynamic etiology of ischemia by kinking of the vessel is very rare due to the usually good collateral supply in the anterior current region, a scattering of wall adherent thrombi from the kinked area seems to be more possible. A prerequisite for this, however, is the presence of a vascular inner layer lesion, as is to be expected in the long-term course of mechanically stressed kinking. The frequent occurrence of vascular dissections in kinkings (Kim et al. 2016) also supports this assumption. Relevant wall damage, however, can only be expected in the presence of a circumscribed kinking or stenosis with a thickened vessel wall, while elongations and coilings can be classified with some probability as harmless accidental findings. There seems to be a connection to the development of intracranial arteriosclerosis (Kim et al. 2015).

Kinkings and Carotid Interventions

If carotid operations or stent implantations are performed without angiography solely on the basis of the ultrasound findings, it is important for the surgeon whether the stenosis is in the area of a kinking formation or whether an elongated vessel course is present poststenotically, which has a significant influence on the decision on therapy. Anomalies in the course of the disease represent a high-risk situation for the provision of a stent (Morgan et al. 2014).

Summary

Curved vascular courses are frequent findings on the carotids, their probability increases with increasing age. "Normal" elongations must be distinguished from kinkings and coilings. An increased risk of stroke is only to be expected in the case of pronounced defects due to lesions of the inner wall of the vessels. Color coded duplex sonography allows the detection of kinking formations, provided they are not located too far cranially below the skull base. Kinking stenoses are to be assessed primarily on the basis of flow disturbances.

20.2 Hypoplasia of the Carotid Artery

Pronounced congenital hypoplasia of the carotid artery and its branches are very rare, so that when they occur, doubts are always raised as to whether this is an acquired constriction of the vessel due to an upstream or downstream flow obstruction (Sect. 14.2.1) or a long-distance dissection (Sect. 18.1). Slighter differences in calibre in the range around 10% are more common. Here, the left carotid artery is usually the vessel with the larger caliber.

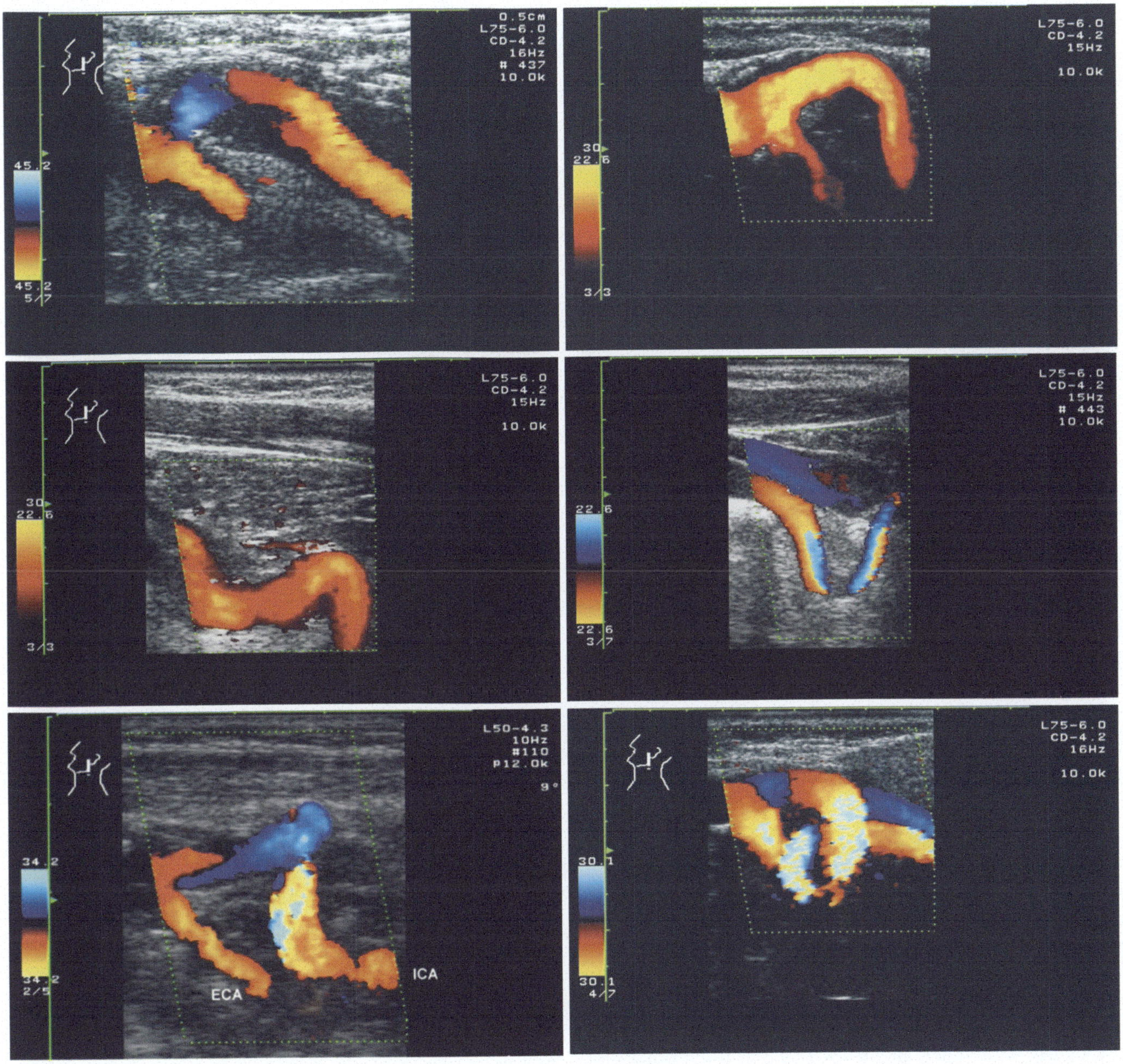

Fig. 20.2 Longitudinal sections of buckling formations of the internal carotid artery

20.2.1 Sonographic Assessment

Of course, the diagnosis of hypoplasia of the internal carotid artery can only be made on the basis of duplex sonography; Doppler sonography does not provide clear results. However, differential diagnosis is difficult (see overview below) and is usually only possible indirectly on the basis of the absence of pathological flow phenomena in the brain base and periorbital arteries.

Differential Diagnostic Considerations for Suspected "Hypoplasia" of the Internal Carotid Artery

- Occlusion of the internal carotid artery with the branch of the external carotid artery leading to the cranial side
- Longer distance of a dissection, extending caudally to the bifurcation
- "Collapsed" vessel with high-grade flow obstruction in the further course of the vessel

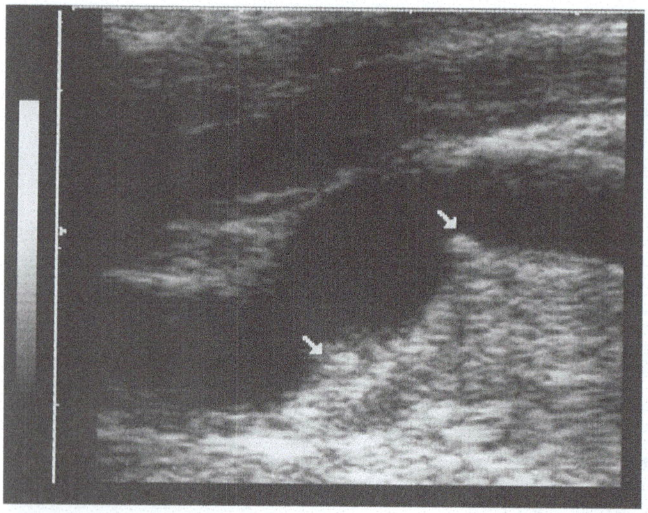

Fig. 20.3 Example of a not yet very pronounced kinking of the internal carotid artery (at least in the current head position), which, however, suggests wall lesions at the kink points

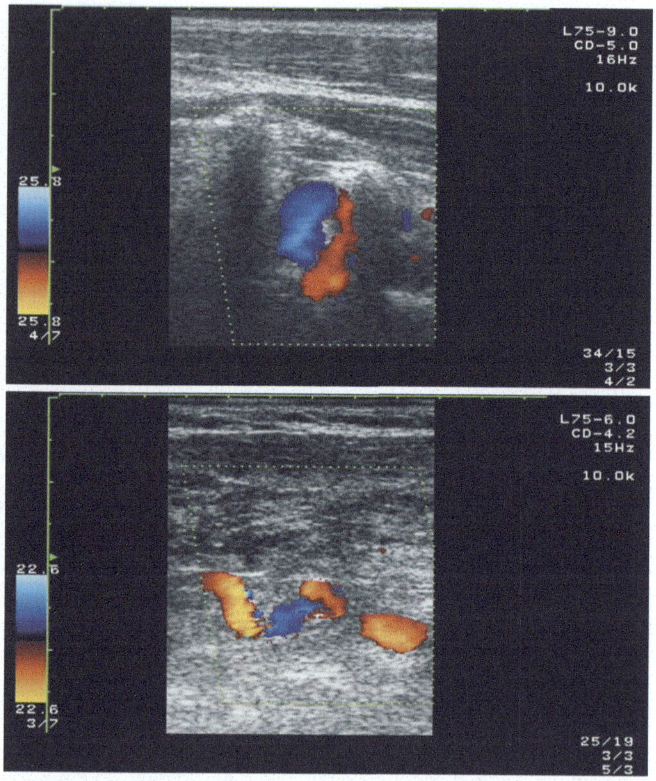

Fig. 20.4 Kinking (above) and elongation (below) of the vertebral artery in the V2 section

Aplasias of an internal carotid artery are a rarity. In this case, the sectional ultrasound view typically shows the external carotid artery running solitary along the neck. The differentiation from an occlusion of the internal carotid artery is usually not difficult to make, since the recognizable vessel has no diameter fluctuation in the entire course of the neck and especially no **carotid bulb** (Fig. 20.6). In carotid aplasia, the periorbital arteries are almost always perfused inconspicuously from the inside to the outside.

20.2.2 Clinical Significance

Congenital hypo- and aplasias of the carotid artery are generally a random finding and as such have no clinical significance. According to experience in Japan, where such anomalies are apparently more frequent, they are often associated with other anomalies (e.g., neurofibromatosis). At an advanced age, such dysplasias can be associated with cerebral ischemia if additional arteriosclerotic changes occur, which further reduce the cerebral blood flow's ability to compensate, which in this case is often limited from birth.

Summary
In the area of the carotid artery, slight differences in calibre are quite common, but more pronounced hypoplasia is rare. In terms of differential diagnosis, long-distance dissections and a "collapsed" vessel should always be taken into consideration in the case of upstream or downstream vascular processes.

20.3 Hypoplasia of the Vertebral Artery

The vertebral arteries show an average diameter of 3.4 mm in adults. The right vertebral artery is usually somewhat smaller (median value right 3.0 mm, left 3.5 mm; Schleyer 2003). However, more pronounced calibre asymmetries are less the exception than the rule, whereby a hypoplastic vertebral artery on one side is usually associated with a "hyperplastic" vessel on the opposite side with a much larger calibre (Fig. 20.7).

20.3.1 Sonographic Assessment

The method of choice for the assessment of vertebral hypoplasia is duplex sonography, with which the diameter of the vessel can be measured directly (Fig. 20.8). Due to the better resolution, the diameter should preferably be determined on the basis of the black and white sectional image in the intertransverse course of the vessel (V2 section). Only in the case of vessel walls that cannot be clearly displayed should the color coded display be used.

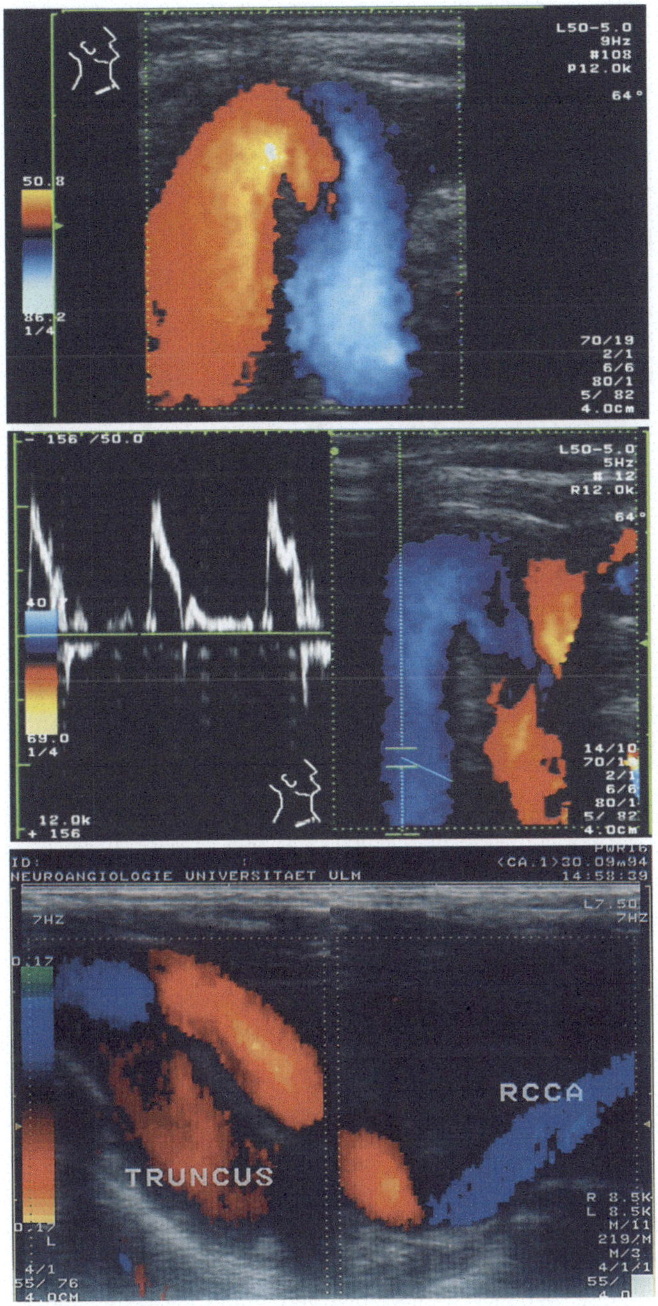

Fig. 20.5 Kinking formations of the subclavian artery (top and middle) and the common carotid artery in the lower part of the neck (bottom)

> **Note**
> **As far as possible, the determination of the vessel diameter of the vertebral artery in the intertransversal course should be carried out using the black and white sectional image.**

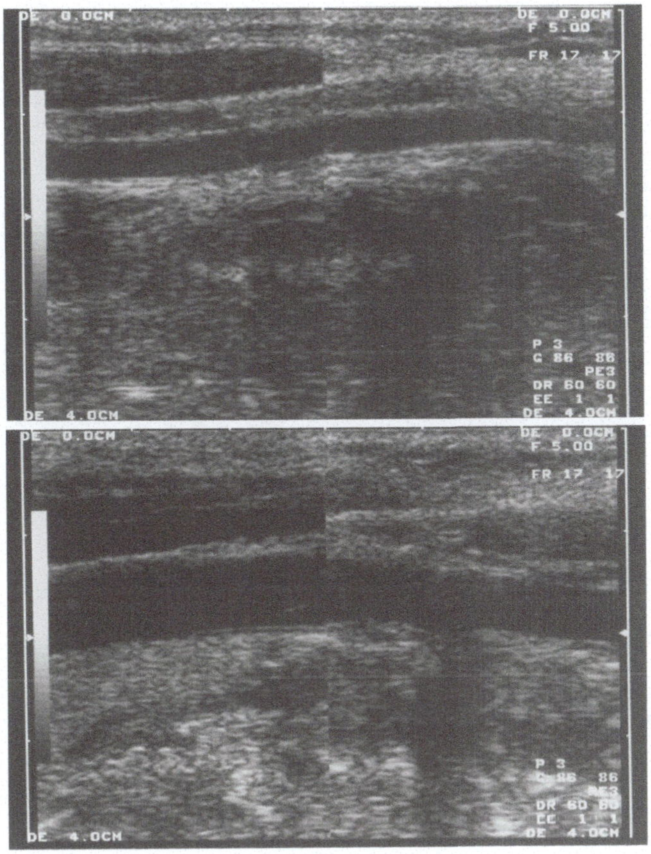

Fig. 20.6 Aplasia of the right internal carotid artery with external carotid artery running solitary along the neck

Definition of Hypoplasia

A hypoplasia is considered to be present if the diameter of an vertebral artery is less than 2.5 mm (Table 20.1; Delcker and Diener 1992). With otherwise normal formation of the vertebrobasilar vascular system the hypoplastic vessel contributes less than 10% to the total vertebrobasilar blood flow in this case (Fig. 15.6). The reason for this disproportionate flow reduction is the paired arrangement of the vertebral arteries with a common final current path, which represents a parallel connection of two flow resistances. Since, according to the law of Hagen-Poiseuille, the vascular resistance is inversely proportional to the vascular diameter in the fourth power (Sect. 15.3.1), even relatively small differences in caliber lead to considerable differences in the flow volumes leading to the brain.

Assessment of Hypoplasia

Unilaterally hypoplastic vertebral arteries with a diameter of less than 2.5 mm supply (with contralateral hyperplasia) mainly – via the spinal arteries – the cervical musculature.

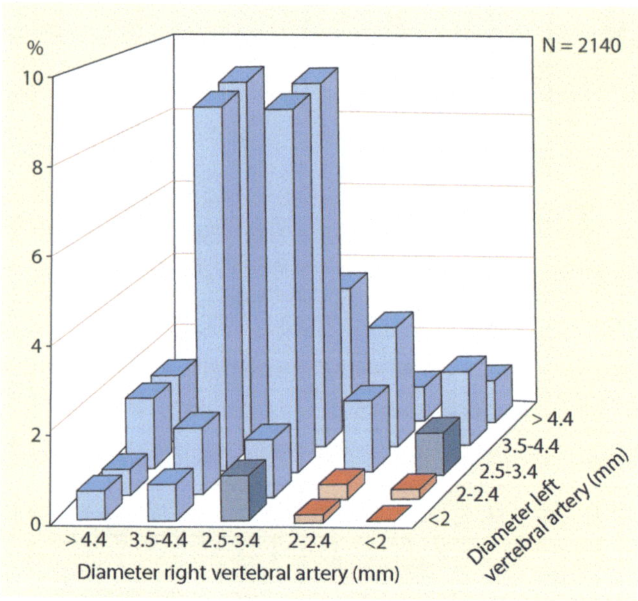

Fig. 20.7 Diameter of the vertebral artery in side comparison in 2140 consecutive patients (Schleyer 2003). In 9% of the cases there was a pronounced hypo- or aplasia of the vertebral artery with a diameter < 2.5 mm and a predominance of the right side (3:2). In 2% of cases both vertebral arteries were massively hypoplastic (sum of diameters <5 mm)

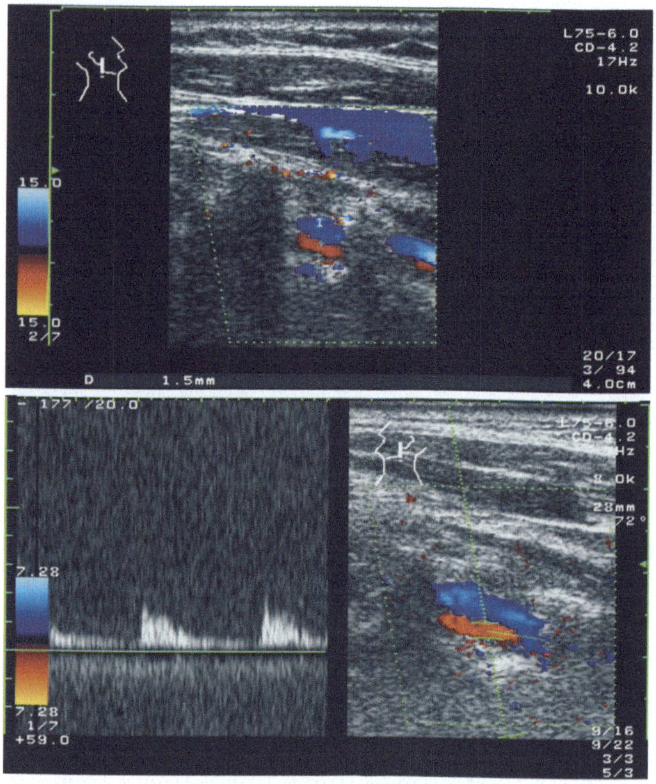

Fig. 20.8 Hypoplasia of the right vertebral artery with a diameter of 1.5 mm with typical reduction of diastolic flow or increased pulsatility with (largely) no connection of the vessel to the basilar artery

Accordingly, intertransversal Doppler drainage of such a vessel shows increased pulsatility. However, since on the other hand, distal occlusion processes of the vessel are also accompanied by increased pulsatility in the upstream section of the vessel, this results in a differential diagnostic problem that cannot be solved in the end.

> **Note**
> **In case of unilateral hypoplasia of the vertebral artery, an increased pulsatility in the affected vessel can only be considered pathological with reservations, since it can also be a physiological flow situation when the vessel is not connected to the basilar artery.**

> **Practical Tips**
> In individual cases, the observation of the "degree" of pulsatility increase is a useful aid in differentiating between distal closure and physiological flow behavior in unilateral vertebral hypoplasia. Thus, a "pendulum flow" or a complete absence of a diastolic flow component (reduce wall filter as much as possible!) can be considered pathological with a high probability, since this finding hardly ever occurs in hypoplastic vertebral arteries.

Assessment of Hyperplasia
A hyperplastic vessel is diagnosed when its diameter significantly exceeds 4 mm. If the vertebral artery on one side is 4.5 mm or more in diameter, hypoplasia of the contralateral vessel is regularly expected.

20.3.2 Clinical Significance

Increased Risk of Cerebral Ischemia
Hypoplasia of one side of the vertebral artery with compensatory hyperplasia of the other side are of particular importance for the cerebral inferior posterior artery (PICA), since this usually emerges from the vertebral artery before the fusion to the basilar artery. In addition to the head rotation-dependent, short-term brain stem syndromes described below when the stronger vessel is clamped, more recent studies have shown that hypoplastic vertebral arteries – especially in bilateral hypoplasia – are associated with an increased risk of brain stem infarction (especially Wallenberg syndrome) (Gaigalaite et al. 2016, Mitsumura et al. 2016). The basilar artery is mostly bent to the side of the hyperplastic vertebral artery and this position variant seems to lead to an increase in basilar artery infarctions in addition to the increase in PICA

Table 20.1 Evaluation of calibre differences of the vertebral arteries

Diameter	Evaluation
>4 mm	Hyperplasia
3–4 mm	Normal caliber
2.5 mm	Borderline hypoplasia
<2.5 mm	Hypoplasia

infarctions, probably because small perforators are pulled out and their supply is disturbed (Zhu et al. 2016).

Head Rotation Dependent Circulatory Disorders

Bends of an vertebral artery in certain head positions are considered physiological and are "absorbed" by the paired attachment of the two vertebral arteries. Failure symptoms of the posterior cerebral circulation can, however, occur in individual cases when one vertebral artery is distinctly hypoplastic and the other, hyperplastic vessel is already compressed during "normal" head rotations due to osteochondrotic changes occurring with age (Case Study 20.1). The specific term for this kind of stroke is "**Bow Hunter's Stroke**." This is spoken in the context of the word "archery," since archery involves a powerful rotation of the head (Duan et al. 2016) and can cause transient as well as permanent ischemic symptoms.

Clinically, a corresponding suspicion must be expressed if reproducible (!) attacks of rotational vertigo with nystagmus occur at defined head rotations, which – also reproducible – disappear completely within a few seconds after turning back the head (Strupp et al. 2000; see overview). An interventional or surgical consequence should only occur after multimodal confirmation and confirmation of the diagnosis by means of DSA (Duan et al. 2016).

Indications of an Intermittent Compression Syndrome of the Vertebral Artery

- Reproducible attacks of vertigo in certain head postures
- Nystagmus and possibly further brain stem failures during the attacks
- Disappearance of symptoms within a few seconds after turning the head back
- One of the two vertebral arteries clearly hypoplastic

"Vertebrobasilar Insufficiency"

Although the diagnosis of a "vertebrobasilar insufficiency" in dizziness and syncope is still made today, it is usually an embarrassing diagnosis without factually substantiated vascular findings and should be avoided. It should always be remembered that the leading symptom of vertigo has considerably more non-vascular than vascular causes. Last but not least, the term "vertigo" is extremely ambiguous and ranges from acute attacks of rotary vertigo with nausea and vomiting to diffuse feelings of insecurity.

Until now, however, little attention has been paid to the fact that for hemodynamics in the posterior cerebrovascular region, the question of unilateral hypoplasia with hyperplasia of the opposite side is less important than the interaction of the two vertebral arteries. Assuming a total cross-sectional area of both vertebral arteries of usually about 18 mm^2 and a total flow volume of 160–180 ml/min, the linear relationship between cross section and flow volume (Sect. 5.3.3) results in a drop in vertebral blood flow below 100 ml/min if the cross-sectional area is 10 mm^2 is undercut. This situation affects 1–2% of the population.

Case Study 20.1: Head Rotation-dependent Compression of the Vertebral Artery

A 46-year-old roofer recently suffered from a provocative massive rotation vertigo when his head was turned to the right. Syncopations also occurred several times.

Sonography demonstrated a stenosis of the left vertebral artery at the origin of the artery and an occlusion of the right vertebral artery. Turning the head to the right resulted in a reproducible stoppage of blood flow in the area of the left atlas loop (Fig. 20.10).

Angiography confirmed a kinking stenosis at the origin of the left vertebral artery, which led to a "damming up" of contrast medium in the further course of the vessel when turning the head. After the interventional insertion of a stent, the symptoms ceased (Fig. 20.9).

In cases with such anomalies posterior cerebrovascular hemodynamics is provided to a considerable extent via the internal carotid artery and via embryonic hyperplastic posterior communicating arteries. The very thin-calibre basilar artery with its numerous branches represents the border zone between the anterior and posterior current region. Although it has not yet been proven by prospective studies, it is highly probable that this area is particularly vulnerable to blood pressure fluctuations (Case Study 20.2) and – due to the low flow velocity – there may also be an increased tendency to thrombus formation (Fig. 20.11).

Since the calculation of the total cross-sectional area is quite "unwieldy," in practice an addition of the vessel

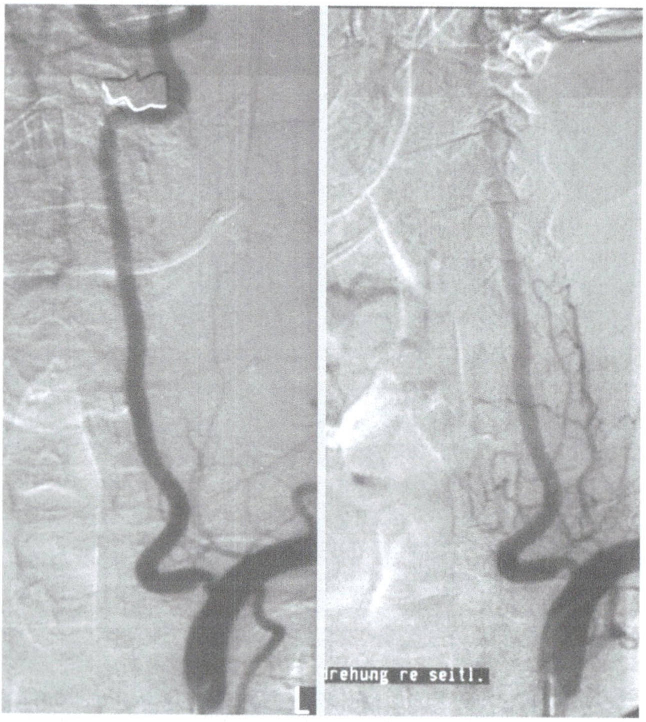

Fig. 20.9 Stenosis of the left vertebral artery at the origin of the artery. When turning the head to the right (right picture) the contrast medium is stopped

diameters of the vertebral arteries is sufficient for a first impression. Normally the sum of the vessel diameters is 6–8 mm (Table 20.2). If the sum of the diameters falls below a value of 4–5 mm, a pronounced vertebrobasilar hypoplasia has to be assumed, which affects the entire posterior circulation including the basilar artery. In this case the posterior cerebral arteries are regularly supplied by the anterior current region, which can be impressively demonstrated in the color coded duplex sonogram (see Case Study 20.2).

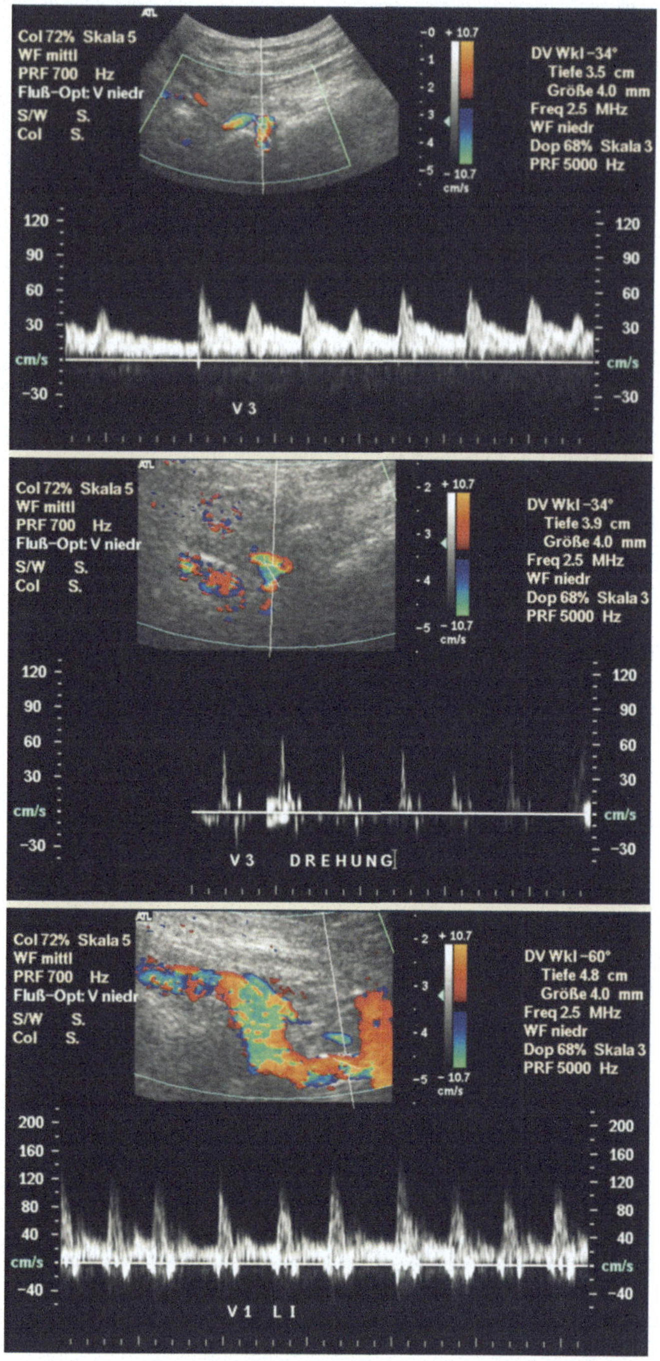

Fig. 20.10 Left vertebral artery in the area of the atlas loop without (top) and with (middle) head rotation. Below: Discharge of the left vertebral artery (due to the almost 90° angle of incidence no measurement of the flow velocity possible)

Case Study 20.2: "Vertebrobasilar Insufficiency" in Severe Vertebral Hypoplasia

The 51-year-old businessman suffered an amnesic episode lasting several hours on a hot summer's day after a long car journey. A migraine was not known, there was no seizure disorder, an open foramen ovale and a vascular dissection could be excluded.

The only abnormality investigated by duplex sonography was a pronounced hypoplasia of the vertebrobasilar system with a diameter of the vertebral artery of 1.5 mm on the right and 2.4 mm on the left (total diameter 3.9 mm, total cross sect. 6.3 mm^2) (Fig. 20.12 above). The posterior cerebral artery was (predominantly) supplied on both sides by the internal

Case Study 20.2 (continued)

carotid artery (Fig. 20.12 bottom), which could also be confirmed by MRI. The basilar artery could not be reliably visualized either transnuchally or

(continued)

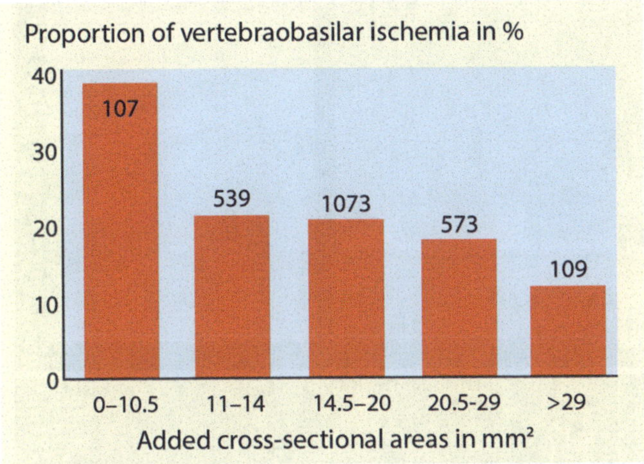

Fig. 20.11 Proportion of vertebrobasilar ischemias in patients with cerebral infarctions in the posterior (n = 491) and anterior (n = 1908) stream

Case Study 20.2 (continued)
transtemporally. In the absence of other diseases and known hypotension, a drop in blood pressure with temporary border zone ischemia in basal brain structures is assumed to be the most likely cause of the symptoms.

Note
If the sum of the vertebral artery diameters does not exceed 5 mm, a vertebrobasilar hypoplasia with an embryonic version of the posterior cerebral artery can be assumed.

Summary
An asymmetrical diameter of the vertebral artery is the rule rather than the exception. Hypoplasia of the vertebral artery with a diameter of 2.5 mm and less is found in 5–10% of the population, the contralateral vessel is then mostly hyperplastic. Bilateral hypoplasia of the vertebral artery may play a role in the development of transient and permanent ischemia in the posterior current region.

20.4 Arteriovenous Malformations and Fistulas

Arteriovenous short circuits **(Angiomas, AV fistulas)** can occur in the context of a congenital vascular malformation or connective tissue weakness, but also traumatically or spontaneously for no apparent reason. In principle, they can occur at any point of the vascular system.

20.4.1 Sonographic Assessment

The sonographic assessment of arteriovenous short circuits focuses primarily on the assessment of the supplying vessels (**"feeder"**). The findings to be determined here are ultimately identical for all localizations (overview below). The special features going beyond this are listed in the description of the most frequent clinical constellations.

Sonographic Findings in the Feeder Vessels of Arteriovenous Fistulas and Angiomas

- Significantly increased flow volume
- Frequent dilatation of the upstream vessel sections
- Turbulence due to hyperperfusion
- Decreased pulsatility due to the reduction of the peripheral resistance
- In the case of intracerebral angiomas, markedly reduced or completely eliminated cerebrovascular reactivity
- Strongly perfused veins with arterial flow character

20.4.2 Clinical Significance

Extracranial Carotid Jugular Fistula

Arteriovenous short-circuits between the carotid artery including its extracranial branches (especially the superior thyroid artery) and the jugular artery are almost always the result of a lesion of the vessel wall caused by a central venous catheter. The main clinical symptoms are, in addition to the typical history, a palpable buzzing in the neck and an auscultable, usually high-frequency stenotic noise over the affected region.

Sonographically, an AV fistula must be suspected if the ultrasound scan of the cervical vessels reveals massive flow disturbances at points that cannot be clearly assigned to a

Table 20.2 Evaluation of the diameter sum of the vertebral arteries

<4 mm	4.0–5.5 mm	6–8 mm	8.5–9 mm	>9 mm
Distinctive hypoplasia	Moderate hypoplasia	Normal findings	Moderate hyperplasia	Distinctive hyperplasia

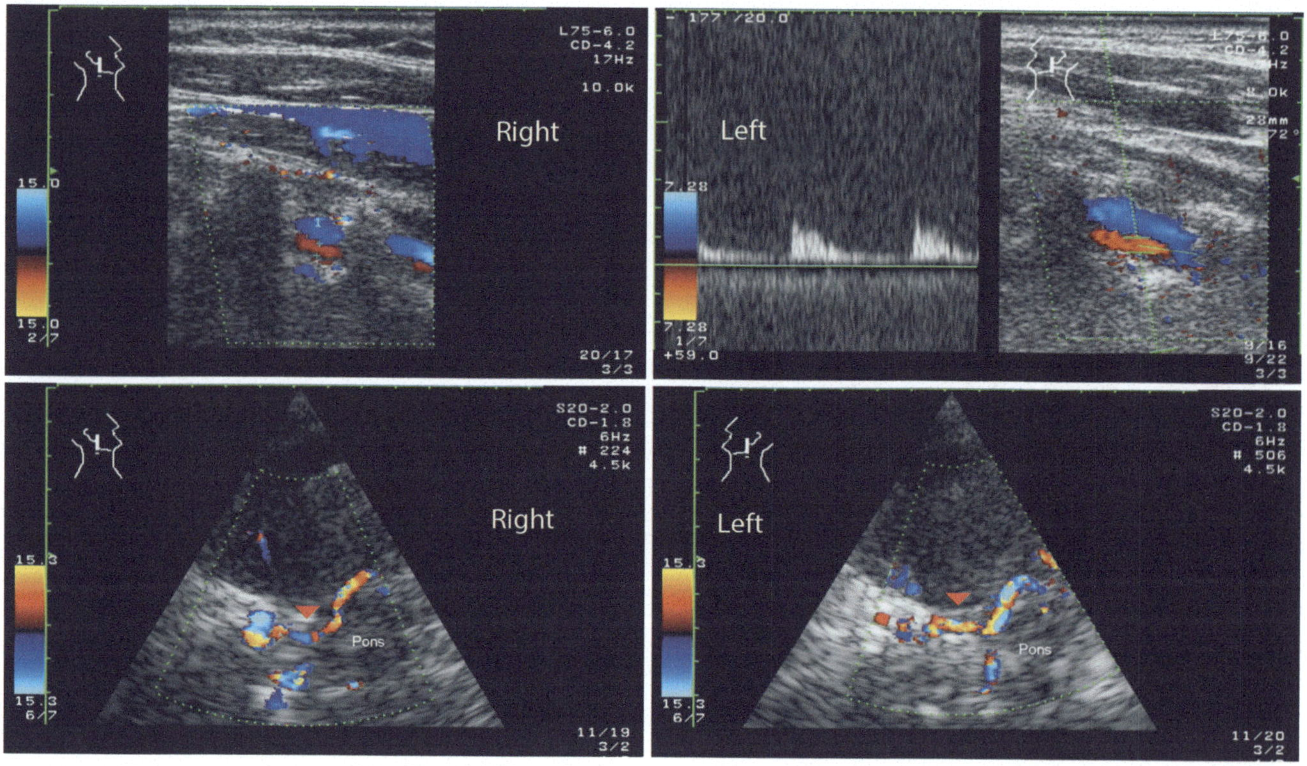

Fig. 20.12 Hypoplastic vertebrobasilar vascular system

stenosis. When searching in detail with color coded duplex sonography, the fistula canal is usually directly detectable. A comparison with the flow volume of the contralateral carotid artery allows statements to be made about the fistula volume.

Dural AV Fistulas of the Skull Base

Whenever a pulse-synchronous ringing in the ears occurs, in addition to stenoses in the area of the carotid siphon, an arteriovenous fistula must always be considered (following overview), which typically lies in the area of the dura mater at the base of the skull (Arning et al. 1997). Such vascular short-circuits usually occur spontaneously without any recognizable cause by dilation of pre-existing arteriovenous microshunts. Only in individual cases a connection can be established with sinus vein thrombosis, possibly in the context of a flu-like infection, but also with prolonged exposure of the unprotected head to cold, for example, when skiing.

Frequent Causes of Pulse Synchronous Ear Noises (after Pegge et al. 2017; Thie et al. 1993)

- **Local causes** in the ear, for example, tumors of the inner ear
- **Stenoses** the arteries supplying the brain, for example, dissections near the base of the skull, fibromuscular dysplasia, carotid siphon disease
- **Hyperfusion,** for example, dural AV fistulas (mostly dura, more rarely pia or cervical), carotid-cavernous fistulas, glomus tumors of the base of the skull
- **Other causes** for example, sinus vein thrombosis, pseudotumor cerebri with intracranial hypertension.

The treatment is usually carried out via branches of the external carotid artery, whereby the occipital artery, the posterior auricular artery, the medial meningeal artery and the ascending pharyngeal artery with their end branches are particularly affected. Only in rare cases are there also connections from the vertebral artery (Arning et al. 1999). The outflow is usually into the sinus transversus or sigmoid and from there into the jugular vein. The diagnosis can often be made clinically if a local vascular noise can be auscultated when the stethoscope is positioned in the area of the mastoid and the tinnitus, which is often perceived as very disturbing by the patient, becomes less or even disappears when local pressure is applied with the finger. Only in passing, it should

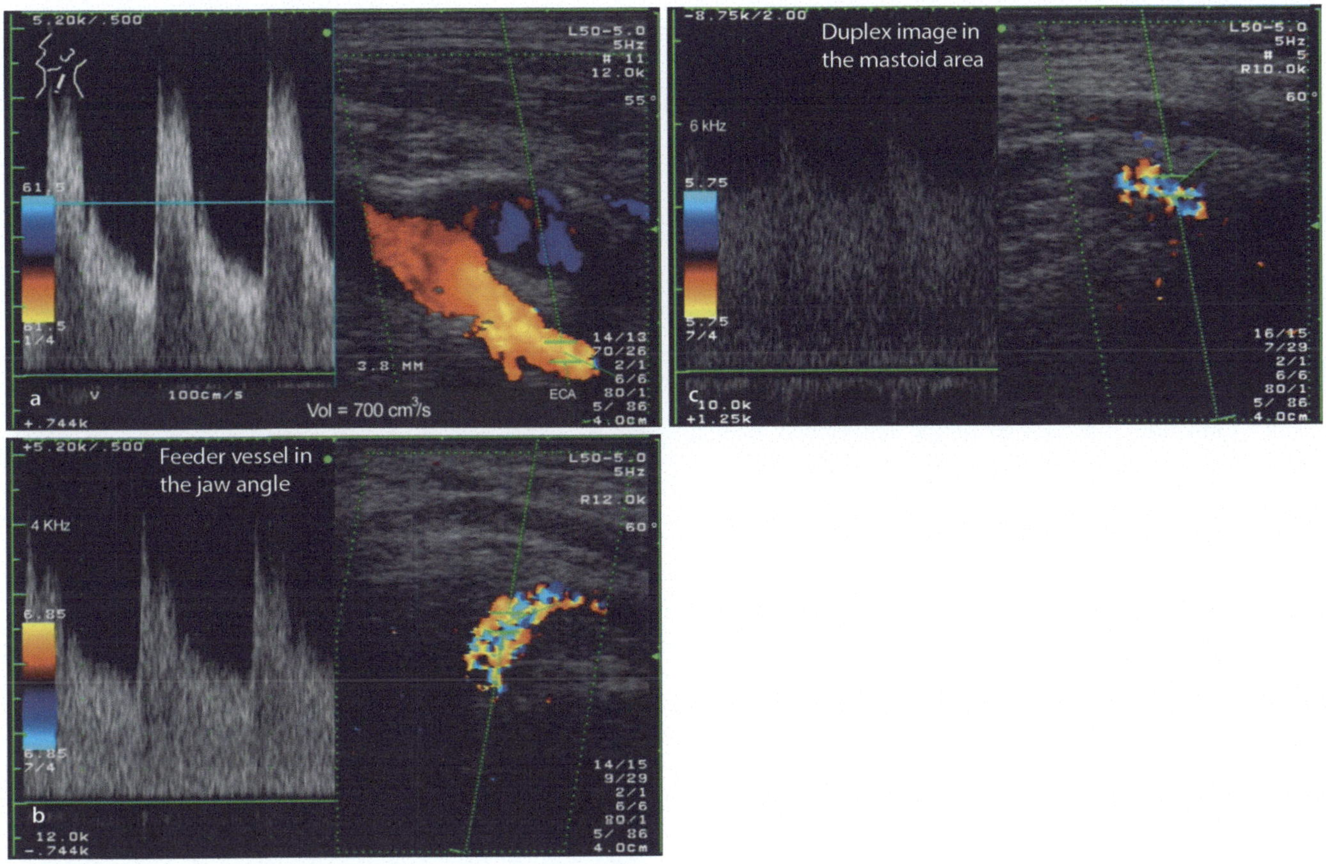

Fig. 20.13 Arteriovenous fistula at the skull base. Duplex sonography of the ipsilateral external carotid artery shows a considerable flow volume of 700 ml/min (**a**). Derivation of a feeder vessel (probably retroauricular artery) in the region of the jaw angle (**b**). Parts of the dural fistula at the lower base of the skull with typically reduced pulsatility of the flow signal (**c**)

be mentioned that this maneuver can also lead to spontaneous closure in the case of smaller fistulas.

Sonographically, the local findings and the abnormalities in the "feeder vessels" of such fistulas must be differentiated.

Local Findings

In the area of the skull base there are usually numerous vessels running in alternating directions with high Doppler frequency and pronounced flow disturbance. Often there is also a **seagull cry phenomenon** detectable (Fig. 5.8). Due to the greater penetration depth, the CW Doppler probe is usually better suited than duplex sonography for the detection of such fistula vessels. The color coded display does not generally provide any significant additional aspects, since individual vessels cannot be differentiated due to the pronounced flow disturbance. ◀

Findings in Feeding Vessels

The determination of flow volume in the external carotid artery in side comparison is of essential importance for the therapeutic considerations (Case Study 20.3). The difference gives an approximate indication of the shunt volume and thus of the cardiac load. A relevant load can be assumed if the shunt volume reaches about 500 ml/min and more. ◀

Case Study 20.3: Retroauricular AV Fistula

The 33-year-old doctor noticed a left-sided, pulse-synchronous ear noise from complete well-being, which increased considerably in volume over the course of a few weeks.

At clinical examination the noise could be confirmed by auscultation with maximum behind the left ear. Sonographically a pronounced hyperperfusion with a flow volume of 700 ml/min (right 150 ml/min) was observed in the left external carotid artery (Fig. 20.13a). A strong vessel was found in the left mandibular angle, which could be traced to below the mastoid (Fig. 20.13b). Several vessels with a high diastolic flow signal could be derived there (Fig. 20.13c). Given this constellation of findings,

(continued)

Case Study 20.3 (continued)
there was no doubt about the presence of a retroauricular AV fistula. Due to the high fistula volume, the indication for an interventional procedure was given. An initial attempt at therapy by embolization failed and led to complications in the form of an initially complete peripheral facial nerve palsy. Only after extensive operative skeletonization could a far-reaching closure of the fistula be achieved.

Carotid Cavernous Fistulas

Fistula formations on passage of the intracranial internal carotid artery through the cavernous sinus ("direct carotid-cavernous fistulas") usually occur as a result of craniocerebral injuries, but can also occur spontaneously. Due to the often considerable shunt volume, they often represent a urgent indication for interventional procedures. Here too, the suspected diagnosis can be made clinically – due to the usually pronounced ringing in the ears and the positive auscultation findings, especially when the stethoscope is positioned over the eye bulb. Due to the local increase of blood pressure in the draining veins there is often also a protrusion of the eye bulb with pulsating injection of sclera and chemosis. Sonographically, three findings can be recorded.

Intracranial Local Findings

The transtemporal examination of the brain basal arteries secures the suspected diagnosis of a direct carotid-cavernous fistula, if multiple "color dots," which cannot be assigned to any single vessel, with signs of a massive flow disturbance in the Doppler spectrum can be detected at a depth of 60–70 mm. The middle cerebral artery and the anterior cerebral artery, on the other hand, can usually be detected with a completely unremarkable flow signal. ◀

Findings in the Periorbital Arteries

Due to the extremely low peripheral resistance in the intracranial current area, the periorbital arteries show almost always a retrograde flow, whereby a differentiation from the also massively perfused veins of the orbital cavity is often hardly possible. ◀

Extracranial Duplex Findings

As in the case of dural fistulas, the main purpose of the duplex examination is to estimate the shunt volume by quantitatively determining the amount of flow in the internal carotid artery in side by side comparison. ◀

Intracerebral Vascular Malformations

In the diagnosis of the mostly congenitally existing **angiomas** and **cavernomes**, the contribution of Doppler and duplex sonography is only marginal, since these can be diagnosed with a much lower detection limit by CT and MRI. If the diameter of the angioma is larger, the supplying vessels (**feeder**) are hyperperfused compared to standard values and often show turbulences by Doppler insonation. A differentiation of increased Doppler frequencies in stenoses can be made on the basis of the reaction to hyperventilation: Due to the decoupling of the angioma from cerebral autoregulation, the flow drop in the supply vessels during hyperventilation is significantly lower than normally expected. Postoperatively, as expected, the perfusion in the affected vessels decreases and the cerebrovascular reserve capacity increases.

Summary
Arteriovenous fistulas can occur congenitally, traumatically or spontaneously. Fistulas between the carotid artery and the jugular vein after central venous puncture can be clearly diagnosed by duplex sonography. More difficult is the direct detection of dural fistulas in the area of the skull base, which often lead to a disturbing pulsatile tinnitus in the ear. The determination of flow volume in the external carotid artery provides evidence of the cardiac load. Fistulas between the intracranial internal carotid artery and the cavernous sinus can be clarified sonographically together with the appropriate clinical symptoms. The fistula volume can be estimated by comparing the extracranial internal carotid artery of both sides. In the case of intracerebral angiomas, Doppler and duplex sonography are not of major importance in view of the more informative imaging methods.

References

Arning C, Grzyska U, Lachenmayer L (1997) Laterale kraniale Durafistel. Nachweis mit Doppler- und Duplexsonographie Nervenarzt 68:139–146

Arning C, Grzyska U, Hammer E, Lachenmeyer L (1999) Spontane vertebrale arteriovenöse Fistel. Nachweis und Therapiekontrolle mit der farbkodierten Duplexsonographie. Nervenarzt 70:359–362

Delcker A, Diener HC (1992) Die verschiedenen Ultraschallmethoden zur Untersuchung der A. vertebralis – eine vergleichende Wertung. Ultraschall Med 13:213–220

Duan G, Xu J, Shi J, Cao Y (2016) Advances in the pathogenesis, diagnosis and treatment of Bow Hunter's syndrome: a comprehensive review of the literature. Interv Neurol 5:29–38

Gaigalaite V, Vilimas A, Ozeraitiene V, Dementaviciene J, Janilionis R, Kalibatiene D, Rocka S (2016) Association between vertebral artery hypoplasia and posterior circulation stroke. BMC Neurol 26(16):118

Kamenskiy AV, Pipinos II, Carson JS, MacTaggart JN, Baxter BT (2015) Age and disease-related geometric and structural remodeling of the carotid artery. J Vasc Surg 62:1521–1528

Kim BJ, Kim SM, Kang DW, Kwon SU, Suh DC, Kim JS (2015) Vascular tortuosity may be related to intracranial artery atherosclerosis. Int J Stroke 10:1081–1086

Kim BJ, Yang E, Kim NY, Kim MJ, Kang DW, Kwon SU, Kim JS (2016) Vascular Tortuosity May Be Associated With Cervical Artery Dissection 47:2548–2552

Macchi C, Gulisano M, Giannelli F, Catini C, Pratesi C, Pacini P (1997) Kinking of the human internal carotid artery: a statistical study in 100 healthy subjects by echocolor Doppler. J Cardiovasc Surg Torino 38:629–637

Mitsumura H, Miyagawa S, Komatsu T, Hirai T, Kono Y, Iguchi Y (2016) Relationship between vertebral artery hypoplasia and posterior circulation ischemia. J Stroke Cerebrovasc Dis 25:266–269

Morgan CE, Lee CJ, Chin JA, Eskandari MK, Morasch MD, Rodriguez HE, Helenowski IB, Kibbe MR (2014) High-risk anatomic variables and plaque characteristics in carotid artery stenting. Vasc Endovasc Surg 48:452–459

Pegge SAH, Steens SCA, Kunst HPM, Meijer FJA (2017) Pulsatile tinnitus: differential diagnosis and radiological work-up. Curr Radiol Rep 5:5

Schleyer A (2003) Hypoplasien der A. vertebralis – ein Risikofaktor für Hirninfarkte im hinteren Stromgebiet? Dissertation Universität Ulm

Strupp M, Planck JH, Arbusow V, Steiger HJ, Brückmann H, Brandt T (2000) Rotational vertebral artery occlusion syndrome with vertigo due to "labyrinthine excitation". Neurology 54:1376–1379

Thie A, Goosens Merkt H, Freitag J, Spitzer K, Zeumer H, Kunze K (1993) Pulsatile tinnitus: clinical and angiological evaluation. Cerebrovasc Dis 3:160–167

Zhu W, Wang YF, Dong XF, Feng HX, Zhao HQ, Liu CF (2016) Study on the correlation of vertebral artery dominance, basilar artery curvature and posterior circulation infarction. Acta Neurol Belg 116: 287–293

21 Ultrasound Diagnostics in Acute Stroke

Bernhard Widder and Gerhard F. Hamann

Since mechanical thrombectomy has become an evidence-based therapy for acute cerebral infarction (Rodrigues et al. 2016), the question of whether there is an occlusion of the large basal arteries of the brain, especially of the proximal middle cerebral artery (M1) and the distal internal carotid artery (ICA), is even more important in acute cerebral infarction than before. Despite the now widely available CT and MR imaging, including the possibilities of the associated non-invasive or semi-invasive vessel imaging (CTA, MRA), neurovascular ultrasound diagnostics continues to play an important role in stroke diagnosis and therapy. Ultimately, a distinction must be made between three periods in the course of stroke care:

Thrombolysis Phase
In the first 30–60 min after admission of acute stroke patients until the beginning of a possible intravenous thrombolysis ("door to needle time") ultrasound diagnostics generally has no significance and its use would only delay the start of a possible lysis therapy. Methods of choice here are CT and MR diagnostics, if possible immediately supplemented by a visualization of the large brain-supplying arteries (CTA, MRA) to localize a causative vascular occlusion.

Intervention Phase
Following the determination of the indication and, if necessary, the start of a possible intravenous thrombolysis, an emergency sonographic diagnosis is of importance if there has been no previous imaging of the vessels or if this has not led to usable results, and if the detection of an occlusion of the large cerebral arteries would lead to a (supplementary) mechanical thrombectomy. Although ultrasound diagnostics requires the examiner to have a certain amount of experience with the method, it is more suitable than any other method as a fast "bedside" method when limited to a few examination steps, in order to recognize the vascular processes, which often are dynamically, and to follow their course. The method of choice here is color coded duplex sonography with a "state of the art" equipment. Due to methodological limitations, extra- and transcranial Doppler sonography is not important in acute situations. The indication for an ultrasound examination exists mainly in the following situations:

- Patients with contraindications against the administration of contrast medium (thus no CTA possible)
- Patients with massive claustrophobia (thus no MRI possible)
- Patients who reject CTA and/or MRA based on previous experience
- Restless patients who cannot undergo neuroradiological imaging
- Inconclusive results due to technical problems (insufficient bolus tracking in CTA) or patient-related problems (no sufficient vessel contrast imaging due to severe heart failure)
- pregnant patients.

Post-Acute Phase
The main significance of neurovascular ultrasound diagnostics, however, lies in the post-acute phase, when the cause of the brain infarct is to be clarified and further strokes should be prevented. Due to the combination of imaging and hemodynamic parameters, color coded duplex sonography - often not as the sole method, but in the context of CT and/or MR angiography - is able to provide essential information for differential diagnosis and for further interventional or conservative procedures. Ultrasound diagnostics is thus an essential component of stroke care, and comprehensive ultrasound examination of the extra- and intracranial arteries in the first

B. Widder (✉)
Expert Opinion Institute, District Hospital, Guenzburg, Germany
e-mail: bernhard.widder@bkh-guenzburg.de

G. F. Hamann
Clinic of Neurology and Neurological Rehabilitation, District Hospital, Guenzburg, Germany

B. Widder, G. F. Hamann (eds.), *Duplex sonography of the brain-supplying arteries*, https://doi.org/10.1007/978-3-662-65566-5_21

24 hours after a cerebral infarction still appears to be urgently indicated.

In summary, Table 21.1 shows the advantages and disadvantages of the three main modalities used for vascular diagnostics in acute stroke.

21.1 Emergency Diagnostics

21.1.1 Special Features of Emergency Diagnostics

The "primary diagnosis" of acute stroke is characterized by a number of special features compared to sonographic "routine diagnosis" (overview).

Limited Examination Time
In view of the short therapeutic time window of only a few hours, the complete diagnostics including computer tomography, cardiovascular monitoring and emergency laboratory must be carried out in an optimally managed stroke unit within a maximum period of 45–60 minutes. This means that a maximum of 10–15 minutes are available for the ultrasound examination.

Note
Multiple, sometimes redundant single examinations or examination procedures - often recommended in sonographic "routine diagnostics" to increase the reliability of the findings - should be avoided in favor of the method most suitable for answering the question.

Difficult Examination Conditions
The majority of patients examined with acute symptoms are only slightly cooperative and in some cases also considerably restless. Overall, the conditions for conducting a reliable examination are unfavorable.

Practical Tips
In patients with neglect and/or spontaneous head rotation, it is recommended that the examination is performed as far as possible while maintaining the head rotation assumed by the patient himself.

Increased Pressure for a Diagnostic Decision
It should not be underestimated that the result of the sonographic examination can have immediate therapeutic consequences, which are interventional and can lead to a worsening of the clinical situation if wrongly indicated (Sect. 21.1.4). A review of the findings at a later time by another examiner - which is quite common in "routine" sonographic diagnostics - is not possible due to the short time window.

Special features of primary emergency diagnostics after acute stroke

- Intracranial vessel occlusion as the most common pathological finding
- Localization of occlusion and extent of cerebral underperfusion as essential questions
- Limited examination time
- Difficult examination conditions
- Increased diagnostic decision-making pressure

In summary, the ultrasound examination in the primary diagnosis of acute stroke ("intervention phase") requires an examination procedure adapted to the examination situation with, in particular, targeted selection of the most suitable sonographic procedure and limitation to the most important questions.

21.1.2 Selection of the Sonographic Method

The limited examination time in primary emergency diagnostics after an acute stroke does not allow a validation of findings through several individual examinations, which is frequently used in "routine diagnostics." The method of choice is extra- and intracranial color coded duplex sonography. Examinations with the CW Doppler pen probe are only useful in individual cases to differentiate the localization of the occlusion (Sect. 21.1.3).

21.1.3 Localization Diagnostics

Sonographic Examination of the Anterior Circulation

Occlusion of the Proximal Internal Carotid Artery

The diagnosis is made "prima vista" with color coded duplex sonography. If the periorbital arteries are retrogradely perfused, it can be assumed that the artery is still open above the ophthalmic artery origin, which speaks against the presence of a carotid T-occlusion as the "worst case" of disturbed cerebral perfusion. The ability to visualize the middle cerebral artery and the A1 segment of the anterior cerebral artery, the latter usually with retrograde flow direction and turbulent flow in the anterior communicating artery, ensures the diagnosis. ◀

Table 21.1 Advantages and disadvantages of various examination procedures for clarifying the vascular status in acute cerebral infarction

	Advantages	Disadvantages
CT angiography (CTA)	Fast, robust, widely available, high resolution, complementary perfusion diagnostics "mismatch diagnostics" (CBV/CBF) possible	X-rays, iodine-containing contrast medium with possible problems with kidney and thyroid dysfunction, artifacts due to vascular calcification, frequent reconstruction artifacts in routine diagnostics
MR angiography (MRA)	If limited to the brain base arteries, MR angiography without contrast medium (time-of-flight, TOF) possible, vascular calcifications unproblematic, in addition with DWI/PWI sequences "mismatch diagnostics" possible, DWI sequence shows acute infarction most reliably, especially in the posterior circulation	Problematic in restless and unstable patients, complete vascular status requires the use of contrast medium, overall more time-consuming and more susceptible to artifacts than CTA (e.g., imaging of supra-aortic vascular branches), lower resolution than CTA, contraindications for example, for pacemakers
Color coded duplex sonography	Fast, non-invasive, available at bedside, can be repeated as often as required (follow-up under therapy)	Requires experience, only useful as an additional examination to CT or MRI, if no CT/MR angiography is available, extracranial artifacts due to vascular calcification and problems in obese, "short-necked" patients, transcranially not feasible without contrast medium in about 20% of patients

Occlusion of the Distal Internal Carotid Artery

In this situation, which is frequent in carotid dissections, the extracranial internal carotid artery shows a characteristic residual blunt signal (Fig. 21.1). The periorbital arteries are retrograde, antegrade or not derivable, depending on the location of the occlusion. If the cerebral arteries are not affected, the conditions found in the middle and anterior cerebral artey correspond to the above mentioned situation in proximal carotid artery occlusion. ◄

Carotid T-occlusion

If the occlusion is located above the ophthalmic artery origin, the extracranial internal carotid artery shows a more or less reduced flow signal, but normally no blunt signal (Fig. 21.1). The periorbital arteries then characteristically have an antegrade flow. Transcranially no flow signal is found in the carotid T-region (A1 segment of the anterior cerebral artery and M1 segment of the middle cerebral artery). A distinction from an artifact due to an insufficient temporal ultrasound window is possible, if the basal brain structures can be clearly recognized in the B-Mode image (Fig. 21.2), and at least parts of the contralateral circulation and/or the ipsilateral posterior cerebral artery are visible. ◄

Practical Tips

In the absence of an at first glance pathological extracranial residual blunt signal, the most reliable parameter for the prediction of an intracranial occlusive process is the side-by-side comparison of flow volume in the extracranial internal carotid artery. If this is reduced by 50% or more compared to the contralateral vessel, there is almost certainly a greater intracranial flow obstruction.

Main Stem Occlusion of the Middle Cerebral Artery

A middle cerebral artery which cannot be visualized under sufficient examination conditions when all other ipsilateral arteries of the anterior circulation are displayed, allows the "prima vista" diagnosis of a main stem middle artery occlusion (Fig. 21.3). ◄

Distal Main Stem Occlusion or Multiple Branch Occlusions of the Middle Cerebral Artery

If the middle cerebral artery, or at least its initial section, can be visualized, its flow signal provides additional

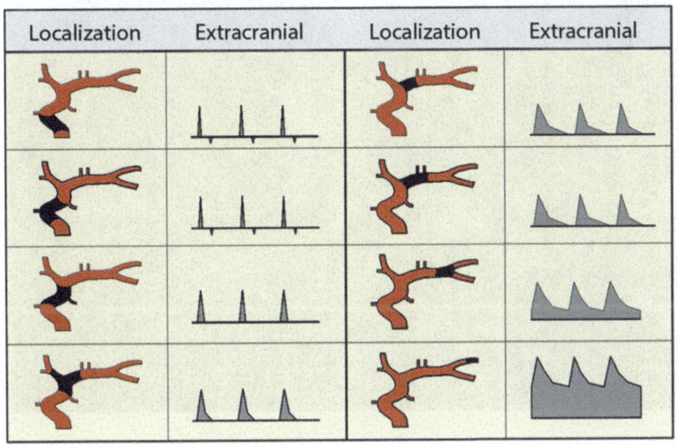

Fig. 21.1 Extracranial Doppler/duplex findings in the internal carotid artery as a function of intracranial occlusion localization

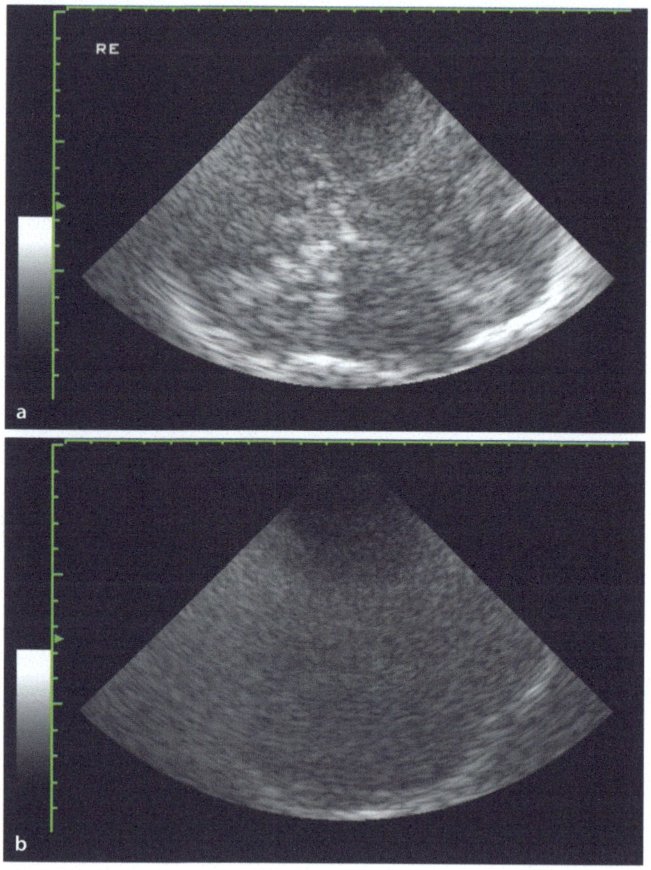

Fig. 21.2 (**a, b**) Evaluation of the temporal ultrasound window on the basis of the visibility of intracranial lead structures (brain stem, clivus, sphenoid bone) in B-mode imaging of the brain. Sufficient (**a**) and insufficient (**b**) investigation conditions

information with regard to a more distal occlusive process. Absolute values of flow velocity as well as side comparisons are indicative. The side comparison can be performed using the asymmetry index (Sect. 10.5.5). Mean intensity-weighted flow velocities (mean) <40 cm/s or a side difference > 20% according to the (modified) asymmetry index indicate an occlusion of a main branch of the middle cerebral artery, velocities <20 cm/s or a (modified) asymmetry index >50% indicate a distal main stem occlusion (Table 14.6). ◄

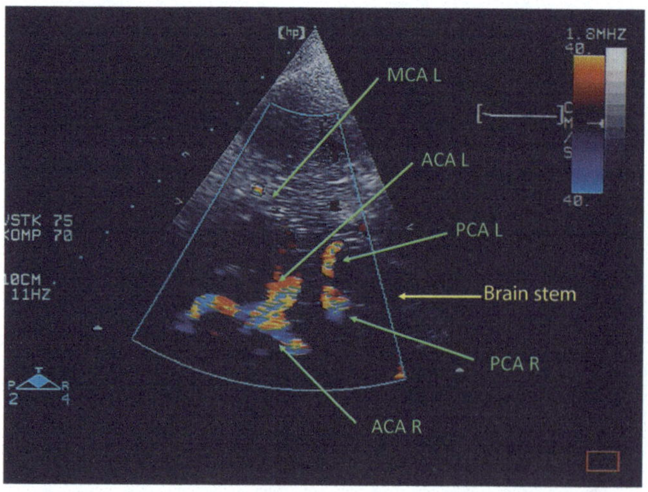

Fig. 21.3 Right main mediastinal vascular occlusion in a 37-year-old female patient with acute hemiparesis of the left side. Minimal residual flow in the left middle cerebral artery

However, this requires that upstream flow obstacles (e.g., occlusion of the internal carotid artery) are excluded, as they can also cause corresponding changes in flow velocity and asymmetry index. A reduced pulsatility can serve as an indirect sign in these cases. Furthermore, since the asymmetry index primarily classifies neither flow velocity as normal or pathological, the interpretation of a pathological index as an ipsilateral flow reduction (compared to a contralateral increase) is only possible in a normal contralateral blood flow situation.

Sonographic Examination of the Posterior Circulation
The following constellations of findings are relevant.

Occlusion of the Proximal Vertebral Artery (V1/2 Segment)

Isolated occlusive processes of the vertebral artery in the V1/2 segment normally do not lead to an increased hemodynamic risk due to the numerous possibilities of collateralization (extracranial collaterals from the external carotid artery, Sect. 1.8.2, paired vertebral arteries and posterior communicating arteries). Sonographically, it is not difficult to detect such an occlusion if the vessel itself is visible by B-mode imaging, and a collateral filling via spinal vessels can be detected in the further course of the vessel. ◄

Occlusion of the Distal Vertebral Artery (V3/4 Segment)

The combination of a visible vertebral artery in B-mode imaging, a typical oscillating or blunt flow in the vessel and corresponding clinical symptoms (Wallenberg's syndrome) enables the certain diagnosis of an occlusion in the distal part of the vertebral artery (Fig. 21.4). ◄

Basilar Artery Occlusion

A bilateral oscillating flow in the extracranial vertebral arteries in the case of an acute disturbance of consciousness leaves no doubt about the diagnosis of a basilar artery thrombosis. As high as the positive predictive value is, however, the negative predictive value is also low, especially for thrombosis of the middle and distal basilar arteries, that is, an inconspicuous extracranial ultrasound finding does not reliably rule out basilar artery occlusion. This is caused by intact inferior posterior cerebral arteries,

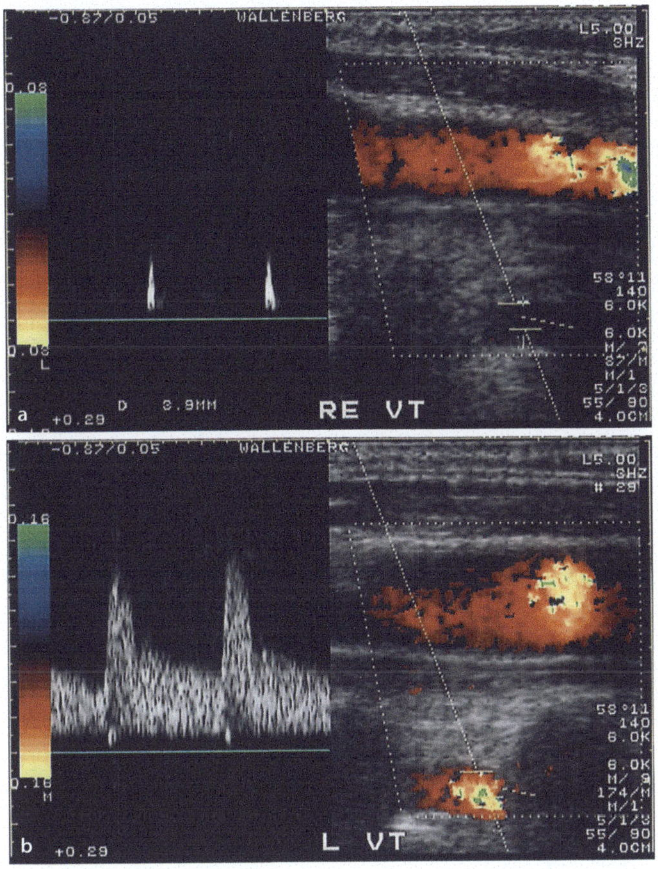

Fig. 21.4 (**a, b**) Distal vertebral artery occlusion right with blunt signal (**a**) in the clearly visible right extracranial vertebral artery compared to normal flow velocity left (**b**) in a patient with acute right-sided Wallenberg syndrome

a possible collateralization via cerebellar arteries as well as by anatomical variants. ◀

Conversely, basilar artery occlusion can be largely ruled out with the help of transnuchal examination. The decisive diagnostic criterion is the continuous (!) visualization of the typical Y of the brainstem vessels up to a depth of about 100 mm without breaks and without conspicuous alias phenomena. If this situation is present and an inconspicuous flow signal is found at the distal end of the basilar artery, there is no basilar thrombosis with high reliability (see overview).

Basilar artery occlusion can be excluded by color duplex sonography if the vertebrobasilar junction (vertebrobasilar Y) can be visualized

- continuously,
- to a depth of approx. 100 mm,
- without conspicuous alias phenomena and
- can be derived at the top of the basilar with a normal Doppler signal.

21.1.4 Clinical Significance

Color coded duplex sonography is a fast procedure that allows an assessment of the cerebrovascular situation even in restless patients when neither CT nor MR angiography is available or does not provide sufficient image quality. It should be noted that MR angiography in particular is highly motion-dependent and thus less suitable for uncooperative patients. There are two main limiting factors of ultrasound: On the one hand, an assessment of the cerebral arteries is not possible in about 20% of patients due to insufficient ultrasound transmission through the temporal bone ("temporal window"), which could only be overcome by the use of ultrasound contrast medium, which is, however, comparably expensive to CT and MRI contrast media, and, on the other hand, the performance of the examination requires some experience. If limited to the symptomatic side with presentation of the internal carotid artery and middle cerebral artery ("**Fast Track Ultrasound**"), however, even a physician in training should, after 50–100 of his own sonographic examinations, be able to perform such an examination in no more than 5 minutes.

Summary

In contrast to the usual routine sonographic diagnostics, the emergency investigation in acute stroke has several special features: The available examination time is limited to 10–15 minutes at most, the examination conditions are difficult and there is a high pressure to make a decision. The examination therefore concentrates on the detection and localization of an occlusion of a large artery supplying the brain as a probable cause of cerebral misperfusion. This detection can regularly only be carried out using color coded duplex sonography, the simple Doppler technique has no significance either extra- or transcranially.

21.2 Monitoring

In addition to clinical monitoring, emergency diagnostics at the stroke unit is followed by basic monitoring of general cardiovascular functions and specific monitoring of cerebrovascular and cerebral processes. Sonographic follow-up examinations can be used to control the success of a recanalizing therapy and to detect secondary cerebrovascular complications such as hyperperfusion and an increased intracranial pressure.

21.2.1 Recanalization of Vascular Occlusions

It goes without saying that revascularization also include monitoring the success of the therapy. Ultrasound diagnostics is the method of choice here due to its non-invasiveness and low cost. However, recanalizations of the middle cerebral artery also occur spontaneously and are the rule rather than the exception in the first 14 days after fresh closure of the vessel. About half of the recanalizations occur within the first 48 hours (Alexandrov et al. 1994).

TIBI Graduation

Thrombolysis In Brain Infarction (TIBI) graduation was introduced as a measure for a semi-quantitative recording of recanalization using transcranial Doppler sonography (Burgin et al. 2000; Demchuk et al. 2001). It is based on the method widely used in interventional cardiology as **Thrombolysis In Myocardial Infarction** (TIMI) graduation (Table 21.2).

However, the TIBI-graduation - in contrast to the TIMI-graduation at the coronaries - does not represent the course of flow condition during recanalization of a main stem of the middle cerebral artery. Thus, the criteria listed under TIBI grades 1–3 are characteristic for a flow signal at an upstream or downstream middle cerebral artery occlusion and are not correlated with a recanalization of this artery.

Additional Information

Another limiting factor is that the extracranial vascular status was not systematically investigated in the investigations underlying the classification and that MR, CT and digital subtraction angiographies were used as reference methods with different sensitivity and specificity for individual occlusion processes. In addition, the median time interval between the reference method and transcranial Doppler sonography was <3 h, but in about 1/4 of the examinations it was 3–24 h and > 24 h respectively.

Despite these limitations, especially if a normal Doppler sonographic flow signal can be detected under monitoring in the middle cerebral artery (grade 5), where previously under comparable conditions no or only a minimal signal could be derived (grade 0 or 1), a recanalization of an initial arterial occlusion can be assumed. However, the inclusion of both the intermediate grades and the interpretation of a change from one degree to the next as progressive recanalization is problematic. The differently reduced signals rather speak for different occlusion localizations and changes can be explained by other causes than recanalization in the actual sense.

Clinical Significance

Especially sonographic monitoring after acute stroke has contributed significantly to the understanding of the pathophysiology of acute vascular occlusion and the effect and efficacy of lysis therapy.

A rapid recanalization of occlusions of large cerebral arteries (carotid T, main stem of the middle cerebral artery) is practically not observed spontaneously, whereas an intravenous thrombolysis leads to a recanalization in 50% of cases within the next 2 hours. In contrast, branch occlusions (also multiple) spontaneously show an early recanalization rate in the same order of magnitude (Gerriets et al. 2000). By intravenous thrombolysis within the 3 h time window, the recanalization rate in patients with cardiogenic embolism can be quadrupled within the first 6 h after stroke compared to the spontaneous course. After this time, no more lysis-related recanalizations are to be expected (Molina et al. 2001).

21.2.2 Hyperperfusion

In the course of recanalization, Doppler sonography often shows a significantly increased flow velocity in the affected vessel. This can indicate an incomplete recanalization with still persistent stenosis or a hyperperfusion with dilated arterioles. The distinction between these two causes is of therapeutic importance, since hyperperfusion is associated with an increased risk of bleeding and can increase intracranial pressure. In this case, the perfusion pressure should rather be lowered, whereas the opposite is indicated for stenoses.

The differentiation between hyperperfusion and stenosis is not unproblematic from a sonographic point of view, but there are three aids to differentiation (Sect. 14.3.3).

Height of the Flow Acceleration

Since there is a linear relationship between flow volume and flow velocity and the flow volume hardly ever doubles during hyperperfusion, in this situation a doubling of the flow velocity compared to standard values can be expected (up to a maximum of 160–180 cm/s). In contrast, higher flow velocities are only achieved in stenoses, since there is a quadratic relationship to the degree of stenosis (Sect. 14.3.3).

Table 21.2 Thrombolysis in brain infarction (TIBI) graduation of the Doppler sonographic flow signal in the middle cerebral artery to describe the phases of flow restitution under thrombolysis. (According to Burgin et al. 2000; Demchuk et al. 2001)

TIBI degree	Flow signal	
0	Missing	No regular pulsatile flow signal despite background noise
1	Minimal	Systolic peaks (also on both sides of the zero line) or low systolic signal without diastole
2	Pseudovenous	Reduced systolic flow velocity and pulsatility, delayed systolic rise
3	Diminished	Reduced flow velocity (in side comparison >30%), normal flow characteristics
4	Accelerated	Increased flow velocity (in side comparison >30% or mean > 80 cm/s), turbulence
5	Normal	Normal flow velocity and signal

Short- Versus Long-Distance Flow Acceleration

A typical characteristic of hyperperfusion is that it affects the entire vascular segment and does not only occur locally, as is the case with some stenoses. However, this distinguishing feature is not generally applicable, as stenoses (or vasospasms, Sect. 22.2) can also be very long in individual cases.

MCA/ICA Index

Under normal circumstances and also in the case of hyperperfusion, the quotient between the maximum systolic flow velocity in the middle cerebral artery (MCA) and the internal carotid artery (ICA) of the same side is in the range of 1.0–2.0. The more the MCA/ICA index exceeds the value of 2, the greater the likelihood of an intracranial stenosis. A value of 3 or higher is considered to ensure a high grade stenosis (overview below).

Use of the MCA/ICA Index

1.0–2.0: Normal/hyperperfusion.
2.0–3.0: Intracranial stenosis possible.
>3.0: Intracranial stenosis safe.

Summary

In the monitoring phase following the emergency diagnosis, sonography is suitable for monitoring the course of drug-induced and spontaneous vascular recanalizations. In addition, specific neurological complications, for example, cerebral hyperperfusion, can be detected. The most important parameter for differentiating between hyperperfusion and residual stenosis after recanalization is the level of local flow velocity.

21.3 Etiologic Assessment

After completion of the primary emergency diagnosis and usually already during the acute monitoring phase, the stroke unit treatment focuses on the prevention of stroke relapse in the following 24–48 hours. The main aim is to identify the cause of the stroke (overview).

Questions to be clarified sonographically in acute cerebral infarction with already existing CT or MR angiography

- Extracranial carotid artery
  - Cardiac thrombus
  - Floating thrombus
  - Character of a dissection
  - Generalized arteriosclerosis
  - Graduation of carotid stenoses
  - Signs of vasculitis
- Cerebral arteries
  - Graduation of intracranial stenoses
  - Monitoring of progress
  - Assessment of collateral ways
  - Determination of the cerebrovascular reserve capacity
  - Detection of the vertebrobasilar system
  - Hypoplasia or dissection
  - Signs of vasculitis
  - Assessment of hemodynamics in proximal occlusions of the vertebral artery.

A comprehensive, well-documented ultrasound examination of the extra- and intracranial brain-supplying arteries should be performed as early as possible in the stroke unit or neurological intensive care unit. Special attention should be paid to patients with a non-conclusive, artifact-disturbed or technically inadequate initial CT or MR angiography as well as those with competing embolism sources or clinical worsening. Actual or "device-related" changes in vascular status may result in relevant and immediate modifications of the therapeutic strategy (e.g., high-grade stenosis vs. occlusion).

21.3.1 Differential Diagnosis of Stroke Etiology

- **Arterial embolization.** The ultrasound B-mode image of the carotid artery provides much better information than other imaging techniques about generalized arteriosclerotic changes in the vascular system, which indicate an arterial-embolic cause of brain infarcts. An intima-media or plaque thickness of ≥1.5 mm is most likely associated with generalized arteriosclerotic changes also in the aortic arch. Furthermore, ultrasound provides a surrogate marker for the progression of arteriosclerosis and the control of vascular risk factors.
- **Cardiac embolization.** A carotid occlusion that appears homogeneous in the ultrasound image without obvious arteriosclerotic changes indicates a cardiogenic thrombus. The same applies to floating thrombi in the area of the carotid bifurcation, which are much easier to detect than with other imaging techniques.
- **Dissection.** A tapering internal carotid artery ("string sign") is highly predictive for the presence of a vascular dissection. In addition, the visible original vascular lumen helps to distinguish between primary hypoplasia and dissection-related narrowing in the course of the vertebral artery.
- **Vasculitis.** A homogeneously low-echogenic, concentric thickening of the vessel wall ("halo effect") in the extracranial vessels indicates the presence of vasculitis.

21.3.2 Hemodynamic Assessment

- **Grading of stenosis.** The graduation of stenoses based on the visible narrowing of the flow or contrast medium band is associated with uncertainties in all available imaging techniques for physical reasons. Due to the possibility of Doppler sonographic measurement of the flow velocity, however, ultrasound diagnostics has the essential advantage that it can be used to (additionally) graduate extra- and intracranial vascular stenoses on the basis of hemodynamic parameters. Most studies on interventions for carotid stenosis are based on such hemodynamic criteria, so that ultrasound diagnostics is indispensable for determining the indication for such interventions.
- **Stenosis-occlusion differentiation.** In intracranial occlusive processes, both CT and MR angiography often do not allow a clear differentiation between high-grade stenosis and collateralized occlusion. The detection of a Doppler sonographic stenosis signal contributes to such differentiation.
- **Progress monitoring.** Due to its risk-free and cost-effective repeatability, ultrasound diagnostics is suitable for monitoring the course of both extra- and intracranial vascular occlusions and stenoses. Rapidly recanalizing vascular processes indicate a cardiac embolus or dissection, while experience shows that arteriosclerotic changes show a static or progressive course. Even in the case of acutely inserted extra- or intracranial stents as part of stroke treatment, ultrasound can be used to monitor as often as desired.
- **Low flow situation.** A frequent cause of secondary deterioration after ischemic events are "low-flow situations" behind vascular occlusion with development of thrombi. Ultrasound diagnostics is more suitable than any other method for making statements about a thrombogenic "low-flow situation" in the corresponding vessel section by quantitatively assessing the blood flow distal to outlet occlusions, particularly of the common carotid artery or vertebral artery, which are often partially collateralized via skin and muscle branches.
- **Assessment of the hemodynamics.** The determination of the flow volume in the extracranial carotids and vertebral arteries enables - not least in the context of observations of the course of the disease - quantitative statements about cerebral perfusion in intracranial occlusive processes. The presence of sufficient intracranial collaterals can be estimated by examining the flow direction and velocity in the anterior and posterior commnicating arteries as well as in the downstream arterial sections. In addition, the determination of cerebrovascular reserve capacity distal to vascular stenoses and occlusions provides a quick overview of the - albeit rather rare - risk of suffering hemodynamically induced infarction in the case of a drop in blood pressure.

Summary

The essential domain of neurovascular ultrasound diagnostics lies in its contribution to the differential diagnosis of brain infarcts and the hemodynamic assessment of extra- and intracranial vascular stenosis and occlusion.

References

Alexandrov AV, Bladin CF, Norris JW (1994) Intracranial blood flow velocities in acute ischemic stroke. Stroke 25:1378–1383

Burgin WS, Malkoff M, Felberg RA, Demchuk AM, Christou I, Grotta JC, Alexandrov AV (2000) Transcranial doppler ultrasound criteria for recanalization after thrombolysis for middle cerebral artery stroke. Stroke 31:1128–1132

Demchuk AM, Burgin WS, Christou I, Felberg RA, Barber PA, Hill MD, Alexandrov AV (2001) Thrombolysis in brain ischemia (TIBI) transcranial Doppler flow grades predict clinical severity, early recovery, and mortality in patients treated with intravenous tissue plasminogen activator. Stroke 32:89–93

Gerriets T, Postert T, Goertler M, Stolz E, Schlachetzki F, Sliwka U, Seidel G, Weber S, Kaps M (2000) DIAS I: duplex-sonographic assessment of the cerebrovascular status in acute stroke. A useful tool for future stroke trials. Stroke 31:2342–2345

Molina CA, Montaner J, Abilleira S, Arenillas JF, Ribó M, Huertas R, Romero F, Alvarez-Sabín J (2001) Time course of tissue plasminogen activator-induced recanalization in acute cardioembolic stroke: a case-control study. Stroke 32:2821–2827

Rodrigues FB, Neves JB, Caldeira D, Ferro JM, Ferreira JJ, Costa J (2016) Endovascular treatment versus medical care alone for ischaemic stroke: systematic review and meta-analysis. BMJ 353:1754

Cerebral Vasospasms

22

Bernhard Widder and Gerhard F. Hamann

22.1 Spontaneous Vasospasms

Vasospasms during manipulation of a vessel (e.g., during digital subtraction angiography) or in its vicinity (e.g., during ENT surgery) have been known for many years, but spontaneous vasospasms in the context of migraine have also been demonstrated (Arning et al. 1998; Schlüter and Kissig 2002). In the latter case, it is now more likely that these are manifestations of a RCVS (reversible vasoconstriction syndrome, Chap. 19) (Ducros and Wolff 2016), especially since triptans are known triggers of RCVS and are frequently used in migraine. Thus, a pathophysiological as well as therapeutic connection can be assumed.

Sonographic Assessment
Characteristic Doppler ultrasound findings of vasospasm are rapidly fluctuating stenoses or even occlusions of the extra- and/or intracranial brain-supplying arteries (Case Study 22.1).

Clinical Significance
The main clinical significance lies in the recognition that spontaneous vasospasms of larger arteries are obviously possible. In case of fluctuating findings, the possibility of such a situation should therefore be considered.

Case Study 22.1 (After Arning et al. 1998)
In the 32-year-old woman multiple episodes of a left-sided amaurosis fugax and a transient hemiplegia on the right side were found in the medical history. The MRI revealed a left border zone cerebral infarction, but color coded duplex examination did not reveal any correlating pathological findings. During the inpatient rehabilitation a new visual disturbance occurred. An immediately performed ultrasound examination showed a filiform stenosis 4 cm above the origin of the left internal carotid artery as well as indirect indications of a higher grade stenosis located further cranially in the right internal carotid artery. A control 18 h later, however revealed completely normal findings. Six weeks later, a further attack with visual disturbance occurred showing again a rapidly reversible stenosis of the left internal carotid artery. After treatment with a calcium antagonist, the patient was unremarkable for a period of 12 months with the exception of three very short attacks with visual disturbances.

Summary
Spontaneous vasospasms with fluctuating occlusive processes of the brain-supplying arteries are probably more frequent than previously assumed, especially in connection with migraine.

22.2 Vasospasms in Subarachnoid Hemorrhages

In addition to secondary bleeding, vasospasms are the most important and most frequent complication of spontaneous and traumatic subarachnoid hemorrhages (SAH). They

B. Widder (✉)
Expert Opinion Institute, District Hospital, Guenzburg, Germany
e-mail: bernhard.widder@bkh-guenzburg.de

G. F. Hamann
Clinic of Neurology and Neurological Rehabilitation, District Hospital, Guenzburg, Germany

B. Widder, G. F. Hamann (eds.), *Duplex sonography of the brain-supplying arteries*, https://doi.org/10.1007/978-3-662-65566-5_22

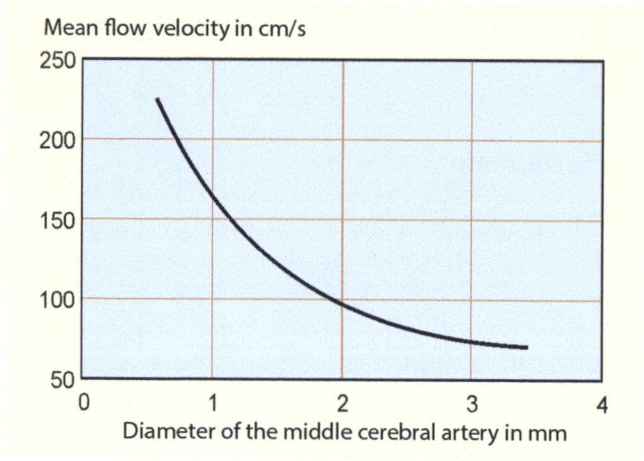

Fig. 22.1 Effect of vasospasm-induced diameter changes of the middle cerebral artery on the Doppler sonographically measured flow velocity

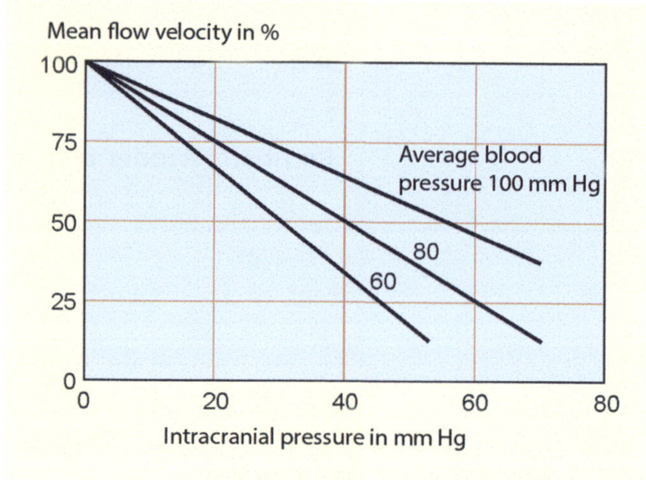

Fig. 22.2 Influence of increases in cerebral pressure on the flow velocity in the middle cerebral artery as a function of systemic blood pressure (according to Klingelhöfer et al. 1991)

generally develop with a latency of 3–5 days after the event and are caused by exposure to vasoconstrictive blood degradation products. This leads to segmental vasoconstriction with a Doppler-sonographically detectable increase in flow velocity (Fig. 22.1). Delayed neurological deficits may occur due to the deficient blood flow caused by the stenosis. Although ultrasound diagnostics for vasospasm detection is required in the American guidelines, it is not consistently implemented in the reality of care (Kumar et al. 2017).

22.2.1 Basic Methodological Problems

Already in the 1980s a large number of publications have been published describing the value of transcranial Doppler sonography in the detection of vasospasms after subarachnoid hemorrhages and in therapy control after the administration of calcium antagonists. In the 1990s, however, increasingly skeptical statements were added (Grosset et al. 1993; Laumer et al. 1993; Lennihan et al. 1993). In particular three problems were mentioned:

- Lack of correlation between increased Doppler frequencies and the occurrence of a neurological deficit
- Lack of correlation between increased Doppler frequencies and the occurrence of critical vasospasms
- Lack of accuracy of Doppler examination in the detection of vasospasms.

Prediction of a Neurological Deficit

The fact that there is only a marginal connection between the Doppler frequency increase and the occurrence of a neurological deficit is not surprising given the experience with arteriosclerotic stenoses. Depending on the extent of collateral supply, even relatively high-grade stenoses have only an insignificant hemodynamic effect, and stenotic thrombus formation depends more on the coagulation situation than on the degree of stenosis. However, ultrasound diagnostics has a relatively good predictive value for the development of secondary neurological deficits after SAB, the so-called "delayed cerebral ischemia" (DCI, Kumar et al. 2017). A sensitivity of 90% was found with a specificity of 71%, a positive predictive value of 57% and a negative predictive value of 92%. The sonographic detection of vasospasms after SAB thus indicates the patient's risk for the development of DCI; conversely, a normal ultrasound finding after SAB seems to predict a favorable clinical development.

Detection of a Critical Vasospasm

The lack of correlation between high Doppler frequencies and the occurrence of "critical" vasospasms may seem surprising at first glance, since for flow physiological reasons there is an inverse quadratic proportionality between flow velocity and vessel diameter (Sect. 2.3). However, this relationship presupposes a peripheral resistance that decreases or at least remains constant with increasing degree of stenosis, as is the case with extracranial stenosis. In subarachnoid hemorrhages, however, this is not necessarily the case, so that misinterpretations in both directions are possible if only the local flow velocity is observed.

Underestimation of Vasospasms

Especially in severe subarachnoid hemorrhages, a relevant increase in intracranial pressure can occur with a resulting increase in peripheral resistance and decrease in flow velocity (Fig. 22.2). Therefore, when assessing vasospasms, it is important to observe not only the flow velocity but also the pulsatility as a criterion for increased intracranial pressure (Sect. 23.1). ◀

Overestimation of Vasospasms

If the previously increased intracranial pressure drops again, there is regularly a disproportionate reduction in peripheral resistance and thus hyperperfusion. A resulting overestimation of vasospasms can easily be avoided by taking into account the MCA/ICA index (Sect. 14.3.3). ◀

Accuracy of the Doppler Examination

The accusation of an overall lack of accuracy of Doppler sonography in the detection of vasospasms is probably due to the fact that the method was uncritically overrated in the early days. In fact, however, there are three limitations to be taken into account, which are well known from the detection of arteriosclerotic stenoses.

Only Direct Assessment Reliable

The accuracy of Doppler and duplex sonography is reduced if the assessment can only be made on the basis of indirect criteria. Vasospasms that are not (yet) associated with very high grade stenosis are therefore only detectable if they affect a vessel segment that is directly accessible by sonography. ◀

Considering Angle Dependence

When examining with the simple transcranial Doppler probe, the angular dependence of the Doppler frequencies must always be taken into account. If color coded duplex sonography is not available, reduced accuracy must therefore be expected when deriving the anterior and posterior cerebral arteries. ◀

Consideration of Collateral Supply

The Doppler and duplex sonographic evaluation of stenoses (and vasospasms) is based on the detection of flow changes. However, with good collateral supply via the anterior common artery, the hemodynamic effect of a spasm in the A1 segment of the anterior cerebral artery can be eliminated (Fig. 22.3). However, a well collateralized vasospasm will not lead to hemodynamic problems. ◀

Summarizing the points of criticism, one comes to the ultimately banal conclusion that ultrasound diagnostics – as in the case of its application in arteriosclerotic vascular lesions – is of course not capable of doing the physically impossible. If, however, one observes the limitations described in the basic part of this book, very reliable statements can be made on the basis of the method, especially about vasospasms in the main stem of the middle cerebral artery.

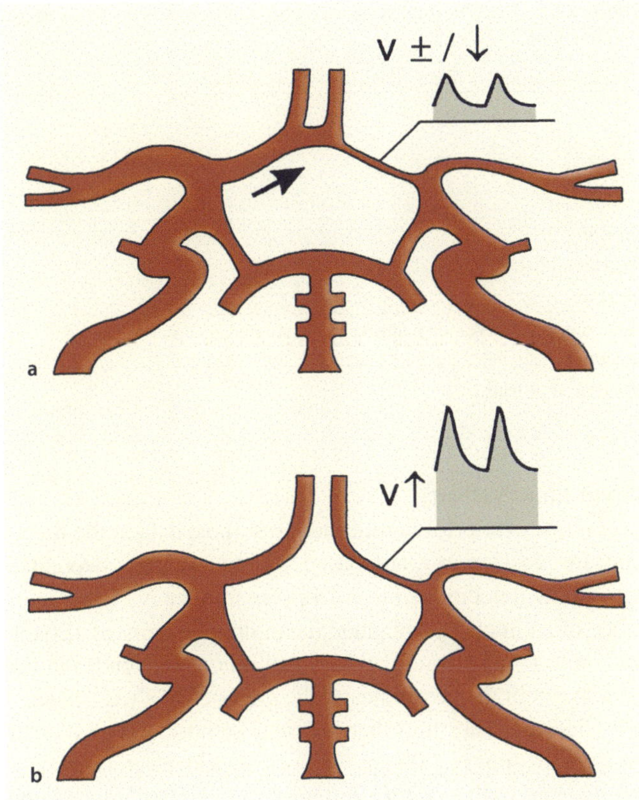

Fig. 22.3 (**a, b**) Problems with the Doppler sonographic detection of vasospasms in the A1 segment of the anterior cerebral artery depending on the position of the anterior communicating artery. With well-developed anterior communicating artery and corresponding collateral supply, flow velocity in the vasospastic A1 segment is normal or even reduced (**a**). Only in hypoplastic or also vasospastic anterior communicating artery an increased flow velocity occurs in the A1 segment (**b**)

22.2.2 Sonographic Assessment

Since vasospasms are equivalent to arteriosclerotic stenoses with regard to their hemodynamic effect, the criteria already mentioned in Sect. 14.3.2 apply in principle. In the following, therefore, the most important findings will only be briefly described again in summary form and the essential special features of vasospasm diagnostics will be dealt with (Table 22.1).

Table 22.1 Doppler/duplex sonographic characteristics of vasospasms in the middle cerebral artery (frequency data related to a transmission frequency of 2 MHz)

Increased Doppler frequencies or flow velocities	Mean value	≥120 cm/s (≥3 kHz) = borderline
		≥160 cm/s (≥4 kHz) = significant
		≥200 cm/s (≥5 kHz) = critical
	Maximum value	≥160 cm/s (≥4 kHz) = relevant
		≥220 cm/s (≥6 kHz) = critical
and/or		
Increased MCA/ICA index	MCA/ICA >3.0	
and/or		
Increase in flow velocity during the first week	50%/day or 40 cm/s (1 kHz) per day	
and/or		
Increased pulsatility	Pulsatility index (PI) >1.0	
	Resistance index (RI) >0.6	

Blood Flow Velocity

In contrast to arteriosclerotic stenoses, most data in the literature for vasospasms are based on the intensity-weighted mean flow velocity or mean Doppler frequency. The occurrence of an intensity-weighted mean flow velocity of 120 cm and more (=3 kHz at 2 MHz transmission frequency) in the middle cerebral artery indicates the presence of a vasospasm – provided there are no other vascular stenoses on any other basis; from approx. 200 cm/s, a critical vasospasm is present. With regard to the anterior and posterior cerebral arteries, the values indicated should be reduced by 20–25%. The diagnosis can be regarded as confirmed in particular if such a Doppler signal can only be derived on one side. However, if the intracranial pressure also increases at the same time, there is no increase in flow velocity (Fig. 22.4).

In relation to the **maximum systolic flow velocity** the rule known from arteriosclerotic stenoses applies, according to which 160 cm/s (=4 kHz related to 2 MHz transmission frequency) indicate a relevant constriction. Critical flow velocities – also analogous to arteriosclerotic lesions – are to be expected from a maximum flow velocity of approx. 220 cm/s (= 6 kHz at 2 MHz transmission frequency).

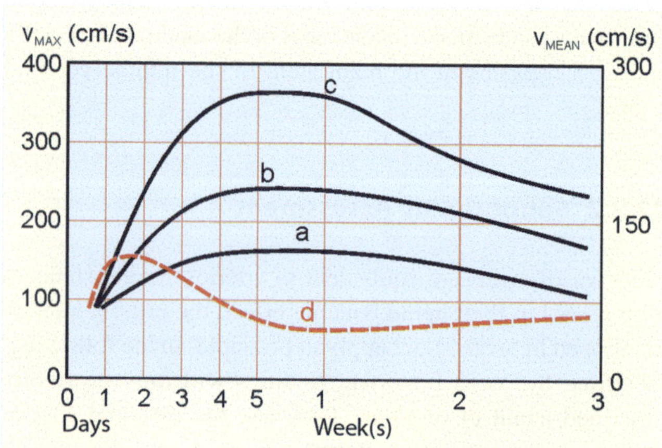

Fig. 22.4 (**a**–**d**) Course of flow velocity in the large cerebral arteries with varying degrees of vasospasm. (**a**) Moderate, (**b**) significant, (**c**) critical increase in flow velocity; (**d**) short-term increase, followed by an often dramatic drop in flow velocity when intracranial pressure is increased

MCA/ICA Index

The quotient of the Doppler frequencies between the middle cerebral artery and the internal carotid artery (MCA/ICA index) is particularly suitable for differentiating between hyperperfusion and vasospasm. As already described in Sect. 14.3.3, this is normally (and in the case of hyperperfusion) 2.0 or less. Values >3.0 indicate a relevant vasospasm.

Increase in Flow Velocity

An increase in mean flow velocity of about 50% or 40–50 cm/s per day during the first 4–6 days after subarachnoid hemorrhage indicates a developing vasospasm.

Pulsatility

As expected, the highest predictive value for the occurrence of neurological complications is the observation of pulsatility. As explained in Chap. 23, an increase in pulsatility indicates the presence of increased intracranial pressure regardless of the absolute level of blood flow velocity. A pulsatility index (PI) of 1.0 and a resistance index (RI) of 0.6 should be assumed as limit values (Klingelhöfer et al. 1991). Such increased values are regularly associated with intracranial pressure of 20 mmHg and more. It goes without saying that the patient must be (largely) in a state of normocapnia and have a "normal" heart rate. Since pulsatility can also be influenced by cardiac factors (e.g., aortic insufficiency) in individual cases, the temporal course of the systolic-diastolic relationship should be observed in particular.

Summary
Vasospasms are significant complications of subarachnoid hemorrhage, which develop with a latency period of 3–5 days after bleeding. They indicate with relatively high accuracy the risk of developing ischemic complications. Hemodynamically, they are equivalent to arteriosclerotic stenoses, so that the well-known Doppler sonographic criteria apply for their detection. The accuracy is very high in the middle cerebral artery, but only moderate in the anterior cerebral artery due to anatomical variations. With simultaneous intracranial pressure increase, the flow velocity decreases, which can lead to misinterpretations. In this case, the increase in pulsatility of the flow signal points the way forward. Hyperperfusion can be distinguished from vasospasm by the MCA/ICA index.

22.3 Vasospasms in Inflammatory Brain Diseases

One of the complications of inflammatory brain diseases – especially in the context of purulent meningitis – are vasospasms of the vessel walls. The corresponding diagnostic criteria are discussed in the case of cerebral vasculitides (Sect. 17.4.1).

References

Arning C, Schrattenholzer A, Lachenmayer L (1998) Cervical carotid artery vasospasmus causing cerebral ischemia: detection by immediate vascular ultrasonographic investigation. Stroke 29:1063–1066

Ducros A, Wolff V (2016) The typical thunderclap headache of reversible cerebral vasoconstriction syndrome and its various triggers. Headache 56:657–673

Grosset DG, Straiton J, McDonald I, Cockburn M, Bullock R (1993) Use of transcranial Doppler sonography to predict development of a delayed ischemic deficit after subarachnoid hemorrhage. J Neurosurg 78:183–187

Klingelhöfer J, Sander D, Holzgräfe M, Bischoff C, Conrad B (1991) Cerebral vasospasm evaluated by transcranial Doppler sonography at different intracranial pressures. J Neurol 75:752–758

Kumar G, Albright KC, Donnelly JP, Shapshak AH, Harrigan MR (2017) Trends in transcranial Doppler monitoring in aneurysmal subarachnoid hemorrhage: a 10-year analysis of the nationwide inpatient sample. J Stroke Cerebrovasc Dis 26:851–857

Laumer R, Steinmeier R, Gonner F, Vogtmann T, Priem R, Fahlbusch R (1993) Cerebral hemodynamics in subarachnoid hemorrhage evaluated by transcranial Doppler sonography. Part 1: reliability of flow velocities in clinical management. Neurosurgery 33:1–8

Lennihan L, Petty GW, Fink ME, Solomon RA, Mohr JP (1993) Transcranial Doppler detection of anterior cerebral artery vasospasm. J Neurol Neurosurg Psychiatry 56:906–909

Schlüter A, Kissig B (2002) MR angiography in migrainous vasospasm. Neurology 59:1772

Diagnostics for Increased Cerebral Pressure and Cerebral Circulatory Arrest

23

Georg Gahn and Bernhard Widder

Detection and measurement of increased intracranial pressure based on changes in pulsatility and flow velocity in the cerebral basal arteries were one of the first clinical applications of transcranial Doppler sonography. In the meantime, this determination has gained great importance in the diagnosis of cerebral circulatory arrest in the context of brain death diagnostics. Furthermore, increased intracranial pressure can also be detected by changes in the diameter of the optic nerve sheath (Sect. 26.2).

23.1 Assessment of Elevated Cerebral Pressure

Increased intracranial pressure values have a hemodynamic effect like increased peripheral resistance. According to the explanations on flow physiology (Sect. 2.5), changes in intracranial pressure are therefore primarily indicated by a changed pulsatility in the arteries supplying to the brain.

23.1.1 Doppler Sonographic Findings

Pulsatility Index with Increased Intracranial Pressure
A pulsatility index (PI) of 1.0 or more – calculated according to Gosling and King (1974) as

$$\text{Pulsatility index (PI)} = (\text{Systole–Diastole})/\text{Mean}$$

(Sect. 5.2.4) indicates pathologically increased intracranial pressure values of more than 20 mmHg in cardiovascular healthy and (approximately) normocapnic patients with normal pulse rates of 60–80/min. At very high intracranial pressure values the influence of pCO2 is negligible. Under this condition Doppler examination produces clear results even with frequently performed moderate hyperventilation (Homburg et al. 1993).

> Note
> **A pressure increase of 10 mmHg regularly causes an increase in pulsatility index (PI) in the order of 25–50%.**

Flow Curve with Increased Cerebral Pressure
If intracranial pressure values exceed the end-diastolic perfusion pressure, an **oscillating flow pattern** with a cranially directed component during systole and a caudally directed component during diastole (Fig. 23.1). Extreme pressure values cause the oscillating flow to disappear followed by so-called **small systolic spikes** corresponding to the transmitted pulsations without effective blood flow. Systolic spikes appear as relatively narrow, vertical "lines" in the Doppler spectrum. Typically, they do not exceed a flow velocity of 50 cm/s (or 1.0–1.5 kHz at 2 MHz transmission frequency).

> **Sign of massively increased intracranial pressure**
> – "Oscillating flow" with returning pulse wave during diastole
> – "Small systolic peaks" up to 50 cm/s without diastolic flow.

G. Gahn
Department of Neurology, Community Hospital Karlsruhe gGmbH, Karlsruhe, Germany

B. Widder (✉)
Expert Opinion Institute, District Hospital, Guenzburg, Germany
e-mail: bernhard.widder@bkh-guenzburg.de

B. Widder, G. F. Hamann (eds.), *Duplex sonography of the brain-supplying arteries*, https://doi.org/10.1007/978-3-662-65566-5_23

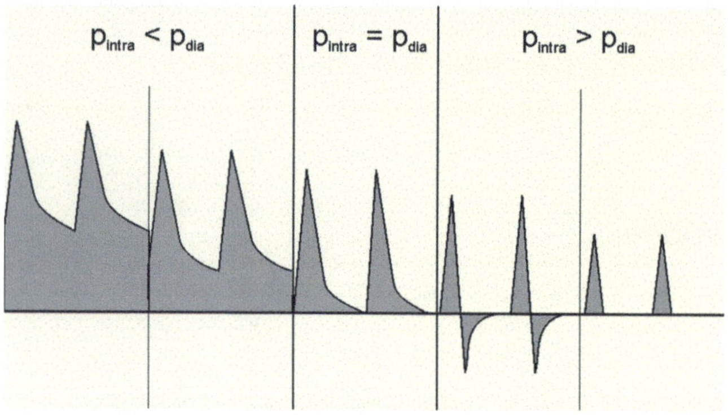

Fig. 23.1 Changes in the pulse curve in the cerebral basal arteries as the intracranial pressure increases from left to right. p_{intra} intracranial pressure; p_{dia} diastolic blood pressure

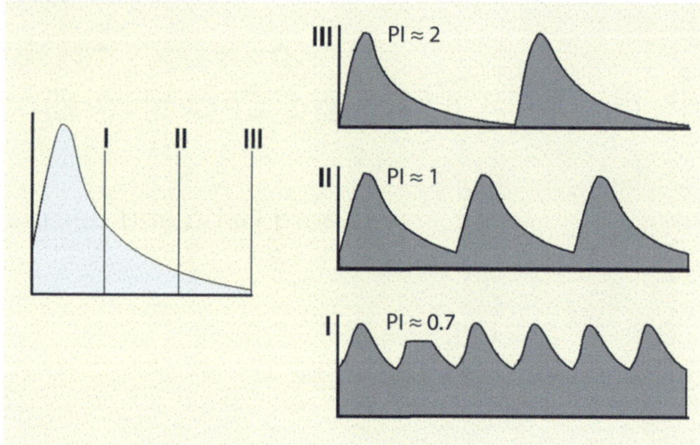

Fig. 23.2 Changes in pulsatility at different heart rates

23.1.2 Influence of Disrupting Factors

Since pulsatility within the cerebral basal arteries depends on numerous individual factors, "normal deviations" of cardiovascular parameters mentioned in Table 23.1 may lead to an incorrect estimation of intracranial pressure values. In presence of such "disturbing variables ," an intracranial pressure measurement is desirable at least once as a reference. If necessary, a current cranial computer tomogram is also sufficient to provide indirect information on current intracranial pressure values.

Abnormal Heart Rate

False-negative findings of the pulsatility index (too low estimated intracranial pressure values) are to be expected in patients with tachycardia above 80–100 heartbeats/min. At least in mildly increased intracranial pressure, diastolic drop in flow velocity cannot be realistically assessed because of a missing drop in pulse curve (Fig. 23.2). Conversely, false-positive results (intracranial pressure values estimated as too high) are possible in bradycardia leading to an apparently increased pulsatility.

Occlusive Processes of Brain-Supplying Vessels

Both false-negative and false-positive values of the pulsatility index (intracranial pressure values estimated as too low or too high) are to be expected, if higher grade occlusive processes of the extra- or intracranial brain-supplying vessels are present at the same time. In this situation, judgement becomes uncertain because of the considerably variable flow patterns in the cerebral basal arteries including the vertebral arteries, which is not to be expected in the case of a generalized increase in intracranial pressure.

23.2 Cerebral Circulatory Arrest

Ultrasound examination of the brain supplying arteries is an established procedure to determine cerebral circulatory arrest in diagnosing brain death. In Germany, the method is included in the recommendations of the Scientific Advisory Board of the German Medical Association and can be used as a so-called "supplementary examination". Irreversibility of loss of brain function by determination of cerebral circulation arrest can be proven in all age groups. Depending on patients age different waiting periods and possibly a repeated examination are required by German guidelines (Walter et al. 2016).

Cerebral circulatory arrest occurs when intracranial pressure exceeds mean arterial pressure (= diastolic pressure + 1/3 × (systolic pressure – diastolic pressure)), assuming normal cardiovascular function. In most cases, cerebral circulatory arrest leads to irreversible loss of brain function. Since typical flow curves occur in the Doppler sonogram of the cerebral basal arteries (Sect. 23.1.1), transcranial Doppler or duplex

Table 23.1 Possible errors in estimating intracranial pressure based on Doppler signal pulsatility

	Misinterpretation of the intracranial pressure as	
Influencing parameter	too high	too low
Blood-pCO_2	Hypocapnia	Hypercapnia
Heart rate/pulse rate	Bradycardia	Tachycardia
Heart valve function	Aortic insufficiency	Aortic stenosis
Cardiac ejection capacity	Diminished	–
Occlusive processes of the brain-supplying vessels	Variable misjudgment depending on stenoses and collateral flow	

examination is suitable for determining irreversible cerebral circulatory arrest in the context of diagnosing brain death. In the current German guideline update, in addition to the proven Doppler sonography, duplex sonography has also been approved as an instrumental procedure for detection of cerebral circulation arrest. Transcranial color coded duplex sonography facilitates identification of cerebral arteries and the corresponding positioning of the measurement volume within the cerebral basal arteries by depicting anatomical structures in the B-scan.

23.2.1 Doppler Sonography Versus Other Procedures

Doppler Versus EEG/EAEP

Compared to the traditional methods of brain wave recording (EEG) and early acoustically evoked potentials (EAEP), ultrasound examination offers the advantage of being independent of possible intoxications and less prone to interference. Furthermore, it can be used equally reliable for supra- and infratentorial as well as for primary and secondary brain damage (following overview). The comprehensive application possibilities of Doppler sonographic enable evaluation of hemispheric as well as vertebrobasilar blood flow . Doppler sonography provides an overview of the supply of the entire brain, whereas EEG and EAEP only consider the cortex and the brain stem respectively.

Last but not least, electrophysiological investigations may be limited by strongly sedating drugs (e.g., barbiturates). The guidelines of the German Medical Association, for example, point out that because of unsecure concentration-effect relationships of these drugs, "in case of doubt" (additional) proof of cerebral circulatory arrest must be requested.

Value of Doppler sonography in the diagnosis of brain death compared to other additional procedures (EEG, EAEP)

- **Advantages**
  - Also applicable for intoxicated patients
  - Less sensitive to interference and artifacts
  - Regardless of the type of cerebral damage
  - No false-positive results if the criteria are strictly observed
- **Disadvantages**
  - Problems with insufficient temporal insonation window
  - Procedural performance requires some experience
  - False-negative findings possible (reperfusion, AV fistula, lack of increased cerebral pressure, calotte defect).

Doppler Versus Angiography/Scintigraphy

Proof of cerebral circulatory arrest may be provided not only by Doppler sonography but also by conventional cerebral angiography, CT angiography and brain perfusion scintigraphy. However, these methods usually require the patient to be transported to the respective examination room. Repositioning and manipulation of the patient can lead to a further increase in a possibly only marginal increase in intracranial pressure leading to additional damage. Furthermore, secondary damage cannot be ruled out by the application of contrast agents in the presence of a disturbed blood-brain barrier.

23.2.2 Doppler and Duplex Sonographic Findings

Doppler/duplex sonographic findings in cerebral circulatory arrest

According to German guidelines, in adults, at an arterial mean pressure of more than 60 mmHg, at least for 30 min

- By Doppler sonography
  a. Intracranially the middle cerebral arteries, internal carotid arteries, and possibly detectable further cerebral basal arteries,
  b. Extracranially the vertebral arteries and, if the corresponding intracranial vessel segments cannot be evaluated, the internal carotid arteries,

  or
- By means of duplex sonography
  a. Intracranially the M1 segments of the middle cerebral arteries, the internal carotid arteries, the V4 segments of the vertebral arteries and the basilar artery as well as possibly detectable further cerebral basal arteries

  be examined and the following findings must be detectable:

(continued)

- Biphasic flow signals (oscillating flow signals) with equally pronounced integral of the ante- and retrograde components
  or
- Early systolic peaks smaller than 50 cm/s and lasting less than 200 ms, with no other flow signal detectable in the remaining cardiac cycle

In the presence of cerebral circulatory arrest, three typical findings are found by Doppler sonography in the cerebral basal arteries – sometimes alternating within a short time (overview).

Doppler sonographic findings in the brain base arteries in the presence of cerebral circulatory arrest

- Oscillating flow
- Small systolic peaks
- Missing flow signal.

Oscillating Flow

This signal is composed of a part directed toward the periphery during systole and toward the heart during diastole (synonymous **biphasic flow** ; Fig. 23.3). According to the guidelines, an equally pronounced integral of the ante- and retrograde components is required, that is, the areas of the antegrade and retrograde components of the Doppler frequency time spectrum within a cardiac cycle must be the same. No exact metrological determination is necessary here, a visual assessment by the examiner is sufficient.

Practical Tips

The backflow component of the oscillating flow can be concealed by the wall filter. For this reason, the wall filter should always be set as low as possible to values of 50 Hz or below – if adjustable on the unit.

Small Systolic Peaks

Small systolic spikes have maximum amplitudes up to 50 cm/s (1–1.5 kHz at 2 MHz transmission frequency) without presence of a diastolic flow signal. These are only small shifts of the blood column and vessel wall movements due to the transmitted pulse wave, which, however, no longer produce a significant flow effect. There are often smooth transitions between oscillating flow and small systolic spikes (Fig. 23.4).

Practical Tips

Frequently, a continuous registration of an intracranial artery during brain death diagnostics shows a respiratory modulation of the flow amplitudes. This indicates a direct dependence of the blood flow on the cerebral pressure and supports the diagnosis of frustrated brain perfusion (Fig. 23.4).

No Usable Doppler Flow Signal

If transcranial ultrasound does not provide blood flow signals in the cerebral basal arteries, this finding can only be considered a reliable sign of cerebral circulatory arrest unless the same examiner, with the same instrument settings, has documented clearly derivable intracranial flow signals in a previous examination or signs of cerebral circulatory arrest are detectable in the extracranial brain-supplying arteries. Ultrasound contrast agents can be used to increase the

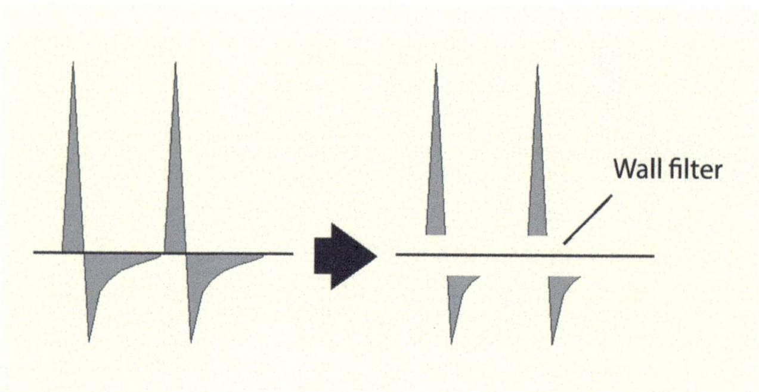

Fig. 23.3 Oscillating flow with nearly equal forward and backward flow (areas above and below zero line) (left)

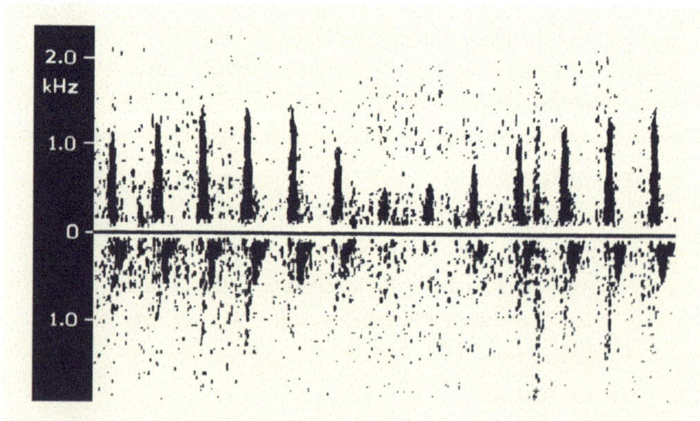

Fig. 23.4 Mixed findings between "small systolic peaks" (maximum Doppler frequency 1.3 kHz) and oscillating flow in the middle cerebral artery in a 2-year-old child after resuscitation following drowning. Note the pronounced respiratory modulation of the pulse curve, which indicates fluctuations in intracranial pressure

Table 23.2 Doppler sonographic detection of cerebral circulatory arrest (according to German guidelines)

Clinical requirements	Arterial mean pressure of more than 60 mmHg
	no major skull bone defect
Device technical settings	Time axis (*sweep*) maximum stretched
	Transmission power (*power*) maximum increased
	Gain (*gain*) increased until screen is filled with artifact dots
	Wall filter ≤50 Hz
	Measurement volume during intracranial examination ≥15 mm
	Envelope faded out
	Examination depth 60–65 mm
Examination procedure	Evidence of cerebral circulatory arrest if oscillating flow or small systolic peaks occur in the following vessels when examined twice at intervals of at least 30 min
	–by Doppler sonography Intracranially middle cerebral arteries, internal carotid arteries and possibly detectable further cerebral arteries Extracranial both vertebral arteries and, if the corresponding intracranial artery segments cannot be evaluated, the internal carotid artery bilaterally or –by means of duplex sonography Intracranially on both sides the M1 segments of the middle cerebral artery, the internal carotid artery, the V4 segments of the vertebral artery and the basilar artery as well as possibly detectable further cerebral arteries

sensitivity of duplex sonography to blood flow signals in the cerebral arteries (Llompart-Pou et al. 2009).

23.2.3 Examination Procedure

Transtemporal Insonation

For the transtemporal examination it is recommended to start in a depth of 60–65 mm (Table 23.2). Since the distal cerebral media often no longer shows any flow at high intracranial pressure values, the examination should be performed as close as possible to the bony carotid siphon. In rare cases, however, due to anatomical variations in this area, no sufficient signal can be found, so that all other depths between 50 and 75 mm must also be evaluated.

Since it can be very difficult to trace small systolic spikes in individual cases, examination should be started at maximum transmission energy. Occasionally this approach can be additionally optimized by maximally increasing the measurement volume, and in some devices also by extending the "ultrasonic signal burst." In addition, the signal amplification of the device should be set as high as diffuse artifact dots appear on the entire screen even without vessel recordings (Fig. 23.4). The latter is also indispensable for documentation. In order to reliably exclude false-positive findings, it is always necessary to avoid suppression of flow curve components with weaker signals.

Practical Tips

If the bone window is insufficient, signal intensity can be improved by raising blood pressure with medication and/or additional intravenous administration of ultrasound signal amplifiers. In the vast majority of cases, after raising arterial pressure with catecholamines or after bolus administration of an ultrasound signal intensifier, at least transmitted vascular pulsations in the Doppler spectrum can be detected as minimal systolic rashes, supporting possible evaluation of cerebral perfusion (Llompart-Pou et al. 2009).

Evaluation of the Vertebrobasilar System

The vertebrobasilar vascular system must always(also) be evaluated, since, especially in patientswith primary supratentorial damage, the assessment of the posterior cerebral circulation allows statements to be made about the failure of the entire cerebral circulation. Current German guidelines place different demands on Doppler and duplex sonography. Doppler sonography only requires extracranial recording of the vertebral arteries, duplex sonography only intracranial recording of the V4 segments of the vertebral arteries and the basilar arteries. At a depth of 65–70 mm at least one vertebral artery can almost always be detected. Due to the common distal course, differentiation of the vertebral arteries is not absolutely necessary. Assuming unfavourable examination conditions in the intensive care unit, frequent hypoplasia of a vertebral artery often permits evaluating only the one with the larger calibre.

Since the vertebral artery can give off branches supplying skin and muscles, "halfway normal" flow signals may occur in this vessel in individual cases, despite an existing cerebral circulatory arrest, (false-negative findings). According to current guidelines, this situation can only be resolved by duplex sonography providing real time imaging of the intracranial sections of the vertebral artery all the way up to the basilar artery.

Practical Tips
In order not to have to turn the patient to the side for transnuchal evaluation of the vertebral and basilar arteries, the back of the head may be placed on the ball of the hand behind the patient. The probe can then be placed and positioned with the fingers in the cavity created between the back of the head and the shoulders. Alternatively, a pillow or bolster can be used to support the head. However, the probe must be inserted and positioned from the side into the abovementioned cavity.

23.2.4 Problems of Transtemporal Assessment

The main problem in Doppler sonographic assessment of cerebral circulatory arrest is an undetectable flow signal from the anterior cerebral basal arteries. Temporary elevation of blood pressure or use of signal amplifiers may be helpful. If the latter are not available or no Doppler signal can be recorded, differentiation between present and absent blood flow or respectively, examination problems due to an insufficient temporal sound window are not possible. According to the current guidelines, prove of cerebral circulation arrest at the extracranial brain-supplying arteries is sufficient.

However, evaluation limited to extracranial examination, provides an increased rate of false-negative findings. Due to increased elasticity of the arteries, in younger patients, a triphasic signal with an antegrade late-diastolic component may occur (Fig. 23.5), which cannot be regarded as evidence of cerebral circulatory arrest with sufficient certainty. Blood flow in the ophthalmic artery also may contribute to the flow signal in the extracranial internal carotid artery. By demonstrating oscillating flow, extracranial duplex examination can ensure cerebral circulatory arrest whereas atypical findings do not permit reliable conclusions.

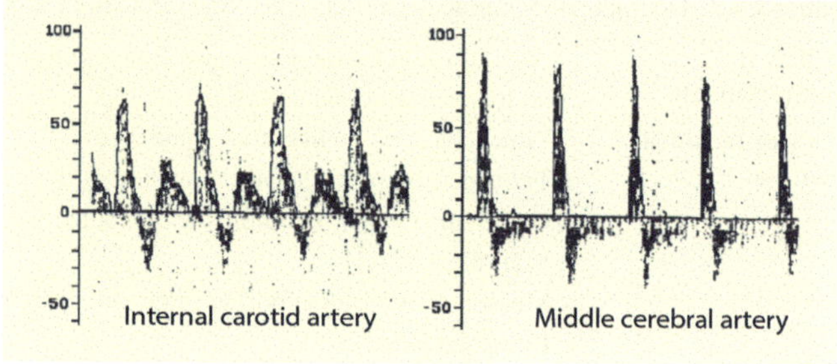

Fig. 23.5 Triphasic flow pattern in the extracranial internal carotid artery (left) in an 18-year-old patient with clear evidence of cerebral circulatory arrest (oscillating flow) during insonation of the intracranial arteries (right)

False-Positive Findings

False-positive results – which are not acceptable in the practical application of the method – can be excluded by strictly applying the criteria mentioned in the Table 23.2. In patients with larger cranial bone defects, caution is recommended, however, even if in this case false-negative findings are to be expected due to the lack of increase in intracranial pressure (Ducrocq et al. 1998). In individual cases a residual flow signals may occur in circumscribed outer brain areas, while the large brain base arteries indicate cerebral circulatory arrest (von Reutern et al. 2009). According to current German guidelines, Doppler or duplex sonography cannot be used to diagnose cerebral circulation arrest in this situation.

False-Negative Findings

False-negative findings are less problematic, since in worst case they lead to an only delayed diagnosis of brain death than would actually have been possible.

Essentially 5 sources of error are to be considered.

Tachycardia

With pronounced tachycardia above approx. 120/min, typical pulse curve forms of cerebral circulatory arrest may no longer be recognizable due to superimposition of the pulse waves, preventing a clear statement (Fig. 23.6). ◄

Arteriovenous Fistulas

Spontaneous or traumatic intracranial AV fistulas can complicate ultrasound assessment, since locally limited flow signal with a high diastolic content may occur

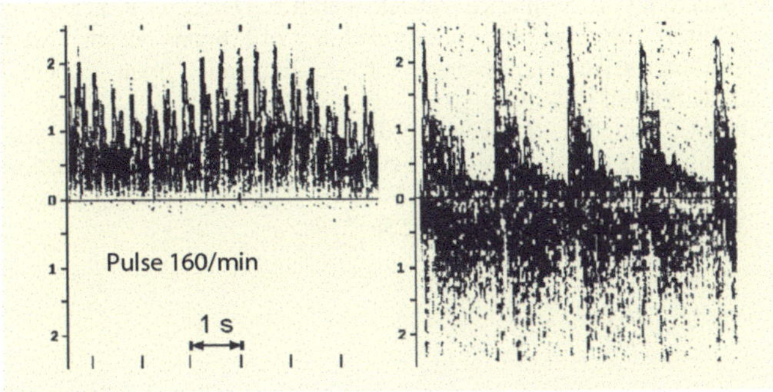

Fig. 23.6 Problem situations of ultrasound examination in cerebral circulatory arrest. Not clearly assessable pulse curve in extreme tachycardia (left). Only the conspicuous respiratory modulation indicates a highly increased intracranial pressure. AV fistula (right) which can be recorded isolated at a depth of 75 mm with simultaneous presence of "small systolic spikes" in the cerebral artery (not shown)

(Fig. 23.6). Even if a clear oscillating flow or "small systolic spikes" can be detected in the distal cerebral artery on both sides, a secure diagnosis of a circulatory arrest cannot be considered according to current guidelines. ◄

Prolonged Brain Death

Finally, there are very rare patients with a long-standing irreversible loss of brain function, in whom cerebral pressure has already fallen after regression of cerebral edema and autolysis of the brain. Cerebral vascular signals may be detectable again. Although these are arteriovenous short circuits without functional results, they make Doppler sonographic (and angiographic) assessment impossible. ◄

Open Fontanel

Transcranial Doppler sonography is not very useful in detecting cerebral circulatory arrest in infants. Due to the still open fontanelles, there is no clear coupling between the functional state of the brain and the cerebral pressure and, respectively the cerebral blood flow in the first months after birth. On the other hand, if the typical Doppler signals of a cerebral circulatory arrest are found in all brain arteries of slightly older infants, this can of course be used as a reliable sign. ◄

Large Open Skull Injuries

The situation with large open skull injuries corresponds to that with open fontanel. The same applies to craniotomized patients, even if the Doppler/duplex criteria of cerebral circulation arrest are met due to stable duraplasty. ◄

23.2.5 Requirements for the Examiner

With regard to the qualification of the examiner the German guidelines demand that: "The examination must be performed by a physician who is specifically experienced in this method".

23.2.6 Requirements for the Status Report

According to German guidelines, the findings report should contain the following information in addition to the usual information (question, description of findings, assessment): Examination time (date, time), blood pressure (arterial mean pressure or systolic and diastolic blood pressure), designation of the displayed arteries with the type of the respective detected flow signals (early systolic spikes, biphasic flow with equally pronounced integral of the antegrade and retrograde components, perfusion obtained, no flow signal detectable); in case of missing transcranial flow signals, if necessary,comparison with the preliminary examination performed by the same examiner; name of the examining/reporting physician and form of archiving the derived flow signals (paper printout or digital). If an organ or tissue donation is performed after determination of brain death (if necessary by performing Doppler or duplex sonography), the findings report (not necessarily the individual original image printouts) has to be archived for 30 years in Germany.

Summary

Transcranial Doppler and transcranial duplex sonography are accepted in Germany as methods for the irreversibility detection of brain function loss according to the guidelines of the German Medical Association. If typical signals (oscillating flow, small systolic peaks) are found in the anterior and posterior arteries supplying the brain when examined twice at 30-minute intervals, evidence of cerebral circulatory arrest has been provided. False-positive findings are not known, false-negative statements are possible in individual cases.

References

Ducrocq X, Hassler W, Moritake K, Newell DW, von Reutern GM, Shiogai T, Smith RR (1998) Consensus opinion on diagnosis of cerebral circulatory arrest using Doppler-sonography. Task Force Group on cerebral death of the Neurosonology Research Group of the World Federation of Neurology. J Neurol Sci 159:145–150

Gosling RG, King DH (1974) Arterial assessment by Doppler-shift ultrasound. Proc R Soc Med 67:447–449

Homburg AM, Jakobsen M, Enevoldsen E (1993) Transcranial Doppler recordings in raised intracranial pressure. Acta Neurol Scand 87: 488–493

Llompart-Pou JA, Abadal JM, Velasco J, Homar J, Blanco C, Ayestarán JI, Pérez-Bárcena J (2009) Contrast-enhanced transcranial color sonography in the diagnosis of cerebral circulatory arrest. Transplant Proc 41:1466–1468

von Reutern GM, Wilms G, Vancalenbergh F, Demaerel P, Dubois B (2009) Angiographic confirmation of brain death after decompressive craniectomy for posttraumatic brain oedema. JBR-BTR 92:78–79

Walter U, Schreiber SJ, Kaps M (2016) Doppler and Duplex Sonography for the diagnosis of the irreversible cessation of brain function ("brain death"): current guidelines in Germany and Neighboring countries. Ultraschall Med 37:558–578

24 Ultrasound in Revascularization Procedures

Bernhard Widder and Gerhard F. Hamann

24.1 Revascularizing Interventions of the Carotid Artery

According to consistent study results, carotid endarterectomy is indicated for symptomatic carotid stenosis with a stenosis degree of more than 70% (German guideline for the diagnosis, therapy and aftercare of extracranial carotid stenosis, AWMF guideline number 004/028). In addition to the diagnosis of stenoses (Chap. 13) to determine the indication for such an intervention, ultrasound diagnostics is of major importance in follow-up examinations after revascularization procedures. In contrast, the benefit of intraoperative sonographic monitoring is rather questionable.

24.1.1 Intraoperative Monitoring in Carotid Surgery

A more recent meta-analysis (Udesh et al. 2017) examined the value of transcranial Doppler sonography for the prediction of perioperative strokes. From 25 studies, almost 5000 patients were evaluated in summary, in which 189 perioperative strokes had occurred. A decrease in the flow velocity as well as the occurrence of microembolic signals in the middle cerebral artery increased the probability of perioperative strokes by a factor of 4. Data on the combination of electrophysiological and ultrasound methods are not available.

The S3 guideline for the diagnosis, therapy, and follow-up care of extracranial carotid stenoses is cautious about the benefits of both electrophysiological and sonographic monitoring:

– Intraoperative neuromonitoring during carotid endarterectomy is not evidence-based, but in case of pathological findings it may help to indicate a shunt during clamping time.
– Since patients with contralateral occlusion are at higher risk of perioperative stroke, they could be operated under regional anesthesia with wakefulness monitoring.

24.1.2 Postoperative Findings

Duplex sonographic checks after carotid artery surgery are standard of care. The method of choice for direct examination of the surgical site is color coded duplex sonography, preferably using relatively low-frequency sound probes due to the frequent swelling of the neck.

Practical Tips
If the carotid bifurcation cannot be assessed with the usual extracranial linear probe in the first postoperative days due to the existing swelling in the neck, the transcranial or an abdominal probe can be used.

Stenoses occurring postoperatively can be reliably detected sonographically, so that contrast-agent-based CT or MRI check-ups are usually unnecessary (Fig. 24.1). Depending on the etiology, the stenoses are presented sonographically differently. Furthermore, the time of their appearance after the operation is characteristic of the underlying cause (Table 24.1).

Practical Tips
According to the German guideline for the diagnosis, therapy and follow-up care of extracranial carotid

(continued)

B. Widder (✉)
Expert Opinion Institute, District Hospital, Guenzburg, Germany
e-mail: bernhard.widder@bkh-guenzburg.de

G. F. Hamann
Clinic of Neurology and Neurological Rehabilitation, District Hospital, Guenzburg, Germany

B. Widder, G. F. Hamann (eds.), *Duplex sonography of the brain-supplying arteries*, https://doi.org/10.1007/978-3-662-65566-5_24

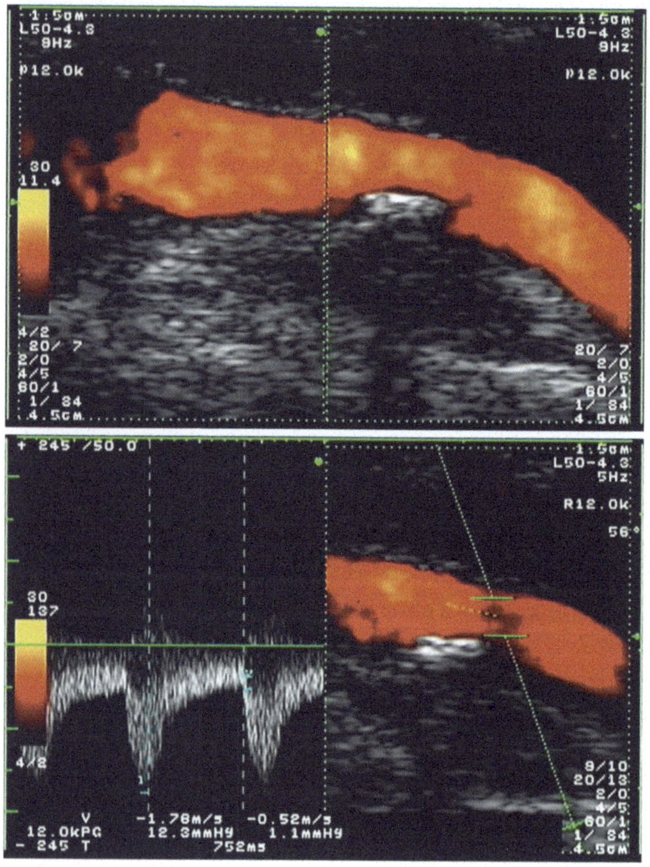

Fig. 24.1 Moderate stenosis due to residual echogenic plaque at the transition of the distal excision area to the internal carotid artery with sonographic control on the fourth postoperative day

stenoses, a non-invasive – preferably sonographic – control after carotid surgery or stent implantation should be performed after 1 month, 6 months and 1 year – thereafter at annual intervals.

Additional Information

In rare cases, duplex sonography can be used to detect a (clinically asymptomatic) occlusion of the internal carotid artery postoperatively. This finding is more frequent in the case of a previously highly stenosed internal carotid artery with post-stenotic constriction and sufficient collateralization, so that a combination of thrombogenic inner vessel wall in the surgical area and a greatly reduced flow velocity must be suspected as the cause.

The expected findings are also determined by the surgical technique used (Fig. 24.2), which will be explained in more detail below (Table 24.2).

Complications After Carotid Endarterectomy with Direct Suture

With this surgical technique, which is rarely performed today, the stenosing intima cylinder is removed after a longitudinal incision of the common-internal transition and the incision is then closed with a direct suture. Postoperatively, the following areas require special attention.

Proximal Border of Resection

Due to the sharp-edged resection border, a step formation or even a dissection of the remaining intima may occur at the proximal edge of the surgical area. Sometimes this leads to a freely floating intima (Fig. 24.3). Since the vessel is quite wide in this area, stenoses caused by this are rare. In contrast, short dissections immediately before the actual surgical area are characteristic for injuries to the vessel wall during clamping of the common carotid artery (Fig. 24.4). In this localization, a higher degree of stenosis can occur up to the mostly spontaneous degradation of the intimal layer. Longer dissections are very rare and can occur, for example, when the shunt is advanced caudally (Fig. 24.5). ◄

Table 24.1 Assessment of the etiology of postoperative stenoses of the carotid artery as a function of the time of their occurrence and duplex sonographic findings

Complication	Verifiability/findings
Residual stenosis	Detectable immediately postoperatively Preferred location at the transition of the distal operating area to the internal carotid artery Stenotic plaque with a sonomorphology comparable to preoperative (Fig. 24.1)
Seam interface retraction	Detectable immediately postoperatively Preferably at the distal patch or suture end for open peeling plastics Very short-stretched ("line-shaped" or "pointy" protruding into the vessel lumen)
Intimal hyperplasia	Detectable within approx. 6–12 months postoperatively, but not immediately postoperatively In the entire operating area, stenosis maximum preferably distal, as the vessel is slimmest here Low echo (only visible in the color coded sectional view)
Arteriosclerotic restenosis	Detectable later than 12 months postoperatively No preferred localization Variable sectional image display

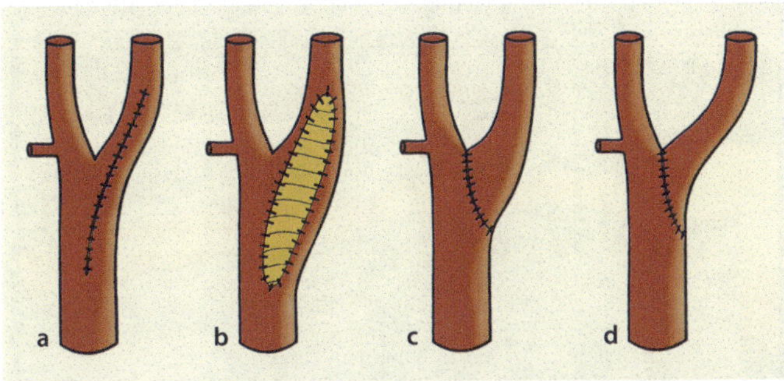

Fig. 24.2 (a–d) Morphological appearance of the carotid bifurcation after surgery. Peeling plastic with direct suture (**a**), peeling plastic with patch (**b**), eversion arterectomy (**c**), shortening operation for buckling (**d**)

Practical Tips

The finding of an intimate flexion floating in the bloodstream confronts the examiner with the difficult question of how to deal with it. Experience shows that small dissections of less than 1 cm in length reattach themselves to the vessel wall or are degraded within 1–2 weeks. Thus, in such cases, despite the impressive findings, it is possible to wait for a while, provided that there is no hemodynamically critical residual stenosis.

Suture Area

Sewing the vessel together does not prevent a slight narrowing of the vessel lumen. Since the carotid bulb is usually significantly wider than the distal internal carotid artery, this rarely results in a relevant stenosis. A suture-related stenosis is when the diameter of the vessel in the exit region of the internal carotid artery falls below that of the distal vessel. ◄

External Carotid Artery

The intima cylinder resected during carotid surgery regularly also includes the outlet of the external carotid artery, but is usually only roughly detached there. This can lead to external stenoses or even occlusions caused by rolled up intimate flews. Although functionally and clinically insignificant, they can cause some confusion during the sonographic examination. As in the case of the common carotid artery (see above), the lip usually reattaches itself or is removed after a few weeks, so that the external carotid artery can be drained again with a normal flow signal during follow-up examinations. ◄

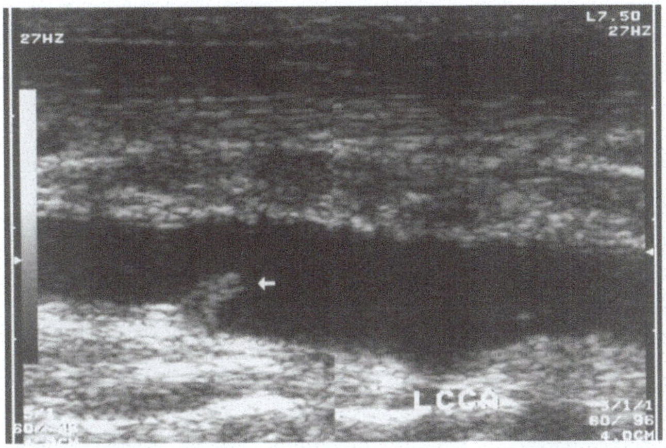

Fig. 24.3 Intimal dissection in the common carotid artery at the proximal end of the operating area with intimal flexion in the bloodstream

Distal End of the Resection

Since a clean cutting edge at the distal end of the excision is technically much more difficult to achieve in the internal carotid artery than in the easily accessible common carotid artery, the risk of recurrent stenosis due to small intimadiscs is highest in this area. Due to the often poorly accessible location below the jaw angle, a clean suture can only be achieved with some effort, so that this is also the predilection site for suture retraction. In addition, this is where the risk of intimal hyperplasia is greatest (Fig. 24.6). Accordingly, special attention must be paid sonographically to the distal end of the excision. To assess the degree of constriction of recurrent stenosis, the sufficiently known sonographic criteria must be used. ◄

Complications After Carotid Artery Endarterectomy with Patch

With this technique, too, the stenosing intima cylinder is first removed after a longitudinal incision of the vessel. In order to avoid operation-related vasoconstriction, however, a strip of

Table 24.2 Sonographically recognizable local complications after surgical measures on the carotid artery

Surgical technique	Carotid artery	Operating area	Internal carotid artery
Direct suture	Intimate level, dissection (also clamping-induced)	Relative stenosis, distal suture retraction	Intimal hyperplasia, step, dissection, kinking
Patch insertion	Intimate level, dissection (also clamping-induced)	Superimposed or floating thrombi, aneurysms ("real," "false," "secondary"), infection, distal suture retraction	Intimal hyperplasia, step, dissection, kinking
Eversionarterectomy	Clamping-induced dissection	Seam retraction	Intimal hyperplasia, step, dissection, kinking
Vessel shortening	Clamping-induced dissection	Seam retraction	Persistent buckling

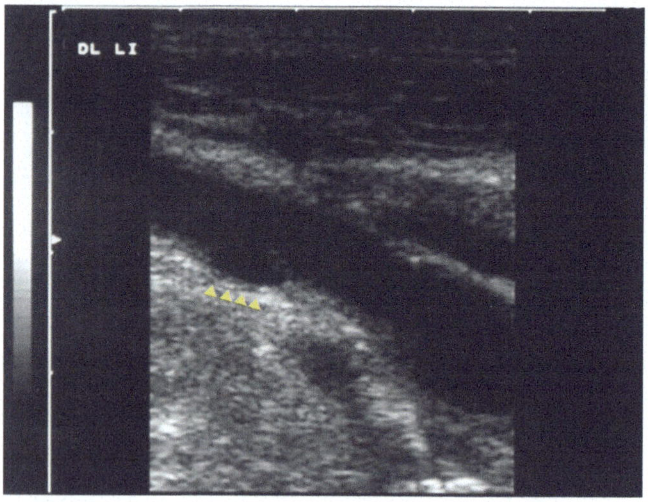

Fig. 24.4 Short-distance intimal dissection in front of the operating area due to clamping-related vascular wall injury

plastic or autologous vein, the so-called **patch,** sewn in. This is usually 2–4 cm long and leads to a certain expansion of the vessel in the operating area. In the sectional image it is regularly clearly visible – provided it is made of plastic – and, as expected, the flow velocity in this area is reduced by Doppler sonography.

Pathological findings at the proximal and distal end of the surgical field are identical to those of the "carotid artery endarterectomy with direct suture" (see above). The following complications may occur due to the patch itself.

Secondary Aneurysm

If the width of the patch is too large (**overpatching**), a considerable aneurysmatic dilatation of the vessel may occur. Due to the resulting reduction of the flow velocity,

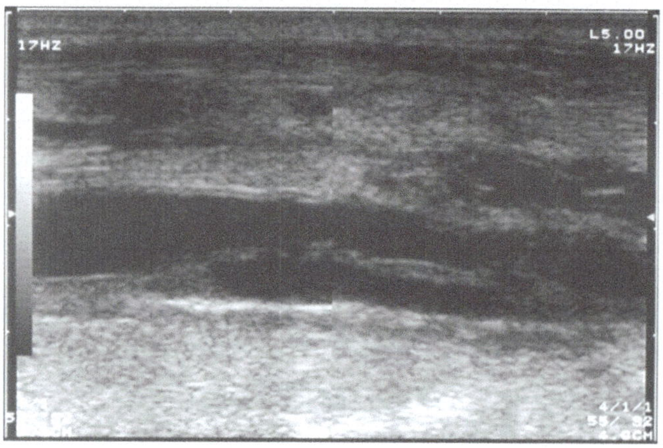

Fig. 24.5 Longer dissection of the common carotid artery, caused by advancing the shunt caudally. Intraoperatively fixed distally to prevent tearing cranially

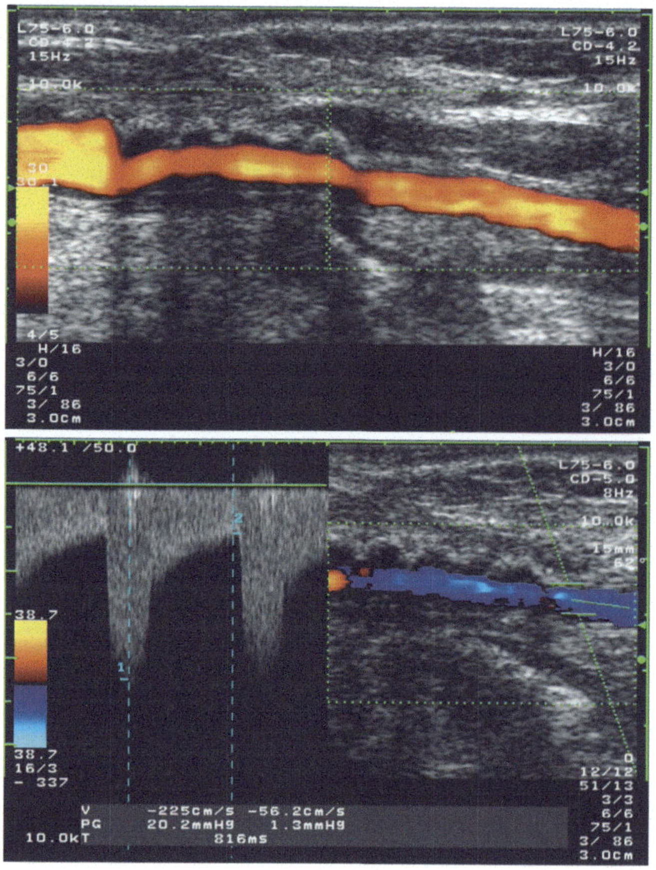

Fig. 24.6 Long-distance residual stenosis of the patch area with stenosis maximum at the distal end of the patch due to intimal hyperplasia. Control after three months postoperatively

thrombotic deposits are not uncommon and can usually be delimited by duplex sonography without difficulty. A vessel diameter of more than 14–15 mm (Sect. 19.3.1) can be classified as pathological. Experience has shown that in most cases the further accumulation of thrombi ceases as soon as the residual flow channel in the patch area has reached the diameter of the internal carotid artery distal to the surgical site, and the findings are not associated with an increased risk of cerebral infarction. ◀

Real Aneurysm

When using a vein patch, an aneurysm develops in rare cases due to the physiological wall weakness of the vein, which can be easily detected by duplex sonography. ◀

False Aneurysm

If the suture is leaking or burst, blood leaks into the adjacent connective tissue. In relatively rare cases, this does not lead to thrombosis of the hematoma, but rather to the formation of a connective tissue pulsating cavity

(continued)

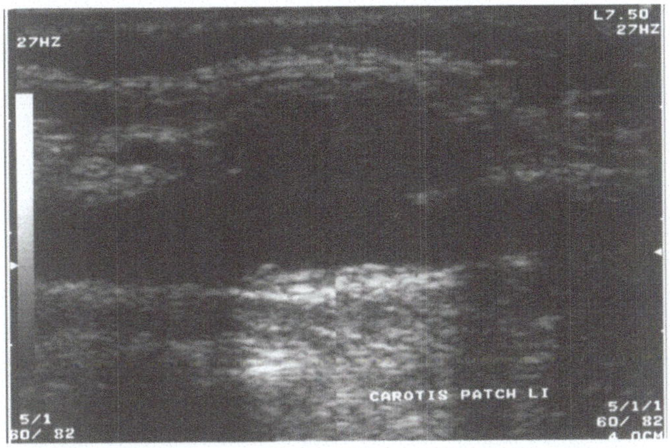

Fig. 24.7 "False" aneurysm (aneurysm spurium) in the area of a vein patch in suture failure. Notice the roundish, low-echo structure above the vascular cord, which can only be delimited from the vessel in a suggestive manner

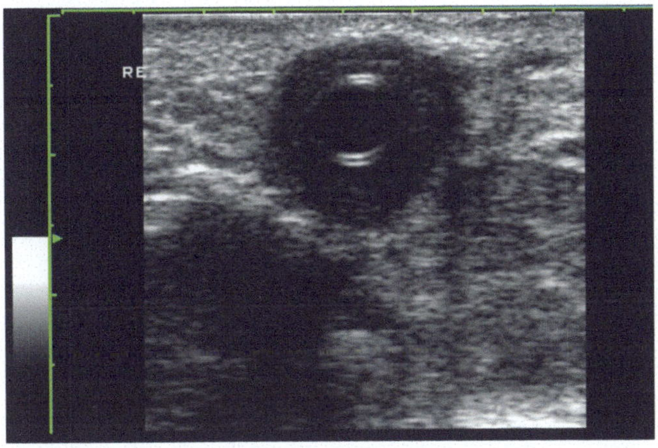

Fig. 24.8 Infected interposition after segmental carotid resection. Mantle-shaped low-echo area around the vascular prosthesis

into which blood flows during systole and out again during diastole. A typical sonographic finding in such a case is a low-echo cavity separated from the original vascular lumen, which is blurred (Fig. 24.7). The original vessel wall is in most cases at least partially still recognizable.

Infected Patch

When using a plastic patch, a septic or even aseptic foreign body reaction occurs in very rare cases. This can be recognized sonographically by the fact that a fuzzily defined, low-echo zone appears on the outside of the patch. In contrast to the "false" aneurysm, this is not hemispherical but elongated and lies like a mantle around the vessel wall (Fig. 24.8). ◀

Kinking Formations

Due to the relatively low elasticity of plastic patches, kinking may occur at the distal end, the extent of which can be easily assessed using color coded duplex sonography. ◀

Complications After Eversion Endarterectomy

In this procedure, the internal carotid artery is severed at its outlet and the outer wall of the vessel is "rolled up" like a stocking over the stenosing intima cylinder. This is finally cut off and the remaining outer wall of the vessel is re-inserted into the internal carotid artery. Compared to open peeling plastic surgery, this procedure has the advantage that suture problems occur less frequently, while step formations and dissections are to be expected more frequently.

Complications After Shortening Surgery

The method of choice for eliminating kink and loop formations of the internal carotid artery is the shortening of the affected vessel. For this purpose, the internal carotid artery is first severed, similar to the eversion arteriotomy. After mobilization of the bent or loop-shaped vessel, an attempt is then made to straighten the vessel and, after appropriate shortening, to reinsert it in a largely stretched state into the common carotid artery.

The most common problem with such shortening operations is the fact that the kink was usually already congenitally present and the vessel wall in the area of the kink is considerably inelastic and thickened. Therefore it can be difficult to achieve an extension of the kinked vessel, so that postoperatively there is a certain increase of the kink angle, but the kink formation as such still exists. Such a situation is to be expected especially if the kink is relatively far distally below the base of the skull and could not be included in the shortening of the vessel. During postoperative ultrasound examination, therefore, persistent kink formations below the base of the skull must be observed. The proximal insertion site is usually not a problem.

Additional Information
Although numerous studies on duplex sonographic controls after carotid reconstruction are now available, almost all of them have in common that only a very global distinction is made between "inconspicuous findings" and the presence of "recurrent stenosis." This procedure is not very helpful for the assessment of surgical results, since – as shown in detail in this chapter – numerous postoperative abnormalities of very different dignity can occur. Since these can

(continued)

generally be recorded by duplex sonography without difficulty, abnormal findings after vascular surgery should always be described in detail in terms of their type, position and extent, as well as their significance for hemodynamics.

24.1.3 Carotid Stenting

Even after carotid stenting, color coded duplex sonography is the method of choice to check the local findings. With the exception of the rare case of a stent with a far cranial end, this method is normally successful in visualizing the dilatation area/stent as well as the caudally and cranially adjacent vascular regions.

Stenoses and Occlusions After Stenting

Since the plaque is not removed, but pressed against the vessel wall, it is not unusual for the lumen or stent to show a certain waist after the procedure. The extent of this is largely determined by the composition of the plaque and is naturally stronger in calcified plaque than in initially atheromatous stenosis. The S3 guideline for the diagnosis, therapy and aftercare of extracranial carotid stenosis therefore requires a control after 4 weeks to exclude an early stent thrombosis (Fig. 24.9).

Probably due to the reduced vascular elasticity in the stent area, the flow velocities measured inside the stent by Doppler sonography are regularly higher than those expected in a healthy vessel. Values of up to 200 cm/s can be detected without residual or recurrent stenosis (Lal et al. 2008; Table 24.3).

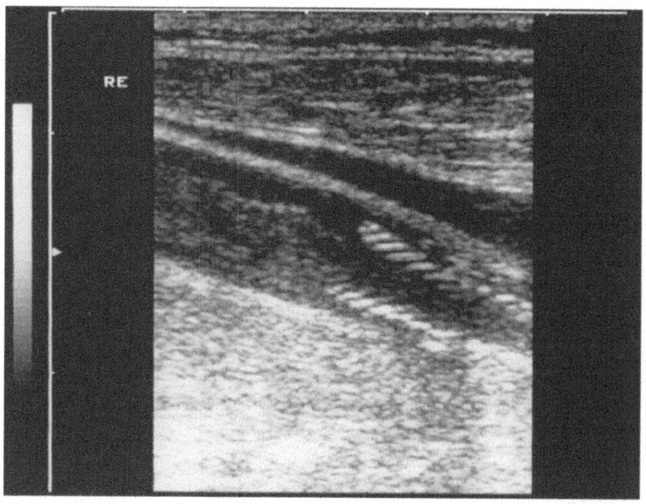

Fig. 24.9 Stent thrombosis 6 days after the interventional procedure in case of initially severe carotid stenosis

Table 24.3 Assessment of increased flow velocities within a carotid stent (according to Lal et al. 2008)

Flow velocity	Degree of stenosis
≥ 220 cm/s	50%
≥ 340 cm/s	70%

Additional Information
Occlusion of the external carotid artery is particularly observed when the stent extends, as regular seen, into the common carotid artery and covers the external outlet. Clinically these remain asymptomatic, as after carotid operations.

Other Postinterventional Complications

Besides general complications, the following complications can be observed sonographically after carotid stenting.

Stent Dislocation

The cause of the rare finding of a stent dislocated distally is usually a disproportion between the width of the expanded stent and the artery. ◀

Stent Fracture

In exceptional cases, fractures within the stent can be observed under high mechanical stress and low flexibility of the selected stent material. ◀

Kinking at the Distal Stent End

With an initially curved course of the internal carotid artery and a relatively long stent, the artery in the stent area may be stretched due to the "stiffness" of the stent with abrupt bending of the vessel at the distal end of the stent. ◀

24.1.4 Hyperperfusion Syndrome

After carotid operations, a normalization of pathological collateral supply can be expected regularly. In some patients, however, the ipsilateral middle cerebral artery immediately after carotid surgery shows a significantly increased perfusion with reduced pulsatility compared to the other side. The frequency of this phenomenon varies widely in the literature, ranging from less than 1% to more than 50%. This may be mainly due to the fact that there is no general consensus on what is meant by such "hyperperfusion." According to the experience of the authors, significant hyperperfusion should only be referred to when the flow velocity increases by 50%

or more compared to normal values – especially when comparing the sides.

The primarily unspecific sonographic findings of hyperperfusion can be compared with the clinical picture of a **"hyperperfusion syndrome"** characterized by severe ipsilateral headaches, epileptic seizures and also cerebral hemorrhages (Wang et al. 2017). It is a rare syndrome affecting only 0.18% of patients. Risk factors are female gender, a major stroke within the last 30 days before surgery, contralateral carotid stenosis over 70% stenosis, coronary heart disease, perioperative blood pressure lability and cardiac complications during surgery. The presence of significant hyperperfusion requires, according to S3 guidelines for diagnosis, therapy and follow-up of extracranial carotid stenosis, timely cerebral imaging (CT) and blood pressure regulation with systolic blood pressure below 140 mm Hg.

Summary
Color coded duplex sonography is the method of choice for postoperative control after reconstructive procedures on the carotid artery. Any abnormalities can be clarified in a differentiated manner (e.g., intimal hyperplasia, dissection, suture retraction, aneurysm). If local examination conditions are unfavorable due to bleeding or edema, indirect sonographic examination procedures are helpful. In the first postoperative days, transcranial Doppler and duplex sonography can be used to rule out possible hyperperfusion.

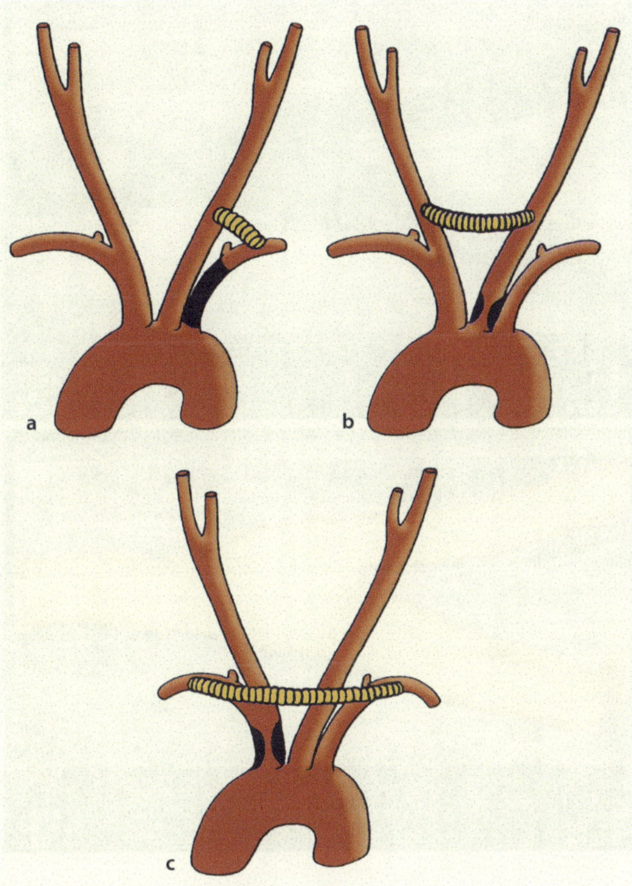

Fig. 24.10 (**a–c**) Most common extracranial bypass types. Carotid-subclavian bypass (**a**), carotid-carotid bypass (**b**), axillo-axillary bypass (**c**)

24.2 Supraaortic Bypass Operations

The primary postoperative control of extracranial bypass types (Fig. 24.10) is performed clinically by comparative pulse palpation. Only secondarily, color coded duplex sonography is added to check the local findings and the effects on the brain-supplying arteries affected.

Sonographic Findings in the Bypass Area

With the exception of the rarely performed bypass operations with direct connection to the aortic arch, a non-physiological flow pattern is typical for all other types, since the blood flow leading to the distal side is redirected proximally at the beginning of the bypass at a more or less acute angle. Accordingly, there is regularly an auscultating noise in this area and, correlating to this, Doppler sonographically pronounced detachment phenomena. The method of choice for assessing the suture points is sectional sonography, which generally produces clear results even without the color coded technique (Fig. 24.11).

Effects on Brain-Supplying Arteries

The effects of a bypass operation on the blood flow in the arteries supplying the brain can be easily assessed by duplex sonography if the subclavian or axillary arteries are also affected. Due to the disturbed flow at the site of the bypass and the associated loss of pressure, an only slight improvement in blood flow in the vertebral arteries compared to the preoperative findings, for example, the transformation of a complete into an incomplete steal effect, is not unusual and should not be considered pathological. A definite pathological finding is only present if a subclavian steal effect is detectable postoperatively to an unchanged or even increased degree.

Summary
When controlling bypass operations near the aorta, the assessment of the suture points in the sectional image is the main focus. Flow disturbances at the exit of the bypass are not to be considered pathological and occur regularly.

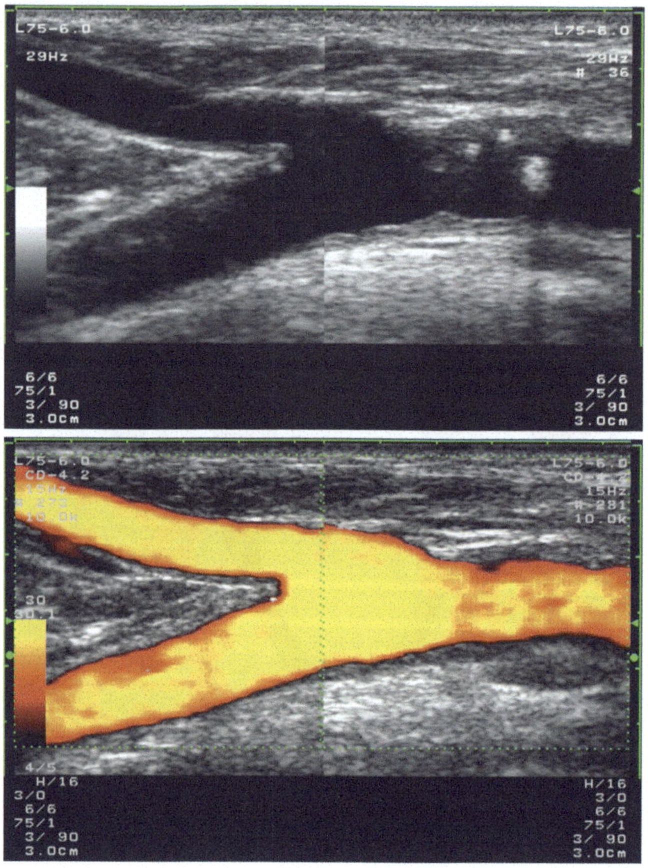

Fig. 24.11 Sonographic image of a carotid-subclavian vein bypass. Secondary findings: tangentially incised, non-stenosing plaque in the common carotid artery cranial of the bypass

24.3 Extra-intracranial Bypass Surgery

Extracranial to intracranial bypass surgery (EC-IC), which was introduced in the 1960s, is intended to improve the blood supply to the affected hemisphere in patients with severe constrictions of the intracranial internal carotid artery and/or middle cerebral artery. In the "classical" technique, a branch of the superficial temporal artery is microsurgically connected to a branch of the cerebral artery in the M2/M3 segment (so-called STA-MCA bypass) through a small drill hole in the area of the temporal scale as an end-to-side anastomosis (Fig. 24.12).

Due to the negative results of a large randomized study (EC/IC Bypass Study Group 1985), this technique disappeared from the surgical repertoire of most neurosurgical clinics in the mid-1980s. As a case-by-case decision, however, such procedures are still performed in some neurosurgical centers (Neff et al. 2004; Sandow et al. 2013). The indication has to be set very strictly, since an EC-IC bypass study conducted with modern methods of patient selection (Powers et al. 2011) also yielded a negative result.

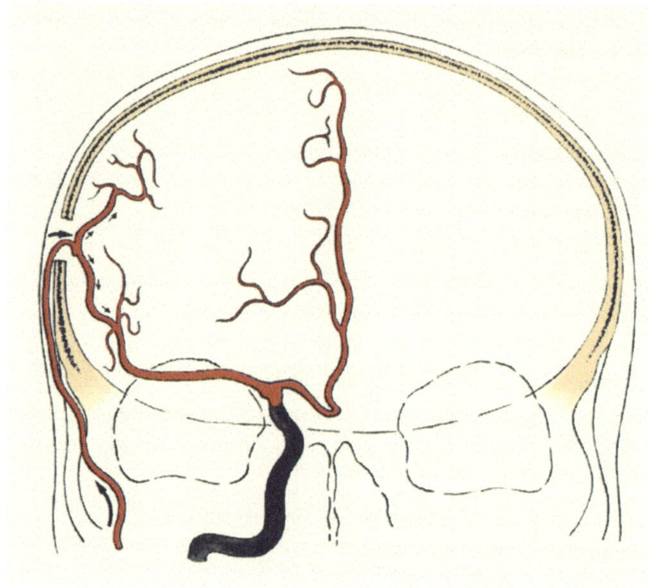

Fig. 24.12 Technique of extra-intracranial bypass surgery by connecting the superficial temporal artery to a branch of the cerebral artery

24.3.1 Preoperative Diagnostics

Sonographic Assessment

The indication for extra-intracranial bypass surgery can be supported sonographically by three examination findings.

Evidence of Hemodynamic Failure

The Doppler sonographic determination of the cerebrovascular reserve capacity (Chap. 12) can be used as a basic filter to determine the extent to which an extra-intracranial bypass may be useful and necessary. ◀

Evidence of an Intact External Carotid Artery

The basic prerequisite for the creation of an extra-intracranial anastomosis is an intact external carotid artery without high-grade stenoses. The assessment is carried out according to the criteria mentioned in Chap. 13 ◀

Evidence of a Large Caliber Superficial Temporal Artery

Another basic requirement for the hemodynamic benefit of an STA-MCA bypass is a sufficiently large caliber superficial temporal artery. This assessment can easily be made using color coded duplex sonography. The vessel is shown in longitudinal section immediately in front of the ear and can be followed cranially into the parietal branch, which is usually of a larger caliber, and more rarely into the frontal branch. ◀

Clinical Significance

All three sonographic criteria mentioned contribute to the indication of an extra-intracranial bypass. Of particular

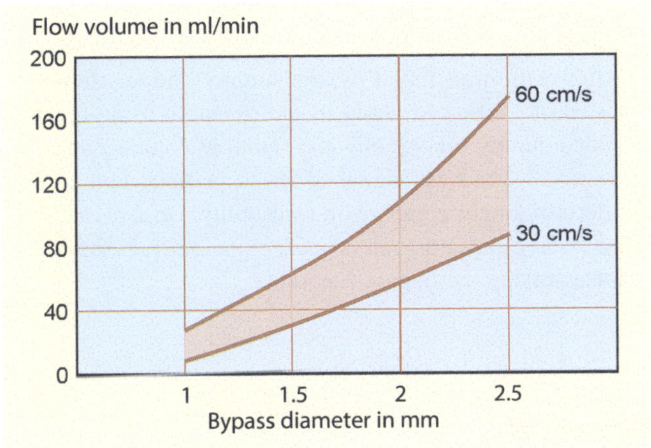

Fig. 24.13 Flow volumes to be expected in an extra-intracranial bypass in relation to the diameter of the anastomosis vessel, based on average flow velocities of 30–60 cm/s

importance is the evaluation of the superficial temporal artery as a donor vessel, which has hardly been considered in the literature so far. For obvious hemodynamic reasons, such an anastomosis can only contribute significantly to cerebral perfusion if a relevant amount of blood reaches the brain via the bypass. Based on the fact that the hemispheric blood flow is usually 200–250 ml/min and the anterior communicating artery can achieve 150–200 ml/min of collateral flow with good functional capability, a relevant contribution of extra-intracranial anastomosis can only be expected for flow physiological reasons if the diameter of the superficial temporal artery is 1.8–2 mm (Fig. 24.13).

24.3.2 Postoperative Findings

Sonographic Assessment

3 parameters are available for sonographic examination of the function of extra-intracranial anastomoses.

Assessment of Pulsatility

In functional anastomoses, the supplying superficial temporal artery (predominantly) becomes a brain-supplying vessel. In preauricular derivation there is therefore a significantly reduced pulsatility in the Doppler spectrum, which is typical for the brain arteries. ◀

Measurement of Flow Volume

With the help of color coded duplex sonography, the bypass in the area of the borehole can be followed regularly from the outside to the inside (Fig. 24.14). Using the usual criteria, local constrictions can be detected and,

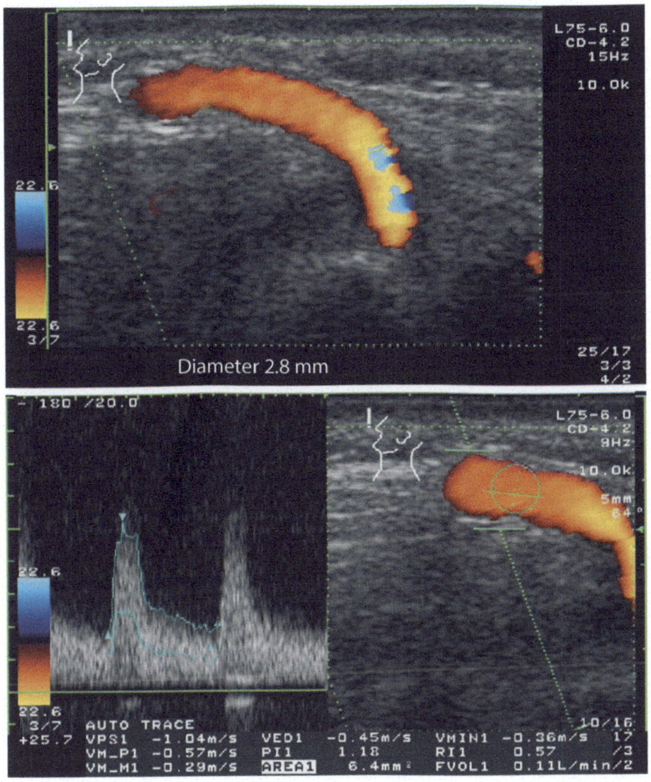

Fig. 24.14 Control examination after extra-intracranial bypass surgery. If discharged in the area of the drill hole, strong visualization of the bypass with a diameter of approx. 2.0 mm and a flow volume of approx. 110 ml/min

above all, the flow volume in the bypass can be measured. Although the accuracy is not very high due to the small vessel diameter of usually approx. 2 mm (Sect. 5.3.3), it is sufficient to check the development of the anastomosis during the course of the procedure. Experience has shown that the attainable flow volume will not exceed 100–200 ml/min even in the final state, but in the best case it will be of the order of magnitude that would be expected from an anterior communicating artery muscle with an intact circle of Willis. ◀

Assessment of the Intracranial "Watershed"

Due to the existing bone defect, the examination conditions are particularly favorable for transcranial color coded duplex sonography. The color coded directional detection makes it possible to regularly determine the "watershed" between the blood flow from the outside via the bypass and the blood flow from the inside via collateral vessels and to check this in the course of the examination (Fig. 24.15). ◀

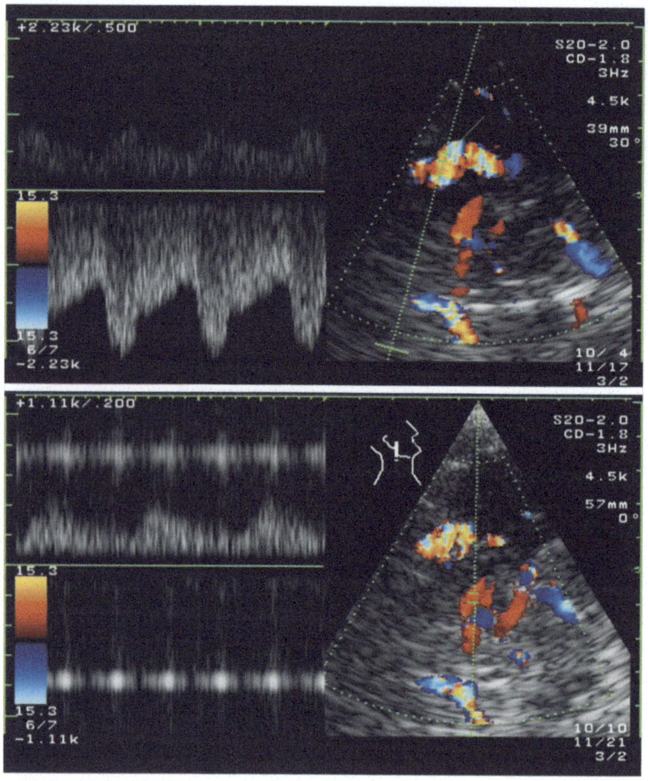

Fig. 24.15 Transcranial axial color duplex image after extra-intracranial bypass surgery in the case of an occlusion of the ipsilateral internal carotid artery. In the vicinity of the bypass a strongly perfused vessel is visible (top). In contrast, the ipsilateral middle cerebral artery shows (unchanged) only a flattened, low flow signal (approx. 20 cm/s systolic) (bottom)

Note

Due to the increased ultrasound energy radiation into the brain tissue in the case of bone defects, the examination time with the transcranial Doppler and duplex probe after bypass operations should be kept as short as possible and the transmission power reduced.

Summary

After extra-intracranial bypass surgery, the anastomosis can be followed along its entire length using color coded duplex sonography and the flow volume can be assessed. The flow signal of the superficial temporal artery in lateral comparison (pulsatility, cerebrovascular reserve capacity) can be used as an indirect criterion for assessing the bypass function.

References

EC/IC Bypass Study Group (1985) Failure of extracranial-intracranial arterial bypass to reduce the risk of ischemic stroke. Results of an international randomized trial. N Engl J Med 313:1191–1200

Lal BK, Hobson RW 2nd, Tofighi B, Kapadia I, Cuadra S, Jamil Z (2008) Duplex ultrasound velocity criteria for the stented carotid artery. J Vasc Surg 47:63–73

Neff KW, Horn P, Dinter D, Vajkoczy P, Schmiedek P, Düber C (2004) Extracranial-intracranial arterial bypass surgery improves total brain blood supply in selected symptomatic patients with unilateral internal carotid artery occlusion and insufficient collateralization. Neuroradiology 46:730–737

Powers WJ, Clarke WR, Grubb RL Jr, Videen TO, Adams HP Jr, Derdeyn CP, COSS Investigators (2011) Extracranial-intracranial bypass surgery for stroke prevention in hemodynamic cerebral ischemia: the Carotid Occlusion Surgery Study randomized trial. JAMA 306:1983–1992

Sandow N, von Weitzel-Mudersbach P, Rosenbaum S, König S, Buchert R, Mehl SR, Garbe A, Vajkoczy P (2013) Extra-intracranial standard bypass in the elderly: perioperative risk, bypass patency and outcome. Cerebrovasc Dis 36:228–235

Udesh R, Natarajan P, Thiagarajan K, Wechsler LR, Crammond DJ, Balzer JR, Thirumala PD (2017) Transcranial Doppler monitoring in carotid endarterectomy: a systematic review and meta-analysis. J Ultrasound Med 36:621–630

Wang GJ, Beck AW, DeMartino RR, Goodney PP, Rockman CB, Fairman RM (2017) Insight into the cerebral hyperperfusion syndrome following carotid endarterectomy from the national Vascular Quality Initiative. J Vasc Surg 65:381–389

25 Cardiac Right-Left Shunt

Bernhard Widder and Gerhard F. Hamann

Cardiac right-left shunts, which are found in the diagnostic work-up of verebrovascular diseases, are almost without exception caused by atrial septum anomalies, that is, a patent foramen ovale or an atrial septal defect. Ventricular septal defects as well as large atrial septal defects that extend to the valve level and involve the mitral valve usually become symptomatic in infancy and childhood due to their hemodynamic effects in the pulmonary and body circulation. The frequency and importance of non-cardiac right-left shunts, especially intrapulmonary shunts, can only be speculated. Although thcsc non-cardiac shunts are regularly suspected when left-atrial contrast medium is detected without echocardiographically visible intracardiac contrast medium passage, they are rarely verified directly.

25.1 Anatomy and Pathophysiology

An patent foramen ovale (PFO) as a residual of the prepartum fetal circulation is found in 34% of adolescents and young adults according to extensive sectional statistics. In middle age the incidence is 25%, while in old age (>80 years) a PFO can only be detected in about 20% of cases (Hagen et al. 1984). The size varies between 1 and 11 mm, increases with age and is 5 mm in the median.

In the literature the term open foramen ovale sometimes also includes an atrial septal defect. Even if the morphological differences seem to be rather small, the functional differences are considerable:

- **Atrial septal defect (ASD).** Missing overlap between septum secundum and septum primum in an area of the atrial septum with the consequence of a permanently open shunt.
- **Patent foramen ovale (PFO).** The septum primum spans the fossa ovalis and overlaps the septum secundum in the entire rim area, but has not (sufficiently) grown on it (Fig. 25.1). This results in a valvsalva mechanism which becomes effective when the right atrial pressure is increased.

The occurrence of a right-left shunt in the presence of an PFO thus presupposes a short-term or chronic increase in pressure in the right atrium. Thrombi, for example, as a result of deep vein thrombosis of the leg, can thus enter the arterial system and lead to a cerebral embolism (**paradoxical embolism**).

25.2 Clinical Significance

For many years there was considerable controversy as to whether the closure of a PFO in "cryptogenic" stroke is capable of preventing further stroke recurrences. Previous studies did not provide clear results in this regard. In 2017, three studies have been published which prove the benefit of implanted closure systems.

The CLOSE study (Mas et al. 2017) enrolled 663 patients, two thirds of whom had a PFO with a large shunt. In the approximately 5-year follow-up period, none of the patients suffered a further event after PFO closure, whereas this was the case in 14 patients under medical therapy. Most strokes occurred in patients who had both a PFO and an atrial septal aneurysm.

Also in the Gore REDUCE study (Søndergaard et al. 2017) with 664 patients and a proportion of 80% with medium to large PFO, 20% of them with atrial septal aneurysm, a benefit of PFO occlusion compared to platelet aggregation inhibition alone was shown with a reducing the risk of

B. Widder (✉)
Expert Opinion Institute, District Hospital, Guenzburg, Germany
e-mail: bernhard.widder@bkh-guenzburg.de

G. F. Hamann
Clinic of Neurology and Neurological Rehabilitation, District Hospital, Guenzburg, Germany

B. Widder, G. F. Hamann (eds.), *Duplex sonography of the brain-supplying arteries*, https://doi.org/10.1007/978-3-662-65566-5_25

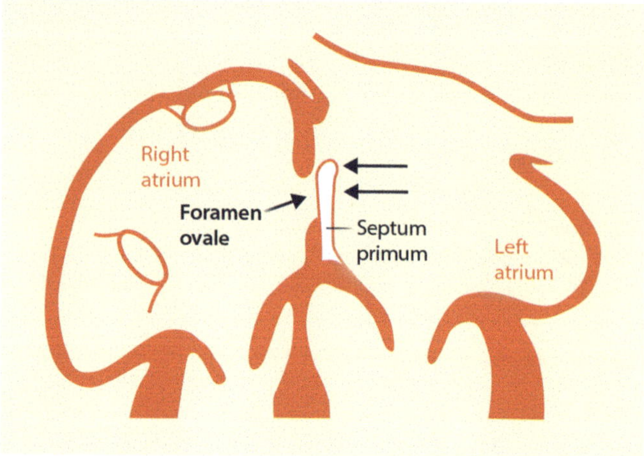

Fig. 25.1 Anatomy of the foramen ovale. The fetal open connection between the two atria normally closes postpartum during the first year of life by fusion of the septum primum with the surrounding tissue

stroke in the course of the approximately 3-year follow-up by 50%.

Comparable results were ultimately also found in the RESPECT study (Saver et al. 2017), which had not yet shown a significant benefit of PFO closure in 980 patients in the primary analysis after 2 years. In the follow-up over 4 years, however, a risk reduction of 45% was found in the intervention group.

25.3 Detection by Echocardiography

To detect a cardiac right-left shunt, transesophageal echocardiography (TEE) is the method of choice (Homma et al. 2016). Its advantage over transcranial Doppler sonography is the direct detection of the shunt and cause of the shunt and the detection of possible other cardiac pathologies. In contrast, transthoracic echocardiography (TTE) is of no importance in the detection of right-left shunts, since it does not have sufficient accuracy (Belkin et al. 1994; Di Tullio et al. 1993).

In clinical practice, however, swallowing disorders, aphasia, neglect or somnolence in patients with stroke can present significant obstacles to transesophageal echocardiography. Additional problems in performing Valsalva maneuvers may be a lack of cooperation by sedation, but also incomplete glottal closure when the esophageal probe is in place. This makes the examination quite complex, relatively uncomfortable for patients and not always reliable.

25.4 Detection by Transcranial Doppler sonography (PFO Test)

Transcranial Doppler sonography is an easy to perform alternative to transesophageal echocardiography with high sensitivity and specificity. The results are also only slightly dependent on the examiner. Only right-left shunts of small magnitude are overlooked in individual cases, but this does not significantly limit the usefulness of the method.

25.4.1 Ultrasonic Contrast Medium

The detection of a PFO in transcranial Doppler sonography requires the intravenous injection of a ultrasound contrast medium which is not able to passage the lung vascular bed. At present, agitated saline solution is the most suitable method. Here, 6–7 ml of isotonic 0.9% saline solution is mixed with 1–2 ml of the patient's own blood and 0.2 ml of room air between two syringes until a dense foam forms and no individual air bubbles are visible. The blood portion serves to stabilize the air microbubbles that have formed, which are retained over a period of 30–60 s, thus improving the reliability of the test (Gentile et al. 2014).

Practical Tips
When preparing the ultrasonic contrast medium, it is recommended to use disposable syringes with screw thread. Otherwise, when the solution is forced to move back and forth between the syringes, their connecting cone can slip out of the three-way stopcock, causing hygiene problems.

25.4.2 Doppler Sonographic Settings

Doppler derivation during transcranial contrast medium Doppler sonography is most reliable with simultaneous derivation of both middle cerebral arteries in the main trunk region (60–65 mm depth) by 2 probes fixed to the head. In clinical routine, however, one-sided measurement with a hand-held probe seems sufficient, but in this case a helper is required for the application of the contrast medium. For unilateral examinations, the drainage of the left middle cerebral artery is recommended, since microbubbles flow preferentially into the left carotid for anatomical reasons (Devuyst et al. 1997). Alternatively, color coded duplex sonography can of course also be used as a method for recording the Doppler signal (Blersch et al. 2002).

25.4.3 Performing the PFO Test

Immediately after preparation, at least 5 ml of the ultrasound contrast medium is administered intravenously as a bolus within a maximum of 2–3 s via a sufficiently thick cannula to achieve the highest possible contrast medium density in the right atrium. The patient should lie down and the arm with the injection cannula should be at body height.

Additional Information
Studies by Hamann et al. (1998) show that the sensitivity of the test is better when the contrast agent is injected into the femoral vein than when it is applied into the arm vein. This is due to the direct flow from the inferior vena cava to the foramen ovale. For reasons of practicability, however, this procedure is rarely used. However, as the "second-best" method, care should be taken to inject into the right arm, as this allows a greater density of contrast medium to be achieved in the right atrium. In any case, the PFO test should be performed with at least two passes with different sequences (see overview below).

PFO Test During Valsalva Maneuver
To activate the valvsalva effect in an open foramen oval, the right-atrial pressure should be increased significantly. 10 s after application of the contrast agent bolus, the patient is asked to perform a Valsalva maneuver with holding air and pressing for a period of about 5 s. In the case of a cardiac right-left shunt, the microembolic signals caused by the injected vesicles usually occur within a few seconds after the end of the maneuver. If no microembolic signals appear in the first run, the same procedure should be repeated in the second run with a latency reduced to 5 s between the injection of contrast medium and the start of the Valsalva maneuver.

Practical Tips
In contrast to echocardiography, coughing during the Valsalva maneuver is less appropriate for the PFO test, since the probe artifacts that occur during this procedure cause difficulties in identifying microembolic signals and lead to a lower specificity of the test.

PFO Test Under Normoventilation
If microembolic signals appear after the Valsalva maneuver, it is necessary to clarify in the second run whether the shunt is effective without increasing the right-atrial pressure. Here the patient is asked to breathe evenly and calmly. In a positive case, microembolism signals usually appear in the Doppler sonogram of the drained basal brain artery about 5–10 s after contrast medium injection.

Procedure of the Transcranial PFO Test
- Preparation
  - Lying position of the patient
  - Explanation and practice of the Valsalva maneuver
  - Preferred measurement of the left cerebral media in the outflow area from the internal carotid artery (60–65 mm depth)
  - Preferred puncture of the right antecubital vein in the area of the elbow
  - Preparation of at least 10 ml ultrasound contrast medium
- First pass
  - Bolus injection of 5 ml contrast medium
  - 10 s after injection, perform the Valsalva maneuver previously practiced with the patient
  - 5 s Duration of the Valsalva maneuver
  - 20–25 s Observation time after injection
- Second pass, if many microembolic signals occur during the first pass
  - Bolus injection of 5 ml contrast medium
  - Let patients breathe calmly
  - 20–25 s Observation time after injection
- Second pass, if no microembolic signals occur in the first pass
  - Repeat the procedure as in the first round, but start the Valsalva maneuver already 5 s after contrast injection

Additional Information
It is crucial for the success of the Valsalva maneuver that it begins as precisely as possible when the maximum contrast density in the right atrium has been reached. In the case of a cubital injection site and the exclusion of cardiac insufficiency with relevant venous congestion, this is the case approx. 10 s after the start of the injection (Heinel 1999; Fig. 25.2).

Practical Tips
Effective execution of the Valsalva maneuver can be checked by means of the Doppler sonographic flow curve by decreasing the flow speed and increasing the pulse frequency during the pressing process and opposite reactions at the beginning of the subsequent normoventilation.

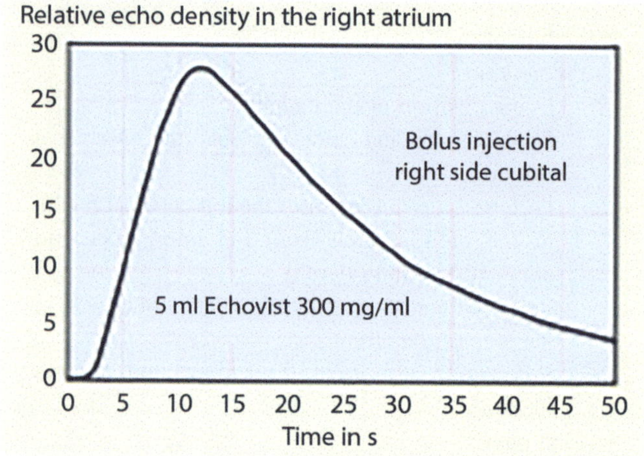

Fig. 25.2 Average increase in right atrial echo density relative to baseline density (relative echo density) after right-cubital bolus injection of 5 ml Echovist 300 mg/ml

25.4.4 Doppler Sonographic Findings

Detection of a Right-Left Shunt

Even the occurrence of a single microembolic signal formally indicates the presence of a right-left shunt, even if this finding is functionally and clinically irrelevant.

Very small, exceptionally longer persisting vesicles can enter the arterial system by passage of the pulmonary capillary network – even without postulating a pulmonary shunt. Since only single microbubbles are involved, it is not to be expected that a functionally relevant shunt will be diagnosed false positive. False-negative findings can occur if the Valsalva maneuver starts too early or too late and the contrast medium has not yet or has already passed the right atrium. A sufficiently exact "timing" of the maneuver and, if necessary, repetition with altered latencies is therefore recommended. This should at least allow the diagnosis of larger shunts for which a connection with cerebral ischemia can be suspected.

PFO and/or ASD as Shunt Cause

Based on the assumption that microbubbles reach the cerebral vascular system earlier via an intracardiac shunt than especially via an intrapulmonary shunt, short latencies between contrast agent injection and the occurrence of microembolic signals are evaluated as an indication of a PFO and/or an atrial septal defect. However, since the latency times for such cardiac and pulmonary shunt causes overlap to a not inconsiderable extent, no reliable differentiation is possible in individual cases (Horner et al. 1997). Taking this limitation into account, a detection time of 20–25 s after contrast medium injection is recommended for the detection of a cardiac shunt (Droste et al. 1999).

Extent of a Right-Left Shunt

On the basis of the detected microembolic signals the shunt extent can be estimated semi-quantitatively (Table 25.1, Fig. 25.3). A continuous "shower" of microembolic signals without individually delimitable signals is referred to in the Anglo-American literature as **curtain** (Jauss and Zanette 2000). Microembolic signals even without Valsalva maneuvers additionally indicate a permanent shunt, for example, in the case of an atrial septal defect.

There are no investigations on the relationship between the Doppler sonographic estimated shunt size and the size of an underlying open foramen ovale.

Table 25.1 Evaluation of the shunt extent using the microembolic signals detected in a middle cerebral artery during Valsalva maneuvers. (after Jauss and Zanette 2000)

Quantity the microembolic signals	Shunt size
≤10	Minimal
>10, but still individually countable	Medium
Full-length "shower." not more individually countable	Large

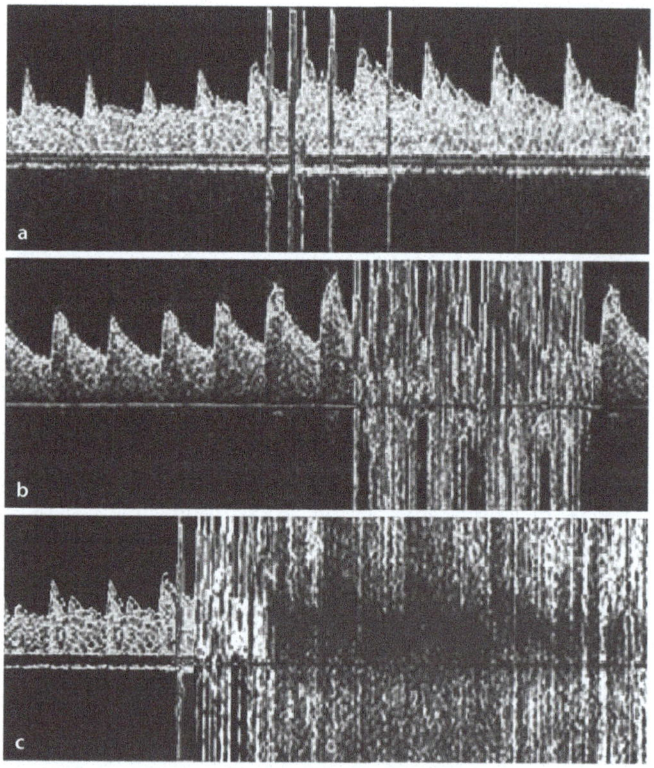

Fig. 25.3 Different degrees of microembolic signals in the middle cerebral artery. (**a**) single bubbles, (**b**) just single count "bubbles," (**c**) continuous "shower"

25.4.5 Side Effects

A risk has not yet been identified. In the case of the ultrasound contrast media produced in-house, a risk must always be discussed if larger air bubbles enter the arterial circulation. Complications of this kind have not been described in the literature to date, but have also been little studied. In animal experiments no pathological findings in rabbit brains could be detected after injection of agitated saline solution with small amounts of air into the internal carotid artery (Görtler et al. 1995).

Summary
Transcranial contrast agent Doppler sonography is comparable to transesophageal echocardiography in its accuracy in the clarification of a right-left shunt. If a right-left shunt exists, microembolic signals in the basal arteries of the brain appear a few seconds after intravenous bolus administration of a self-made ultrasound contrast medium made of agitated saline solution and subsequent Valsalva maneuver. The number of detectable microembolic signals provides information about the hemodynamic relevance of a PFO, which is the underlying pathology in most cases. Up to 10 microembolic signals are considered unspecific. The presence of a hemodynamically relevant right-left shunt is considered a risk factor for the occurrence of cerebral ischemia, as this can cause thrombi and gas bubbles (e.g., in diverse and during neurosurgical procedures in a seated position) to pass from the venous to the arterial vascular system.

References

Belkin RN, Pollack BD, Ruggiero ML, Alas LL, Tatini U (1994) Comparison of transesophageal and transthoracic echocardiography with contrast and color flow Doppler in the detection of patent foramen ovale. Am Heart J 128:520–525

Blersch W, Draganski B, Holmer S, Koch H, May A, Bogdahn U, Hölscher T, Schlachetzki F (2002) *Transcranial duplex sonography* in the detection of patent foramen ovale. Radiology 225:693–699

Devuyst G, Despland PA, Bogousslavsky J, Jeanrenaud X (1997) Complementarity of contrast transcranial Doppler and contrast transesophageal echocardiography for the detection of patent foramen ovale in stroke patients. Eur Neurol 38:21–25

Di Tullio MR, Sacco RL, Venketasubramanian N, Sherman D, Mohr JP, Homma S (1993) Comparison of diagnostic techniques for the detection of a patent foramen ovale in stroke patients. Stroke 24: 1020–1024

Droste DW, Kriete JU, Stypmann J, Castrucci M, Wichter T, Tietje R, Weltermann B, Young P, Ringelstein EB (1999) Contrast transcranial Doppler ultrasound in the detection of right-to-left shunts. Comparison of different procedures and different contrast agents. Stroke 30:1827–1832

Gentile M, De Vito A, Azzini C, Tamborino C, Casetta I (2014) Adding blood to agitated saline significantly improves detection of right-to-left shunt by contrast-transcranial color-coded duplex sonography. Ultrasound Med Biol 40:2637–2641

Görtler M, Niethammer R, Khatib Y, Widder B, Pieper KS, Herrmann M (1995) Ultrasound contrast agents: iatrogenic emboli which can Couse focal dilatations or microaneurysms in cerebral arterioles? Stroke 26:732–732

Hagen PT, Scholz DG, Edwards DW (1984) Incidence and size of patent foramen ovale during the first 10 decades of life: an autopsy study of 965 normal hearts. Mayo Clin Proc 59:17–20

Hamann GF, Schatzer-Klotz D, Frohlig G, Strittmatter M, Jost V, Berg G, Stopp M, Schimrigk K, Schieffer H (1998) Femoral injection of echo contrast medium may increase the sensitivity of testing for a patent foramen ovale. Neurology 50:1423–1428

Heinel G (1999) Standardisierung der transkraniell-dopplersonographischen Erkennung des offenen Foramen ovale. Dissertation, Universität Ulm

Homma S, Messé SR, Rundek T, Sun YP, Franke J, Davidson K, Sievert H, Sacco RL, Di Tullio MR (2016) Patent foramen ovale. Nat Rev Dis Primers 21(2):15086

Horner S, Ni XS, Weihs W, Harb S, Augustin M, Duft M, Niederkorn K (1997) Simultaneous bilateral contrast transcranial Doppler monitoring in patients with intracardiac and intrapulmonary shunts. J Neurol Sci 150:49–57

Jauss M, Zanette EM, for the Consensus Conference (2000) Detection of right-to-left shunt with ultrasound contrast agent and transcranial Doppler sonography. Cerebrovasc Dis 10:490–496

Mas JL, Derumeaux G, Guillon B, Massardier E, Hosseini H, Mechtouff L et al. for the CLOSE Investigators (2017) Patent foramen ovale closure or anticoagulation vs. antiplatelets after stroke. N Engl J Med 377:1011–1021

Saver JL, Carroll JD, Thaler DE, Smalling RW, MacDonald LA, Marks DS, Tirschwell DL et al. for the RESPECT Investigators (2017) Long-term outcomes of patent foramen ovale closure or medical therapy after stroke. N Engl J Med 377:1022–1032

Søndergaard L, Kasner SE, Rhodes JF, Andersen G, Iversen HK, NielsenKudsk JE et al. for the Gore REDUCE Investigators (2017) Patent foramen ovale closure or antiplatelet therapy for cryptogenic stroke. N Engl J Med 377:1033–1042

Transorbital Sonography

26

Max Nedelmann

Transorbital sonography of the optic nerve, optic sheath, papilla and central retinal artery is a relatively simple examination technique that can provide important diagnostic information for various diseases. The determination of the diameter of the liquor-filled optic nerve sheath as well as the question of the presence of papilledema in diseases with increased intracranial pressure is of particular importance. A further field of application is the diagnosis of central retinal artery occlusion.

26.1 Examination Procedure

The transorbital ultrasound examination is performed on the lying patient. Gel is applied to the closed upper lateral eyelid and the sound probe is placed in a transversal plane. For better standardization and to avoid bulb movements, the patient may be asked to keep the gaze in the direction of his feet.

Linear array probes used for extracranial vascular diagnostics are also suitable for transorbital ultrasound, but higher frequency probes (>12 MHz) may lead to an improved image quality. In order to exclude a possible danger to the eye, especially the lens, due to thermal or mechanical effects, the transmitting power must be reduced to a mechanical index between 0.1 and 0.3.

> **Note**
> **For transorbital sonography, always reduce the MI to ≤0.3. For examination of the central retinal artery, "low flow" settings are required for color coded duplex sonography.**

M. Nedelmann (✉)
Regio Kliniken GmbH, Clinic for Neurology, Pinneberg, Germany
e-mail: info-regiokliniken@sana.de

26.1.1 B-Scan of the Optic Nerve and Optic Sheath

The low-echo optic nerve is searched for in a longitudinal view, which is regularly successful in its end section. It is surrounded by a structure rich in echo, the liquor-filled optic nerve sheath, which in turn is usually separated from the surrounding tissue by a narrow low-echo seam. The hyperechogenicity of the optic sheath is explained by reflections from a trabecular meshwork (Killer et al. 2011).

Since the subarachnoid space of the optic nerve sheath communicates directly with the intracranial CSF spaces, intracranial pressure changes caused by changes in the diameter of the optic nerve sheath (hereinafter ONSD – "optic nerve sheath diameter") and by the appearance of a papilledema can be detected sonographically.

ONSD is determined by convention at a depth of 3 mm behind the retina (Fig. 26.1). Since certain measurement inaccuracies cannot be excluded, the measurement should be repeated three times and the median value should be used. The zoom function can help. For healthy subjects, ONSD was determined at 5.4 ± 0.6 mm (Bäuerle et al. 2012) – with good agreement with MR tomography (Bäuerle et al. 2013a). In healthy subjects the papilla cannot be delimited.

26.1.2 Imaging of the Central Artery

The central retinal artery as a branch of the ophthalmic artery enters the optic nerve together with the central retinal vein about 10 mm from the bulb and runs centrally until it branches off at the papilla. Within the optic nerve, the artery and the opposite vein can be reliably visualized by color coded duplex sonography (Fig. 26.1).

Care should be taken to set the pulse repetition frequency as low as possible while maintaining a high gain ("low flow" settings). The central retinal artery is located using the color

B. Widder, G. F. Hamann (eds.), *Duplex sonography of the brain-supplying arteries*, https://doi.org/10.1007/978-3-662-65566-5_26

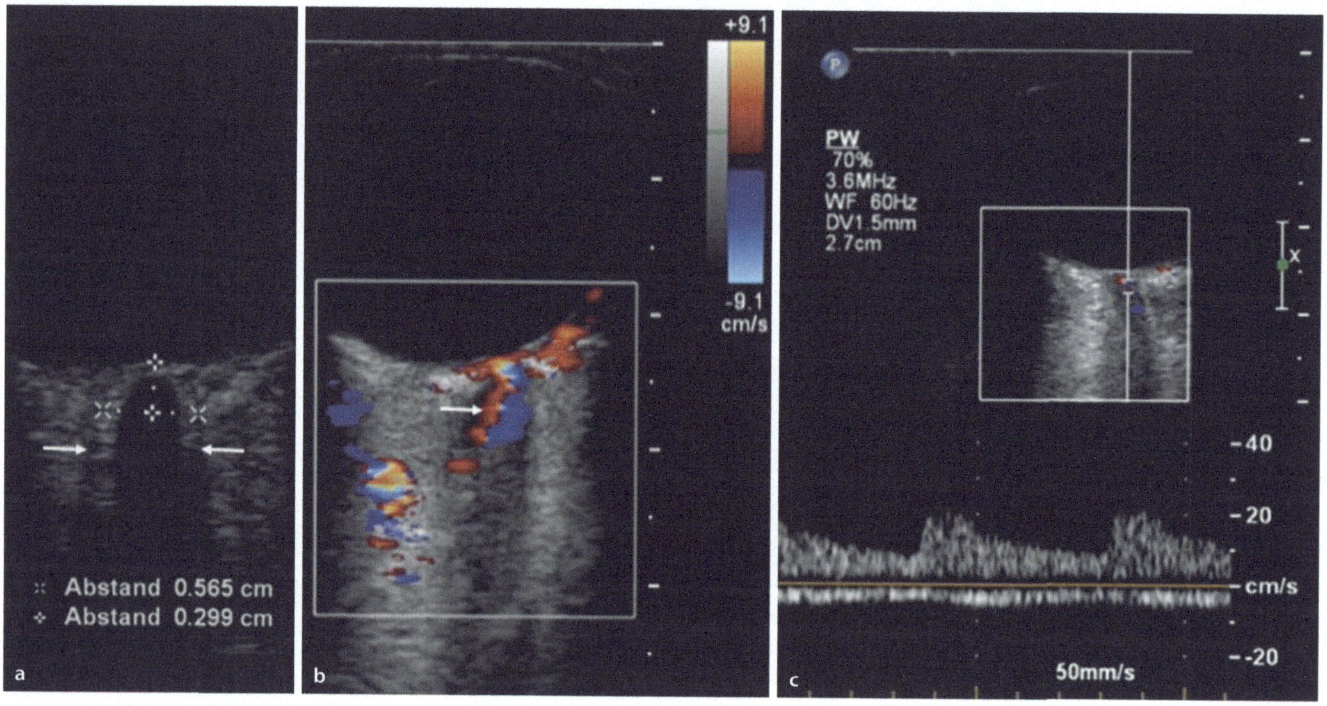

Fig. 26.1 Normal findings of the optic nerve and the central retinal artery. (**a**) Optic nerve (low-echo) and optic nerve sheath rich in echoes, which in turn delimits itself echo-free from the surrounding tissue (arrows). By convention, the diameter of the optic nerve sheath at a depth of 3 mm (vertical pair of measurement points) is determined in the transverse diameter (horizontal pair of measurement points). (**b**, **c**) in the distal course of the optic nerve, the central retinal artery (arrow) and the accompanying (opposite) central retinal vein are regularly shown

Doppler function and the sample volume of the PW-Doppler is placed there. The systolic flow velocity is usually around 10–20 cm/s.

26.2 Increased Intracranial Pressure

Acute and chronic diseases associated with an increase in intracranial pressure lead to an increase in ONSD regardless of their cause (e.g., cerebral pseudotumor, craniocerebral trauma, space-occupying infarcts or bleeding). Patients with cerebral pseudotumor have average values around 6.4 ± 0.6 mm (Bäuerle and Nedelmann 2011), rarely over 8 mm. Other diseases show values in a similar order of magnitude.

A threshold value to differentiate between normal findings and pathologically extended ONSD is given in various studies as 5.8–5.9 mm, with a sensitivity of 90% and a specificity of 85% (Dubourg et al. 2011). The differentiation of pathological findings from normal findings is therefore not always successful; the clinical context is therefore needed.

A papilledema can also be sonographically displayed and its elevation measured. In the clear case, a papilledema is easy to recognize, but comparative work on ophthalmoscopy for borderline cases is missing.

Of particular interest are the temporal dynamics of changes in the optic nerve and papilla. The ONSD shows a prompt reaction after the occurrence and after the removal of the cerebral pressure-increasing event. In the case of the cerebral pseudotumor, a decrease in ONSD can be observed in many patients immediately after therapeutic CSF removal. Sonographically detectable changes in the papilla, on the other hand, develop slowly over a period of several days and regress correspondingly slowly. The method is therefore ideally suited for follow-up examinations under pressure-lowering therapy, for example, for controls after therapeutic lumbar puncture for cerebral pseudotumor or after surgical treatment (Fig. 26.2).

It is interesting to note that in individual cases ONSD may not normalize, so that repeated pressure reliefs, for example, repeated CSF withdrawals, may be necessary until treatment is successful. As a possible explanation for this phenomenon, an opticus compartment syndrome has been postulated, which could be explained by narrow anatomical conditions of the optic nerve sheath in the optic canal (Killer et al. 2011).

26.3 CSF Hypotension

Pathologically reduced CSF pressure is found in dural leakage as a result of fractures of the skull base, neurosurgical interventions, post-puncture or in spontaneous CSF hypotension syndrome. In addition to the typical clinical presentation (e.g., position-dependent headache), the determination of

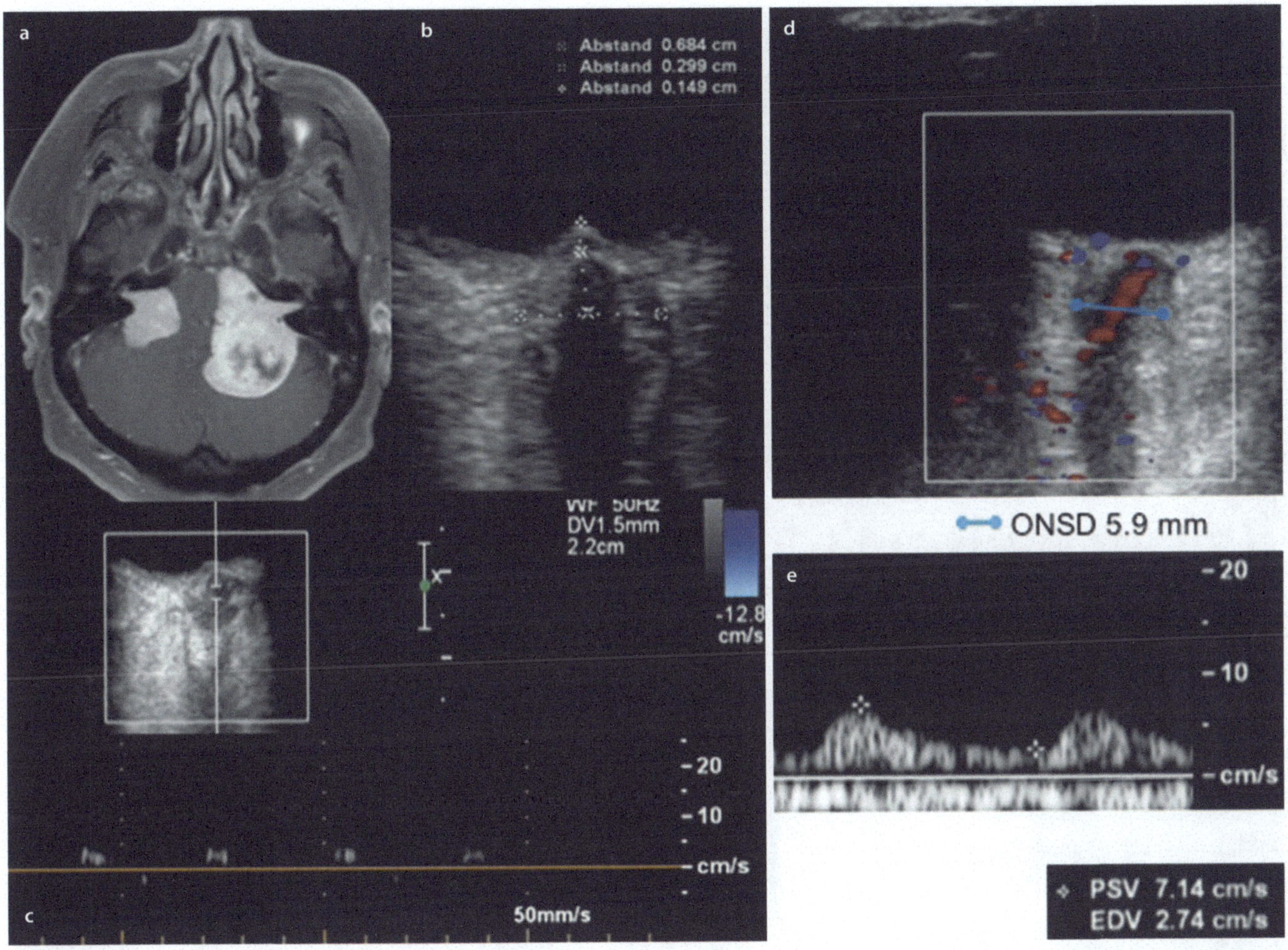

Fig. 26.2 Changes in the optic nerve as a consequence of hydrocephalus occlusus in neurofibromatosis type 2. left: (**a**) The MRI shows extensive acoustic neuroma, which in the patient leads to signs of intracranial pressure and a rapidly progressive reduction in visual acuity (visual acuity around 0.1) (MRI: Klinik für Neuroradiologie, UKE, Hamburg). (**b**, **c**) transorbital ultrasound reveals the typical consequences of an increased intracranial pressure with significant dilatation of the optic nerve sheath and a considerable papilledema, explaining the reduction in visual acuity. An additional consequence of the pressure changes at the optic nerve was a clearly reduced blood flow in the central retinal artery with a Doppler spectrum reduced to systolic peaks. On the right side: (**d**, **e**) following emergency extirpation of the left-sided tumor a rapid reconstitution of visual acuity occurred. The ultrasound showed a regression of the papilledema and the ONSD, as well as normalization of the Doppler signal in the central retinal artery

ONSD as a complementary procedure to other imaging techniques can be helpful and also help to monitor the success of therapy (Bäuerle et al. 2013b; Dubost et al. 2011).

The optic nerve sheath may collapse and be presented with a reduced diameter, but in individual cases the distinction from normal findings may be difficult. Dynamic measurements with comparison in a lying and standing position can then help, whereby the change of position in patients leads to a further reduction of ONSD of 10% on average (Fichtner et al. 2016).

26.4 Central Retinal Artery Occlusion

By use of color coded Doppler sonography, the central retinal artery can be reliably located in healthy persons. Therefore, if sufficient experience is available, the absence of a color coded Doppler signal and absence of a pw Doppler signal at the typical location, in combination with the appropriate clinical syndrome, reliably indicates central retinal artery occlusion (in the following CRAO) (Fig. 26.3). Occasionally, an occlusion signal can also be detected in the central artery; the central vein can still be displayed occasionally. In the course of time, a reopening of the artery after successful treatment or spontaneous recanalization can be well documented (Nedelmann et al. 2015).

B-scan sonography can detect a so-called retrobulbar “spot sign” in a proportion of embolically caused CRAO. This is a dot-like echo rich signal in the central retinal artery that can be easily distinguished from the otherwise low-echo optic nerve (Ertl et al. 2014).

The etiology of the “spot sign” is not clearly explained. There is much to suggest that it is a calcified part of the embolus, as it persists over time (also in the case of a

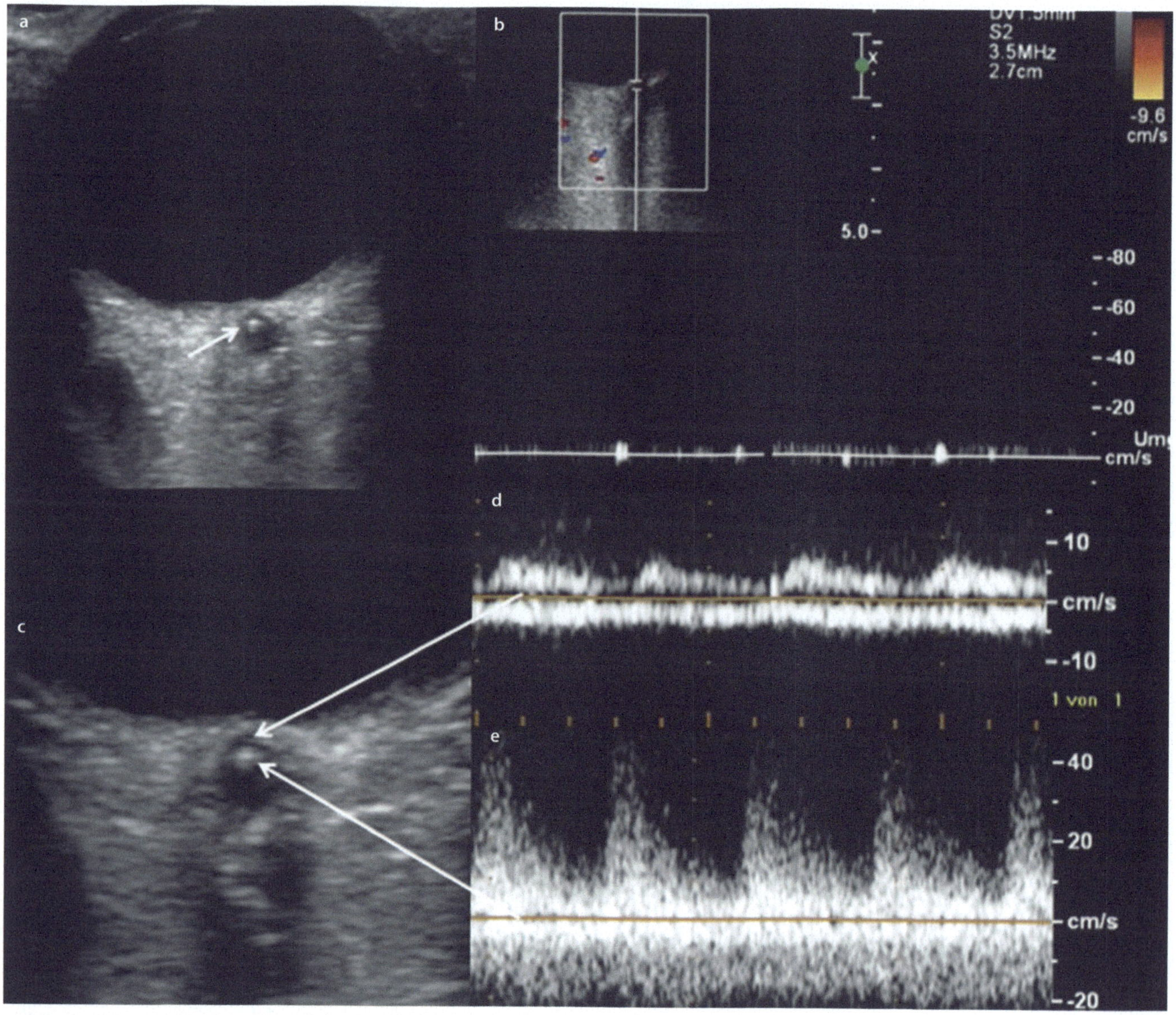

Fig. 26.3 The patient developed a central retinal artery occlusion with persistent loss of vision in the left eye after twice having experienced amaurosis fugax. The typical finding of a retrobulbar spot sign (arrow) in projection on the central retinal artery (**a**), at the same time the occlusion of the artery (**b**). Immediately after successful systemic thrombolysis with complete recovery of visual acuity the spot sign can still be detected (**c**), but Doppler sonography shows a recanalized central artery (**d**), with formation of a stenosis at the level of the spot sign (**e**). The findings were unchanged after 6 months

recanalized artery; Fig. 26.3; Altmann et al. 2015), is more common in atherosclerotic embolism and is a negative predictive marker for the success of thrombolysis. It is not found in vasculitic CRAO, so that the detection of a spot sign in case of CRAO speaks against a vasculitic etiology (Ertl et al. 2012).

Note

The retrobulbar "spot sign" is found in a proportion of embolically caused central retinal artery occlusions, but not in vasculitic etiology. The detection of a spot sign thus largely rules out vasculitic etiology.

Summary
An intracranial pressure increase regularly leads to a dilatation of the optic nerve sheath and to a detectable papilledema. A central retinal artery occlusion can be detected by Doppler sonography, in addition, a so-called "spot sign" is often found in the B-scan. The transorbital findings can be useful in the initial diagnosis to differentiate between vasculitic and embolic etiology as well as in the course of follow-up examinations and therapy control.

References

Altmann M, Ertl M, Helbig H, Schömig B, Bogdahn U, Gamulescu MA, Schlachetzki F (2015) Low endogenous recanalization in embolic central retinal artery occlusion – the retrobulbar "spot sign". J Neuroimaging 25:251–256

Bäuerle J, Nedelmann M (2011) Sonographic assessment of the optic nerve sheath in idiopathic intracranial hypertension. J Neurol 258: 2014–2019

Bäuerle J, Lochner P, Kaps M, Nedelmann M (2012) Intra- and interobserver reliability of sonographic assessment of the optic nerve sheath diameter. J Neuroimaging 22:42–45

Bäuerle J, Schuchardt F, Schroeder L, Egger K, Weigel M, Harloff A (2013a) Reproducibility and accuracy of optic nerve sheath diameter assessment using ultrasound compared to magnetic resonance imaging. BMC Neurol 13:187

Bäuerle J, Gizewski ER, von Stockhausen K, Rosengarten B, Berghoff M, Grams AE, Kaps M, Nedelmann M (2013b) Sonographic assessment of optic nerve sheath collapse and transorbital monitoring of treatment effects in a patient with spontaneous intracranial hypotension. J Neuroimaging 23:237–239

Dubost C, Le Gouez A, Zetlaoui PJ, Benhamou D, Mercier FJ, Geeraerts T (2011) Increase in optic nerve sheath diameter induced by epidural blood patch: a preliminary report. Br J Anaesth 107:627–630

Dubourg J, Javouhey E, Geeraerts T, Messerer M, Kassai B (2011) Ultrasonography of optic nerve sheath diameter for detection of raised intracranial pressure: a systematic review and meta-analysis. Intensive Care Med 37:1059–1068

Ertl M, Altmann M, Torka E, Helbig H, Bogdahn U, Gamulescu MA, Schlachetzki F (2012) The retrobulbar "spot sign" as a discriminator between vasculitic and thrombo-embolic affections of the retinal blood supply. Ultraschall Med 33:E263–E267

Ertl M, Barinka F, Torka E, Altmann M, Pfister K, Helbig H, Bogdahn U, Gamulescu MA, Schlachetzki F (2014) Ocular color-coded sonography – a promising tool for neurologists and intensive care patients. Ultraschall Med 35:422–431

Fichtner J, Ulrich CT, Fung C, Knüppel C, Veitweber M, Jilch A, Schucht P, Ertl M, Schömig B, Gralla J, Z'Graggen WJ, Bernasconi C, Mattle HP, Schlachetzki F, Raabe A, Beck J (2016) Management of spontaneous intracranial hypotension – transorbital ultrasound as discriminator. J Neurol Neurosurg Psychiatry 87:650–655

Killer HE, Jaggi GP, Miller NR, Huber AR, Landolt H, Mironov A, Meyer P, Remonda L (2011) Cerebrospinal fluid dynamics between the basal cisterns and the subarachnoid space of the optic nerve in patients with papilloedema. Br J Ophthalmol 95:822–827

Nedelmann M, Graef M, Weinand F, Wassill KH, Kaps M, Lorenz B, Tanislav C (2015) Retrobulbar spot sign predicts thrombolytic treatment effects and etiology in central retinal artery occlusion. Stroke 46:2322–2324

Part V

Glossary and Standard Values

Glossary of Sonographic Terms

27

Bernhard Widder and Gerhard F. Hamann

Summary
The following compilation provides an overview of the most frequently used special terms in Doppler and duplex sonography.

Acoustic energy	Mechanical energy that is converted into a sound wave. Unit: Joule = Watt × second.
Acoustic shadow	Deletion of ultrasonic signals by sound-impermeable (calcified) structures.
Aliasing	Incorrect measurement of Doppler frequency shift if it exceeds half the pulse repetition frequency (PRF) in pulsed Doppler systems.
Aliasing threshold	Upper limit of Doppler frequency shift that is still correctly displayed in pulsed Doppler and color coded duplex systems.
A-mode (amplitude mode)	Representation of the amplitudes of echo signals as a function of the transit time between echogenic structures and transducer: abscissa= time axis, ordinate = axis of the amplitude of the echo signal. The distance on the time axis indicates the location of the reflection according to the transit time of the echoes.
Amplitude	Peak to peak extension of an oscillating wave.
Angio-mode	Vessel imaging by color coded duplex sonography; see power mode.
Angle correction	Adjustment of the angle between the Doppler sound beam and the vessel axis using a rotatable bar visible in the duplex image (for flow velocity measurements).
Array	Spatial arrangement of ultrasound transducer elements: Linear, annular, and circular
Artifact	False echo signals, usually caused by reverberation, mirroring or blooming
Axial resolution	Minimum discrimination distance between two reflectors in the propagation direction of ultrasound; also called depth resolution or longitudinal resolution, mainly depending on transmission frequency.
B-Flow technique	Method for detecting blood flow by subtracting consecutive ultrasound images.
Bidirectional	Describes the property of Doppler devices to differentiate between flow toward or away from the probe.
B-mode imaging (brightness mode)	Two-dimensional ultrasound image by displaying echo signals on the screen, the amplitude being reproduced by brightness modulation in a gray-scale.
Border zone reflection	Normally narrow, echogenic structure by orthogonal insonation of a vessel defining the vessel vall. See Intima Media Thickness.
Broadband transducer	Transducer with very short sound pulses and a resulting broad spectrum (frequency band) of transmission frequencies.
Color capture	Summation of color coded images taken one after the other for the projection of threedimensional structures in one imaging plane (see also persistence).
Color coded duplex sonography	B-mode imaging with inherent flow information in a color window.
Color window	Box within the B-mode image, in which flow information is displayed color coded

(continued)

B. Widder (✉)
Expert Opinion Institute, District Hospital, Guenzburg, Germany
e-mail: bernhard.widder@bkh-guenzburg.de

G. F. Hamann
Clinic of Neurology and Neurological Rehabilitation, District Hospital, Guenzburg, Germany

B. Widder, G. F. Hamann (eds.), *Duplex sonography of the brain-supplying arteries*, https://doi.org/10.1007/978-3-662-65566-5_27

Confetti effect	Cloudy dots of different colors appearing behind high-grade stenoses in color coded imaging due to vibration effects in the surrounding tissue.
Continuous wave (CW) Doppler	Doppler technique in which sound waves are continuously emitted and received; it works with two piezoelectric crystals (transmitter/receiver).
Curved-array transducer	Transducer with curved arrangement of adjacent piezo crystals, resulting in a trapezoidal image field.
CW Doppler	Continuous transmission and reception of ultrasound in simple extracranial Doppler devices.
Decibel (dB)	Relative measure of the strength two physical signals: Intensity ratio (dB) = 10 * log I1/I2
Degree of carotid artey stenosis	Different classifications for assessing the degree of carotid artery stenoses: Local degree of stenosis: % stenosis=(1 [c/b]) * 100, distal degree of stenosis: % stenosis=(1 [c/a]) * 100. a=poststenotic lumen, b = original lumen in the stenosis area, c = lumen in the stenosis. The experimentally based mathematical formula for conversion between local and distal stenosis degree is; distal stenosis (%) = 1,67 * local stenosis (%), local stenosis (%) = 0.6 * distal stenosis (%).
Delayed systolic rise	Delayed rise of the Doppler pulse curve during systole behind very high grade stenoses (see also Delta signal).
Delta signal	Low-frequency, triangular flow signal without diastolic flow component behind highest-grade stenoses (see also delayed systolic rise)
Depth compensation	Electronic compensation, which compensates for attenuated reflection from deeper tissue layers.
Diastolic ratio	Relative proportion of enddiastolic flow, compared to the systolic value (parameter for assessing peripheral resistance).
Distal color filling	Filling of the entire vessel lumen with color coded flow information behind a high-grade stenosis.
Doppler effect	Frequency shift that occurs when there is relative movement between the transmitter and receiver of a wave front.
Doppler shift	Difference between transmitted and received frequency.
Duplex sonography	Combination of B-mode imaging and Doppler technique.
Dynamic focusing	Variable adjustment of focal points in the ultrasound image.
Early diastolic backflow	Early diastolic retrograde flow component in vessels with high peripheral resistance.
Far field	Range of the sound field beyond the focus.
Fast Fourier transformation (FFT)	Calculation rule for rapid frequency analysis.
Filter	Electronic circuit for suppressing signals of certain frequencies.
Filter, high pass	Device for selecting frequencies above a defined cut-off frequency; such an electrical filter is integrated in a Doppler system, for example, to delimit artifacts in the low-frequency range (e.g., wall movements).
Flow disturbance	Deviation of the flow filaments, distributed over the vessel cross section from the physiological, rotationally symmetrical ("laminar") profile.
Flow profile	Flow profiles are composed of several adjacent flow filaments in a three-dimensional space; physiologically, the flow is lowest in the area of the vessel wall (see Laminar flow); in pathological processes, considerable changes can occur.
Flow separation	Flow disturbance by deflection of flow filaments, for example, in case of vessel dilatations, branches and bends.
Focus	Area of maximum lateral resolution in the field of an ultrasound transducer.
Fourier transformation	Mathematical algorithm for analysing the frequency spectrum of Doppler signals.
Frame rate	Number of new gray-scale or color coded ultrasound images generated within one second.
Frequency	Number of oscillations per second a wave (unit: Hz Hertz; kHz Kilohertz, MHz Megahertz; 1 cycle/s = 1 Hz).
Frequency density spectrum	Representation of the frequency density distribution of the Doppler spectrum at a specific time of the cardiac cycle.
Frequency time spectrum	Display of the Doppler frequency spectrum over time.
Gain	Amplification of the reflected ultrasonic signal.
Gray scale	Brightness-modulated display of ultrasounds echos in several gray scales.
Impedance	Sound resistance of different tissues.
Insonation angle	Angle between the Doppler sound beam and the longitudinal axis of the vessel under examination.
Intima-media thickness (IMT)	Distance between the two echogenic lines, which limit the vessel lumen inward by B-mode imaging.
Laminar flow	Parabolic, rotationally symmetrical flow profile in vessels.
Lateral resolution	Minimum distance between two reflective structures perpendicular to the sound beam that can still be discriminated.
Linear array transducer	Ultrasound transducer with straight arrangement of the piezo elements; a rectangular field of view results.
Low-flow setting	Special setting parameters of color coded duplex sonography for the detection of low blood flow.
Macaroni sign	Concentric, homogeneous, relatively low-echo thickening of the vessel wall indicating the presence of arteritis.
Mean (value)	Intensity weighted average flow velocity in a vessel.

(continued)

Mechanical index (MI)	Parameter of the acoustic transmission power of ultrasonic devices.
Mirror artifact	Mirror artifacts occur with reflectors lying in the sound axis, which act as a mirror and display structures not located in the sectional plane
M-Mode (motion mode)	Display of the amplitudes of a one-dimensional sound beam in a brightness-coded manner over time, particularly used in cardiology.
Multifrequency sound transducer	Possibility to shift the nominal frequency of an ultrasonic transducer (see also broadband transducers).
Multigate Doppler	Several sample volumes are placed along the sound beam and analyzed independently of each other.
Near field	Range of the ultrasonic field from the transducer to the focus.
Oscillating flow	During the cardiac cycle unphysiologically changing antero−/retrograde flow, for example, in a subclavian steal effect.
Persistence	Superimposing successive color coded images for better representation of color coded flow information (see also color capture),
Phased-array transducer	Transducer with crystal elements building up a sector-shaped image.
Pourcelot index (resistance index)	Resistance Index (RI) according to Pourcelot to assess peripheral vascular resistance.
Power	Transmitted ultrasound power of the ultrasonic device.
Power mode	Displaying intensity changes of the color coded duplex signal, widely independent of the direction of flow and flow velocity.
Pseudo-vein	Arterial flow signal with distinctly reduced pulsatility behind very high-grade stenoses resembling a veinous flow signal.
Pseudo-occlusion	Subtotal stenosis with hardly any blood flow left.
Pulsatility	Systolic-endiastolic ratio of the Doppler flow curve.
Pulsatility index	Pulsatility index (PI) according to Gosling to assess peripheral vascular resistance.
Pulse repetition frequency (PRF)	Frequency of emitted ultrasonic pulses in kHz.
Pulsed wave Doppler	Ultrasound pulses are emitted discontinuously with a variable pulse repetition frequency (PRF) and a sample volume can be defined where the Doppler spectrum is to be measured.
PW-Doppler method	Pulsed Doppler technique in which the ultrasound transducer alternately sends and receives ultrasound pulses (in transcranial Doppler sonography and in duplex sonography).
Resistance index (RI)	Parameter to assess the peripheral resistance in arteries.
Reverberation	"Ping-pong" artifacts in B-mode imaging, when two strong reflectors are facing each other in parallel.
Reynolds number	Indicates mathematically the transition from laminar to turbulent flow.
Sample volume	Window shiftable along the sound axis of the Doppler beam for selective detection of Doppler spectrum in investigator definable tissue depths.
Scan lines (synonymous with color lines)	"Virtual" Doppler sound beams, identifiable by the position and orientation of the color window in color coded duplex sonography.
Scattering	In contrast to reflection, scattering describes a diffuse reflection of ultrasound due to interaction with tissue structures.
Seagull cry phenomenon	Harmonic frequency components in the Doppler spectrum at extremely high flow velocities.
Sectional view	Two-dimensional imaging of tissue structures using the echo pulse method (see B-mode imaging).
Sector-array transducer	Ultrasound transducer to generate a sector-shaped image section.
Ultrasound beam	Simplified term for the ultrasonic field emitted by an ultrasonic transducer.
Energy	Mechanical energy that is transported in the form of a sound wave. Unit: Joule = Watt × second.
Power	Sound energy that is transported per time in the form of a wave. Unit: Joule/second = Watt.
Sound velocity	Sound frequency [Hz] x wavelength [m].
Spectrum broadening	Broadening of the Doppler frequency density spectrum, due to the occurrence of low frequency components in case of flow disturbances.
Spectrum width	Defined differently by different authors as an indication of turbulence.
String sign	Tapered diameter distal to the carotid bulb as an indication of a dissection.
Systolic deceleration	Short-term reduction of flow velocity occurring during systole, for example, in case of an incomplete steal effect.
Systolic maximum frequency	Maximum frequency occurring during systole in the Doppler frequency spectrum (synonymous peak frequency).
Systolic peaks	Small systolic signals of low amplitude at extremely high intracranial pressure values.

(continued)

Systolic window	Physiological predominance of higher frequency components during systole in the Doppler frequency spectrum.
Tandem stenosis	Two (or more) successive stenoses occurring in one vessel.
Temporal bone window	Relatively thin bone located at the temporal bone that allows the transmission of ultrasound.
Time gain compensation (TGC)	Transit-time-dependent increase in gain in ultrasound imaging to compensate for attenuation losses in body tissue.
Tissue harmonic imaging (THI)	Evaluation of harmonics of reflected ultrasound signals to improve lateral resolution and image contrast.
To-and-fro-sign	Unphysiologically simultaneous forward-backward flow, mainly caused by aneurysms.
Transducer	Piezoelectric crystals (transducer elements) used to convert electrical energy into mechanical energy and vice versa in ultrasound devices
Transmission frequency	Frequency of the sound waves emitted by a transducer.
Turbulence	Flow disturbance when the Reynolds number is exceeded (in stenosis or hyperperfusion).
Ultrasound	Frequencies above the human hearing range (16,000 Hz). In examinations of biological tissue, frequencies of about 1–20 MHz are used.
Ultrasound contrast agents	Intravenously applied contrast agents to improve the Doppler signal analysis.
Ultrasound probe	One (pulsed Doppler) or two (continuous Doppler) piezoelectric crystals used in Doppler pin probes.
Variance	Parameter describing the width of the frequency density spectrum, used for the quantification of flow disturbances.
Velocity mode	Color coded vessel imaging depending on the mean value of the measured Doppler frequency shift.
Wall filter	High-pass filter that filters out Doppler shifts in the low-frequency range caused by wall movements.

Standard Values

28

Bernhard Widder and Gerhard F. Hamann

The knowledge of standard values is the prerequisite for the definition of pathological findings. Especially from the beginning of Doppler and duplex sonographic diagnostics there are numerous studies available.

The following compilation of the literature does not claim to be complete and is essentially limited to works with larger numbers of investigations. Furthermore, in the extracranial area it is limited to information on the inner vessel diameters, the maximum systolic velocities measured by duplex sonography, and the flow volumes. Doppler frequencies are not described because their range of fluctuation is too large due to the variable insonation angle. Transcranially, both the systolic maximum frequencies measured by Doppler sonography and the systolic maximum velocities determined with the aid of transcranial color coded duplex sonography and corrected by the insonation angle are mentioned. The description of end-diastolic Doppler frequencies and flow velocities has generally been omitted, as they are of no significance in practice with few exceptions. Furthermore, information on pulsatility (PI) and mean value is only given if their determination is relevant, for example, in the assessment of increased intracranial pressure values. Further details may be found in the cited original literature.

As far as possible, age-adapted standard values are given in the tables. The values marked with ± always represent the 1 standard deviation. The graphs attached at the end summarize the available data and serve for quick orientation.

28.1 Extracranial Duplex Sonography

28.1.1 Common Carotid Artery

Diameter (inside)	n	Age	[mm]
Schöning et al. 1994	48	35 ± 12	6.3 ± 0.9
Polak et al. 1996, male.	2017	73 ± 6	6.3 ± 0.9
Polak et al. 1996, female	2722	72 ± 4	5.7 ± 0.7
Mannami et al. 2000, male.	237	30–44	6.3 ± 0.5
	377	45–54	6.4 ± 0.6
	573	55–64	6.5 ± 0.7
	568	65–74	6.6 ± 0.8
	278	75–89	6.7 ± 0.8
Mannami et al. 2000, female	293	30–44	5.8 ± 0.4
	554	45–54	5.9 ± 0.5
	708	55–64	6.1 ± 0.6
	575	65–74	6.2 ± 0.6
	224	75–89	6.4 ± 0.7
Diameter (inside)	n	Age	[mm]
Scheel et al. 2000	24	20–39	6.0 ± 0.7
	24	40–59	6.1 ± 0.8
	30	60–85	6.2 ± 0.9
Systolic maximum speed	n	Age	[cm/s]
Schöning et al. 1994	48	35 ± 12	96 ± 25
Scheel et al. 2000	24	20–39	101 ± 22
	24	40–59	89 ± 17
	30	60–85	81 ± 21
PI	n	Age	Measured value
Schöning et al. 1994	48	35 ± 12	1.7 ± 0.5
Scheel et al. 2000	24	20–39	1.9 ± 0.4
	24	40–59	1.5 ± 0.4
	30	60–85	1.7 ± 0.3
Flow volume	n	Age	[ml/min]
Schöning et al. 1994	48	35 ± 12	470 ± 120
Scheel et al. 2000	24	20–39	426 ± 99
(average both pages)	24	40–59	434 ± 111
	30	60–85	373 ± 80

B. Widder (✉)
Expert Opinion Institute, District Hospital, Guenzburg, Germany
e-mail: bernhard.widder@bkh-guenzburg.de

G. F. Hamann
Clinic of Neurology and Neurological Rehabilitation, District Hospital, Guenzburg, Germany

B. Widder, G. F. Hamann (eds.), *Duplex sonography of the brain-supplying arteries*, https://doi.org/10.1007/978-3-662-65566-5_28

28.1.2 Internal Carotid Artery

Diameter	n	Age	[mm]
Schöning et al. 1994	48	35 ± 12	4.8 ± 0.7
Scheel et al. 2000	24	20–39	4.8 ± 0.6
	24	40–59	4.7 ± 0.5
	30	60–85	4.9 ± 0.8
Systolic maximum speed	n	Age	[cm/s]
Schöning et al. 1994	48	35 ± 12	66 ± 16
Scheel et al. 2000	24	20–39	72 ± 18
	24	40–59	65 ± 10
	30	60–85	58 ± 11
PI	n	Age	Measured value
Schöning et al. 1994	48	35 ± 12	1.1 ± 0.3
Flow volume	n	Age	[ml/min]
Schöning et al. 1994	48	35 ± 12	265 ± 62
Scheel et al. 2000	24	20–39	277 ± 49
	24	40–59	254 ± 57
	30	60–85	224 ± 43

28.1.3 External Carotid Artery

Diameter	n	Age	[mm]
Schöning et al. 1994	48	35 ± 12	4.1 ± 0.6
Scheel et al. 2000	24	20–39	4.0 ± 0.4
	24	40–59	4.1 ± 0.7
	30	60–85	4.3 ± 0.7
Systolic maximum speed	n	Age	[cm/s]
Schöning et al. 1994	48	35 ± 12	83 ± 17
Päivänsalo et al. 1996	553	59	77 ± 37
Scheel et al. 2000	24	20–39	86 ± 14
	24	40–59	85 ± 18
	30	60–85	81 ± 30
PI	n	Age	Measured value
Schöning et al. 1994	48	35 ± 12	2.2 ± 0.5
Flow volume	n	Age	[ml/min]
Schöning et al. 1994	48	35 ± 12	160 ± 66
Scheel et al. 2000	24	20–39	145 ± 31
	24	40–59	175 ± 73
	30	60–85	170 ± 51

28.1.4 Vertebral Artery

Diameter	n	Age	[mm]
Schöning et al. 1994	48	35 ± 12	3.4 ± 0.6
Seidel et al. 1999, right	50	56 ± 14	3.4 ± 0.6
Seidel et al. 1999, left	–	–	3.7 ± 0.6
Scheel et al. 2000	24	20–39	3.3 ± 0.3
	24	40–59	3.2 ± 0.4

(continued)

Diameter	n	Age	[mm]
	30	60–85	3.6 ± 0.4
Systolic maximum speed	n	Age	[cm/s]
Schöning et al. 1994	48	35 ± 12	48 ± 10
Seidel et al. 1999, right	50	56 ± 14	46 ± 14
Seidel et al. 1999, left	–	–	51 ± 13
Scheel et al. 2000	24	20–39	52 ± 6
	24	40–59	47 ± 8
	30	60–85	45 ± 11
PI	n	Age	Measured value
Schöning et al. 1994	48	35 ± 12	1.3 ± 0.4
Flow volume	n	Age	[ml/min]
Schöning et al. 1994	48	35 ± 12	85 ± 33
Seidel et al. 1999, right	50	56 ± 14	77 ± 30
Seidel et al. 1999, left	–	–	105 ± 46
Scheel et al. 2000	24	20–39	86 ± 20
(Average both pages)	24	40–59	73 ± 18
	30	60–85	77 ± 29

28.2 Transcranial Doppler Sonography

28.2.1 Middle Cerebral Artery

Systolic maximum frequency	n	Age	[kHz]
Arnolds and others Reutern 1986	51	<40	2.4 ± 0.5
	–	>40	2.1 ± 0.5
Hennerici et al. 1987	50	<40	2.4 ± 0.4
	–	40–60	2.3 ± 0.4
	–	>60	2.0 ± 0.4
Mean frequency value	n	Age	[kHz]
Hennerici et al. 1987	50	<40	1.5 ± 0.2
	–	40–60	1.5 ± 0.3
	–	>60	1.2 ± 0.3

28.2.2 Anterior Cerebral Artery

Systolic maximum frequency	n	Age	[kHz]
Arnolds and others Reutern 1986	51	<40	1.8 ± 0.4
	–	>40	1.7 ± 0.3
Hennerici et al. 1987	50	<40	1.9 ± 0.4
	–	40–60	2.2 ± 0.5
	–	>60	1.9 ± 0.5

28.2.3 A Cerebri Posterior

Systolic maximum frequency	n	Age	[kHz]
Arnolds and by Reutern 1986	51	<40	1.5 ± 0.3

(continued)

Systolic maximum frequency	n	Age	[kHz]
	–	>40	1.3 ± 0.2
Hennerici et al. 1987	50	<40	1.4 ± 0.3
	–	40–60	1.5 ± 0.5
	–	>60	1.3 ± 0.3

28.2.4 Basilar Artery

Systolic maximum frequency	n	Age	[kHz]
Arnolds and by Reutern 1986	51	<40	1.6 ± 0.3
	–	>40	1.3 ± 0.2
Hennerici et al. 1987	50	<40	1.4 ± 0.2
	–	40–60	1.5 ± 0.4
	–	>60	1.3 ± 0.5

28.3 Transcranial Color Coded Duplex Sonography

28.3.1 Middle Cerebral Artery (M1 Segment)

Systolic Maximum speed	n	Age	[cm/s]
Schöning et al. 1993a	96	35 ± 12	107 ± 18
Schöning et al. 1993b	64	2–10	142 ± 19
	–	11–18	130 ± 19
Martin et al. 1994	82	20–39	113
	58	40–59	106
	53	>60	92
Krejza et al. 1999	182	20–40	120 ± 28
	–	41–60	109 ± 28
	–	>60	92 ± 17
Shambal et al. 2003	290	0–2	104 ± 20
	–	3–13	151 ± 22
	–	14–18	127 ± 22
	–	19–39	116 ± 20
	–	40–59	97 ± 16
	–	60–69	95 ± 17
	–	70–91	93 ± 14
PI	n	Age	Measured value
Martin et al. 1994	82	20–39	0.84
	58	40–59	0.81
	53	>60	0.97

28.3.2 Anterior Cerebral Artery (A1 Segment)

Systolic maximum speed	n	Age	[cm/s]
Schöning et al. 1993b	64	2–10	120 ± 27
	–	11–18	107 ± 20

(continued)

Systolic maximum speed	n	Age	[cm/s]
Schöning et al. 1993a	94	35 ± 12	91 ± 17
Martin et al. 1994	77	20–39	91
	49	40–59	88
	42	>60	79
Krejza et al. 1999	182	20–40	82 ± 21
	–	41–60	80 ± 22
	–	>60	72 ± 13
Shambal et al. 2003	290	0–2	85 ± 21
	–	3–13	117 ± 23
	–	14–18	108 ± 22
	–	19–39	87 ± 16
	–	40–59	84 ± 19
	–	60–69	81 ± 16
	–	70–91	96 ± 16

28.3.3 (P1 Segment)

Systolic maximum speed	n	Age	[cm/s]
Schöning and Walter 1992	98	35 ± 12	70 ± 13
Schöning et al. 1993b	64	2–10	94 ± 18
	–	11–18	85 ± 12
Martin et al. 1994	84	20–39	81
	56	40–59	71
	54	>60	66
Krejza et al. 1999	182	20–40	75 ± 16
	–	41–60	74 ± 17
	–	>60	62 ± 12
Systolic maximum speed	n	Age	[cm/s]
Shambal et al. 2003	290	0–2	69 ± 17
	–	3–13	84 ± 15
	–	14–18	77 ± 14
	–	19–39	72 ± 16
	–	40–59	61 ± 12
	–	60–69	53 ± 11
	–	70–91	56 ± 11

28.3.4 Vertebral Artery (V4 Segment)

Systolic Maximum speed	n	Age	[cm/s]
Schöning and Walter 1992	87	35 ± 12	60 ± 16
Martin et al. 1994	94	20–39	66
	69	40–59	59
	63	>60	52
Shambal et al. 2003	290	0–2	54 ± 19
	–	3–13	79 ± 15
	–	14–18	70 ± 13
	–	19–39	66 ± 14
	–	40–59	56 ± 14
	–	60–69	52 ± 13
	–	70–91	56 ± 13

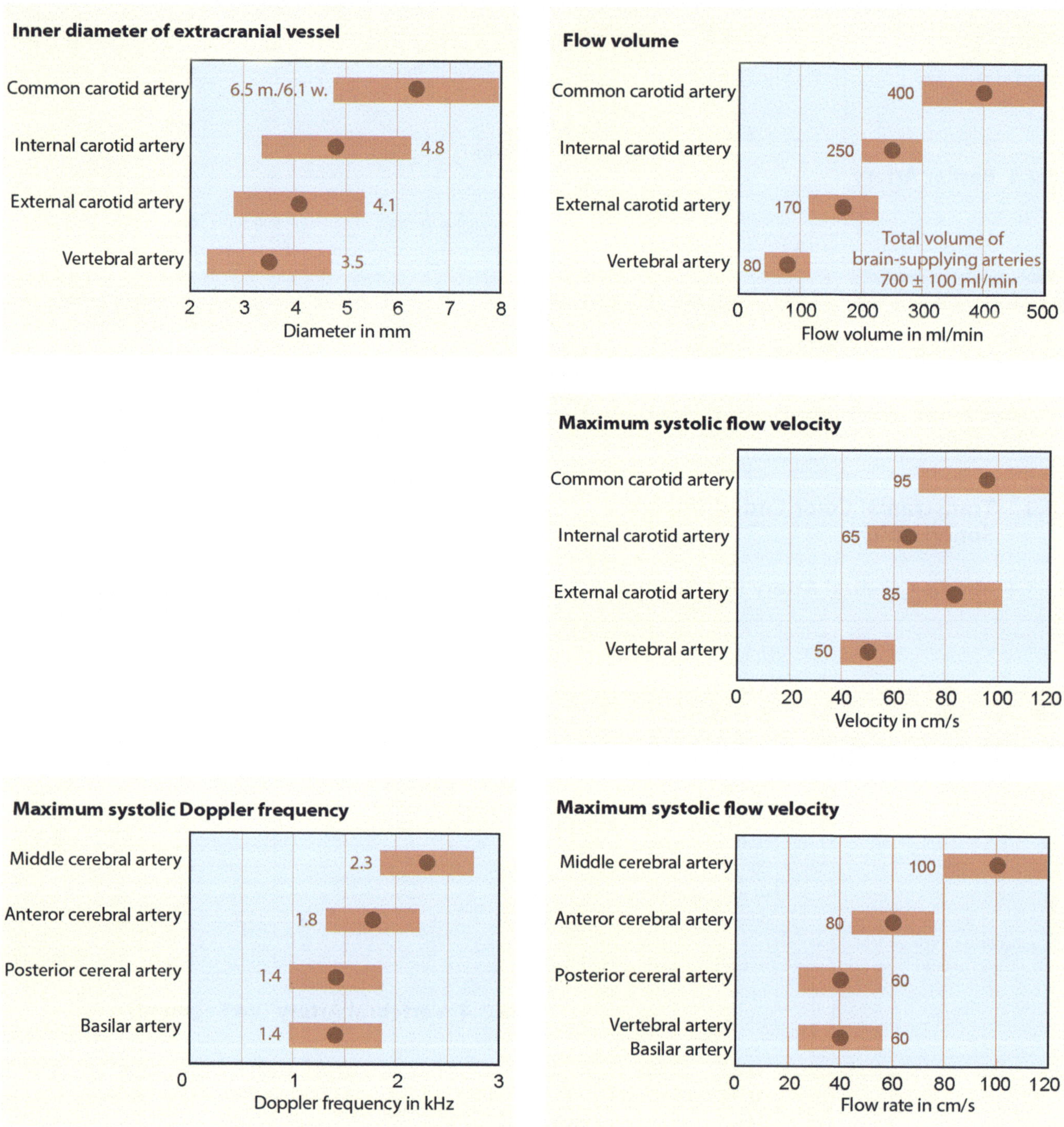

Fig. 28.1 Summary of important standard values

28.3.5 Basilar Artery

Systolic maximum speed	n	Age	[cm/s]
Schöning and Walter 1992	45	35 ± 12	67 ± 15
Martin et al. 1994	45	20–39	74
	31	40–59	63
	30	>60	54
Shambal et al. 2003	290	0–2	73 ± 19
	–	3–13	98 ± 21
	–	14–18	86 ± 20
	–	19–39	70 ± 12
	–	40–59	62 ± 15
	–	60–69	60 ± 16
	–	70–91	64 ± 18

28.4 Summary of Important Standard Values

The following graphs (Fig. 28.1) serve as a quick orientation in daily practice. They refer to the usually investigated age segment over 50 years. The information is given under consideration of the simple standard deviation.

References

Arnolds BJ, von Reutern GM (1986) Transcranial Doppler sonography. Examination technique and normal reference values. Ultrasound Med Biol 12:115–123

Hennerici M, Rautenberg W, Sitzer G, Schwartz A (1987) Transcranial Doppler ultrasound for the assessment of intracranial arterial flow velocity—Part 1. Examination technique and normal values. Surg Neurol 27:439–448

Krejza J, Mariak Z, Walecki J et al (1999) Transcranial color Doppler sonography of basal cerebral arteries in 182 healthy subjects: age and sex variability and normal reference values for blood flow parameters. Am J Roentgenol 172:213–218

Mannami T, Baba S, Ogata J (2000) Strong and significant relationships between aggregation of major coronary risk factors and the acceleration of carotid atherosclerosis in the general population of a Japanese city: the Suita Study. Arch Intern Med 160:2297–2303

Martin PJ, Evans DH, Naylor AR (1994) Transcranial color-coded sonography of the basal cerebral circulation. Reference data from 115 volunteers. Stroke 25:390–396

Päivänsalo M, Leinonen S, Turunen J et al (1996) Quantification of carotid artery stenosis with various Doppler velocity parameters. Röfo 164:108–113

Polak JF, Kronmal RA, Tell GS et al (1996) Compensatory increase in common carotid artery diameter. Relation to blood pressure and artery intima-media thickness in older adults. Cardiovascular Health Study. Stroke 27:2012–2015

Scheel P, Ruge C, Schöning M (2000) Flow velocity and flow volume measurements in the extracranial carotid and vertebral arteries in healthy adults: reference data and the effects of age. Ultrasound Med Biol 26:1261–1266

Schöning M, Walter J (1992) Evaluation of the vertebrobasilar-posterior system by transcranial color duplex sonography in adults. Stroke 23:1280–1286

Schöning M, Buchholz R, Walter J (1993a) Comparative study of transcranial color duplex sonography and transcranial Doppler sonography in adults. J Neurosurg 78:776–784

Schöning M, Staab M, Walter J, Niemann G (1993b) Transcranial color duplex sonography in childhood and adolescence. Age dependence of flow velocities and waveform parameters. Stroke 24:1305–1309

Schöning M, Walter J, Scheel P (1994) Estimation of cerebral blood flow through color duplex sonography of the carotid and vertebral arteries in healthy adults. Stroke 25:17–22

Seidel E, Eicke BM, Tettenborn B, Krummenauer F (1999) Reference values for vertebral artery flow volume by duplex sonography in young and elderly adults. Stroke 30:2692–2696

Shambal S, Grehl H, Zierz S, Lindner A (2003) Age dependence of Doppler parameters in the basal cerebral arteries evaluated by transcranial color-coded duplex sonography. Reference data from 290 volunteers. Fortschr Neurol Psychiatr 71:271–277

Index

B. Widder, G. F. Hamann (eds.), *Duplex sonography of the brain-supplying arteries*, https://doi.org/10.1007/978-3-662-65566-5

G

H

I

T

U

V

The manufacturer's authorised representative in the EU is Springer Nature Customer Service Centre GmbH, Europaplatz 3, 69115 Heidelberg, Germany. If you have any concerns regarding our products, please contact ProductSafety@springernature.com

Printed and bound by CPI Group (UK) Ltd, Croydon, CR0 4YY
28/09/2026
02224097-0002